Behavioral Medicine and Integrated Care

Melanie P. Duckworth • William T. O'Donohue
Editors

Behavioral Medicine and Integrated Care

Efficient Delivery of Effective Treatments

Springer

Editors
Melanie P. Duckworth
Department of Psychology
University of Nevada, Reno
Reno, NV, USA

William T. O'Donohue
Department of Psychology
University of Nevada, Reno
Reno, NV, USA

ISBN 978-3-030-06565-2 ISBN 978-3-319-93003-9 (eBook)
https://doi.org/10.1007/978-3-319-93003-9

This Springer imprint is published by the registered company Springer Nature Switzerland AG
The registered company address is: Gewerbestrasse 11, 6330 Cham, Switzerland

Contents

Part I
Behavioral Medicine and Integrated Care: Efficient Delivery of Effective Treatments

Chapter 1
Introduction

Melanie P. Duckworth and William T. O'Donohue

Healthcare delivery systems and health insurance are in a state of crisis in the United States (Wendel, Serrett, & O'Donohue, 2018). This has been true for several decades and, as the controversies surrounding the Affordable Care Act make obvious, solutions are not easily forthcoming. Most healthcare professionals and patients are not satisfied with the quality of current healthcare. Many individuals do not have acceptable access to healthcare, with large differences in access contributing to disparities that center around socioeconomic status, race, and geography. The healthcare delivery system is both inefficient and costly, with current healthcare costs accounting for approximately 19% of gross domestic product (GDP), a GDP amount nearly four times that observed in 1960. Advances in medical technology are considered one of the most important drivers of escalating healthcare costs (Wendel et al., 2018). Historically, as one aged, there was little one could do about joint deterioration. Now there are multiple options for managing joint deterioration such as hip replacement, knee replacement, and shoulder replacement. The aging United States population and the advances in medical technology ensure that such growth in healthcare costs will be unsustainable. Using the classic "guns versus butter" model of macroeconomics, one can confidently predict that current expenditures in the healthcare sector will reduce spending across other vital economic sectors. There are problems with the extent to which evidence-based treatments are used. There is the problem of medical errors—errors that occur at such frequency that one healthcare economist has concluded that it is safer to mountain climb than to spend time in a hospital (Wendel et al., 2018). There are questions about the financial model (e.g., for profit versus nonprofit, one payor versus multiple payors, and federally-controlled versus state-controlled) that, when applied, would best ensure that heathcare systems are fiscally sound. There are basic questions about why the healthcare system is divided and even siloed between physical health and mental health.

M. P. Duckworth (✉) · W. T. O'Donohue
Department of Psychology, University of Nevada, Reno, Reno, NV, USA
e-mail: melanied@unr.edu

M. P. Duckworth, W. T. O'Donohue (eds.), *Behavioral Medicine and Integrated Care*,
https://doi.org/10.1007/978-3-319-93003-9_1

Finally, there are critiques that suggest our healthcare delivery system needs to be reoriented into a wellness system instead of a system that simply reacts to illness.

It is estimated that 50% of adults in the United States are experiencing the symptoms and consequences of medical illness (Ward, Schiller, & Goodman, 2014). More alarming are the health statistics that indicate that as many as 32% adults and 12% children are attempting to manage the healthcare requirements and functional limitations imposed by multiple chronic conditions (Clark et al., 2015; Zhong et al., 2007). Integrated care can be considered one of the more ambitious and far-reaching efforts to redefine both the primary targets of healthcare and the points along the health-disease continuum that will serve to maintain the good health of many persons while reducing the disease burden borne by others (O'Donohue, Cummings, Cucciare, Runyan, & Cummings, 2005). The effectiveness of all healthcare integration efforts will require clear delineation of the pathways involved in: maintaining good health; accurately identifying behavioral health problems and their relationship to physical problems; modifying disease risk; managing the biological and psychosocial demands associated with diagnosed medical conditions; and behaving to reduce the associated compromise to function and overall quality of life (Duckworth & Iezzi, 2010). When these healthcare integration efforts are successful, the patient is allowed the experience of "one-stop shopping" in their primary care physician's office. Because of the relative plenitude of primary care offices across the United States, integrated care is thought to have the advantage of both decreasing access problems and reducing stigma for mental health problems. However, this also highlights a workforce shortage in both primary care physicians and integrated care behavioral health providers (O'Donohue & Maragakis, 2014)

Behavioral medicine is the discipline that may credited with first locating healthcare efforts at the nexus between the physical and psychosocial demands of disease management (Agras, Kazdin, & Wilson, 1979). This discipline emerged in the 1970s and helped focus the attention of psychologists on psychological factors impacting physical health presentations. The targets of behavioral medicine traditionally have included those health behaviors—obesity and other eating disorders, exercise, nutrition, sleep, smoking, stress, substance use, and treatment noncompliance—that contribute significantly to disease risk and to disease morbidity and mortality. Behavioral medicine was also the first mental health subdiscipline to target chronic pain, a symptom that is now thought to be one of the "vital signs" that are to be routinely assessed and prioritized. The need to effectively and efficiently integrate applied behavioral medicine into integrated care systems cannot be questioned. What must be questioned is the "what" and the "how" involved in making evidence-based behavioral medicine standard practice in those primary care medical settings that will serve as the homes for integrated healthcare.

In the integrated care context, behavioral assessment and behavioral management are best guided by the biopsychosocial model (Engel, 1977; Suls & Rothman, 2004; Tovian, 2006). This model views physical disease as an experience that is influenced by the interplay of biological, psychological, and social factors. Successful management of such diseases requires that all aspects of the illness experience are addressed. The assessment and management of patients with single and multiple medical conditions usually begins in the primary care setting. The primary care setting has been regarded as the de facto mental health system as most behavioral health is being diagnosed (accurately or inaccurately) there and treated there. Primary care providers (PCPs) are responsible for obtaining a patient's verbal report of symptoms and conducting a physical examination. PCPs initially focus on establishing the type, intensity, and duration of the patient's symptoms and relating the reported symptoms to some acute environmental circumstance, to some newly occurring medical circumstance, or to some already diagnosed condition. The PCP's goals for medical evaluation include determining whether further diagnostic testing is indicated, establishing a medical diagnosis, determining if medical findings can account for the patient's report of symptoms, and forwarding treatment recommendations (Duckworth, Iezzi, & Carlson, 2018). However, most PCPs are less comfortable diagnosing and treating behavioral health problems than medical problems. Certainly, their training in behavioral health has increased in recent years; however, it is still the case that PCPs usually welcome a behavioral health specialist as part of their primary care team (Wamsley et al., 2016).

As part of an integrated approach to disease management, PCPs often serve as "the point person" for integrating delivery of the patient's required healthcare across a team of providers, including medical specialists, nurses, physiotherapists, nutritionists, and occupational and rehabilitation therapists (Duckworth et al., 2018). One of the most important roles of the PCP is that of communicator of disease information, treatment recommendations, and detailed, patient-tailored, self-management instructions. In the chronic pain context, for example, the PCP is required to oversee all prescribed treatments, including the prescription and use of pain medications and patient engagement in and benefit from various rehabilitation efforts. In the absence of a complete response to these pain management efforts, and in the presence of persistent pain, the most function-preserving message from the PCP to the patient is to maintain as normal and active a life as possible in spite of pain and to moderate expectations for pain reduction (Duckworth, Iezzi, & Sewell, 2009). In addition, the PCP needs to provide reassurance about the patient's prognosis, be especially conservative in recommending pharmacotherapy or other invasive pain treatments, and avoid overmedicalizing or overpathologizing the pain patient, thereby preventing the development of a host of other problems (e.g., medication abuse; Duckworth et al., 2018; Duckworth et al., 2009).

As patients experience an increase in the number of diagnosed conditions, the level of burden and cost associated with managing these comorbid conditions increase dramatically (Gerteis et al., 2014). In the context of multiple chronic conditions, patients' self-management regimens become increasingly complex and require more effort, more time, and mastery of skills sets aimed at managing the medical conditions, managing care systems, and managing the personal and interpersonal stress and distress that occurs in the face of chronic illness. In the current era of healthcare, with its emphasis on efficient, integrated case management *and* cost containment, stepped and collaborative case management in integrated care settings is becoming the new standard for management of chronic conditions (O'Donohue & Draper, 2010). Stepped care models are designed to optimize the match between identified healthcare needs and the interventions deployed to effectively manage those needs, all while minimizing care costs. The stepped care model maximizes patient-provider interactions by using assurance, education, and self-activation during the earliest stages of disease management and by providing care management and support from other systems when necessary. The most effective stepped care approaches share an emphasis on sequenced intervention that (1) addresses patients' disease-related worries and concerns and provides psychoeducation aimed at imparting accurate information about the patient's diagnosis and correcting misconceptions, (2) provides structured support for self-management efforts such as physical exercise and activity engagement, (3) provides more intensive psychological intervention aimed at addressing clinically significant emotional distress and lifestyle impairment as frequent concomitants of disease diagnosis and management, and (4) provides prevention and wellness options to help bring patients to higher levels of health and functioning (Duckworth et al., 2009).

Although the vision of integrated care has gained wide acceptance and many integrated care settings exist, there are numerous problems with this movement. First, integrated care has many different meanings. It can mean that the services of behavioral health providers are available but can only be accessed by virtue of travel to a site other than that of the medical provider. The term can be used to describe the co-location of healthcare providers from different disciplines in the absence of any true team-based integration of care. Ideally, the term integrated care is used to reference healthcare systems in which interdisciplinary teams of healthcare providers and allied health professions contribute jointly to the assessment, diagnosis and management of those physical, psyhchological and sociocultural factors that are most relevant to health maintenance and recovery from ill health. Efforts to effectively implement and determine the costs associated with integrated care are also complicated by the fact that the health conditions that are targeted and the assessment protocols and interventions that are deployed in the context of integrated care can vary dramatically from setting to setting. Integrated care can imply the use of a comprehensive care model such as the screening, brief intervention and referral to treatment (SBIRT) model; it can imply the use of a stepped care approach or the use of eHealth and it can imply that supportive psychotherapy is being offered or that more targeted, evidence-based treatment procedures are being employed. Integrated care can mean that only a select few behavioral health problems are targeted—depression being a one of the most common of these—or that a wider array of behavioral health problems are targeted. Finally, integrated care can indicate the assessment of only a limited number of health risk factors, problems, and outcomes or it can indicate an assessment approach that comprehensively evaluates risk, disease, and treatment response along with patient satisfaction, provider satisfaction, and medical cost offsets. The phrase "integrated care" has become an honorific that represents a diversity of delivery models.

Perhaps such diversity of kind can be seen as salutary—one can systematically determine what works best across a variety of care contexts. However, a key problem is that the implementation of all these "integrated care" systems outstrips the evidence base. We have too little psychometric information on behavioral health screening instruments and too little information related to the efficacy (and safety) of brief integrated care treatments. We have too little information on the financial impact of integrated care—do these integrated care models result in cost savings? And if they do, how large are the savings? We have too little information pertaining to the delivery of integrated care in a patient-centered manner. The challenges related to the implementation of integrated care reduce to two major problems: (1) too many healthcare systems implement integrated care in ways that are not data-based or data-generating; and (2) medical care systems are now importing all the problems that specialty mental healthcare has suffered, including allegiance to a theoretical perspective in the absence of supportive data or in the face of competing data; use of assessment instruments for which psychometric properties are unknown or insufficient; implementation of interventions that are not evidence-based or implementation of evidenced-based interventions by care providers who are without sufficient training and/or experience treating patients with complex and interacting medical and psychological conditions; and the proffer of broad claims about the financial impact of integrated care that are not substantiated with data.

This book identifies many of the challenges involved in the delivery of effective integrated care, highlights some of the gaps that are present in the research literature pertaining to the application of behavior change strategies to both health and illness in the primary care context, and provides readers with relevant information regarding potential solutions to these problems in healthcare delivery. Although there are texts that independently address issues relevant to integrated care and behavioral health, this book is uniquely structured to provide healthcare professionals with expert guidance in translating and streamlining evidence-based, behavioral medicine treatment strategies into a set of robust and executable health management skills that can be easily implemented in the context of integrated care.

The book is organized into four sections, with book sections and chapters organized to provide (1) an overview of the pathways and specific skills involved in integrating behavioral medicine and primary care medicine in a manner that enhances disease prevention, disease risk modification, and disease management and (2) specific recommendations for addressing the challenges of effective healthcare integration at the level of the patient, at the level of the provider, and at the level of the administrative system that undergirds all patient-provider interactions. In the first section of the book, an introduction to the text, an overview of the role of behavioral medicine in integrated care settings is provided and current estimates for the prevalence of medical diseases and the lifestyle behaviors that serve as risk factors for these diseases are reviewed. In the second section of the book, some of the key problems in healthcare service delivery are delineated, with chapters addressing the need for provider training, patient screening, and the use of evidence-based treatments. The third section of the book addresses some of the key challenges to healthcare integration, emphasizing the electronic health record as a technology that has the potential to transform healthcare delivery. Also addressed in this section are healthcare constructs such as health literacy, shared decision-making, and patient-centered care; these constructs are often neglected in the larger contexts of care delivery and cost containment. In the fourth section of the book, healthcare cost containment is discussed from the perspectives of medical regimen adherence, health risk behavior management, and the challenge of providing coordinated care to those with multiple chronic conditions. In the final section of the book, step-by-step guides are provided for the application of behavioral health treatment strategies to some of the most medically and personally demanding and costly medical conditions, including cancer, chronic pain, and dementia.

References

Agras, S., Kazdin, A., & Wilson, G. T. (1979). *Behavior therapy*. New York, NY: W.H. Freeman.

Clark, N. M., Lachance, L., Benedict, M. B., Little, R., Leo, H., Awad, D., & Wilkin, M. K. (2015). The extent and patterns of multiple chronic conditions in low-income children. *Clinical Pediatrics, 54*, 515–524.

Duckworth, M. P., & Iezzi, T. (2010). Physical injuries, pain, and psychological trauma: Pathways to disability. *Psychological Injury and Law, 3*, 241–253.

Duckworth, M. P., Iezzi, T., & Carlson, G. C. (2018). Stepped care for chronic pain in integrated care settings. In A. Maragakis & T. W. O'Donohue (Eds.), *Principle-based stepped care and brief psychotherapy for integrated care settings*. New York, NY: Springer.

Duckworth, M. P., Iezzi, T., & Sewell, T. (2009). Assessing and managing chronic pain in the primary care setting. In L. James & W. T. O'Donohue (Eds.), *The primary care consultant toolkit: Tools for behavioral medicine* (pp. 183–197). New York, NY: Springer Press.

Engel, G. L. (1977). The need for a new medical model: A challenge for biomedicine. *Science, 196*, 129–136.

Gerteis, J., Izrael, D., Deitz, D., LeRoy, L., Ricciardi, R., Miller, T., & Basu, J. (2014). *Multiple chronic conditions chartbook*. Rockville, MD: Agency for Healthcare Research and Quality Publications.

O'Donohue, W., Cummings, N., Cucciare, M., Runyan, T., & Cummings, J. (2005). *Integrated behavioral healthcare*. Boston, MA: Humanity Books.

O'Donohue, W., & Draper, C. (2010). *Stepped care and e-health*. Hoboken, NJ: Springer.

O'Donohue, W., & Maragakis, A. (2014). Healthcare reform means training reform. *Journal of Online Education, 1*, 73–87.

Suls, J., & Rothman, A. (2004). Evolution of the biopsychosocial model: Prospects and challenges for health psychology. *Health Psychology, 23*(2), 119–125.

Tovian, S. M. (2006). Interdisciplinary collaboration in outpatient practice. *Professional Psychology: Research and Practice, 37*(3), 268–272.

Wamsley, M. A., Steiger, S., Julian, K. A., Gleason, N., O'Sullivan, P. S., Guy, M., & Satterfield, J. M. (2016). Teaching residents screening, brief intervention, and referral to treatment (SBIRT) skills for alcohol use: Using chart-stimulated recall to assess curricular impact. *Substance Abuse, 37*(3), 419–426.

Ward, B. W., Schiller, J. S., & Goodman, R. A. (2014). Multiple chronic conditions among US adults: A 2012 update. *Preventing Chronic Disease, 11*, E62–E66.

Wendel, J., Serrett, T., & O'Donohue, W. (2018). *Understanding healthcare economics* (2nd ed.). Hoboken, NJ: Springer.

Zhong, W., Finnie, D. M., Shah, N. D., Wagie, A. E., Sauver, J. L., Jacobson, D. J., & Nassens, J. M. (2007). Effect of multiple chronic diseases on the health care expenditures in childhood. *Journal of Primary Care & Community Health, 6*, 2–9.

Chapter 2
The Role of Behavioral Medicine in Integrated Healthcare

Dawn K. Wilson and Allison M. Sweeney

Introduction

The United States has the highest costs associated with healthcare expenditures per capita and has been shown to have poorer health outcomes compared to other industrialized countries (Woolf & Aron, 2013). Improving the quality of healthcare and population health has recently become a national public health priority (Stoto, 2013). Although medical treatments are often considered a critical component of healthcare, they explain a relatively small amount of variability in physical health outcomes. For example, when examining the factors that contribute to premature death, investigators have estimated that access to healthcare explains 10% of the variance in outcomes (Schroeder, 2007). Alternatively, behavioral patterns explain 40% of the variance, with the remaining variance being explained by environmental exposure (5%), social circumstances (15%), and genetic predispositions (30%). Furthermore, the Oxford Alliance for Health has suggested that most chronic diseases can be traced to a limited set of modifiable health behaviors, including tobacco smoking, alcohol consumption, physical activity, and diet (Suhrcke, Nugent, Stuckler, & Rocco, 2006). Such findings suggest that interventions focused on improving engagement in healthy lifestyle habits may be a highly effective approach for both treating and preventing the development of chronic illness. Thus, the field of behavioral medicine has the potential to play a fundamental role in reducing healthcare utilization and costs by improving lifestyle habits that have been related to the prevention of chronic diseases.

This research was supported in part by the National Institute of Child Health and Human Development (R01HD072153).

D. K. Wilson (✉) · A. M. Sweeney
Department of Psychology, Barnwell College, University of South Carolina,
Columbia, SC, USA
e-mail: wilsondk@mailbox.sc.edu; sweeneam@mailbox.sc.edu

M. P. Duckworth, W. T. O'Donohue (eds.), *Behavioral Medicine and Integrated Care*,
https://doi.org/10.1007/978-3-319-93003-9_2

Effectiveness of Lifestyle and Self-Management Interventions

Converging evidence from randomized controlled trials suggests that improving self-regulation through behavior change techniques is an effective approach for promoting changes in health-related behaviors across the life span. For example, self-monitoring, which involves prompting people to keep a record of a specified behavior (e.g., in an electronic or written diary), is considered to be one of the most effective strategies for eliciting changes in diet and physical activity (Michie, Abraham, Whittington, McAteer, & Gupta, 2009). Other common strategies include prompting specific goal setting, including planning details such as the frequency, intensity, or duration of a behavior, as well as specifying when, where, and how the goal will be carried out (Gollwitzer, 1999). Furthermore, action planning, including prompting people to identify potential barriers to performing a behavior and planning ways to overcome them, is another frequently used strategy (Ayotte, Margrett, & Hicks-Patrick, 2010; Bandura, 2004). In this section, we review interventions in which various professionals, including teachers, primary care physicians, and community members, were trained to use behavior change strategies as a method for improving health-related behaviors among high-risk populations.

Children-Focused Randomized Controlled Interventions

The Child and Adolescent Trial for Cardiovascular Health (CATCH; Perry et al., 1997) was a multi-site intervention that examined the role of the elementary school environment, school-based health education, and home-based health education. Across four states, 96 elementary schools were randomly assigned to implement (1) a school-based program (including a school food service modification, PE intervention, and a behaviorally oriented health skills training), (2) a school-based program plus a home-based program, or (3) the usual health curriculum. School cafeteria lunches were modified to provide healthier meals with less fat and salt, and PE classes were modified to encourage more vigorous physical activity. The classroom education program was teacher-led and implemented across three academic school years. The primary goals of the intervention were to teach students to identify and choose healthy food, to engage in regular physical activity, and to avoid tobacco use. The program emphasized behavioral skill development around healthy eating and physical activity, including encouraging students to set behavior change goals and receiving feedback from teachers and support from peers. The home-based intervention was designed to complement the behavioral skills learned at school. Students were instructed to complete additional skill-building education activities with their parents and were encouraged to attend family fun nights, school-based evening events in which families could spend time together engaging in physical activity and eating healthy snacks. On average, 58% of the students attended the family fun nights, bringing two other family members with them. Overall, 69% of the students participated in the home curricula each year, but, on average, only 43% completed the entire home curricula. On average, 79% of the parents of students in family intervention schools participated in some of the home curricula.

The results of the trial showed that compared to the control group, participants in the two intervention groups reported significantly greater dietary knowledge; greater perceived parental, friend, and social reinforcement for food choices; lower daily total energy intake; lower daily energy intake from fat; and more minutes of daily physical activity (Luepker et al., 1996). Although the intervention groups were more effective than the control group on several outcomes, few differences were observed between the school-based and school plus family-based intervention. Additionally, blood pressure, body mass index, heart rate, and cholesterol did not differ significantly between groups. Taken together, the CATCH trial demonstrated that providing children with behavioral skills training and an environment that supports a healthy lifestyle (e.g., healthy school lunch choices, PE class activities) is an effective approach for helping children to maintain a healthy diet and engage in regular physical activity.

School-based behavioral interventions have also been found to be an effective approach for changing health-related behaviors among middle school students. The Active by Choice Today (ACT) trial was a multi-site randomized trial that aimed to increase intrinsic motivation and improve behavioral skills for engaging in regular physical activity (Wilson et al., 2008). Twenty-four middle schools in South Carolina (matched by size, percentage of minority students, percentage of free or reduced lunch, and urban vs. rural) were randomly assigned to implement a motivational and behavioral skills intervention or a general health education program. Students in the intervention group participated in a 17-week after-school program which consisted of (1) a 10-min snack break, (2) 60 min of physical activity of the student's choice, (3) a 20-min motivational and behavioral skills training session, and (4) 30 min of homework assistance.

The skills training sessions focused on a variety of behavioral skills designed to increase self-efficacy, behavioral competency, and social support for engaging in physical activity (from parents and peers); these skills included goal setting (completed in a group setting), communication skills, and providing and seeking support outside of the program. Additionally, students in the intervention group completed two video-taped sessions in which they described positive coping strategies for increasing physical activity outside of the program days with family and friends. The purpose of these sessions was to help students develop increased motivation and a positive self-concept for physical activity. Alternatively, students in the general health education program completed a 17-week after-school program in which they received information about nutrition, stress management, drug prevention, and dropout prevention.

To examine whether the behavioral skills training facilitated greater moderate to vigorous physical activity, all students were instructed to wear an accelerometer for 7 consecutive days prior to the intervention, mid-intervention, and 2 weeks post-intervention. At mid-intervention, students in the intervention group engaged in greater physical activity than students in the control group (Wilson et al., 2011).

However, 2 weeks after the intervention was completed, there was no longer a significant difference in physical activity between the two groups. In post-intervention focus groups, students reported several environmental barriers that prevented them from engaging in physical activity outside of school including interfering demands at home, a lack of motivation without the support of teachers, and a lack of support or involvement from parents. These results suggest that providing students with behavioral skills training is effective at increasing school-based physical activity; however, additional support and training is needed to help students cope with barriers in the home environment that interfere with physical activity maintenance.

In addition to demonstrating changes in health-related behaviors, there is evidence that behavioral skill-oriented health sessions can lead to a reduction in the prevalence of obesity. In the Planet Health trial, ten middle schools were randomly assigned to implement the Planet Health educational program or the usual curriculum and PE classes (Gortmaker et al., 1999). The Planet Health program aimed to implement four behavioral changes: reducing television viewing to 2 h/day, increasing physical activity, decreasing consumption of high-fat foods, and increasing consumption of fruits and vegetables. Teachers were trained to implement an interdisciplinary curriculum approach so that the intervention materials were integrated into students' major subject courses and PE over 2 academic years. More specifically, the curriculum was designed to provide students with the behavioral and cognitive skills to enable behavior change (e.g., problem-solving, self-monitoring), opportunities to practice skills to increase perceived competence in carrying out new behaviors, and behavior change support from multiple teachers.

After 2 years, there was a significantly greater reduction in the prevalence of obesity among female students in the intervention group compared to the control group. Among male students, obesity declined in both the intervention and control group, with no significant difference shown between these groups. Both male and female students in the intervention demonstrated a significant reduction in television viewing time relative to the control group. Among female students only, there was a significant increase in fruit and vegetable consumption and a significant decrease in total energy intake relative to the control group. Reduced television watching mediated the effect of the intervention on the reduction in obesity among female students, such that each hour reduction in television viewing predicted a reduced odd of being obese. Female students appear to have been more responsive to the intervention, which suggests that the causal processes guiding weight loss may be different for male and female students. Although the findings did not generalize to all students, the Planet Health trial was the first randomized controlled field trial to provide evidence that a school-wide behavioral skills program can be successful at helping to reduce the prevalence of obesity.

Another approach to reducing obesity among adolescents is to provide parents with the behavioral skills and motivation to help their children change their health-related behaviors. Motivational interviewing (MI) is a patient-centered counseling style designed to decrease ambivalence and increase patients' motivation for behavioral change (Miller & Rose, 2009). Rather than providing overt advice or educational information, MI aims to elicit the motivation to change from the patients themselves by using strategies such as reflective listening and shared decision-making. The early stages of MI counseling focus on building motivation, whereas the later stages can be adapted to incorporate behavioral skills training, including helping patients to identify goals, create an action plan, anticipate potential barriers, and engage in self-monitoring (Resnicow & McMaster, 2012). Previous studies have integrated MI with behavioral skills techniques (Wilson et al., 2015). There is ample evidence that MI is an effective strategy when coupled with behavioral skills training for helping overweight and obese adults lose weight (for a review, see Armstrong et al., 2011) and an effective strategy for helping parents to facilitate weight loss among their overweight or obese children (Spear et al., 2007).

In a recent randomized controlled trial, BMI^2, Resnicow et al. (2015) provided MI and behavioral skills training to pediatricians and registered dieticians (RD). Pediatric offices were then randomly assigned to provide parents of overweight or obese adolescents with (1) usual care, (2) four MI sessions with a pediatrician (pediatrician only), or (3) four MI sessions with a pediatrician and six MI sessions with a dietician (pediatrician + RD). At a 2-year follow-up, patients in the integrated healthcare group (pediatrician + RD) demonstrated the lowest body mass index. The integrated healthcare group was significantly different from the usual care group, but there was no significant difference in BMI between the usual care and pediatrician only group. These findings provide one example of how a well-established counseling strategy, coupled with behavioral skills training, can be improved further by incorporating an integrated team of healthcare professionals.

Middle Age Adult-Focused Randomized Controlled Interventions

Primary care offices present a good opportunity to identify and intervene with patients who may be high risk for developing a chronic health problem (e.g., those who are physically inactive and/or overweight). For example, the Activity Counseling Trial (King et al., 1998) tested the effectiveness of primary care-based physical activity counseling across a 2-year period. Sedentary adults (M_{age} = 51 years) were randomly assigned to (1) a standard care group, (2) a staff-assistance group, or (3) a staff-counseling group. All participants were given the same recommendations for physical activity and written materials from their primary care provider. The staff-assisted group received additional behavioral skills training including meeting with a health counselor to form an individualized physical activity plan, self-monitoring physical activity with an accelerometer, receiving personalized feedback about overcoming barriers via mail, and structured counseling sessions during naturally occurring doctor visits. The staff-counseling intervention group received the same treatment as the staff-assistance group, plus additional resources including frequent phone-based behavioral skills counseling (e.g., to evaluate success at meeting their physical activity goals, develop solutions for dealing with barriers, and provide social support), in addition to in-person counseling sessions and behavior skills training classes.

After 2 years, there was no significant difference in self-reported physical activity; however, both intervention groups demonstrated significantly greater cardiorespiratory fitness than the standard care group, as measured by maximal oxygen uptake (Simons-Morton et al., 2001). Follow-up analyses revealed that several demographic, physiological, environmental, and psychosocial variables influenced the effectiveness of the intervention. Specifically, among patients in the assistance group, those with relatively low income and worse health at baseline were less likely to maintain their physical activity goal past the first year. Among participants in the counseling group, those who reported seeing other walkers/exercisers in their neighborhood and relatively high self-efficacy for overcoming barriers at baseline were significantly more likely to meet their physical activity goals at the 2-year time point. Taken together, these findings indicate that educational information alone is insufficient for improving adherence to physical activity goals. Behavioral counseling that incorporates self-monitoring and personalized feedback appears to be an effective approach, but it is important also to account for individual differences in responsivity.

In addition to working individually with patients in primary care offices, there may also be opportunities to instill behavioral skills training at the community level. For example, the Positive Action for Today's Health (PATH) trial was a randomized trial that tested whether increasing perceptions of safety and access for physical activity, and using social marketing to address motivators for walking, was effective at increasing neighborhood walking (Wilson et al., 2010, 2015). Across three low-income communities in South Carolina (matched by crime, ethnicity, physical activity, and income), communities were randomly assigned to implement an intervention combining a police-patrolled walking program with social marketing strategies for increasing physical activity, a police-patrolled walking program only, or a general health education program (control group). The intervention focused on African American adults (M_{age} = 51.0 years) residing in the targeted low-income communities who were capable of engaging in regular walking (i.e., no disabling medical conditions). In both intervention groups, participants had the opportunity to engage in scheduled neighborhood trail walks during weekday evenings and Saturday mornings. The scheduled walks were organized through local community centers, led by a walking leader trained in CPR and safety prevention, and were patrolled by a police officer. Alternatively, the general health education program included general health events highlighting chronic disease prevention.

Participants in the full intervention program also received social marketing materials aimed at addressing individual-, interpersonal-, and community-level barriers for neighborhood walking. This information was delivered through a 1-year calendar, with each month focusing on one of the following objectives: (1) beliefs about safety and access to local walking trails, (2) beliefs and attitudes toward increasing physical activity, (3) beliefs and attitudes about improving mental health and well-being, (4) building self-efficacy for engaging in regular walking, and (5) improving community connectedness. The calendar was designed to give participants the opportunity to practice several behavioral strategies, including goal setting, self-rewards, and progress tracking. The calendar was intended to increase self-efficacy, promote the five objectives of the program, and provide logistics about the scheduled community walks.

To test whether the intervention was effective at increasing physical activity, all participants were instructed to wear an accelerometer for 7 consecutive days. Accelerometer-assessed moderate to vigorous physical activity was measured pre-intervention, at the end of the 1-year intervention, 6 months after the end of the intervention, and 12 months after the end of the intervention. Additionally, attendance was recorded at each scheduled PATH walk to index the total number of monthly participants. Across the 24-month follow-up period, there was no significant difference in moderate to vigorous physical activity between the three groups. However, walking attendance in the full intervention group increased significantly from 40 walkers per month to 400 walkers by 9 months, with a sustained average of about 200 walkers per month after 18 and 24 months. This change in trail walking was not observed in the community that received only the police-patrolling support. Furthermore, a follow-up analysis showed an intervention effect of the full intervention program on accelerometry estimated moderate-to-vigorous PA among older adults in the PATH trial (Sweeney, Wilson, & Van Horn, 2017). Results from the PATH trial suggest that behavioral skills training delivered through social marketing campaigns can be effective for influencing neighborhood walking; these findings further highlight the importance of taking into account physical and social and environmental factors (e.g., perceptions of safety) when designing behavior change interventions.

Behavioral interventions have been shown to be effective for changing health-related behaviors, including physical activity and diet. Extending these findings, there is further evidence that changes in health-related behaviors can reduce or delay the onset of chronic disease. A seminal example highlighting the utility of lifestyle interventions for preventing chronic illness is the Diabetes Prevention Program (DPP; DPP Group, 1999, 2002). The DPP was a 27-center randomized controlled trial that compared the effectiveness of a lifestyle intervention relative to pharmacological therapy and a placebo control group for preventing the onset of type 2 diabetes, among high-risk individuals (M_{age} = 50.6). Participants in the lifestyle-intervention group set weight-loss and physical activity goals. They worked individually with a case manager who delivered a series of core-curriculum sessions, which consisted of a weigh-in, review of self-monitoring records, presentation of educational information, continuous identification of barriers to weight loss and physical activity, and the development of a weekly action plan for meeting the physical activity and weight-loss goals. These sessions were tailored based on the individual's specific needs and his or her cultural background.

Across a 3-year follow-up period, diabetes incidence was lowest among the lifestyle-intervention group, with the lifestyle-intervention group showing a reduced risk of onset of 58% and the medication group showing a reduced risk of 31%, relative to the control group. In a follow-up study, to examine the long-term maintenance of these effects, participants from all three groups were recontacted and offered the opportunity to participate in a group-based lifestyle intervention (DPP Group, 2009). Ten years after the original assignment to the DPP, the cumulative incidence of diabetes remained lowest among individuals assigned originally to the lifestyle-intervention group.

In line with research suggesting that chronic illnesses cluster (Suhrcke et al., 2006), the lifestyle changes made by participants in the DPP appear to have also influenced their risk for developing cardiovascular disease (DPP Research Group, 2013). Specifically, over the 10-year follow-up period, all three groups showed a significant reduction in systolic blood pressure, diastolic blood pressure, and LDL cholesterol; however, the lifestyle-intervention group demonstrated the lowest use of lipid and blood pressure medication. These findings suggest that participants who made lifestyle changes, with less medication, achieved a similar long-term reduced risk of cardiovascular disease than participants in the medication and control groups. Since the DPP, several other randomized controlled trials have reported positive effects of lifestyle interventions as a strategy for preventing diabetes (Pan et al., 1997; Tuomilehto et al., 2001). There is converging evidence, then, that promoting healthy lifestyle habits is an effective strategy for reducing people's risk for developing chronic illness.

Elderly Adult-Focused Randomized Controlled Interventions

In addition to preventing the onset of chronic illness, behavioral lifestyle changes may also improve health outcomes among patients already living with chronic illnesses. The Look AHEAD study ("Action for Health in Diabetes"; Look AHEAD Research Group, 2006) was the first randomized controlled trial to provide direct evidence for the longitudinal health benefits of lifestyle changes (i.e., weight loss) among patients with a chronic illness. The Look AHEAD study tested whether intentional weight loss among overweight or obese individuals with type 2 diabetes led to a reduction in cardiovascular morbidity and mortality (M_{age} = 59.0 years). Participants were randomly assigned to complete a diabetes support and education program (control group), or an intensive lifestyle-intervention program, designed to help patients lose at least 7% of their initial weight and to increase their physical to at least 175 min/week.

The lifestyle intervention drew upon the methods used in the DPP but was adapted for individuals already diagnosed with type 2 diabetes. Phase 1 of the program aimed to help patients achieve initial weight loss through weekly on-site sessions with a lifestyle counselor during the first 6 months and three sessions per month during months 7–12. Through a mixture of group and individual sessions, participants received educational information about behavioral weight control including topics such as the importance of self-monitoring and methods of physical activity. Participants were instructed to track their daily caloric intake and were provided with a portion-controlled meal plan. Additionally, they were instructed to gradually increase their weekly minutes of physical activity and were offered opportunities to participate in supervised activity classes. Among patients struggling to meet the dietary and physical activity recommendations, individualized support was offered to help patients identify problem behaviors, provide a list of solutions, and develop a written plan with specific goals and action plans.

During years 2–4, Phase 2 of the program aimed to help patients maintain their weight loss and consisted of bimonthly individual sessions in which a lifestyle counselor would reinforce strategies introduced in year 1 (e.g., reviewing self-monitoring records, problem-solving, goal setting). Participants had the opportunity to participate in a refresher group program and a reunion group program to reconnect with acquaintances from Phase 1. During Phase 3 of the program (year 5 and beyond), participants were encouraged to attend monthly, individual on-site sessions with a lifestyle counselor. The purpose of these sessions was to help review successes and challenges in maintaining weight and physical activity goals and to provide support for dietary and physical activity lapses and weight regain. Participants were followed for 13.5 years (median follow-up of 9.6 years; Look AHEAD Research Group, 2014a, 2014b).

The lifestyle-intervention group was effective at helping patients to lose weight. The largest change in body weight was observed in the first year, such that the intervention group had an average weight loss of 8.6%, whereas the control group has an average weight loss of 0.7% (Look AHEAD Research Group, 2007). By the end of the fifth year, patients in the intervention group had gradually regained about half of their lost weight and tended to remain at that weight for the rest of the trial (Look AHEAD Research Group, 2013, 2014a). The control group displayed small decreases in weight across all years; however, at each time point, the intervention group displayed a greater change in weight loss than the control group. Importantly, patients in the intervention group reported greater practice of critical physical activity and weight control behaviors, including increasing self-reported physical activity, reducing caloric intake and fat intake, using meal replacements, and weighing themselves on a regular basis (Look AHEAD Research Group, 2014a). These results suggest that the successful weight loss of the intervention group may be attributable, in part, to the self-monitoring skills acquired during the individual and group sessions of the intervention.

Although the intervention was successful at helping patients to achieve and maintain weight loss, there was no difference in cardiovascular deaths between the intervention and control groups (Look AHEAD Research Group, 2013). However, participants in the intervention group benefited in a number of other ways including improved metabolic control, blood pressure, and lipid profile (Look AHEAD Research Group, 2013). Participants in the intervention group reported a greater reduction in the use of glucose-lowering and antihypertensive medicine, were less likely to be diagnosed with metabolic syndrome, and displayed a greater rate of remission of type 2 diabetes (Look AHEAD Research Group, 2007, 2013). Furthermore, patients who completed the lifestyle intervention spent fewer days in the hospital and required less medication relative to patients in the control group, yielding savings of approximately $600 per year (Look AHEAD Research Group, 2014b). Thus, results from the Look AHEAD trial support the use of lifestyle interventions that emphasize self-monitoring as a cost-effective strategy for improving weight-related health outcomes among patients with chronic illness.

In addition to providing chronic illness patients with the information and skills to change their dietary and physical activity tendencies, behavioral interventions may be strengthened further by providing patients with information about how to self-manage their chronic conditions. Self-management education programs aim to provide patients with information about managing their symptoms and improving their quality of life. Such programs often incorporate a structured learning experience that aims to increase patients' knowledge about (1) the medical management of their health condition; (2) changing or maintaining new behaviors, including adopting health lifestyle habits; and (3) coping with the emotional challenges of chronic illness (Corbin & Strauss, 1988; Lorig & Holman, 2003). Randomized controlled trials have provided ample evidence that self-management programs are effective for helping patients with a variety of chronic conditions, including asthma (Lorig, Gonzalez & Ritter, 1999), coronary heart disease (Clark, Dodge et al., 1997), and chronic pain (LeFort, Gray-Donald, Rowat, & Jeans, 1998).

One example of an effective self-management approach is the Chronic Disease Self-Management Program (CDSMP), a community-based self-management intervention (Lorig et al., 1999). Patients with at least one chronic illness (including heart disease, lung disease, stroke, arthritis) were randomly assigned to complete a 7-week educational program or to a control group (M_{age} = 62.2 years). The education program was led by trained lay leaders, many of whom had a chronic disease, and covered a range of topics including physical activity, the use of cognitive symptom management techniques, nutrition, fatigue and sleep management, dealing with negative emotions, communication with health professionals, and problem-solving. The sessions incorporated a variety of techniques designed to increase self-efficacy for managing one's chronic illness, such as the use of weekly action plans and feedback.

At a 6-month follow-up, compared to the control group, patients who completed the CDSMP demonstrated a significantly greater change in minutes of physical activity, the practice of cognitive symptom management, and improved communication with their physicians. Additionally, the treatment group reported greater health, less disability, fewer limitations in their social activities, greater energy, less health distress, and fewer nights spent in the hospital. Additionally, participants who had originally participated in the control group were later offered the opportunity to complete the CDSMP. Six months after completing the program, similar to the original treatment group, these patients reported a significant increase in physical activity, a greater use of cognitive symptom management, less health distress, fewer limitations in their social activities, and fewer nights spent in the hospital. Furthermore, 2 years after completing the CDSMP, relative to their baseline status, patients continued to show reduced health distress, greater self-efficacy for managing their chronic illness, and fewer visits to their physician/ER (Lorig et al., 2001). The positive effects of the CDSMP have been replicated with diverse populations (Lorig, Ritter, & Gonzalez, 2003) and using Internet-based delivery (Lorig et al., 2008). Thus, the additional studies demonstrated the generalizability and translational aspects of the CDSMP approach to long-term lifestyle change.

Summary of Critical Components of Behavioral Interventions

The randomized controlled trials reviewed in this section represent a diverse range of approaches to promoting changes in health-related behaviors. Table 2.1 highlights some of the key features of these trials including information about the environment in which the study took place, primary goals, the type of behavioral strategies used, and main findings from the study. These interventions incorporated a range of behavioral skills training, with the majority of studies reporting that these strategies were aimed at increasing self-efficacy. Social cognitive theory proposes that self-efficacy, or an individual's belief in his or her capacity to carry out behaviors needed to attain a desired outcome, plays a central role in how people approach goals (Bandura, 1986). Specifically, people high in self-efficacy tend to be more likely to believe that they can master challenging problems and recover quickly from setbacks, skills which may be especially important among people seeking to change health behaviors (Bandura, 2004).

Although it is evident that many of the trials included in this section focused on similar types of behavioral skills, including goal setting, action planning, self-monitoring, and problem-solving, there is likely considerable variability in how these skills were defined and implemented (Abraham & Michie, 2008). For example, goals can vary on a number of dimensions, including specificity, time span, and feasibility. Similarly, self-monitoring strategies may range from the use of objective tools such as an accelerometer to keeping behavioral logs to greater conscious awareness of one's actions. Variability in these constructs may be critical for understanding when and why behavioral skills training is likely to be most effective for changing health behaviors (for a similar critique, see Sheeran, Klein, & Rothman, 2016). Relatedly, although behavioral skills training is presumed to increase self-efficacy, trials rarely report manipulation checks to confirm whether behavioral skills training engendered higher levels of self-efficacy among the intervention (relative to the control) group. Future research may consider incorporating more explicit definitions describing how behavioral skills are being defined and implemented and provide evidence that these skills are having positive effects on people's level of self-efficacy. For an example of explicit definitions and taxonomy of behavioral change techniques, see Abraham and Michie (2008).

In summary, greater standardization of implementation of behavioral interventions is needed to advance the effectiveness of health promotion interventions in integrated healthcare settings. Critical factors include addressing self-monitoring, receiving feedback, action plans, problem-solving, and goal setting. Engaging significant others such as family members, parents, teachers, and healthcare providers in the process may increase the likelihood of successful implementation and improvements in youth health-related outcomes.

Table 2.1 Summary of randomized control trials

Trial	Participants	Environment	Length of study	Primary goals	Behavioral training skills	Primary results for the intervention group
Child and Adolescent Trial for Cardiovascular Health (CATCH)	Children (M_{age} = 8.76 years)	Elementary school, classroom-based program	3 academic years	Teach students to identify and choose healthy food, engage in regular physical activity, and avoid tobacco-use	Modeling by cartoon characters, food preparation, monitoring, goal setting, perceived support	Greater dietary knowledge; Greater perceived support for food choices; Lower daily total energy intake; Lower daily energy intake from fat; More minutes of daily physical activity
Active by Choice Today (ACT)	Children (M_{age} = 11.34 years)	Middle school, after-school program	17 weeks	Increase intrinsic motivation and improve behavioral skills, so as to increase physical activity	Goal-setting, developing communication skills, providing and seeking support outside of the program, developing a positive self-concept	Greater physical activity mid-way through the intervention; Participants encountered environmental barriers outside of the program that prevented physical activity maintenance
Planet Health	Children (M_{age} = 11.70 years)	Middle school, classroom-based program	2 academic years	Reduce television viewing to 2 h/day, increase physical activity, decrease consumption of high-fat foods, and increase consumption of fruits and vegetables	Goal-setting, self-monitoring, perceived support	Reduction in television viewing time; Reduction in the prevalence of obesity (female students only); Increase in fruit and vegetable consumption and a decrease in total energy intake (female students only)
BMI[2]	Parents and children (M_{age} adults = 5.1 years)	Primary care office	2 years	Increase intrinsic motivation and teach behavioral skills to parents, so as to decrease BMI among adolescents	Goal-setting, action planning, problem-solving, self-monitoring	The group who received the intervention from both a physician and a dietician had the lowest BMI

Activity Counseling Trial	Adults (M_{age} = 51.0 years)	Primary care office	2 years	Increase and maintain physical activity and cardiorespiratory fitness among sedentary adults	Planning, self-monitoring with an accelerometer, goal-setting, problem-solving solutions for barriers	No significant difference in self-reported physical activity; Greater cardio-respiratory fitness (as measured by maximal oxygen uptake)
Positive Action for Today's Health (PATH)	Adults (M_{age} = 51.0 years)	Community-based	2 years	Increase perceptions of safety and access for physical activity, so as to increase physical activity	Goal-setting, self-rewards, self-monitoring	No significant difference in accelerometer-assessed physical activity; Significant increase in number of walkers on neighborhood trails
Diabetes Prevention Program (DPP)	Adults (M_{age} = 50.6 years)	Clinical centers	3 years; also completed 10 year follow-up	Prevent or delay the onset of type 2 diabetes through changes in physical activity and diet	Self-monitoring, planning, goal-setting, problem-solving solutions for barriers	Lower incidence of diabetes
Look AHEAD study (Action for Health in Diabetes)	Adults (M_{age} = 59 years)	Clinical centers	Three phases across 5 years; followed for 13.5 years	Test whether intentional weight loss leads to a reduction in cardiovascular morbidity and mortality	Self-monitoring, planning, problem-solving for barriers	Significant reduction in weight loss, but no significant difference in cardiovascular deaths; Significant improvement in metabolic control, blood pressure, and lipid profile; Less likely to be diagnosed with metabolic syndrome and displayed a greater rate of remission of type 2 diabetes

(continued)

Table 2.1 (continued)

Trial	Participants	Environment	Length of study	Primary goals	Behavioral training skills	Primary results for the intervention group
Chronic Disease Self-Management Program (CDSMP)	Adults (M_{age} = 62.2 years)	Community-based	2 years	Health behaviors, health status, and health service utilization	Generating weekly action plans, modeling behaviors, problem-solving, goal-setting	Greater change in minutes of physical activity, the practice of cognitive symptom management, and improved communication with physicians; Greater health, less disability, fewer limitations in their social activities, greater energy, less health distress, and fewer nights spent in the hospital.

Multidisciplinary Approaches to Healthcare and Cost-Effectiveness

While behavioral skills training interventions have been effectively delivered by clinical and health psychologists, interventions that have been offered by physicians have been shown to produce relatively small effects. For example, a meta-analysis of 17 randomized controlled trials found that brief advice from a physician (compared to no advice) was associated with a small but significant increased probability of quitting smoking (relative risk (RR) 1.66, 95%; *CI* = 1.42–1.94 (Stead, Bergson, & Lancaster, 2008). Similarly, a recent meta-analysis found that relative to control settings, behavioral lifestyle interventions implemented in primary care settings were effective for reducing body mass index among adolescents, but the overall effect size was small in magnitude (*d* = 0.26; Mitchell, Amaro, & Steele, 2016). In general, while physician-based interventions have shown small effects on improving health behaviors, more research is needed to compare the integration of behavioral interventions in healthcare settings with behavioral health experts and to evaluate the cost-effectiveness of effectively implementing behavioral interventions in the healthcare setting.

An increasing number of trials are providing cost-effectiveness analyses that further support the benefits of integrating behavioral interventions into part of the integrated care treatment plan. The DPP trial conducted cumulative undiscounted per capita direct medical costs analyses of the interventions over 10 years (DPP Research Group, 2012). The cumulative combined total direct medical costs of care were least for lifestyle outside of the DPP trial ($26,810 lifestyle vs. $27,384 pharmacological therapy vs. $29,007 placebo). The cumulative quality-adjusted life years were greatest for lifestyle (6.89) than pharmacological therapy (6.79) or placebo (6.74). When costs and outcomes were discounted at 3% and adjusted for survival, lifestyle cost $12,878 per quality-adjusted life years and pharmacological therapy had slightly lower costs and nearly the same quality-adjusted life years as placebo. These results suggest that from a payer perspective, lifestyle and pharmacological therapy interventions provided marginally more cost savings compared to placebo.

The Look AHEAD Research Group (2014b) assessed the relative impact of the intensive lifestyle intervention on use and costs of healthcare in the Look AHEAD trial. Overweight and obese adults were randomized to the intensive lifestyle intervention or a diabetes support and education comparison program. The intensive lifestyle intervention resulted in reductions in annual hospitalizations, hospital days, and number of medications and resulted in a cost savings for hospitalization and medication producing a relative per-person 10-year cost savings of $5280. However, these cost savings were not demonstrated for those with a history of cardiovascular disease. Lorig et al. (2001) have also estimated that the savings accrued by fewer visits to the hospital and emergency rooms across a 2-year period is at least three times greater than the cost of providing the CDSMP.

Taken together, the results from these cost-effectiveness studies suggest that providing patients with self-management and behavioral lifestyle programs not only improves their ability to manage and cope with their chronic illnesses, but it is also a cost-effective approach that can ultimately lead to reductions in national healthcare costs. As evidenced by a recent special issue, there is an increased need for developing standardized approaches to cost-effective analyses for the evaluation of behavioral interventions (Wilson, Christensen, Jacobson, & Kaplan, 2018).

Summary and Conclusions

In this chapter we reviewed the evidence from randomized controlled trials that demonstrate the importance of integrating behavioral interventions for improving lifestyle behaviors (e.g., physical activity, healthy diet, weight management) for preventing and treating a variety of chronic diseases. Critical components of effective interventions included targeting self-regulation and self-efficacy through strategies such as self-monitoring, developing action plans, and utilizing effective goal setting strategies across the life span. While limited research exists on comparing the effectiveness of integrating behavioral health experts into the integrated care team, the effects of traditional randomized trials show the consistent effectiveness of implementing behavioral interventions with a high fidelity of delivery. Furthermore, there is a growing literature that supports the cost-effectiveness of behavioral interventions on reducing hospital utilization and medication usage. Overall, cost savings are potentially substantial and have important implications for reducing national healthcare costs.

References

Abraham, C., & Michie, S. (2008). A taxonomy of behavior change techniques used in interventions. *Health Psychology, 27*, 379–387.

Armstrong, M. J., Mottershead, T. A., Ronksley, P. E., Sigal, R. J., Campbell, T. S., & Hemmelgarn, B. R. (2011). Motivational interviewing to improve weight loss in overweight and/or obese patients: A systematic review and meta-analysis of randomized controlled trials. *Obesity Reviews, 12*, 709–723.

Ayotte, B. J., Margrett, J. A., & Hicks-Patrick, J. (2010). Physical activity in middle-aged and young-old adults the roles of self-efficacy, barriers, outcome expectancies, self-regulatory behaviors and social support. *Journal of Health Psychology, 15*, 173–185.

Bandura, A. (1986). *Social foundations of thought and action: A social cognitive theory*. Englewood Cliffs, NJ: Prenctice-Hall, Inc.

Bandura, A. (2004). Health promotion by social cognitive means. *Health Education & Behavior, 31*, 143–164.

Clark, N. M., Janz, N. K., Dodge, J. A., Schork, M. A., Wheeler, J. R., Liang, J., ... & Santinga, J. T. (1997). Self-management of heart disease by older adults: Assessment of an intervention based on social cognitive theory. *Research on Aging, 19*, 362–382.

Corbin, J. M., & Strauss, A. (1988). *Unending work and care: Managing chronic illness at home*. San Francisco, CA: Jossey-Bass.

Diabetes Prevention Program Outcomes Study Research Group, Orchard, T. J., Temprosa, M., Barrett-Connor, E., Fowler, S. E., Goldberg, R. B., … Watson, K. E. (2013). Long-term effects of the Diabetes Prevention Program interventions on cardiovascular risk factors: A report from the DPP Outcomes Study. *Diabetic Medicine, 30*, 46–55.

Diabetes Prevention Program Research Group. (1999). The Diabetes Prevention Program: Design and methods for a clinical trial in the prevention of type 2 diabetes. *Diabetes Care, 22*, 623–634.

Diabetes Prevention Program Research Group. (2002). Reduction in the incidence of type 2 diabetes with lifestyle intervention or metformin. *New England Journal of Medicine, 346*, 393–403.

Diabetes Prevention Program Research Group. (2009). 10-year follow-up of diabetes incidence and weight loss in the Diabetes Prevention Program Outcomes Study. *Lancet, 374*, 1677–1686.

Diabetes Prevention Program Research Group. (2012). The 10-year cost-effectiveness of lifestyle intervention or metformin for diabetes prevention: An intent-to-treat analysis of the DPP/DPPOS. *Diabetes, 35*, 723–730.

Gollwitzer, P. M. (1999). Implementation intentions: Strong effects of simple plans. *American Psychologist, 54*, 493–503.

Gortmaker, S. L., Peterson, K., Wiecha, J., Sobol, A. M., Dixit, S., Fox, M. K., & Laird, N. (1999). Reducing obesity via a school-based interdisciplinary intervention among youth: Planet Health. *Archives of Pediatrics & Adolescent Medicine, 153*, 409–418.

King, A. C., Sallis, J. F., Dunn, A. L., Simons-Morton, D. G., Albright, C. A., Cohen, S., … Coday, M. C. (1998). Overview of the Activity Counseling Trial (ACT) intervention for promoting physical activity in primary health care settings. *Medicine & Science in Sports & Exercise, 30*, 1086–1096.

LeFort, S., Gray-Donald, K., Rowat, K., & Jeans, M. (1998). Randomized controlled trial of a community-based psychoeducation program for the self-management of chronic pain. *Pain, 74*, 297–306.

Look AHEAD Research Group. (2006). The look AHEAD study: A description of the lifestyle intervention and the evidence supporting it. *Obesity, 14*, 737–752.

Look AHEAD Research Group. (2007). Reduction in weight and cardiovascular disease risk factors in individuals with type 2 diabetes: One-year results of the look AHEAD trial. *Diabetes Care, 30*, 1374–1383.

Look AHEAD Research Group. (2013). Cardiovascular Effects of Intensive Lifestyle Intervention in Type 2 Diabetes. *New England Journal of Medicine, 369*, 145–154.

Look AHEAD Research Group. (2014a). Eight-year weight losses with an intensive lifestyle intervention: The look AHEAD study. *Obesity, 22*, 5–13.

Look AHEAD Research Group. (2014b). Impact of an intensive lifestyle intervention on use and cost of medical services among overweight and obese adults with type 2 diabetes. *Diabetes Care, 37*, 2548–2556.

Lorig, K., Gonzalez, V. M., & Ritter, P. (1999). Community-based Spanish language arthritis education program: a randomized trial. *Medical Care, 37*, 957–963.

Lorig, K., & Holman, H. (2003). Self-management education: History, definition, outcomes, and mechanisms. *Annals of Behavioral Medicine, 26*, 1–7.

Lorig, K. R., Ritter, P., Stewart, A. L., Sobel, D. S., Brown, B. W., Jr., Bandura, A., … Holman, H. R. (2001). Chronic disease self-management program: 2-year health status and health care utilization outcomes. *Medical Care, 39*, 1217–1223.

Lorig, K. R., Ritter, P. L., Dost, A., Plant, K., Laurent, D. D., & McNeil, I. (2008). The expert patients programme online, a 1-year study of an internet-based self-management programme for people with long-term conditions. *Chronic Illness, 4*, 247–256.

Lorig, K. R., Sobel, D. S., Stewart, A. L., Brown, B. W., Jr., Bandura, A., Ritter, P., … Holman, H. R. (1999). Evidence suggesting that a chronic disease self-management program can improve health status while reducing hospitalization: A randomized trial. *Medical Care, 37*, 5–14.

Luepker, R. V., Perry, C. L., McKinlay, S. M., Nader, P. R., Parcel, G. S., Stone, E. J., ... & Kelder, S. H. (1996). Outcomes of a field trial to improve children's dietary patterns and physical activity: the Child and Adolescent Trial for Cardiovascular Health (CATCH). *Jama, 275*, 768–776.

Michie, S., Abraham, C., Whittington, C., McAteer, J., & Gupta, S. (2009). Effective techniques in healthy eating and physical activity interventions: A meta-regression. *Health Psychology, 28*, 690–701.

Miller, W. R., & Rose, G. S. (2009). Toward a theory of motivational interviewing. *American Psychologist, 64*, 527–537.

Mitchell, T. B., Amaro, C. M., & Steele, R. G. (2016). Pediatric weight management interventions in primary care settings: A meta-analysis. *Health Psychology, 35*, 704–713.

Pan, X. R., Li, G. W., Hu, Y. H., Wang, J. X., Yang, W. Y., An, Z. X., … Howard, B. V. (1997). Effects of diet and exercise in preventing NIDDM in people with impaired glucose tolerance: The Da Qing IGT and diabetes study. *Diabetes Care, 20*, 537–544.

Perry, C. L., Sellers, D. E., Johnson, C., Pedersen, S., Bachman, K. J., Parcel, G. S., ... & Cook, K. (1997). The Child and Adolescent Trial for Cardiovascular Health (CATCH): intervention, implementation, and feasibility for elementary schools in the United States. *Health Education & Behavior, 24*, 716–735.

Resnicow, K., & McMaster, F. (2012). Motivational interviewing: Moving from why to how with autonomy support. *International Journal of Behavioral Nutrition and Physical Activity, 9*, 1–9.

Resnicow, K., McMaster, F., Bocian, A., Harris, D., Zhou, Y., Snetselaar, L., … Hollinger, D. (2015). Motivational interviewing and dietary counseling for obesity in primary care: An RCT. *Pediatrics, 135*, 649–657.

Schroeder, S. (2007). We can do better: Improving the health of the American people. *New England Journal of Medicine, 357*, 1221–1228.

Sheeran, P., Klein, W. M., & Rothman, A. J. (2016). Health behavior change: Moving from observation to intervention. *Annual Review of Psychology* Advance Online Publication.

Simons-Morton, D. G., Blair, S. N., King, A. C., Morgan, T. M., Applegate, W. B., O'Toole, M., ... & Shih, J. H. (2001). Effects of physical activity counseling in primary care: The Activity Counseling Trial: A randomized controlled trial. *JAMA: Journal of the American Medical Association, 286*, 677–687.

Spear, B. A., Barlow, S. E., Ervin, C., Ludwig, D. S., Saelens, B. E., Schetzina, K. E., & Taveras, E. M. (2007). Recommendations for treatment of child and adolescent overweight and obesity. *Pediatrics, 120*, S254–S288.

Stead, L. F., Bergson, G., & Lancaster, T. (2008). *Physician advice for smoking cessation Cochrane review*. London: The Cochrane Library.

Stoto, M. A. (2013). *Population health in the Affordable Care Act era*. Washington, DC: AcademyHealth.

Suhrcke, M., Nugent, R. A., Stuckler, D., & Rocco, L. (2006). *Chronic disease: An economic perspective*. London: Oxford Health Alliance.

Sweeney, A. M., Wilson, D. K., & Lee Van Horn, M. (2017). Longitudinal relationships between self-concept for physical activity and neighborhood social life as predictors of physical activity among older African American adults. *International Journal of Behavioral Nutrition and Physical Activity, 14*(1), 67.

Tuomilehto, J., Lindström, J., Eriksson, J. G., Valle, T. T., Hämäläinen, H., Ilanne-Parikka, P., … Salminen, V. (2001). Prevention of type 2 diabetes mellitus by changes in lifestyle among subjects with impaired glucose tolerance. *New England Journal of Medicine, 344*, 1343–1350.

Wilson, D. K., Kitzman-Ulrich, H., Williams, J. E., Saunders, R., Griffin, S., Pate, R., … Sisson, S. B. (2008). An overview of "The Active by Choice Today" (ACT) trial for increasing physical activity. *Contemporary Clinical Trials, 29*, 21–31.

Wilson, D. K., Trumpeter, N. N., St George, S. M., Coulon, S. M., Griffin, S., Lee Van Horn, M., … Gadson, B. (2010). An overview of the "Positive Action for Today's Health" (PATH) trial for increasing walking in low income, ethnic minority communities. *Contemporary Clinical Trials, 31*, 624–633.

Wilson, D. K., Van Horn, M. L., Kitzman-Ulrich, H., Saunders, R., Pate, R., Lawman, H. G., ... & Mansard, L. (2011). Results of the "Active by Choice Today"(ACT) randomized trial for increasing physical activity in low-income and minority adolescents. *Health Psychology, 30*, 463–471.

Wilson, D. K., Van Horn, M. L., Siceloff, E. R., Alia, K. A., St George, S. M., Lawman, H. G., … Gadson, B. (2015). The results of the "Positive Action for Today's Health" (PATH) trial for increasing walking and physical activity in underserved African-American Communities. *Annals of Behavioral Medicine, 49*, 398–410.

Wilson, D.K, Christensen, A., Jacobson, P., & Kaplan, R.M. (2018). Special Issue on Standards for Economic Analyses for the Field of Health Psychology and Behavioral Medicine. *Health Psychology*.

Woolf, S. H., & Aron, L. (Eds.). (2013). *US health in international perspective: Shorter lives, poorer health*. Bethesda, MD: National Academies Press.

Chapter 3
The Epidemiology of Medical Diseases and Associated Behavioral Risk Factors

Sarah Lindeman, Jon Nolan, and Alexandros Maragakis

Introduction

Drastic improvements in public health paired with advancements in medicine have lowered infant mortality and significantly boosted the average life span (Centers for Disease Control and Prevention (CDC), 2003). As a result, many of the challenges healthcare professionals face have shifted from the treatment of acute illnesses to a focus on the management and prevention of chronic disease (CDC, 2003, 2013). This is partially due to the fact that outbreaks of deadly communicable diseases have been greatly reduced, such as tuberculosis, small pox, and measles. Simultaneously, increased rates of noncommunicable, chronic conditions, as a result of longer life spans and problematic lifestyles, have led to new areas of foci for healthcare professionals.

Changes in the healthcare needs of the general population as well as improved technologies to treat these have produced higher healthcare costs. In 2014, national health expenditures comprised 17.5% of the US gross domestic product (GDP) at $3 trillion. By 2024, these costs are estimated to rise to approximately 19.6% of the GDP (Centers for Medicare and Medicaid Services, 2015). Increased rates of chronic disease such as diabetes and cardiovascular disease contribute to this rise in costs, leading to increased efforts to find affordable methods of risk reduction and improved health outcomes for patients with chronic disease (World Health Organization (WHO), 2016). Ischemic heart disease, stroke, and chronic obstructive pulmonary disease were the top three leading causes of mortality worldwide in 2012 (WHO, 2014), while chronic disease currently contributes to 60% of deaths

S. Lindeman · J. Nolan
Department of Psychology and Counseling, University of Central Arkansas, Conway, AR, USA

A. Maragakis (✉)
Department of Psychology, Eastern Michigan University, Ypsilanti, MI, USA
e-mail: amaragak@emich.edu

M. P. Duckworth, W. T. O'Donohue (eds.), *Behavioral Medicine and Integrated Care*,
https://doi.org/10.1007/978-3-319-93003-9_3

globally (WHO, 2016). By 2020, this number is expected to reach 73%. In the United States, approximately seven in ten deaths are associated with chronic disease (CDC, 2016a).

Behavioral factors play a significant role in the development of chronic diseases and their associated costs. For example, according to the Centers for Disease Control and Prevention (CDC) (2016b), the national cost of smoking reaches $300 billion yearly, with $170 billion in direct medical expenditures. In addition, failure to reach recommended levels of physical activity is estimated to comprise 11.1% of collective healthcare costs after controlling for body mass index (BMI) scores (Carlson, Fulton, Pratt, Yang, & Adams, 2015). Fortunately, opportunities for prevention and treatment are available. Lifestyle factors, such as diet and exercise, greatly contribute to the development of a range of diseases; therefore, behavioral interventions are an avenue for reducing the risk of developing disease and improving quality of life (WHO, 2016). In this chapter, an introductory overview of chronic diseases that will be covered in subsequent chapters in this book, their epidemiology, as well as the behavioral factors that are associated with the disease will be provided. More detailed information regarding the diseases and the specific behavioral treatments used with each disease will be presented later in the book and therefore will not be presented here.

Chronic Diseases and Their Behavioral Factors

Diabetes Mellitus

As carbohydrates are digested, glucose is released into the bloodstream, triggering β-cells in the pancreas to produce insulin, a hormone essential for glucose breakdown (National Institute of Diabetes and Digestive and Kidney Diseases (NIDDKD), 2014; National Health Service (NHS), 2014a). When the body is unable to metabolize glucose, levels remain high in the bloodstream, a condition known as hyperglycemia. This inability to synthesize or effectively use insulin leads to the development of diabetes mellitus, more commonly referred to as diabetes (NIDDKD, 2014; American Diabetes Association (ADA), 2004). Both type 1 and type 2 diabetes symptomology include polydipsia (constantly feeling thirsty), frequent urination, lethargy, polyphagia (increased appetite), inexplicable weight loss, slowly healing wounds, and blurred vision (NHS, 2014a; ADA, 2004). Because biological markers have yet to be identified, plasma glucose, or blood sugar, estimation is the current standard for meeting diagnostic criteria (World Health Organization, 2006).

Once referred to as juvenile diabetes due to its early development, type 1 diabetes is a chronic disease with rapid symptom onset. Characterized as an autoimmune disorder, the body creates antibodies that attack the body's own β-cells. As a result, the process of glucose metabolism is inhibited (NIDDKD, 2014). Type 2 diabetes, previously referred to as adult-onset diabetes, develops at a gradual pace and occurs when (1) the body becomes resistant to insulin, (2) β-cell response to glucose levels fail to produce adequate compensatory levels of insulin, or (3) a mixture of both (NIDDKD, 2014; NHS, 2014a; ADA, 2004). The condition is theorized to be caused by a mixture of a genetic predisposition and environmental risks such as dietary habits and physical activity levels (NIDDKD, 2014). Risk of developing type 2 diabetes increases with age and is higher for those who have close family members with diabetes and those who are overweight (BMI > 24.9) or obese (BMI > 30) (NHS, 2014b).

The development of diabetes leads to an increase of health complications. In 2010, diabetes was ranked the 7th leading cause of death in the United States (American Diabetic Association (ADA), 2013a, 2013b). Increased incidence of cardiovascular, cerebrovascular, and peripheral arterial disease are experienced by people with diabetes (NHS, 2014c; ADA, 2004). Potential long-term complications resulting from hyperglycemia include nephropathy (damage to the kidneys or kidney disease); peripheral neuropathy (loss of sensation), a condition that may lead to foot ulcers and Charcot joints (damage to weight-bearing joints); retinopathy (damage of the retina); and sexual dysfunction (ADA, 2004). If glucose levels remain high, damage to blood vessels, nerves, and organs can occur, even when glucose levels are only mildly raised. Damage to blood vessels in nerves can cause tingling, burning, and numbness. In the digestive system, this damage can lead to nausea, vomiting, diarrhea, and constipation, while damage to blood vessels in the retina can lead to visual damage (NHS, 2014c). In addition, pregnant women with diabetes are more likely to experience miscarriages and stillbirths (NHS, 2014c).

Incidence rates for diabetes have drastically increased from 1980 to 2014, with 493,000 new diagnoses reported in 1980 and 1.4 million newly diagnosed in 2014 (CDC, 2015a; ADA, 2013a). Of adults over age 18, approximately 9% have received a diagnosis of diabetes by a healthcare professional (CDC, 2012a). In seniors (65 or older), diabetes prevalence is even higher at 25.9%. The American Diabetes Association (2013a) found that, of the 29.1 million people in the United States with diabetes, 21 million were diagnosed, while 8.1 million met blood sugar levels that would warrant a diabetes diagnosis but were undiagnosed, indicating that a large portion of the diabetic population may not be receiving treatment for their condition. Among the 29.1 million with diabetes, 1.25 million were diagnosed with type 1, indicating the pervasiveness of type 2 diabetes (ADA, 2013a). In addition, according to the CDC (2016a, 2016b, 2016c), 86 million adults in the United States (over 1 out of 3) meet the criteria for prediabetes, the precursor to type 2 diabetes, which is marked by blood sugar levels ranging from 100 to 125 mg/dL (Mayo Clinic, 2014).

Diabetes has been shown to be negatively correlated with level of education and income level. Of those who have not completed high school, 15% have diabetes, compared to 7% of those who have obtained a minimum of a bachelor's degree (CDC, 2012a). Ethnicity may also play a role in the likelihood of developing the disease. Increased rates of diabetes have been found in African Americans, Alaskan Natives, Native Americans, Hispanics/Latinos, Native Hawaiians, Pacific Islander

Americans, and some Asian Americans, indicating that genetics play a role in the development of diabetes. Susceptibility to diabetes has also been linked to variants of the TCF7L2 gene. People with two copies of the variants have an 80% higher risk of developing diabetes (NIDDKD, 2014). However, given that type 2 diabetes is linked to both genetic and environmental factors, steps can be taken to reduce risk of developing diabetes regardless of socioeconomic, ethnic, or genetic traits (NIDDKD, 2014; NHS, 2014b).

A consequence of increased prevalence rates of diabetes is higher healthcare costs. In 2012, diagnosed cases of diabetes in the United States cost $245 billion, with $176 billion in direct medical costs. The average medical costs of those with diabetes, after controlling for age and gender differences, were 2.3 times that of a nondiabetic person (ADA, 2013a). However, prevention, early detection, and improved treatment have the potential to reduce these costs and increase quality of life for those managing diabetes. Addressing avenues for behavioral changes that will improve health outcomes can provide numerous benefits for diabetic patients.

The accumulation of excess body fat is a significant contributor to the development of type 2 diabetes due to its negative impact on the body's ability to effectively use insulin. As such, weight loss, particularly in the abdominal region, is associated with improvements in blood glucose levels for prediabetic and diabetic patients (NIDDKD, 2014). Even moderate weight loss (5–7% of body weight) lowers the risk of developing diabetes. Because weight gain is the result of excess caloric intake, increased physical activity paired with reduced caloric intake is an ideal option for decreasing the risk of developing this disease (CDC, 2016c). The addition of patient education and a behavioral intervention regarding their condition may improve weight-loss achievement goals. In a study comparing weight loss in 1314 patients with type 2 diabetes, participants in the education and behavioral intervention group lost significant body weight (3.3% body weight loss without medication, 4% with medication (90% of prescriptions were for metformin)), while those in the control group did not (Azar et al., 2015). Maximizing the likelihood of successful weight loss has the potential to improve blood glucose levels and reduce future complications of the disease, leading to decreased healthcare costs and improved treatment outcomes.

Addressing potential roadblocks to success is an essential aspect of achieving desirable treatment outcomes. Stress, for example, has a range of negative effects on the body, including lowering immunity, increasing heart rate, and spiking blood sugar (National Institute of Mental Health (NIMH), n.d.; ADA, 2013b). Strong negative emotions can lead to more impulsive behaviors, including poor dietary choices and decreased treatment adherence (ADA, 2013b). Addressing options for stress management may, therefore, improve treatment outcomes for this population. Simple changes, such as scheduling time for relaxing activities, engaging in physical activity, journaling, or other identified options for patients may improve stress management, thereby improving diabetes management (NIMH, n.d.; ADA, 2013b). Seeking information regarding patient barriers to treatment adherence, such as poor stress management, allows for problem-solving that increases the likelihood of successful intervention.

Obesity

The industrialization of developed countries has led to a wide range of conveniences that have improved everyday life. However, the once adaptive biological drive to consume excess calories to ensure survival in times of famine is no longer compatible with current environmental conditions. Previously rare opportunities to consume and store excess calories have become far more common, while the need for physical activity has drastically decreased (Bellisari, 2008). The culmination of these factors has led to a lower quality of life for many, sparking the need for interventions that address this discrepancy between environment and natural drives.

According to the CDC (2012a, 2012b), becoming overweight or obese occurs when a person's weight exceeds the range considered healthy for a person of their specified height. A common screening method for obesity is calculating patient's body mass index (BMI) using a formula that considers height and weight. While this measure is not a direct measure of body fat, it is correlated with body fat percentage. Considering factors such as muscle mass are important when using the BMI as a screening tool; muscular patients may be falsely flagged as obese due to the higher density of muscle mass (CDC, 2012b; Harvard School of Public Health, 2016). Other affordable methods for examining patient weight status include waist-to-hip ratio, waist circumference, skinfold thickness, and bioelectrical impedance (using electric current to determine body composition) (Dehghan & Merchant, 2008; Harvard School of Public Health, 2016).

More than one-third of adults (36.5%) in the United States are obese (CDC, 2015b). Nationally, prevalence rates of obesity were the highest for non-Hispanic blacks (38.1%), followed by Hispanics (31.3%), and non-Hispanic Whites (27.1%) (CDC, 2015c). A comparison of obesity by education and socioeconomic status found that women with higher incomes are less likely be obese than women with lower incomes, while income was not associated with obesity rates in men; however, among Mexican-American and non-Hispanic black men, obesity was more likely with higher incomes. No connection between obesity rates and education was found in men, while women were less likely to be obese at higher incomes (CDC, 2015b).

The costs associated with obesity are staggering. In 2008, the estimated medical cost of obesity reached $147 billion. Those who are obese experience approximately $1429 in additional annual healthcare costs compared to non-obese patients (CDC, 2015b). Identified conditions related to obesity range from heart disease and stroke to diabetes, cancer, sleep apnea (pauses in, or shallow, breathing while sleeping), and reproductive problems (CDC, 2015b; National Heart, Lung, and Blood Institute (NHLBI), 2012).

In an effort to improve the health status of individuals in the United States, a national health objective of 2010 was to reduce adult obesity rates from 34.3% found by the 2005–2006 National Health and Nutrition Examination Survey to less than 15% (CDC, 2015d). Government and healthcare professionals were not alone in their recognition of need for change. The results of a Gallup Poll showed that, among health ailments, obesity was ranked as the number one "urgent health problem" (Dugan, 2013). Unfortunately, in 2014, no state's obesity prevalence rates fell below 20% (CDC, 2015c). Improved efforts to reduce the prevalence of obesity remain an essential step toward reducing healthcare costs and improving patients' quality of life.

Treatment of obesity can be accomplished via lowering patients' body fat percentage and can be achieved through weight loss (CDC, 2015e). A caloric deficit, or consuming fewer calories than are expended, can be achieved through dietary improvements, increasing energy expenditure, or a combination of both (Mayo Clinic, 2015; CDC, 2015e). While these methods for reaching weight loss are ideal, instructing patients to eat less and exercise more fails to acknowledge the multifaceted endeavor that is weight loss. A variety of environmental factors play a role in adherence to these suggestions, such as larger portion sizes at restaurants, increasingly sedentary work environments, food advertisements, and sugar-laden social events (American Heart Association, 2016). Simple instructions to restrict caloric intake and increase physical activity do not provide information regarding how to successfully engage in healthy behaviors while presented with frequent temptation and fewer opportunities for engagement in physical activity.

Inadequate health-related knowledge may lead to poorer health outcomes. Providing information about options for engaging in health behaviors may increase the likelihood that patients engage in them. Nutritional knowledge has been significantly, positively correlated with engagement in healthy behaviors associated with weight loss, including increased fruit and vegetable intake, lower consumption of sugar, and the replacement of higher-calorie foods with lower-calorie foods in low-income women (Laz, Rahman, Pohlmeier, & Berenson, 2015). Education, therefore, is an important component of weight-loss success. However, knowledge alone may not lead to significant behavior change. In a study comparing the nutritional knowledge and BMI of 500 participants, researchers found a high level of nutritional knowledge overall, but no significant relationship between knowledge and BMI, indicating nutritional knowledge alone may not suffice (O'Brien & Davies, 2007). The addition of behavioral interventions to education efforts has been shown to produce weight loss when compared to those who do not receive a behavioral intervention (Azar et al., 2015).

In addition to targeting risk factors for obesity, such as excess body weight and physical inactivity, identifying patient avenues for social support, addressing sleep hygiene, and improving stress reduction promote weight-loss success via improving the decision-making process (AHA, 2016). Sleep loss is associated with increased self-reported hunger after a single night (Schmid, Hallschmid, Jauch-Chara, Born, & Schultes, 2008); therefore, addressing sleep issues provides an avenue for improving weight-loss outcomes. In addition, the development of stress management skills leads to improved decision-making via a reduction in impulsive, emotionally based decisions, which may contribute to poor health-related choices (ADA, 2013b). Indeed, successful intervention requires a multifaceted approach that ensures clients have the skills and knowledge necessary to adhere to healthy lifestyle choices.

Dementia

As the aging population continues to grow, adults aged 65 and older are estimated to comprise a significantly larger percentage of the population. In 2000, 35 million (12.4%) adults were over age 65 in the United States; this number is projected to reach 71 million (19.6%) in 2030 (Chapman, Williams, Strine, Anda, & Moore, 2006). A rise in the aging population inevitably leads to a rise in age-related diseases and their associated costs. Among these is dementia, an age-linked group of diseases caused by damaged neurons, or nerve cells, in the brain (Alzheimer's Association, 2014). Progressive damage to these neurons can lead to impairment in executive functioning, complex motor skills, memory, judgment, language, attention, perceptual abilities, etc. (Alzheimer's Foundation of America (AFA), 2016; The American Speech-Language-Hearing Association (ASLHA), 2016). Symptom progression can develop slowly over the course of years or rapidly based on the dementia's etiology and eventually leads to an inability to live independently (ADL) (AFA, 2016).

Alzheimer's disease is the most common form of dementia, comprising 60% of all dementia cases for people over age 65 in the United States, and is characterized by the buildup of plaques (protein fragments) and tangles (twisted protein strands) in the brain (AFA, 2016). Other forms of dementia include vascular dementia (caused by stroke or blocked blood supply), dementia caused by Lewy bodies, trauma dementia due to head injury, frontotemporal dementia, and alcohol dementia caused by prolonged alcohol use (AFA, 2016). As the disease progresses, cognitive functioning gradually decreases, making everyday activities such as medication adherence, grooming, cooking, and other self-care practices challenging for patients. Thus, as cognitive functioning declines, dependence on caregivers increases. As such, the average healthcare costs of older adults with dementia compared to those without it are $4134 higher annually, with 75% of this increase in cost attributable to hospitalization and nursing facility fees (Chapman et al., 2006). Current medical costs associated with dementia are approximately $157–215 billion in the United States. As the aging population continues to rise, costs may double by 2040 if prevalence rates and treatment standards remain at their current levels (Lewy Body Dementia Association, 2016).

In the United States, approximately 8.8% of adults over age 65 were reported to have dementia in 2012. These rates indicate a decline in the prevalence of dementia compared to the previous decade's findings (11.6% in 2000). While the cause for this decrease is currently unknown, higher levels of education appeared to be associated with lower rates of dementia onset (National Institute on Aging, 2016). While age may be the foremost risk factor associated with the development of dementia, other risk factors include hypertension, genetics, Down syndrome (associated with early onset), arteriosclerosis (affects blood flow to the brain), smoking, alcohol use, diabetes, and mental illness (National Institute on Aging, 2013). In addition, African American older adults are approximately two times more likely to develop dementia than Caucasian American older adults, while older Hispanic Americans are approximately 1.5 more likely to develop dementia than older Caucasian Americans. In addition, women are more likely to develop dementia than men as a result of a longer average life span (Alzheimer's Association, 2014).

Presently, no cure for dementia exists; therefore, palliative rather than curative treatments are standard (Alzheimer Society Canada, 2015). Treatment goals for palliative care are geared toward improving quality of life and decreasing discomfort associated with disease progression (National Institute of Nursing Research, 2015). Medication aimed toward slowing the progression of the disease may be prescribed but cannot completely stop its progression (Alzheimer Society Canada, 2015). The decreased cognitive functioning associated with disease progression introduces challenges for clinicians and caretakers. McKinney (2015) found that patients with dementia have higher rates of falls, emergency room visits, and poorer medication adherence as well as poor patient and caregiver understanding of their illness. These factors contribute to health complications and lower quality of life for patients with dementia.

For optimal treatment of patients with dementia, both patient and caregiver needs should be addressed. The responsibilities undertaken by caregivers include a wide range of tasks, including, but not limited to, grooming, feeding, shopping, completing chores, movement assistance, medication management, appointment scheduling, transportation, bathing, and managing depressive and aggressive behavior (Alzheimer's Association, 2014). Caregiver burnout is not uncommon and may lead to less effective care for the patient as well as lower quality of life for the caregiver (Chen, Huang, Yeh, Huang, & Chen, 2015; Srivastava, Tripathi, Tiwari, Singh, & Tripathi, 2016). As such, addressing caregiver burnout is an essential aspect of ensuring patients receive adequate care. Teaching coping skills has been a successful technique for reducing burnout (Chen et al., 2015). Relaxation techniques, social support, and a variety of other methods may be used to reduce burnout and improve treatment outcomes. While dementia may be incurable, slowing the onset of the disease and ensuring that patients receive the best care possible can be achieved through palliative care and the use of behavioral interventions aimed toward improving quality of life for patients and caregivers.

Chronic Pain

Pain is a subjective phenomenon defined formally as "an unpleasant sensory and emotional experience associated with actual or potential tissue damage" (International Association for the Study of Pain (IASP), 2014). While acute pain is an adaptive response to harmful environmental stimuli, chronic pain is a maladaptive response to pain in which pain persists when tissue damage is no longer evident. The National Institute of Health (NIH, 2011) defines chronic pain as a chronic disease in which pain persists beyond 3 months, or the time in which the tissue damage associated with the initial pain has healed. That is not to say that the pain an individual with chronic pain is experiencing is "not real" or "all in their head." On the contrary, this is an important concept related to the treatment of chronic pain patients who oftentimes feel invalidated when they are told that there is no biological basis for their pain (Duckworth, Iezzi, & Sewell, 2010).

The experience of pain involves both the peripheral and central nervous systems. Nociceptors throughout the body relay noxious, tissue-damaging environmental inputs to the spine and subsequently the brain. The painful stimuli are then processed in multiple areas of the brain related to sensory discrimination, emotion, motivation, and cognitive evaluation. A response is then set in motion via the production of various neurotransmitters that moderate the experience of pain (NIH, 2016). The experience of chronic pain has been linked with the emotional response and associated cognitive evaluations of pain (Gatchel, McGeary, McGeary, & Lippe, 2014). One's negative cognitive evaluation of pain can lead to a "vicious cycle of nociception, pain, distress, and disability" (p. 120). This cycle is perpetuated when individuals take on a "sick role" and begin to withdraw from normal daily activities out of fear of experiencing or worsening pain (Gatchel et al., 2014). Furthermore, a process of sensitization may also occur in which changes in the nervous system via neuronal plasticity result in individuals becoming hypersensitive to stimuli that otherwise would not result in pain (NIH, 2016).

Chronic pain results in up to $635 billion in total financial costs in the United States (Gaskin & Richard, 2012). As such, pain is the leading contributor to healthcare costs and remains the most common reason for accessing healthcare services (National Institute of Health, 2013). Chronic pain affects more individuals than diabetes, heart disease, and cancer combined with nearly 100 million individuals affected (Gaskin & Richard, 2012). A survey of over 27,000 US individuals revealed that 30.7% of respondents met reported symptoms indicative of chronic experience. Chronic pain prevalence increased with age, was higher for women, and was significantly correlated with unemployment and low household income (Johannes, Le, Zhou, Johnston, & Dworkin, 2010). Furthermore, the incidence of chronic pain is expected to increase as the American population continues to age (Gatchel et al., 2014). Despite the burden chronic pain imposes on the healthcare system, the treatment approach for chronic pain patients remains disjointed and best practices underutilized. Though the primary care setting has become the de facto institution for treating chronic pain, research by Moitra, Sperry, Mongold, Kyle, and Selby (2011) found that PCPs report that dealing with chronic pain patients is both frustrating and time-consuming. The frustration, time consumption, and other complexities associated with treating this disease are compounded with the rise of addiction to prescribed opioids to treat chronic pain patients (Harle et al., 2015). Individuals experiencing chronic pain oftentimes have comorbid depression, anxiety, fatigue, sleep disturbance, and/or decreased appetite due to the persistent emotional component related to the pain experience (NIH, 2011). Individuals with comorbid mental health issues, lower educational levels and employment status, little social support, poor coping strategies, and weight problems typically have a poorer prognosis (Peppin, Cheatle, Kirsh, & McCarberg, 2015). Consequently, a holistic and interdisciplinary approach to the treatment of chronic pain is currently the recommended approach to treating this disease, and early intervention via behavioral strategies is

Table 3.1 Summary of chronic diseases commonly encountered in the healthcare system

Disease	Prevalence	Financial costs	Health complications	Behavioral contributions
Diabetes mellitus	21 million diagnosed (estimated 8.1 million undiagnosed)	245 billion annually	Nephropathy Retinopathy Peripheral neuropathy Cardiovascular disease Sexual dysfunction	Poor diet Sedentary lifestyle Medication adherence
Obesity	36.5% of adults; 17% of children	147 billion annually for medical care	Diabetes mellitus Cardiovascular disease Sexual dysfunction	Poor diet Sedentary lifestyle
Dementia	8.8% of adults over 65	157–215 billion annually for medical care	Higher rates of falls Incontinence Difficulty swallowing Delusions, depression, agitation	Excess alcohol consumption Sedentary lifestyle
Chronic pain	>100 million	635 billion annually	Depression Anxiety Fatigue Sleep disturbance Decreased appetite	Adopting a "sick role" (avoidance behaviors following injury) Low activity levels during acute phase of pain experience
Cardiovascular disease	85.6 million	215 billion annually	Heart attack Stroke Coronary heart disease Blood clots	Poor diet Sedentary lifestyle Cigarette smoking Alcohol
Chronic obstructive pulmonary disease	11 million diagnosed (estimated 24 million undiagnosed)	49.9 billion annually	Shortness of breath Fatigue Heart problems Sleep disturbance Osteoporosis Depression and anxiety Susceptibility to infection	Smoking Secondhand smoke Exposure to air pollution

recognized as a first line of defense against the development and progression of chronic pain (Duckworth et al., 2010; Gatchel et al., 2014) (Table 3.1).

Behavioral interventions are vital and valuable preventive services that reduce the likelihood that acute pain develops into chronic pain (Malmivaara et al., 1995). A review of articles advocating increasing activity in the acute phase of the pain experience revealed significant reductions in pain, the number of pain-related symptoms, and recovery rates in multiple trials (Waddell, Feder, & Lewis, 1997). In a study that analyzed bed rest, exercise, and a return to normal daily activities for individuals with acute lower back pain, it was found that those individuals who were directed to return to normal activities recovered significantly faster than those assigned to bed rest and exercise as measured by the number of sick days taken, pain intensity, ability to work, lumber flexion, and the Oswestry Back Disability Index (Malmivaara et al., 1995). By reassuring individuals of a good prognosis and encouraging a return to everyday behavior, the fear and avoidance associated with the development of chronic pain is addressed (Duckworth et al., 2010).

For individuals who have already developed chronic pain symptoms, goal setting, physical conditioning, acceptance, and pursuit of valued actions are all behavioral interventions aimed at reducing pain avoidance behaviors and sedentary lifestyles that have been shown to increase one's ability to manage their chronic pain (Duckworth et al., 2010; Peppin et al., 2015). Engagement in daily activities and exercise have both been shown to be effective behavioral targets as individuals with more active lifestyles have been shown to have less pain and more musculoskeletal support (Peppin et al., 2015). Setting specific and attainable future goals during intervention is key in ensuring that individuals will adhere to treatment protocols and have been related to increases in mood and functionality (Peppin et al., 2015). Relatedly, self-management (e.g., setting specific goals related to lifestyle changes, exercise, and proper medication adherence), increased via self-management support, has been shown to improve mental health and functional ablement (Kawi, 2014). Finally, assisting individuals in accepting their pain experience while encouraging them to pursue valued actions in spite of their pain has been empirically supported as a means of decreasing anxiety, depression, and functional disability (Duckworth et al., 2010).

Cardiovascular Disease

Cardiovascular disease, or heart disease, is an umbrella term referring to multiple heart and circulation conditions including coronary heart disease (CHD), congestive heart failure, heart attack, arrhythmia, heart valve problems, and congenital heart defects (Mayo Clinic, 2016). Many of the aforementioned heart conditions are the result of a gradual hardening of the arteries, a process known as atherosclerosis (National Heart Lung and Blood Institute (NHLBI), 2015b). Atherosclerosis is the leading cause of heart attack and a major contributor to congestive heart failure and stroke (NHLBI, 2015a). This condition occurs throughout life as plaque consisting of cholesterol and fatty material (atheroma) builds up on the arterial walls. As a result, arteries are narrowed, blood flow is restricted, and the heart must work harder to supply the body with oxygen. Furthermore, plaque may break off the arterial wall and form blood clots (Schobitz, Bauer, & Schobitz, 2010). When a blood clot forms, blood flow can become completely restricted to an area of the body, resulting in a heart attack or stroke. In the case of coronary heart disease (CHD), atherosclerosis occurs inside the heart's coronary arteries, which are responsible for the return of blood to the heart. If a piece of arterial plaque breaks off, a blood clot in the coronary artery may form that completely occludes blood flow in the already narrowed coronary arteries. As a result, ischemia occurs as the heart muscle is starved of oxygen, resulting in permanent damage, a condition known as a heart attack or myocardial infarction. Ischemic strokes occur in a similar manner when blood is not properly supplied to an area of the brain due to the blockage of a blood vessel, typically the result of a blood clot (American Stroke Association (ASA), 2015).

The direct and indirect costs of cardiovascular disease are over $215 billion (AHA, 2015a). Of these conditions, CHD, also referred to as coronary artery disease, has the greatest impact on the healthcare system and contributes to other heart-related conditions such as angina, heart attack, and stroke (AHA, 2015b; NHLBI, 2015b). CHD accounts for 370,000 deaths in the United States each year, representing the nation's leading cause of death and heart attacks (Schobitz et al., 2010). Heart attacks alone account result in a significant amount of hospitalizations as each year approximately 735,000 American individuals experience a heart attack with 525,000 having their first heart attack and 210,000 having had at least one previous heart attack (Mozaffarian et al., 2015). Furthermore, the deleterious effects of CHD are not limited to the United States as CHD remains the leading cause of death globally, affecting around 5% of adults over age 40 in developed countries (Barbero et al., 2016). The seriousness and breadth of this health condition are apparent; however, many concrete behaviors contribute to the incidence and prevalence of CHD, making it a prime candidate for preventive behavioral intervention.

Though certain genetic, psychological, and static factors such as increased age, male sex, high stress levels, and family history of CHD are associated with one's propensity to develop CHD, there are many specific behaviors that contribute to the buildup of arterial fatty tissue that results in and perpetuates CHD (Widmer & Lerman, 2014). Poor dietary choices of foods high in trans fat, sodium, and sugar that contribute to unhealthy blood cholesterol levels, not taking medications as prescribed, low amounts of physical activity, smoking, and alcohol use are all behaviors associated with an increased risk of developing CHD as well as a poorer prognosis following diagnosis (American Heart Association, 2015c; Truthmann et al., 2015; Widmer & Lerman, 2014). Many of these behaviors are directly related to increased stress on a heart receiving poor blood flow (e.g., low amounts of physical activity and poor dietary choices result in obesity, which places strain on the heart) (Schobitz et al., 2010).

Specific behaviors can be targeted to prevent and treat CHD as well as other cardiovascular diseases affected by atherosclerosis (Truthmann et al., 2015). These behaviors include decreasing cigarette and alcohol consumption as well as body weight while increasing physical activity, medication compliance, and healthy dietary behavior. Successful changes in diet have been established in previous research as having a positive impact on cholesterol levels and weight, both of which have been identified as risk factors for CHD (Goodwin, Ostuzzi, Khan, Hotopf, & Moss-Morris, 2016; Cardoso, Moraes, Rosa, & Bello Moreira, 2015). An intensive nutritional intervention for individuals with coronary heart disease found that dietary changes had a significant impact on anthropometric and biochemical markers associated with increased risk for poorer prognosis for individuals diagnosed with the disease (Cardoso et al., 2015). Furthermore, studies regarding the impact of the Mediterranean diet, which consists of high levels of fruit, fish, legumes, whole grains, vegetables, and olive oil as primary source of fat, on heart health have shown a positive impact on blood pressure, endothelial function, and general heart health (Chrysohoou et al., 2010).

Alcohol and cigarette consumption are two lifestyle behaviors that have been shown to increase risk for CHD. Smoking cigarettes has been shown to increase blood pressure and the risk of blood clots while decreasing exercise tolerance and HDL cholesterol (AHA, 2014). Furthermore, cigarette smoking has been cited as the cause of approximately 20% of coronary heart disease cases worldwide (Khan et al., 2012). Alcohol intake may result in a variety of heart-related conditions including cardiomyopathy, arrhythmia, and sudden cardiac death as the ingestion of alcohol may raise the levels of triglycerides in the blood as well as increase blood pressure in addition to the increased, nutritionally void caloric consumption of the alcohol itself (AHA, 2015c). Research following individuals receiving stent placement surgery for CHD found that those who smoked and had high levels of alcohol consumption were significantly more likely to have complications and repeated heart problems in a 7-year follow-up (Yan-Fang et al., 2015). As such, targeting alcohol and cigarette consumption is a generally accepted approach to preventing and reducing the impact of coronary heart and other cardiovascular diseases (Khan et al., 2012).

Finally, increasing physical activity is a viable method of reducing one's risk for CHD and other cardiovascular diseases. Increased activity levels and exercise decrease one's risk for obesity while also decreasing stress levels and promoting general well-being (Yan-Fang et al., 2015). Sedentary lifestyles have been associated with both higher development and poorer prognosis of CHD and other heart problems (Koolhaas et al., 2016; Yan-Fang et al., 2015). A study examining types of physical activity engaged in by older adults in relation to CHD revealed that cycling and domestic work were associated with decreased risk of CHD and are recommended to be promoted in this population to help prevent the development of CHD (Koolhaas et al., 2016). Furthermore, a meta-analysis examining exercise-based cardiac rehabilitation for those with CHD revealed that exercise reduced mortality and increased quality of life across patients and settings (Anderson et al., 2016).

Coronary heart disease as well as other cardiovascular diseases continues to place a burden on the healthcare system. However, the aforementioned behavioral interventions have been shown to both decrease one's risk for developing a heart condition and increase one's quality of life if living with one.

Chronic Obstructive Pulmonary Disease

Chronic obstructive pulmonary disease (COPD) is a progressive lung disease which affects an individual's ability to breathe. This occurs as a result of conditions that affect the lungs' ability to intake and disseminate oxygen, including emphysema, chronic bronchitis, refractory asthma, and bronchiectasis (COPD Foundation, 2016). During the process of respiration, air travels down the windpipe into the bronchial tubes where it is then disseminated into many smaller tubes, known as the bronchioles. At the end of the bronchial tubes are a cluster of small air sacs, known as alveoli, intersected by tiny blood vessels, or capillaries, where the process of gas exchange occurs. The gas exchange occurring in the alveoli involves the passing of oxygen to the blood, from the alveoli into capillaries. The resulting waste gas, carbon dioxide, is subsequently expelled when one exhales (National Heart, Lung, and Blood Institute (NHLBI), 2013a).

In the United States, emphysema and chronic bronchitis are the primary lung conditions that affect the respiration process, thereby resulting in a diagnosis of COPD (NHLBI, 2013b). Chronic bronchitis affects respiration as the inflammation of the bronchial tubes and bronchioles results in an excessive production of mucus. This mucus narrows the air pathway, thus making it more difficult for both oxygen to reach the alveoli and carbon dioxide to be exhaled following gas exchange (National Heart, Lung, and Blood Institue, 2018). Symptoms include a persistent mucus-producing cough lasting at least 3 months over 2 consecutive years. Whereas bronchitis affects the intake of air to the alveoli, emphysema directly affects the alveoli (Mayo Foundation for Medical Education and Research, 2014). Emphysema develops gradually as the alveoli walls are damaged and ruptured. As a result, the surface area of the lungs is reduced, and the amount of oxygen that reaches the bloodstream is decreased due to the malfunctioning alveoli trapping old air in the lungs. The main symptom is shortness of breath made worse during exercise or physical exertion (Mayo Foundation for Medical Education and Research, 2014). The leading cause for COPD is cigarette smoke followed by long-term exposure to other lung irritants (NHLBI, 2013a). Diagnosing COPD and assessing its severity involve methods such as X-ray, CT scans, or spirometry tests (NHLBI, 2013b).

COPD represents the third leading cause of death in the United States. Over 11 million people have been formally diagnosed with COPD, though the prevalence is thought to be much higher, with an estimated 24 million individuals going undiagnosed (NHLBI, 2013a; American Lung Association (ALA), 2016). The economic costs represented by healthcare expenditures, indirect morbidity costs, and indirect mortality costs totaled $49.9 billion in 2010 (ALA, 2013). Much comorbidity (e.g., cardiac disease, diabetes mellitus, hypertension, osteoporosis, and psychological disorders) exists for individuals with COPD due to the impact oxygen deprivation and sedentary lifestyles associated with the disease (Respiratory Health Association, 2016). These comorbidities contribute to COPD being the leading cause of hospitalizations in adults and a rise in the associated healthcare costs (Hill, Gardiner, Cavalheri, Jenkins, & Healy, 2015; Wissam et al., 2008). The incidence per 1000 of COPD as a first-listed diagnosis during the span of 1980–2000 was 45.0 overall, 46.8 for men and 43.4 for women (Mannino, Buist, Petty, Enright, & Redd, 2003). A general trend in the incidence of COPD has emerged since 2001 in which the rates of emphysema and chronic bronchitis diagnoses in women have been consistently higher than in men; the prevalence of COPD in women overtook the prevalence in men in 2011 (ALA, 2013). This is hypothesized to be due to the increase in marketing to women by the tobacco industry in the 1960s, higher vulnerability to lung damage in women due to smaller lungs, the role of estrogen in worsening lung disease, and previous misdiagnoses due to a general conception of COPD being historically a "man's disease" (ALA, 2016).

Though the damage done to the lungs that result in COPD is irreversible, behavioral interventions via lifestyle changes have been shown to improve one's quality of life and slow the progression of the disease (NHLBI, 2013a). For individuals with

COPD who have a history of smoking, smoking cessation should be the first area of intervention. In fact, the only known intervention for slowing further functional decline in the lungs is smoking cessation (Bartlett, Sheeren, & Hawley, 2014). Furthermore, the prevalence of COPD is highest in individuals over 40 with a history of smoking, and 80% of cases are directly linked to the impact smoking has on the lungs (Bartlett et al., 2014). Cigarette smoking irritates the bronchioles and affects the pro- and anti-inflammatory response in the lungs (Chen et al., 2016). The nicotine dependence resulting from years of cigarette smoking results in addiction, with subsequent withdrawal symptoms making this lifestyle change particularly difficult for some individuals (Lavin, 2010). Furthermore, research has found that smoking cessation is reportedly more difficult for individuals with COPD as compared to smokers without the disease (Tashkin & Murray, 2009). However, motivational interviewing techniques, detailed planning, and self-monitoring have all been identified as important active ingredients of behavior change techniques for individuals suffering from COPD (Bartlett et al., 2014; Lavin, 2010).

Sustaining activity levels is another area of behavioral health that must be attended to for individuals with COPD (Hill et al., 2015). COPD affects an individual's ability to engage in normal activities and exercise as their diminished ability to breathe and increased oxygen deprivation result in exertional dyspnea and fatigue. The resulting sedentary lifestyle is associated with increased risks of comorbidities that significantly increase healthcare costs (Hill et al., 2015). Research has shown that individuals with COPD who continue to engage in daily activities and appropriate exercise have both physical and psychological advantages compared with individuals who do not (Emery, Shermer, Hauck, Hsiao, & MacIntyre, 2003; Hill et al., 2015; Walters et al., 2012). Research documenting the physical endurance, cognitive performance, and emotional well-being of individuals diagnosed with COPD a year after a 10-week exercise intervention revealed that individuals who maintained activity and exercise levels following the intervention also maintained the gains in the aforementioned measures (Emery et al., 2003). However, individuals who did not continue their exercise regiments showed decreases in all areas of functioning. Maintaining activity levels following a COPD diagnosis is vital for the improvement and maintenance of the patient's general well-being.

While medications and breathing treatments are common medical interventions, the aforementioned behavioral interventions have been associated with lowered rates of premature death and higher levels of general well-being, making them ideal additions to the treatment of COPD (Hill et al., 2015).

Conclusions

Advancements in the medical field have resulted in effectively controlling a range of acute illnesses and increasing the life span of people worldwide (CDC, 2003). However, the advancements that have accompanied the industrialization of developed countries have not come without a price. Changes in lifestyle in addition to longer life spans have resulted in increased risk of developing chronic disease and subsequent lower quality of life (CDC, 2013; WHO, 2016). As previously mentioned, chronic disease is now the leading cause of death globally, with rates continuing to rise (WHO, 2016). More effective approaches to prevention and treatment of chronic disease are imperative as healthcare professionals continually strive to provide quality, cost-effective treatment.

Fortunately, behavioral interventions provide noninvasive options for addressing the needs of twenty-first-century patients. Contributors to the development of a number of diseases discussed include physical inactivity, poor dietary choices, and other areas of suboptimal engagement in health behaviors (WHO, 2016). As such, increasing engagement with health promoting behaviors may lower the risk of developing certain diseases as well as improving the quality of life for those who have developed a chronic illness. Addressing behavioral contributors to the development of disease will lead to lower healthcare costs and higher quality of life for at-risk populations; therefore, implementing effective behavioral approaches is an ideal avenue for improving health outcomes for patients.

References

Alzheimer Society Canada. (2015). *Treatment options*. Retrieved from http://www.alzheimer.ca/en/About-dementia/Treatment-options.

Alzheimer's Association. (2014). 2014 Alzheimer's disease facts and figures. *Alzheimer's & Dementia, 10*(2), e47–e92 Retrieved from https://www.alz.org/downloads/facts_figures_2014.pdf

Alzheimer's Foundation of America. (2016). *About dementia*. Retrieved from http://www.alzfdn.org/AboutDementia/definition.html.

American Diabetes Association. (2004). Diagnosis and classification of diabetes mellitus. *Diabetes Care, 27*, S5–S10.

American Diabetes Association. (2013a). *Statistics about diabetes*. Retrieved from http://www.diabetes.org/diabetes-basics/statistics/.

American Diabetes Association. (2013b). *Managing stress and diabetes*. Retrieved from http://www.diabetes.org/living-with-diabetes/parents-and-kids/everyday-life/managing-stress-and-diabetes.html.

American Heart Association. (2014). *Smoking and cardiovascular disease*. Retrieved from http://www.heart.org/HEARTORG/HealthyLiving/QuitSmoking/QuittingResources/Smoking-Cardiovascular-Disease_UCM_305187_Article.jsp#.V1Rb6pErK00.

American Heart Association. (2015a). *Direct and indirect costs of cardiovascular disease (CVD) and stroke (in billions of dollars), United States, 2011*. Retrieved from https://www.heart.org/idc/groups/heart-public/@wcm/@sop/@smd/documents/downloadable/ucm_449849.pdf.

American Heart Association. (2015b). *What are heart disease and stroke?* Retrieved from http://www.heart.org/idc/groups/heartpublic/@wcm/@hcm/documents/downloadable/ucm_300313.pdf.

American Heart Association. (2015c). *Alcohol and heart health*. Retrieved from http://www.heart.org/HEARTORG/HealthyLiving/HealthyEating/Nutrition/Alcohol-and-Heart-Health_UCM_305173_Article.jsp#.V1RiX5ErK00.

American Heart Association. (2016). *Understanding the American obesity epidemic*. Retrieved from http://www.heart.org/HEARTORG/HealthyLiving/WeightManagement/Obesity/Understanding-the-American-Obesity-Epidemic_UCM_461650_Article.jsp#.V1SsIZErK00.

American Lung Association. (2013). *Trends in COPD (chronic bronchitis and emphysema): Morbidity and mortality.* Retrieved from http://www.lung.org/lung-health-and-diseases/lung-disease-lookup/copd/learn-about-copd/how-serious-is-copd.html?referrer=https://www.google.com/.

American Lung Association. (2016). *How serious is COPD?* Retrieved from http://www.lung.org/lung-health-and-diseases/lung-disease-lookup/copd/learn-about-copd/how-serious-is-copd.html?referrer=https://www.google.com/.

American Speech-Language-Hearing Association. (2016). *Dementia.* Retrieved from http://www.asha.org/PRPSpecificTopic.aspx?folderid=8589935289&section=Incidence_and_Prevalence.

American Stroke Association. (2015). *Ischemic strokes (clots).* Retrieved from http://www.strokeassociation.org/STROKEORG/AboutStroke/TypesofStroke/IschemicClots/Ischemic-Strokes-Clots_UCM_310939_Article.jsp#.V08_G5ErK00.

Anderson, L., Oldridge, N., Thompson, D. R., Zwisler, A., Rees, K., Martin, N., & Taylor, R. S. (2016). Exercise-based cardiac rehabilitation for coronary heart disease: Cochrane systematic review and meta-analysis. *Journal of the American College of Cardiology, 67*(1), 1–12. https://doi.org/10.1016/j.jacc.2015.10.044

Azar, K. J., Chung, S., Wang, E. J., Zhao, B., Linde, R. B., Lederer, J., & Palaniappan, L. P. (2015). Impact of education on weight in newly diagnosed Type 2 diabetes: Every little bit helps. *PLoS One, 10*(6), e0129348. https://doi.org/10.1371/journal.pone.0129348

Barbero, U., D'Ascenzo, F., Nijhoff, F., Moretti, C., Biondi-Zoccai, G., Mennuni, M., … Gaita, F. (2016). Assessing risk in patients with stable coronary disease: When should we intensify care and follow-up? Results from a meta-analysis of observational studies of the COURAGE and FAME era. *Scientifica, 2016*, 1–10. https://doi.org/10.1155/2016/3769152

Bartlett, Y. K., Sheeran, P., & Hawley, M. S. (2014). Effective behaviour change techniques in smoking cessation interventions for people with chronic obstructive pulmonary disease: A meta-analysis. *British Journal of Health Psychology, 19*(1), 181–203. https://doi.org/10.1111/bjhp.12071

Bellisari, A. (2008). Evolutionary origins of obesity. *Obesity Reviews, 9*(2), 165–180. https://doi.org/10.1111/j.1467-789X.2007.00392.x

Cardoso, D., Moraes, G., Rosa, G., & Bello Moreira, A. S. (2015). Effectiveness of nutritional treatment assessed by the quality of the diet in patients with chronic coronary artery disease. *Nutricion Hospitalaria, 32*(3), 1344–1352. https://doi.org/10.3305/nh.2015.32.3.9175

Carlson, S. A., Fulton, J. E., Pratt, M., Yang, Z., & Adams, K. E. (2015). Inadequate physical activity and healthcare expenditures in the Unites States. *Progress in Cardiovascular Diseases, 57*, 315–323. https://doi.org/10.1016/j.pcad.2014.08.002

Centers for Disease Control and Prevention. (2003). Public health and aging: Trends in aging—United States and worldwide. *Morbidity and Mortality Weekly Report, 52*(06), 101–106 Retrieved from https://www.cdc.gov/mmwr/preview/mmwrhtml/mm5206a2.htm

Centers for Disease Control and Prevention. (2012a). Summary health statistics for U.S. adults: National health interview survey, 2010. *Vital and Health Statistics, 10*(252), 1–207. Retrieved from http://www.cdc.gov/nchs/data/series/sr_10/sr10_252.pdf

Centers for Disease Control and Prevention. (2012b). *Defining adult overweight and obesity.* Retrieved from http://www.cdc.gov/obesity/adult/defining.html.

Centers for Disease Control and Prevention. (2013). *The state of aging and health in America.* Atlanta, GA: United States Department of Health and Human Services Retrieved from http://www.cdc.gov/features/agingandhealth/state_of_aging_and_health_in_america_2013.pdf

Centers for Disease Control and Prevention. (2015a). *Annual number (in thousands) of new cases of diagnosed diabetes among adults aged 18-79 years, United States, 1980–2014.* Retrieved from http://www.cdc.gov/diabetes/statistics/incidence/fig1.htm.

Centers for Disease Control and Prevention. (2015b). *Obesity facts.* Retrieved from http://www.cdc.gov/obesity/data/adult.html.

Centers for Disease Control and Prevention. (2015c). *Obesity prevalence maps.* Retrieved from https://www.cdc.gov/obesity/data/prevalence-maps.html.

Centers for Disease Control and Prevention. (2015d). *Prevalence of overweight, obesity and extreme obesity among adults: United States, trends 1960–62 through 2005–2006*. Retrieved from http://www.cdc.gov/nchs/data/hestat/overweight/overweight_adult.htm.

Centers for Disease Control and Prevention. (2015e). *Strategies to prevent obesity*. Retrieved from http://www.cdc.gov/obesity/strategies/index.html.

Centers for Disease Control and Prevention. (2016a). *Chronic disease prevention and health promotion*. Retrieved from http://www.cdc.gov/chronicdisease/index.htm.

Centers for Disease Control and Prevention. (2016b). *Smoking and tobacco use*. Retrieved from http://www.cdc.gov/tobacco/data_statistics/fact_sheets/fast_facts/.

Centers for Disease Control and Prevention. (2016c). *The surprising truth about prediabetes*. Retrieved from http://www.cdc.gov/features/diabetesprevention/.

Centers for Medicare and Medicaid Services. (2015). *National health expenditure fact sheet*. Retrieved from https://www.cms.gov/Research-Statistics-Data-and-Systems/Statistics-Trends-and-Reports/NationalHealthExpendData/NHE-Fact-Sheet.html.

Chapman, D. P., Williams, S. M., Strine, T. W., Anda, R. F., & Moore, M. J. (2006). Dementia and its implications for public health. *Preventing Chronic Disease, 3*(2), A34 Retrieved from http://www.cdc.gov/pcd/issues/2006/apr/05_0167.htm

Chen, G., Zhou, M., Chen, L., Meng, Z., Xiong, X., Liu, H., … Zhang, J. (2016). Cigarette smoke disturbs the survival of CD8+ Tc/Tregs partially through muscarinic receptors-dependent mechanisms in chronic obstructive pulmonary disease. *PLoS One, 11*(1), 1–11. https://doi.org/10.1371/journal.pone.0147232

Chen, H., Huang, M., Yeh, Y., Huang, W., & Chen, C. (2015). Effectiveness of coping strategies intervention on caregiver burden among caregivers of elderly patients with dementia. *Psychogeriatrics: The Official Journal of the Japanese Psychogeriatric Society, 15*(1), 20–25. https://doi.org/10.1111/psyg.12071

Chrysohoou, C., Panagiotakos, D. B., Aggelopoulos, P., Kastorini, C. M., Kehagia, I., Pitsavos, C., & Stefanadis, C. (2010). The Mediterranean diet contributes to the preservation of left ventricular systolic function and to the long-term favorable prognosis of patients who have had an acute coronary event. *American Journal of Clinical Nutrition, 92*(1), 47–54. https://doi.org/10.3945/ajcn.2009.28982

COPD Foundation. (2016). *What is COPD?* Retrieved from http://www.copdfoundation.org/What-is-COPD/Understanding-COPD/What-is-COPD.aspx.

Dehghan, M., & Merchant, A. T. (2008). Is bioelectrical impedance accurate for use in large epidemiological studies? *Nutrition Journal, 7*, 26. https://doi.org/10.1186/1475-2891-7-26

Duckworth, M. P., Iezzi, T., & Sewell, M. T. (2010). Assessing and managing chronic pain in the primary care setting. In L. C. James & W. T. O'Donahue (Eds.), *The primary care toolkit: Practical resources for the integrated behavioral care provider* (pp. 121–130). New York: Springer.

Dugan, A. (2013, November 21). Americans say cost is top health problem. *Gallup*. Retrieved from http://www.gallup.com/poll/165965/americans-say-cost-top-health-problem.aspx.

Emery, C. F., Shermer, R. L., Hauck, E. R., Hsiao, E. T., & MacIntyre, N. R. (2003). Cognitive and psychological outcomes of exercise in a 1-year follow-up study of patients with chronic obstructive pulmonary disease. *Health Psychology, 22*(6), 598–604. https://doi.org/10.1037/0278-6133.22.6.598

Gaskin, D. J., & Richard, P. (2012). The economic costs of pain in the United States. *The Journal of Pain, 13*(8), 715–724.

Gatchel, R. J., McGeary, D. D., McGeary, C. A., & Lippe, B. (2014). Interdisciplinary chronic pain management: Past, present, and future. *American Psychologist, 69*(2), 119–130. https://doi.org/10.1037/a0035514

Goodwin, L., Ostuzzi, G., Khan, N., Hotopf, M. H., & Moss-Morris, R. (2016). Can we identify the active ingredients of behaviour change interventions for coronary heart disease patients? A systematic review and meta-analysis. *PLoS One, 11*(4), 1–23. https://doi.org/10.1371/journal.pone.0153271

Harle, C. A., Bauer, S. E., Hoang, H. Q., Cook, R. L., Hurley, R. W., & Fillingim, R. B. (2015). Decision support for chronic pain care: How do primary care physicians decide when to prescribe opioids? A qualitative study. *BMC Family Practice, 16*(1), 48–55. https://doi.org/10.1186/s12875-015-0264-3

Harvard School of Public Health. (2016). *From calipers to CAT scans, ten ways to tell whether a body is fat or lean.* Retrieved from https://www.hsph.harvard.edu/obesity-prevention-source/obesity-definition/how-to-measure-body-fatness/.

Hill, K., Gardiner, P. A., Cavalheri, V., Jenkins, S. C., & Healy, G. N. (2015). Physical activity and sedentary behaviour: Applying lessons to chronic obstructive pulmonary disease. *Internal Medicine Journal, 45*(5), 474–482. https://doi.org/10.1111/imj.12570

International Association for the Study of Pain. (2014). *IASP taxonomy.* Retrieved from https://owl.english.purdue.edu/owl/resource/560/10/.

Johannes, C. B., Le, T. K., Zhou, X., Johnston, J. A., & Dworkin, R. H. (2010). The prevalence of chronic pain in United States adults: Results of an Internet-based survey. *The Journal of Pain, 11*(11), 1230–1239.

Kawi, J. (2014). Influence of self-management and self-management support on chronic low back pain patients in primary care. *Journal of the American Association of Nurse Practitioners, 26*(12), 664–673. https://doi.org/10.1002/2327-6924.12117

Khan, S. B., Hafizullah, M., Gul, A. M., Rehman, H. U., Ali, J., Qureshi, M. S., … Abbas Shah, S. F. (2012). Frequency of coronary heart disease risk factors among nurses. *Journal of Postgraduate Medical Institute, 26*(4), 377–385.

Koolhaas, C. M., Dhana, K., Golubic, R., Schoufour, J. D., Hofman, A., van Rooij, F. A., & Franco, O. H. (2016). Physical activity types and coronary heart disease risk in middle-aged and elderly persons. *American Journal of Epidemiology, 183*(8), 729–738. https://doi.org/10.1093/aje/kwv244

Lavin, D. (2010). Smoking. In L. C. James & W. T. O'Donahue (Eds.), *The primary care tool-kit: Practical resources for the integrated behavioral care provider* (pp. 277–289). New York: Springer.

Laz, T. H., Rahman, M., Pohlmeier, A. M., & Berenson, A. B. (2015). Level of nutrition knowledge and its association with weight loss behaviors among low-income reproductive-age women. *Journal of Community Health, 40*(3), 542–548. https://doi.org/10.1007/s10900-014-9969-9

Lewy Body Dementia Association. (2016). *Cost of dementia tops $157 billion annually in the United States.* Retrieved from https://www.lbda.org/content/cost-dementia-tops-157-billion-annually-united-states.

Malmivaara, A., Hakkinen, U., Aro, T., Heinrichs, M. L., Koskenniemi, L., Kuosma, E., … Vaaranen, V. (1995). The treatment of acute low back pain--bed rest, exercises, or ordinary activity. *New England Journal of Medicine, 332*(6), 351–355 Retrieved from http://www.ncbi.nlm.nih.gov/entrez/query.fcgi?cmd=Retrieve&db=PubMed&dopt=Citation&list_uids=7823996\n

Mannino, D. M., Buist, A. S., Petty, T. L., Enright, P. L., & Redd, S. C. (2003). Lung function and mortality in the United States: Data from the first National Health and Nutrition Examination Survey follow up study. *Thorax, 58*(5), 388–393.

Mayo Clinic. (2014). *Tests and diagnosis.* Retrieved from http://www.mayoclinic.org/diseases-conditions/prediabetes/basics/tests-diagnosis/con-20024420.

Mayo Clinic. (2015). *Counting calories: Get back to weight loss basics.* Retrieved from http://www.mayoclinic.org/healthy-lifestyle/weight-loss/in-depth/calories/art-20048065.

Mayo Clinic. (2016). *Heart disease.* Retrieved from http://www.mayoclinic.org/diseases-conditions/heart-disease/basics/definition/con-20034056.

Mayo Foundation for Medical Education and Research. (2014). *Emphysema.* Retrieved from http://www.mayoclinic.org/diseases-conditions/emphysema/basics/definition/CON-20014218?p=1.

McKinney, M. (2015). Building better supports for dementia. *Modern Healthcare, 45*(39), 32.

MedicineNet. (2013). *Bronchitis.* Retrieved from http://www.medicinenet.com/chronic_bronchitis/article.htm.

Moitra, E., Sperry, J. A., Mongold, D., Kyle, B. N., & Selby, J. (2011). A group medical visit program for primary care patients with chronic pain. *Professional Psychology: Research & Practice, 42*(2), 153–159. https://doi.org/10.1037/a0022240

Mozaffarian, D., Benjamin, E. J., Go, A. S., Arnett, D. K., Blaha, M. J., Cushman, M., … American Heart Association Statistics Committee and Stroke Statistics Subcommittee. (2015). Heart disease and stroke statistics-2015 update: A report from the American Heart Association. *Circulation, 131*(24), 535–535.

National Health Service. (2014a). *Type 2 diabetes: Symptoms*. Retrieved from http://www.nhs.uk/Conditions/Diabetes-type2/Pages/Symptoms.aspx.

National Health Service. (2014b). *Type 2 diabetes: Causes*. Retrieved from http://www.nhs.uk/Conditions/Diabetes-type2/Pages/Causes.aspx.

National Health Service. (2014c). *Type 2 diabetes: Complications*. Retrieved from http://www.nhs.uk/Conditions/Diabetes-type2/Pages/Complications.aspx.

National Heart, Lung, and Blood Institute. (2012). *What are the health risks of overweight and obesity?* Retrieved from https://www.nhlbi.nih.gov/health/health-topics/topics/obe/risks.

National Heart, Lung, and Blood Institute. (2013a). *What is COPD.*? Retrieved from http://www.nhlbi.nih.gov/health/health-topics/topics/copd.

National Heart, Lung, and Blood Institute. (2013b). *How COPD is diagnosed.* Retrieved from https://www.nhlbi.nih.gov/health/health-topics/topics/copd/diagnosis.

National Heart, Lung, and Blood Institute. (2015a). *What is atherosclerosis?* Retrieved from http://www.nhlbi.nih.gov/health/health-topics/topics/atherosclerosis.

National Heart, Lung, and Blood Institute. (2015b). *What is coronary heart disease?* Retrieved from http://www.nhlbi.nih.gov/health/health-topics/topics/cad.

National Heart, Lung, and Blood Institue. (2018). Bronchitis. Retrieved from https://www.nhlbi.nih.gov/health-topics/bronchitis.

National Institute of Diabetes and Digestive and Kidney Diseases. (2014). *Causes of diabetes*. Retrieved from http://www.niddk.nih.gov/health-information/health-topics/Diabetes/causes-diabetes/Pages/index.aspx.

National Institute of Health. (2011). *Chronic pain: Symptoms, diagnosis, and treatment.* Retrieved from https://www.nlm.nih.gov/medlineplus/magazine/issues/spring11/articles/spring11pg5-6.html.

National Institute of Health. (2013). *Pain Management*. Retrieved from https://report.nih.gov/nih-factsheets/ViewFactSheet.aspx?csid=57

National Institute of Health. (2016). *Pain in America.* Retrieved from http://www.ninds.nih.gov/disorders/chronic_pain/chronic_pain.htm.

National Institute of Mental Health. (n.d.). *Fact sheet on stress*. Retrieved from http://www.nimh.nih.gov/health/publications/stress/index.shtml.

National Institute of Nursing Research. (2015). *Palliative care*. Retrieved from https://www.nlm.nih.gov/medlineplus/palliativecare.html.

National Institute on Aging. (2013). *Risk factors for dementia.* Retrieved from https://www.nia.nih.gov/alzheimers/publication/dementias/risk-factors-dementia.

National Institute on Aging. (2016). *National study reports decreased dementia prevalence*. Retrieved from https://www.nia.nih.gov/newsroom/announcements/2016/12/national-study-reports-decreased-dementia-prevalence.

O'Brien, G., & Davies, M. (2007). Nutrition knowledge and body mass index. *Health Education Research, 22*(4), 571–575.

Peppin, J. F., Cheatle, M. D., Kirsh, K. L., & McCarberg, B. H. (2015). The complexity model: A novel approach to improve chronic pain care. *Pain Medicine, 16*(4), 653–666. https://doi.org/10.1111/pme.12621

Respiratory Health Association. (2016). *Understanding COPD: Comorbidities.* Retrieved from http://www.lungchicago.org/understanding-copd-comorbidities/.

Schmid, S. M., Hallschmid, M., Jauch-Chara, K., Born, J., & Schultes, B. (2008). A single night of sleep deprivation increases ghrelin levels and feelings of hunger in normal-weight healthy men. *Journal of Sleep Research, 17*(3), 331–334. https://doi.org/10.1111/j.1365-2869.2008.00662.x

Schobitz, R. P., Bauer, L. L., & Schobitz, E. P. (2010). Behavioral health consultation for coronary heart disease. In L. C. James & W. T. O'Donahue (Eds.), *The primary care toolkit: Practical resources for the integrated behavioral care provider* (pp. 121–130). New York: Springer.

Srivastava, G., Tripathi, R. K., Tiwari, S. C., Singh, B., & Tripathi, S. M. (2016). Caregiver burden and quality of life of key caregivers of patients with dementia. *Indian Journal of Psychological Medicine, 38*(2), 133–136. https://doi.org/10.4103/0253-7176.178779

Tashkin, D. P., & Murray, R. P. (2009). Smoking cessation in chronic obstructive pulmonary disease. *Respiratory Medicine, 103*(7), 963–974.

Truthmann, J., Busch, M. A., Scheidt-Nave, C., Mensink, G. M., Gößwald, A., Endres, M., & Neuhauser, H. (2015). Modifiable cardiovascular risk factors in adults aged 40-79 years in Germany with and without prior coronary heart disease or stroke. *BMC Public Health, 15*(1), 1–7. https://doi.org/10.1186/s12889-015-1929-5

Waddell, G., Feder, G., & Lewis, M. (1997). Systematic reviews of bed rest and advice to stay active for acute low back pain. *British Journal of General Practice, 47*, 647–652.

Walters, J. E., Cameron-Tucker, H., Courtney-Pratt, H., Nelson, M., Robinson, A., Scott, J., … Wood-Baker, R. (2012). Supporting health behaviour change in chronic obstructive pulmonary disease with telephone health-mentoring: Insights from a qualitative study. *BMC Family Practice, 13*(1), 55–61. https://doi.org/10.1186/1471-2296-13-55

Widmer, J. R., & Lerman, A. (2014). Endothelial dysfunction and cardiovascular disease. *Global Cardiology Science & Practice, 2014*(3), 1–33. https://doi.org/10.5339/gcsp.2014.43

World Health Organization. (2006). *Definition and diagnosis of diabetes mellitus and intermediate hyperglycemia*. Retrieved from http://www.who.int/diabetes/publications/Definition%20and%20diagnosis%20of%20diabetes_new.pdf.

World Health Organization. (2014). *Top 10 causes of death*. Retrieved from http://www.who.int/mediacentre/factsheets/fs310/en/.

World Health Organization. (2016). *Integrated chronic disease prevention and control*. Retrieved from http://www.who.int/chp/about/integrated_cd/en/.

Yan-Fang, W., Xiao-Li, M., Chen, Y., Ling, F., Jing, Y., & Jun, Z. (2015). Impact of daily lifestyle on coronary heart disease. *Experimental and Therapeutic Medicine, 10*(3), 1115–1120. https://doi.org/10.3892/etm.2015.2646

Part II
Key Problems in Healthcare Service Delivery

Chapter 4
Provider Training: Recognizing the Relevance of Behavioral Medicine and the Importance of Behavioral Health Consultation and Referral

Ronald R. O'Donnell

The clinical case for behavioral medicine as a critical component of primary care integrated health is firmly established (Fisher et al., 2011). Behavioral conditions such as depression, anxiety and substance use disorder, stress and adjustment disorders, and lifestyle habits such as smoking, overeating, and lack of exercise all contribute to worse outcomes and higher costs for patients with chronic medical conditions (Kathol et al., 2005). Behavioral conditions such as depression, anxiety, substance-related disorders, and trauma are highly comorbid with NCDs, representing more than 40% of patients seen in primary care (Wang et al., 2007). Behavioral treatments such as the Diabetes Prevention Program for prediabetes (Diabetes Prevention Program Research Group, 2011), the Primary Care Behavioral Health (PCBH) for behavioral conditions (Robinson & Reiter, 2016), and the Collaborative Care Model (CCM) for comorbid medical and behavioral chronic conditions (Ratzliff, Unutzer, Katon, & Stephens, 2016) have proven effective in improving medical (e.g., blood sugar, blood pressure) and patient-reported behavioral (e.g., depression, anxiety) clinical outcomes.

The business case for behavioral medicine is growing, with evidence that behavioral interventions designed to prevent and improve the management of NCDs and behavioral conditions can lead to cost savings attributed to decreased utilization of high-cost healthcare services such as emergency department visits and hospital admissions (Katon et al., 2012). The basis for the business case is research showing the high cost of behavioral risk factors and conditions that contribute to poor outcomes for NCDs. Behavioral conditions, such as depression, anxiety, and somatic symptom disorders, and lifestyle habits, such as smoking, poor nutrition, and lack of physical activity, all contribute to worse outcomes and higher costs for patients

R. R. O'Donnell (✉)
College of Health Solutions, Arizona State University, Phoenix, AZ, USA
e-mail: Ronald.odonnell@asu.edu

M. P. Duckworth, W. T. O'Donohue (eds.), *Behavioral Medicine and Integrated Care*,
https://doi.org/10.1007/978-3-319-93003-9_4

with chronic medical conditions (Kathol et al., 2005). Evidence shows that targeted, focused behavioral interventions delivered in primary care settings improve both health outcomes and reduce medical costs by lowering patterns of high utilization of healthcare services (Chiles, Lambert, & Hatch, 2002).

NCDs represent a global epidemic, with about 38 million global deaths in 2012, expected to increase to 52 million by 2030 (Zimmet, 2003). Major NCDs are primarily caused by four behavioral health risks: physical inactivity, poor nutrition, tobacco use, and excessive alcohol use (Milani et al., 2016). Research demonstrates that the preventive effects of increased physical activity and improved nutrition can prevent about 1.3 million chronic disease-related deaths and about 18 million deaths caused by obesity, cardiovascular disease, and diabetes, respectively (Milani et al., 2016). This business case for integrated behavioral medicine is based on identifying and targeting these complex patients systematically and improving the health of the entire population targeted, with the assumption that as these patients become healthier utilization and associated costs of care will decrease.

Despite the strong clinical and business case for behavioral medicine in integrated care, substantial challenges remain. First, the supply of clinicians proficient in behavioral medicine and integrated behavioral health is not sufficient to meet the demand for patients in need of behavioral health in primary care and other medical settings. A report by the US Department of Health and Human Services on the supply of and demand for behavioral health providers projected significant shortages by 2025 (HRSA, 2015). This widening gap between supply and demand is driving by the increased emphasis on treating behavioral conditions in primary care (Modern Healthcare, 2016). A report by the American Hospital Association (2016) highlighted related challenges in the gap between supply and demand for behavioral health providers. In terms of education and training, behavioral health students are siloed in education programs at the undergraduate and graduate level that do not focus on primary care behavioral health (AHA, 2016). There is a lack of behavioral training for primary care physicians, advanced practice registered nurses (APRNs), physician assistants (PAs), and nurse practitioners (NPs) even though these providers have assumed responsibility for primary care behavioral health (AHA, 2016). Education and training programs are needed to train both the medical and specialty behavioral health workforce in behavioral medicine in primary care in order to meet the patient demand.

A second challenge lies in the focus of current models of education, training, and delivery of behavioral medicine in integrated primary care. Kathol, deGruy, and Rollman (2014) argue that behavioral medicine must transition to become a value-based, financially sustainable component of primary care. The nationwide movement from fee-for-service to value-based payment requires that providers and administrators deliver value-based behavioral medicine that delivers highest quality of care with the most efficient resources at the lowest cost (Bao et al., 2017). Kathol and associates (2014) argue that current models of primary care behavioral medicine are not based on systematic, evidence-based, and value-based models of behavioral medicine. Instead, behavioral consultants arrive in primary care and apply psychotherapy approaches not tailored to primary care. While these approaches may result in high provider and patient satisfaction, they are not value-based.

Value-Based Behavioral Medicine and the Predominant Models of Behavioral Medicine: The Collaborative Care Model (CCM) and Primary Care Behavioral Health (PCBH)

Kathol and colleagues (2014) make seven programmatic recommendations for value-based behavioral medicine in primary care:

First, the BHCs are part of a medical network and paid through medical benefits under a single budget.

Second, a consolidated electronic health record (EHR) patient registry to identify complex patients for behavioral interventions, rather than universal screening for behavioral risks/conditions.

Third, fully trained interprofessional teams in primary care working together to improve medical and behavioral outcomes that will result in reduced need for high-cost services such as emergency department and hospital care, leading to cost savings.

Fourth, stepped care, matching level of treatment intensity to patient condition severity and systematic follow-up to manage treatment failures.

Fifth, define desired medical and behavioral outcomes and treat to target, resulting in efficient use of limited resources for complex patients, which should produce cost savings.

Sixth, apply evidence-based behavioral treatment algorithms with routine outcome assessment that target patient clinical, quality of life, and satisfaction goals.

Seventh, a defined care manager role, cross-trained in medical and behavioral, whole-person care to provide care coordination and guide complex patients to condition self-management (Kathol et al., 2014).

In summary, only by dedicating human resources to provide behavioral medicine interventions targeted to complex cases will the promise of improved health, reduced utilization, and cost savings be realized.

Kathol and colleagues (2014) are critical of integrated behavioral medicine programs that screen and assess primarily behavioral conditions such as depression in primary care or only comorbid medical and behavioral conditions. These approaches may neglect the medically complex patients that require lifestyle behavioral medicine to prevent or reverse cardiovascular risks and NCDs. This approach has implications for training in the two predominant models of integrated behavioral medicine, the Primary Care Behavioral Health (PCBH) model (e.g., Robinson & Reiter, 2016) and the Collaborative Care Model (CCM) as exemplified by the AIMS Center (Ratzliff et al., 2016). The CCM is consistent with the value-based approach and has a significant body of research showing evidence of improved medical and behavioral outcomes and reduced utilization and associated costs of care (Katon et al., 2012). The collaborative care model of chronic disease management is based on a multidisciplinary, primary care, team-based approach in which primary care physicians, behavioral health professionals, and care managers work together to provide evidence-based interventions for comorbid medical and behavioral conditions (Katon et al., 2012). A care manager, usually a nurse, plays a critical role in educating patients and family caregivers about the medical and behavioral conditions, using motivational enhancement to improve engagement and retention, developing and monitoring a treatment plan, and tracking outcomes systematically (Katon et al., 2012).

The PCBH is more widely used and there is greater variability in the approaches to patient screening, assessment, and treatment (Hall et al., 2015). Many PCBH approaches do not use the critical components of complex patient case identification and treat to target care management (e.g., Robinson & Reiter, 2016). The PCBH model may be easier to implement since it does not require a patient registry, a dedicated care manager role, and systematic follow-up based on treat to target goals. It is associated with high provider and patient satisfaction and is often well-suited to fee-for-service reimbursement and sustainability (Robinson & Reiter, 2016). The CCM model is more challenging to implement and less well-suited to FFS reimbursement, since many components such as care management are not consistently tied to reimbursement billing codes. However, with the shift to value-based payment, there will be a growing demand for behavioral medicine based on the approach outlines by Kathol and associates (2014).

The position of this author is that the value-based, PCBH and CCM approaches are compatible, and must be combined to meet the demand for value-based services outlined by Kathol and associates (2014). This chapter will review the competencies and associated training needs for primary care behavioral medicine with an emphasis on value-based, financially sustainable components that are designed to achieve the triple aim of improved patient experience, improved population health, and decreased cost by reducing the use of high-cost medical services as targeted, complex patients improve their health and quality of life. Practical examples of existing training and education programs will be highlighted. In addition, this chapter will introduce the role of health information technology and new workforce solutions to improving efficiency and effectiveness for more patients while maintaining financial sustainability.

Behavioral Medicine Competencies and Value-Based Care

Approaches to training providers in behavioral medicine in integrated care have evolved early efforts to define the field and scope of behavioral medicine (Fisher et al., 2011) to competencies for behavioral health consultants in primary care (Hall et al., 2015) and now in the patient-centered medical home (PCMH) model of primary care (Kazak, Nash, Hiroto, & Kaslow, 2017). These recent competencies include behaviorally anchored examples, robust training materials, and strategies for how to implement training. In addition, there is an emerging framework of interprofessional education in integrated care, recognizing the need for providers of diverse disciplines to work together effectively in primary care (APA, 2016).

McDaniel and colleagues (2014) identified six clusters of primary care psychology and associated competencies that are consistent with behavioral medicine: (1) science based on biopsychosocial model, research, and evaluation; (2) interdisciplinary systems, including leadership, administration, and advocacy; (3) professionalism in values, cultural diversity, primary care ethics, and reflective practice that emphasizes self-care; (4) building sustainable primary care, interprofessional relationships; (5) applications of practice management, screening and assessment, intervention, and consultation; and (6) education in teaching and supervision. McDaniel and associates (2014) identified essential components of knowledge, skills, and attitudes for each cluster, each with sample behavioral examples. Clinical vignettes were used to demonstrate competencies in practice. These clusters are important in moving beyond clinical competencies to the leadership, practice management, focused on sustainability necessary for value-based behavioral medicine.

Kazak and colleagues (2017) described the roles, evidence, opportunities, and challenges for psychologists in PCMHs. The authors provided principles for integrated behavioral medicine based on the Joint Principles of the PCMH (AAFP, 2007): (1) a personal physician committed to the health of each patient; (2) PCP-directed, team-based medical practice; (3) whole-person orientation that integrated physical, behavioral, and social aspects of patient health; (4) coordinated medical and behavioral care; (5) quality and safety reflected in patient registries, EHRs, medical record documentation, shared decision-making, and responsibility for patient treatment planning; (6) enhanced access to care by including BHCs in care plans; (7) payment that recognized value-added behavioral medicine interventions; and (8) access to behavioral medicine resources for providers, patients, and families. The authors also described the multitude of roles for the BHC in integrated care: clinician, consultant, teacher/supervisor, manager/team leader, and researcher (Table 4.1) (Kazak et al., 2017).

Kazak and colleagues (2017) assert that training models must incorporate research on the effectiveness of integrated care, workforce development, finance, and accountability in leadership and advocacy. They also note that FFS reimbursement does not include support for nonreimbursable services such as team-based consultation and education, program development and evaluation. These competencies are closely aligned with the value-based model of behavioral medicine outlined by Kathol and associates (2014). They note the importance of population health and cost savings and the importance of BHCs to advocate for behavioral medicine with clinical, research, and workforce components that are financially sustainable.

Hall and colleagues (2015) studied how organizations prepare clinicians to work together in integrated primary care settings in 19 practices. Recruiting BHCs was difficult because most clinicians were not trained sufficiently for primary care behavioral medicine. For the practice's new to integration, this problem was exacerbated by a lack of experienced leaders to provide training. These practice leaders often failed to recognize the time and resources necessary to train a new workforce on key competencies. The training strategies ranged from hiring consultants to train, sending staff to external training programs, hosting residency training programs, or creating their own programs. Onboarding new staff was accomplished by reviewing

Table 4.1 Roles, responsibilities, and activities of psychologists in patient-centered medical homes

Roles	Responsibilities	Activities
Clinician	Provides whole-person assessment, diagnosis, referral-specific conceptualization; evidence-based interventions	Screen for psychosocial and behavioral health problems; change health behaviors; implement brief evidence-based interventions; provide preventive interventions; treat couples/families; manage complex patients in collaboration with team to address complex biopsychosocial needs
Consultant	Responds to requests for patient care issues promptly with practical recommendations	Coach primary care provider on methods to facilitate health behavior change; provide treatment recommendations
Teacher/ supervisor	Teaches and provides supervision to trainees in psychology and other fields	Train psychology and other healthcare providers (e.g., medicine, nursing, pharmacy) by developing curricula and providing supervision and training; foster collaborative team work
Administrator/ team lead	Facilitates management of behavioral and behavioral health service; promotes collaboration between/across sites; and enhances team functioning	Lead efforts to build behavioral health services within PCMH; network with outside agencies to foster collaborative care in the medical neighborhood; provide interventions to enhance team functioning; increase access to care; develop interprofessional behavioral health group protocols in chronic pain, depression, and diabetes management; collaborate in system redesign
Researcher	Applies research methods to quality improvement practices in support of PCMH goals	Lead quality improvement projects; review cultural sensitivity of approaches to determine the sensitivity and specificity for a given population; develop program evaluation tools to determine efficacy of interventions; evaluate efficacy of PCMH model and attend to implementation and dissemination of care models

From Kazak et al. (2017)
Note. PCMH patient-centered medical home

training manuals, shadowing experienced staff, and ensuring that new hires had sufficient time to study and receive mentoring and support (Hall et al., 2015). The authors concluded that a lack of training capacity and applied, experiential learning activities is a major barrier to developing the integrated primary care workforce.

Beachum et al. (2017) focused on the need to prepare psychologists for leadership in the PCMH. The demand for BHCs to lead integrated care behavioral medicine in the PCMH far exceeds the supply of trained professionals, creating an opportunity for psychologists and other professionals (Beachum et al., 2017). The authors note that in addition to clinical competencies, BHCs must be skilled in practice management, program development and evaluation, quality improvement, and interprofessional collaboration. Beachum et al. (2017) propose a taxonomy for competency-based training for BHCs in the PCMH, organized by training resources

Table 4.2 Training activities by level of intensity and program resources

Level of training intensity	Program resources	Possible training activities
Exposure	Modest	Reading assignments in existing courses Trainees belong to relevant listservs for discussions of timely topics and threads Dissemination of PCMH information and resources Health psychology course that includes assignment in interprofessional and/or PCMH assignments Attend clinical didactics/colloquia by PCMH experts Shadow PCMH providers in clinic Directed readings; discussion groups
Experience	Moderate	Primary care psychology course or modules PCMH training for interested faculty members Practicum/rotation in PCMH setting Assignments in PCMH program development and outcomes evaluation
Emphasis	Substantial	Multiple PCMH clinical placements Peer supervision opportunities Collaboration with PCMH practice team and administration on: Outcomes evaluation Quality improvement
Major	Immersion	Half- to full-time PCMH clinical placements, including clinical service delivery and administrative functions Supervision of predoctoral and internship trainees as well as other health professionals Population health research (including system and broad population)Demographic, medical, and social epidemiological perspectives on population health Quality improvement Policy development related to PCMH formative and summative outcomes relative to system, community, and broader population

From Beachum et al. (2017)
Note. PCMH patient-centered medical home

and intensity from lowest to highest, with degree of program resources required and possible training activities (Table 4.2). First, and least intensive, is *exposure* through readings, coursework, or observation/shadowing, such as learning the NCQA's PCMH recognition program (NCQA, 2014). Second is *experience* in the form of in vivo or real-world work experience shadowing or joining meetings in the PCMH such as a practicum rotation. This experience should include structured, programmatic activities to build competencies. Third, *emphasis* is defined as a major rotation of 16–40 h/week time commitment for a structured and in-depth learning experience. Fourth, the *major area of study* is the most comprehensive training program, defined as 2- or more 40-h/week rotations, such as an internship or postdoctoral fellowship (Beachum et al., 2017). Table 4.2 includes detailed competencies for each level of training intensity. Leadership in integrated primary care behavioral medicine is critical for the BHC to promote the value-based behavioral medicine model with PCPs, other clinicians, and senior leadership.

In summary, these recent approaches to competencies for behavioral medicine in primary care now incorporate many of the value-based healthcare dimensions outlined by Kathol and associates (2014). The challenge is to identify training and education programs that are consistent with value-based behavioral medicine competencies, widely available for both new students entering undergraduate and graduate degree programs, for practicing medical providers, and for specialty behavioral health providers interested in practicing in primary care.

Exemplar Training and Education Programs

One of the most comprehensive training resources for the BHC in integrated care is the Curriculum for an Interprofessional Seminar on Integrated Primary Care (IS-IPC) (APA Interprofessional Seminar on Integrated Primary Care Work Group, 2016). This is a course syllabus comprised of eight modules with outline content and resources (links to white papers, web pages, videos, etc.). The seminar may be used by practice leaders for new and existing BHCs and includes (1) introduction to interprofessional education and healthcare, (2) integrated primary care, (3) population health, (4) ethics, (5) leadership, (6) quality improvement, (7) health finance, and (8) health policy and advocacy (APA, 2016). Each module includes topic-specific learning outcomes and competencies, an outline of didactic content and sample classroom activities, web-based resources and references, and recommended learning assessment approaches (APA, 2016). The IS-IPC is designed for trainers to incorporate all or a subset of modules and training content, based on the individual needs of each practice. The IS-IPC appears well-suited to meet the challenge noted by Hall and colleagues (2015) of detailed, evidence-based training content to help new and existing integrated care practices develop internal training strategies. In addition, the IS-IPC is consistent with value-based care as evidenced by competencies in population health, leadership, quality improvement, and finance.

Exemplar Integrated Care Behavioral Medicine Training Programs

Integrated care behavioral medicine training and education programs are available at the graduate degree and certificate level. Graduate degree programs are well-suited to students entering the field, and certificate programs are a feasible approach for training and education of practicing medical and specialty behavioral health providers. The extent to which existing programs address all of the components of value-based care (Kathol et al., 2014) varies significantly. However, it appears that increasingly training and education programs are moving from basic clinical competencies to practice management, leadership, and business competencies also. The following is a selective list of exemplar programs.

The University of Massachusetts Medical School Center for Integrated Primary Care (UMASS CIPC) offers certificate courses in the PCBH model, motivational interviewing, and integrated care management (http://www.umassmed.edu/cipc/pcbh/overview/). The UMASS CIPC certificate courses are available as short courses or full certificate programs. The course content includes video recordings and live online sessions for some programs. The courses are taught by faculty who are experienced in integrated health behavioral medicine.

The Arizona State University Doctor of Behavioral Health (DBH) online degree program is an interdisciplinary degree open to master's degree-level professionals interested in practicing at the doctoral level (https://www.chs.asu.edu/programs/schools/doctor-behavioral-health). Clinical and management concentrations are available. The DBH clinical concentration prepares licensed master's degree-level clinicians such as social workers, counselors, nurses, and physician assistants to provide integrated behavioral health in primary care. The DBH management concentration prepares master's degree professionals to design, implement, and evaluate integrated care programs. The DBH includes an internship program in which students practice in primary care clinics in their local community while consulting with a small group on a webinar platform led by an experienced doctoral consultant. The DBH program has recently added a Master of Integrated Healthcare designed to prepare future managers to lead integrated care programs and an online continuing education program designed for physicians, nurses, physician assistants, and specialty behavioral health clinicians. The DBH degree and continuing education programs are focused on all of the key areas of value-based behavioral health outlined by Kathol and associates (2014). In addition to the PCBH and CCM approaches, there is an emphasis on practice management, quality improvement, financial management, and return on investment.

The National Register of Health Service Psychologists recently announced an "Integrated Healthcare Training Series" (https://www.nationalregister.org/ihts/). The series includes 41 videos that cover models of integrated behavioral healthcare delivery in primary care. The videos are grouped into categories of models and concepts, implementation, practice, medical management, pharmacological management, and psychosocial management, all delivered by experts in each topic. The National Register training series does address many of the value-based healthcare components outlined by Kathol et al. (2014), but lacks detail on topics such as population health, cost savings, and return on investment.

The AIMS (Advancing Integrated Mental Health Solutions) Center provides a wealth of resources useful for training and education on the CCM (https://www.aims.uw.edu). The website is a resource center rather than a formal training and education program, although consultation services are available. The AIMS Center content is consistent with value-based healthcare, including topics such as team structure, financing and building the business case, and accountable care and value-based purchasing strategies. A Financial Modeling Workbook is available to help build a financial sustainable integrated behavioral health delivery model.

In addition to these exemplar programs, the American Psychological Association maintains a directory of education and training for psychology in primary care. The directory includes doctoral degree programs, internship, and postdoctoral training programs for primary care psychology (http://www.apa.org/ed/graduate/primary-care-psychology.aspx). These programs are largely doctoral psychologist degree, internship, and postdoctoral programs with an emphasis on primary care behavioral health. Many of these programs focus on psychologist training with additional courses on primary care behavioral health.

In summary, primary care behavioral medicine training and education programs are available to meet the demand for educating new students as well as current practitioners. These programs share a strong emphasis on models and clinical delivery of behavioral medicine interventions in primary care. Many lack the value-based content recommended by Kathol and associates (2014). It is likely that value-based healthcare will be added to doctoral degree programs currently lacking that emphasis. The more immediate need to train current medical and behavioral providers will likely require selecting from two or more existing certificate or continuing education programs to develop a comprehensive training program that includes these value-based components. Examples of this approach follow.

Exemplar Approaches to Implementing Integrated Care Behavioral Medicine Training Programs

Dobmeyer and colleagues (2016) described the training program for integrated care and behavioral health in a large healthcare system, the Department of Defense (DoD). They studied the DoD experience in training BHCs in PCBH model primary care clinics globally. The training curriculum was a phased model that included preparatory self-learning, classroom training and role-play exercises, in vivo training during a site visit, and sustainment training using consultation calls and continuing education units over time (Table 4.3).

Dobmeyer and colleagues used the Tri-Service BHC Core Competency Tool (CCT) adapted from the Air Force BHC Core Competency Tool (USAF, 2011) and based on the PCBH model of integrated care developed by Kirk Strosahl and Patricia Robinson of Mountainview Consulting Group (2017), like the competencies published in Robinson and Reiter (2016). The CCT is based on the six clusters common to BHC core competency research: (1) clinical practice, (2) practice management, (3) consultation, (4) documentation, (5) team performance, and (6) administrative, with specific behaviors or attributes were added to each (Table 4.4).

The pre-training phase self-guided learning activities were spread over 1–2 months, prior to enrolling in the classroom phase. In addition to learning activities, trainees participated in primary care meetings, huddles, and shadowed

Table 4.3 BHC training phases and curriculum topics

Pre-training (orientation)
Duration: 1–2 months, from time of hire at site until start of Phase I classroom training
Topics
Independent review of relevant policy documents and practice manual
Attend clinic meetings and huddles
Shadow primary care providers
Military cultural competency ([a]added later)
Phase I (Classroom)
Duration: 3½–4 days (~13 h on didactic topics, 14 h for patient care role plays, 5 h for hands-on medical record training)
Topics
Overview of Primary Care Behavioral Health (PCBH)
Roles and core competencies of behavioral health consultants (BHCs)
Assessment
Documentation
Ethics and integrated care
Demonstration of initial BHC appointment
Behavioral Health Measure-20 (BHM-20) ([a]added later)
Working together with the behavioral health care facilitator ([a]added later)
Service-specific policies and programs
Simulated patient care (role plays) and evaluation of core competencies (14 h)
Hands-on electronic medical record training using BHC module (5 h) ([a]added later)
Phase II (site visit)
Duration: 1–2 days
Topics
Trainer observes BHC providing patient care and consultation (1/2 to 2 days)
Review of topics, as indicated (e.g., documentation, assessment tools, strategies to increase referrals, practice management, etc.)
Evaluation of core competencies
Leadership meeting with recommendations
Sustainment training
Duration: once per month, or more if needed
Topics
Consultation calls with service program manager (monthly)
Webinar series (monthly); primarily focused on chronic medical conditions (e.g., diabetes, obesity, chronic pain) and maladaptive health behaviors (e.g., tobacco use, alcohol misuse) ([a]added later)

From Dobmeyer et al. (2016)

[a]Topics that were not part of the original curriculum but were added at a later date to address identified gaps

PCPs. The phase 1 classroom was a 4-day in-person training based on didactics, demonstration, role-play, and EHR hands-on training (Table 4.3). Topics included the PCBH model, basic clinical competencies, outcome assessment, and ethical considerations (Dobmeyer et al., 2016). The simulated patient care role-play scenarios were conducted in small groups under the guidance of one trainer. The scenarios were clinical case studies based on actual patients. At the completion of 2 days, each trainee was evaluated by the trainer and had to achieve a pass on a subset of test items to be allowed to begin work with patients. The phase 2 clinical site training

Table 4.4 Tri-Service BHC core competencies

Dimension	Element	Attribute
I. Clinical practice and knowledge skills	I.a. Role definition	Says introductory script smoothly, conveys the BHC role to all new patients, and answers patient's questions
	I.b. Problem identification	Identifies and defines the presenting problem with the patient within the first half of the initial 30-min appointment
	I.c. Assessment	Focuses on current problem, functional impact, and environmental factors contributing to/maintaining the problem; uses tools appropriate for primary care
	I.d. Problem focus	Explores whether additional problems exist, without excessive probing
	I.e. Population-based care	I.e.1. Understands the difference between population-based and case-focused approach I.e.2. Provides care along a continuum from primary prevention to tertiary care; develops/uses pathways to routinely involve BHC in care of chronic conditions[a]
	I.f. Biopsychosocial approach	Understands relationship of medical and psychological aspects of health[a]
	I.g. Use of evidence-based interventions	Utilizes evidence-based recommendations/interventions suitable for primary care for patients and PCPs
	I.h. Intervention design	I.h.1. Bases interventions on measurable, functional outcomes and symptom reduction I.h.2. Uses self-management, home-based practice I.h.3. Uses simple, concrete, practical strategies, based on empirically supported treatments for primary care
	I.i. Multi-patient intervention skill	Works with PCPs to provide classes and/or groups in format appropriate for primary care (e.g., drop-in stress management class, group medical visit for a chronic condition)[a]
	I.j. Pharmacotherapy	Can name basic psychotropic medications; can discuss common side effects and common myths; abides by recommendation limits for non-prescribers. Consults with EBHC when needed[a]
II. Practice management skills	II.a. Visit efficiency	30-min visits demonstrate adequate introduction, rapid problem identification and assessment, and development of intervention recommendations and a plan
	II.b. Time management	Stays on time when conducting consecutive appointments[a]

(continued)

Table 4.4 (continued)

Dimension	Element	Attribute
	II.c. Follow-up planning	Plans follow-up for 2 weeks or 1 month, instead of every week (as appropriate); alternates follow-ups with PCPs for high-utilizing patients
	II.d. Intervention efficiency	Completes treatment episode in four or fewer visits for majority of patients; structures behavioral change plans consistent with time-limited treatment[a]
	II.e. Visit flexibility	Appropriately uses flexible strategies for visits: 15 min, 30 min, phone contacts, secure messaging[a]
	II.f. Triage	Attempts to manage most problems in primary care, but does triage to mental health, chemical dependency, or other clinics or services when necessary
	II.g. Case management	II.g.1. Utilizes patient registries (if they exist); takes load off of PCP (e.g., returns patient calls about behavioral issues); advocates for patients[a] II.g.2. Refers and coordinates with BHCF and EBHC[a]
	II.h. Community resource referrals	Is knowledgeable about and makes use of community resources (e.g., refers to community self-help groups, etc.)[a]
III. Consultation skills	III.a. Referral clarity	Is clear on the referral questions; focuses on and responds directly to referral questions in PCP feedback
	III.b. Curbside consultation	Successfully consults with PCPs on demand about a general issue or specific patient; uses clear, direct language in a concise manner[a]
	III.c. Assertive follow-up	Ensures PCPs receive verbal and/or written feedback on patients referred; interrupts PCP, if indicated, for urgent patient needs[a]
	III.d. PCP education	Delivers brief presentations in primary care staff meetings (PCP audience; focus on what BHC can do for them, what PCPs can refer, what to expect, how to use BHC optimally, etc.)[a]
	II.e. Recommendation usefulness	Recommendations are tailored to the pace of primary care (e.g., interventions suggested for PCPs can be done in 1–3 min)
	III.f. Value-added orientation	Recommendations are intended to reduce PCP visits and workload (e.g., follow-up with BHC instead of PCP)
	III.g. Clinical pathways	Participates in team efforts to develop, implement, evaluate, and revise pathway programs needed in the clinic[a]

(continued)

Table 4.4 (continued)

Dimension	Element	Attribute
IV. Documentation skills	IV.a. Concise, clear charting	Clear, concise notes detail: referral problem specifics, functional analysis, pertinent history, impression, specific recommendations, and follow-up plan[a]
	IV.b. Prompt PCP feedback	Written and/or verbal feedback provided to PCP on the day the patient was seen[a]
	IV.c. Appropriate format	Chart notes use SOAP four-section format (subjective, objective, assessment, plan)[a]
V. Administrative knowledge and skills	V.a. BHC policies and procedures	Understands scheduling, templates, codes for primary care work, criticality of accurate medical coding[a]
	V.b. Risk management protocols	Understands limits of existing BHC practices; can describe and discuss how and why informed consent procedures differ, etc.[a]
	V.c. Coding documentation	Routinely and accurately completes coding documentation[a]
VI. Team performance skills	VI.a. Fit with primary care culture	Understands and operates comfortably in fast-paced, action-oriented, team-based culture[a]
	VI.b. Knows team members	Knows the roles of the various primary care team members; both assists and utilizes them[a]
	VI.c. Responsiveness	Readily provides unscheduled services when needed (e.g., sees patient during lunch time or at the end of the day, if needed)[a]
	VI.d. Availability	Provides on-demand consultations by beeper or cell phone when not in the clinic; keeps staff aware of whereabouts[a]

From Dobmeyer et al. (2016)

BHC behavioral health consultant, *PCP* primary care provider, *EBHC* external behavioral health consultant, *BHCF* behavioral health care facilitator

[a]Attribute that is rated only in Phase II (site visit) training

started about 3–6 months after completion of phase 1. Each BHC visited his or her local clinic and practiced advanced competencies. The trainer evaluated the remaining competencies by shadowing the BHC in the clinic, reviewing documentation, and observing BHC–PCP consultations and team huddles. Sustainment training included scheduled distance learning, such as monthly group phone calls to review cases, practice issues, and new learning (Dobmeyer et al., 2016).

Serrano, Cos, Daub, and Levkovich (2017) developed simulated patient scenarios to evaluate the competencies of BHCs working in PCBH model in Federally Qualified Health Centers. A simulated patient is an actor or volunteer that receives training on being a patient in a role-play scenario. The trainee interacts with the simulated patient and is rated on target competencies by experts (Serrano et al., 2017). They developed a simulated BHC encounter using standardized patients that was repeated twice over 2 years. Next, the authors developed a BHC competency tool, the Behavioral Health Consultant Observation Rating Scale (BHC-

ORS). In addition, they used the Working Alliance Inventory (WAI), a validated measure of BHC performance based on patient ratings of therapeutic alliance (Munder, Wilmers, Leonhart, Linster, & Barth, 2010). BHCs also completed a satisfaction survey to evaluate their experience with the simulated patient encounter (Serrano et al., 2017).

The results of the Serrano study (2017) were marred by changes in research design over the course of the 2 years. The BHC-ORS scoring was changed to improve interrater reliability, and experimenter bias was a problem given the dual role of trainer and evaluator. The target BHC competencies generally improved once identified as training needs in year 1 of the simulation. Patient feedback on the WAI showed average treatment alliance for BHCs. The BHCs rated the experience as helpful for training. These results were used by practice leadership for ongoing strategic planning for training. In sum, the authors concluded that the results support the use of simulated patient scenarios as they are useful and feasible and recommended changes to the research approach based on this pilot (Serrano et al., 2017).

Emerging Value-Based Competencies

There are several new areas of professional competency relevant to value-based healthcare and integrated behavioral medicine. The aging of the population, increased burden of NCDs, and new medical technologies are resulting in rising healthcare costs that are a challenge for funding (Gentry & Badrinath, 2017). There are more effective treatments options available than can be afforded in limited budgets. In response to this challenge of limited resources, Kathol and associates (2014) recommend a strategy of using BHCs in primary care to target complex patients in order to achieve cost savings by reducing utilization of high-cost services such as emergency department and hospital care. Value-based healthcare is based on the quality of care over cost and time (Badash et al., 2017). For patients, this means safe, effective care at reasonable costs; for providers it means utilizing evidence-based treatments that consider patient decision-making and attitudes (Dartmouth-Hitchcock, n.d.).

There are three emerging areas especially relevant to behavioral medicine in the PCMH. First, several lines of research demonstrate that nonprofessional lay workers or lower-level medical assistants can be trained to delivery population health interventions at lower cost than licensed BHCs, adding value by reducing costs and enabling more patients to receive treatments (Kim et al., 2016). Second, there is emerging evidence that health technologies such as mobile phone apps (mHealth) and wearable sensors are useful in helping patients to prevent and better manage health risks and NCDs (Milani & Franklin, 2017). These new health technologies can extend the impact of the BHC role in behavioral medicine from the clinical practice to the home and workplace of the patient, improving outcomes and efficiency. Third, new value-based payment models are emerging that will be critical for BHCs in integrated primary care to develop sustainable behavioral medicine programs (Bao et al., 2017).

Community Health Worker, Lay and Medical Assistant Behavioral Medicine Workforce Development

Most patients with behavioral conditions do not have access to evidence-based behavioral interventions due to barriers such as lack of trained providers and human resources shortages (WHO, 2008). An emerging solution to this barrier in low- and middle-income countries is to train and supervise nonspecialist healthcare workers to deliver transdiagnostic behavioral treatments (Bennett-Levy et al., 2010; Patel, Chowdhary, Rahman, & Verdeli, 2011). In rural areas, frontline health workers usually provide care in their local community and work in roles such as community health worker or nurse, delivering low-cost, effective, evidence-based interventions to meet the needs of the patients in the community (Patel et al., 2011).

A systematic review was conducted by Kim and associates (2016) of community-based health workers to improve chronic disease management among vulnerable populations. The authors reviewed 67 studies that met their selection criteria, all but 4 conducted in the United States. Compared to no intervention of other treatments, community behavioral health worker interventions resulted in increased screening for breast, cervical, and colorectal cancers; lowered blood pressure, blood glucose, and weight; and increased physical activity (Kim et al., 2016). The community health worker interventions were also associated with cost savings. Djuric and associates (2017) evaluated the effectiveness of health coaching by medical assistants in primary care to help patients to improve healthy lifestyle behaviors. Subjects who completed the study at 12 weeks had significant weight loss, improvements in diet, and physical activity. Patients and providers were highly satisfied and valued the availability of health coaching.

Behavioral interventions by supervised lay health workers are a potential solution that is gaining attention as part of the global behavioral health research agenda. The World Health Organization (WHO), as part of its Mental Health Gap Action Programme, has produced a series of manualized behavioral interventions adapted for delivery by lay health workers (Dawson et al., 2015). Dawson et al. (2015) describe one such intervention, Problem Management Plus (PM+) (WHO, 2016). PM+ is a manualized, transdiagnostic treatment manual that includes evidence-based, low-intensity interventions such as motivational interviewing and stress management, designed to enhance patient engagement and enhance patient ability to cope with stress and improve conditions such as anxiety and depression. The M+ intervention was adapted for use in primary care in Pakistan, and the results showed that the intervention was feasible and effective in reducing symptoms of posttraumatic stress disorder and improving functioning in a conflict-ridden area of Peshawar, Pakistan (Rahman et al., 2016).

Taken together, these studies show that lay persons or lower-level health professionals with appropriate training can deliver effective behavioral medicine interventions to at-risk populations. These interventions appear especially useful in providing help to underserved, vulnerable populations and in reducing health disparities (Kim et al., 2016). These findings point to an opportunity for BHCs to develop, implement, and maintain lay or medical assistant health coaches based on population health management approaches such as the CCM. This workforce may be utilized to target complex patients as recommended by Kathol and associates (2014) or to target other patient populations that are at risk but with lower levels of complexity, such as prediabetes patients. It is recommended that workforce development based on community health workers, medical assistants, or other nonprofessionals be added to the key competencies for BHCs to extend the reach of behavioral medicine with effective interventions at lower cost with high patient satisfaction, hallmarks for value-based care.

Health Technologies and Behavioral Medicine: Apps and Wearables

There is a rapid proliferation of health information technology designed to introduce devices such as mobile phone apps, remote telemonitoring, and wearable sensors to improve patient self-management of chronic conditions (Lucas, 2014). A recent review concluded that mHealth interventions are effective in promoting physical activity and healthy eating in developing countries (Muller, Alley, Schoeppe, & Vandelanote, 2016). Smartphone mHealth tools can lead to improved health outcomes and reduced overall costs for chronic conditions by providing physicians and BHCs with real-time patient data on health indicators, autoadministered therapies, adherence, and treat-to-target goals. With this information healthcare providers can utilize approaches such as shared decision-making and encourage patient condition self-management.

Incorporating smartphone apps and wearables into integrated care behavioral medicine interventions is consistent with value-based care. The mHealth resources are highly efficient and low cost relative to the human resource capital needed to staff a PCMH. Low-cost, efficient treatments that are effective extend the work of the BHC from the clinic to the patient home. These tools are also consistent with patient condition self-management, as the patient is encouraged to actively monitor and plan healthier activities.

A study by Block and associates (2015) tested a diabetes prevention and weight loss program, Alive-PD, based on a fully automated behavioral medicine program using email, the Internet, and mobile phone for prediabetes patients. The Alive-PD program improved glycemic control, bmi, waist circumference, TG/HDL ratio, and diabetes risk (Block et al., 2015). The authors conclude that the program has high scalability and has the potential to extend the reach of clinician-delivered diabetes prevention programs to the 86 million US adults with prediabetes and other at-risk groups (Block et al., 2015). Michaelides, Raby, Wood, Farr, and Roro-Ramos (2016) tested the efficacy of a mobile phone version of the Diabetes Prevention Program with human coaching on weight loss for overweight adults. The results of the study showed that the intervention, delivered entirely through a smartphone platform, resulted in a 6-month weight loss comparable to the in-person diabetes prevention program. The program also showed high patient acceptance and feasibility (Michaelides et al., 2016).

Other researchers are comparing or combining mHealth with health coaches. Kowitt and colleagues (2017) developed a population health management intervention, Peers for Progress, that combined lay health coaches and eHealth for patients with type 2 diabetes. Peers for Progress will be studied in a pilot program in collaboration with Horizon Blue Cross Blue Shield and Vanguard Medical Group, a primary care practice in New Jersey (Kowitt et al., 2017). A study by Wayne, Perez, Kaplan, and Rivo (2015) studied a 6-month health coach intervention with and without the use of mobile phone monitoring support for type 2 diabetic patients from a lower-socioeconomic status community. The results showed that health coaching with and without mobile phone support appeared to reduce HbA1c levels and mental health, and that the mobile phone group showed accelerated improvement (Wayne et al., 2015).

These studies show that mHealth behavioral medicine interventions are effective alone or in combination with health coaches in improving health risks and management of NCDs. The mHealth apps are available for general health behaviors, such as nutrition and physical activity, as well as behavioral conditions such as depression (Milani & Franklin, 2017). These mHealth tools may be incorporated into population health management programs; they are popular with patients and show evidence of effectiveness. In summary, mHealth apps can be used to target complex patients consistent with the value-based behavioral medicine approach advocated by Kathol and colleagues (2014) or may be applied to other at-risk populations.

Emerging Value-Based Payment Models and Behavioral Medicine

Many of the competencies and training resources reviewed above include finance and sustainability as key competencies for BHCs delivering behavioral medicine in integrated care (Beachum et al., 2017; Dobmeyer et al., 2016; Kazak et al., 2017). Emerging new models of value-based payment in healthcare are an important competency for BHCs to master in order to develop sustainable behavioral medicine programs. Hubley and Miller (2016) report that while integrated behavioral health programs are rapidly proliferating, there are significant challenges to receiving reimbursement for behavioral medicine programs. A study by Kathol and associates (2010) using key informant interviews with leaders of exemplar integrated behavioral health programs identified disparities in reimbursement for medical versus behavioral interventions as the most significant barrier to financial sustainability. Hubley and Miller (2016) review the status of payment reform for psychologists practicing in integrated care settings, noting both challenges and opportunities. Challenges include the adverse impact of managed behavioral healthcare organization carve-outs that create barriers to fee-for-service reimbursement by BHCs in integrated primary care clinics. Opportunities include alternative payment models such as bundled payment and global capitation. These payment models can provide leaders the discretion to make human resource decisions on value-based decisions rather than solely on fee-for-service reimbursement criteria. It is anticipated that BHCs will be better able to recommend innovative value-based programs such as the CCM, community health or lay health coaches, and mHealth resources under these new payment models.

Summary

In recent years, there has been significant progress in developing competencies and training programs for BHCs to deliver behavioral medicine interventions in integrated primary care settings (Beachum et al., 2017; Dobmeyer et al., 2016; Kazak et al., 2017; Serrano et al., 2017). These new competencies and training programs have moved beyond clinical competencies and now include practice management, quality improvement, health technology, and financial sustainability as key competencies. These new approaches to training BHCs also increasingly incorporate strategies and techniques consistent with the model of value-based behavioral health presented by Kathol and associates (2014), such as population health management. Detailed training resources, such as the APA IS-IPC (APA, 2016), are now available to assist leaders in developing training programs for BHCs based on core, shared competencies.

The emphasis of this chapter is on the value-based context of training the BHC workforce. In addition to the recommendations of Kathol and associates (2014), it is recommended that emerging value-based approaches to promoting behavioral medicine in integrated primary care settings are tested and adopted. The addition of lower-cost community health workers, lay or lower-level medical assistant health coaches, is an excellent example of a value-based enhancement for behavioral medicine. These health workers can reach a larger population at lower cost, with effective results in improving health status. Incorporating mHealth platforms that include apps and wearable sensors is also consistent with value-based healthcare in providing tools that patients can use to manage their health more effectively on their own, with less reliance on in-person clinic visits with BHCs or other health professionals, consistent with shared decision-making and condition self-management. Finally, the rollout of value-based payment models will create opportunities for BHCs to make the business case for behavioral medicine programs that incorporate population health, lower-cost health coach workforce, and mHealth platforms. It is anticipated that BHC competencies and training programs to support behavioral medicine in integrated primary care settings will continue to evolve and adapt these newer competencies and an increased emphasis on value-based care as the healthcare market moves in this direction.

References

American Academy of Family Physicians, American Academy of Pediatrics, American College of Physicians, & American Osteopathic Association. (2007). Joint principles of the patient-centered medical home. Retrieved from: http://www.aafp.org/dam/AAFP/documents/practice_management/pcmh/initiatives/PCMHJoint.pdf

American Hospital Association. (2016). *The state of the behavioral health workforce: A literature review.* Retried from: http://www.aha.org/content/16/stateofbehavior.pdf

American Psychological Association, Interprofessional Seminar on Integrated Primary Care Work Group. (2016). *A curriculum for an interprofessional seminar on integrated primary care.* Retrieved from: http://www.apa.org/education/grad/curriculum-seminar.aspx

Badash, I., Kleinman, N., Barr, S., Jang, J., Rahman, S., & Wu, B. (2017). Redifining health: The evolution of health ideas from antiquity to the era of value-based care. *Cureus, 9*(2), e1018. https://doi.org/10.7759/cureus.1018.

Bao, Y., McGuire, T., Chan, Y., Eggman, A., Ryan, A., Bruce, M., … Unutzer, J. (2017). Value-based payment in implementing evidence-based care: The mental health integration program in Washington state. *AJMC, 23*(1), 48–53.

Beachum, A., Van Sickle, K., Khatri, P., Ali, M., Reimer, D., Farber, E., & Kaslow, N. (2017). Meeting evolving workforce needs: Preparing psychologists for leadership in the patient-centered medical home. *American Psychologist, 72*(1), 42–54.

Bennett-Levy, J., Richards, D., Farrand, P., Christensen, H., Griffiths, K., Kavanagh, D., … Williams, C. (2010). *Oxford guide to low intensity CBT interventions.* Oxford, NY: Oxford University Press.

Block, G., Aar, K., Romanelli, R., Block, T. J., Hopkins, D., Carpenter, H. A., … Block, C. H. (2015). Diabetes prevention and weight loss with a fully automated behavioral intervention by email, web, and mobile phone: A randomized controlled trial among persons with prediabetes. *Journal of Medical Internet Research, 17*(10), E240. https://doi.org/10.2196/jmir.4897

Chiles, J. A., Lambert, M. J., & Hatch, L. (2002). Medical costs offset: a review of the impact of psychological interventions on medical utilization over the past three decades. In N. A. Cummings, W. T. O'Donohue, & K. E. Ferguson (Eds.), *The impact of medical cost offset on practice and research: Making it work for you* (pp. 47–56). Reno, NV: Context Press.

Dartmouth-Hitchcock. What is value-based care? Retrieved from: http://www.dartmouth-hitchcock.org/about_dh/what_is_value_based_care.html on May 15 2017.

Dawson, K., Bryant, R., Harper, M., Tay, A., Rahman, A., Schafter, A., & Van Ommeren, M. (2015). Problem management plus (PM1): A WHO transdiagnostic psychological intervention for common mental health problems. *World Psychiatry, 14*(3), 354.

Diabetes Prevention Program Research Group. (2011). 10-year follow-up of diabetes incidence and weight loss in the diabetes prevention program outcomes study. *Lancet, 374*(9702), 1677–1686.

Djuric, Z., Segar, M., Orizondo, C., Mann, J., Faison, M., Peddireddy, N., … Locke, A. (2017). Delivery of health coaching by medical assistants in primary care. *Journal of American Board of Family Medicine, 30*, 362–370.

Dobmeyer, A., Hunter, C., Corso, M., Nielsen, M., Corso, K., Polizzi, N., & Earles, J. (2016). Primary care behavioral health provider training: Systematic development and implementation in a large medical system. *Journal of Clinical Psychology in Medical Settings, 23*, 207–224. https://doi.org/10.1007/s10880-016-9464-9

Fisher, E., Fitzgibbon, M., Glasgow, R., Haire-Joshu, D., Hayman, L., Kaplan, R., … Ockene, J. (2011). Behavior matters. *American Journal of Professionelle Medicine, 40*(5), e15–e30.

Gentry, S., & Badrinath, P. (2017). Defining health in the era of value-based care: Lessons from England of relevance to other health systems. *Cureus, 9*(3), e1079. https://doi.org/10.7759/cureus.1079

Hall, J., Cohen, D. J., Davis, M., Gun, R., Blount, A., Pollack, D. A., … Miller, B. F. (2015). Preparing the workforce for behavioral health and primary care integration. *Journal of the American Board of Family Medicine, 28*, S41–S51. https://doi.org/10.3122/jabfm.2015.s1.150054

Health Resources and Services Administration/National Center for Health Workforce Analysis; Substance Abuse and Mental Health Services Administration/Office of Policy, Planning and Innovation. (2015). *National projections of supply and demand for behavioral health practitioners: 2013–2025*. Rockville, MD. HRSA.

Hubley, S., & Miller, B. (2016). Implications of healthcare payment reform for clinical psychologists in medical settings. *Journal of Clinical Psychology in Medical Settings, 23*, 3–10. https://doi.org/10.1007/s10880-016-9451

Kathol, R. G., Butler, M., McAlpine, D. D., & Kane, R. L. (2010). Barriers to physical and mental condition integrated service delivery. *Psychosomatic Medicine, 72*(6), 511–518. https://doi.org/10.1097/PSY.0b013e3181e2c4a0

Kathol, R. G., deGruy, F., & Rollman, B. L. (2014). Value-based financially sustainable behavioral health components in patient-centered medical homes. *The Annals of Family Medicine, 12*(2), 172–175. https://doi.org/10.1370/afm.1619

Kathol, R. G., McAlpine, D., Kishi, Y., Spies, R., Meller, W., Bernhardt, T., … Gold, W. (2005). General medical and pharmacy claims expenditures in users of behavioral health services. *Journal of General Internal Medicine, 20*, 160–167.

Katon, W., Russo, J., Lin, E., Schmittdiel, J., Ciechanowski, P., Ludman, E., … Von Korff, M. (2012). Cost-effectiveness of a multicondition collaborative care intervention: A randomized controlled trial. *Archives of General Psychiatry, 69*(5), 506–514.

Kazak, A., Nash, J., Hiroto, K., & Kaslow, N. (2017). Psychologists in Patient-Centered Medical Homes (PCMHs): Roles, evidence, opportunities, and challenges. *American Psychologist, 72*(1), 1–12.

Kim, K., Choi, J., Choi Em Nieman, C., Joo, J., Lin, F., Gitlin, L., & Han, H. (2016). Effects of community-based health worker interventions to improve chronic disease management and care among vulnerable populations: A systematic review. *American Journal of Public Health, 106*(4), e3–e28. https://doi.org/10.2105/AJPH.2015.302977

Kowitt, S., Tang, P., Peples, M., Duni, J., Peskin, S., & Fisher, E. (2017). Combining the high tech with the soft touch: Population health management using eHealth and peer support. *Population Health Management, 20*(1), 3. https://doi.org/10.1089/pop.2016.00

Lucas, H. (2014). New technology and illness self-management: Potential relevance for resource-poor populations in Asia. *Social Science & Medicine, 1*, 9.

McDaniel, S. H., Grus, C. L., Cubic, B. A., Hunter, C. L., Kearney, L. K., Schuman, C. C., … Miller, B. F. (2014). Competencies for psychology practice in primary care. *American Psychologist, 69*(4), 409. https://doi.org/10.1037/a0036072

Michaelides, A., Raby, C., Wood, M., Farr, K., & Roro-Ramos, T. (2016). Weight loss efficacy of a novel mobile diabetes prevention program delivery platform with human coaching. *BMJ Open Diabetes Research and Care 4*, e000264. https://doi.org/10.1136/bmjdrc-2016-000264

Milani, R., Bober, R., Lavie, C. (2016). The role of technology in chronic disease. *Progress in Cardiovascular Diseases, 58*, 579–583.

Milani, R., & Franklin, N. (2017). The role of technology in healthy living medicine. *Progress in Cardiovascular Diseases, 59*, 487. https://doi.org/10.1016/j.pcad.2017.02.001

Modern Healthcare. Demand for mental health services soars amid provider shortage. December 31, 2016. Accessed from: http://www.modernhealthcare.com/article/20161231/TRANSFORMATION03/161229942

Mountain View Consulting Group. About. 2017. Retrieved from https://www.mtnviewconsulting.com/about/

Muller, A., Alley, S., Schoeppe, S., & Vandelanote, C. (2016). The effectiveness of e-&mHealh interventions to promote physical activity and healthy diets in developing countries: A systematic review. *International Journal of Behavioral Nutrition and Physical Activity, 13*, 109.

Munder, T., Wilmers, F., Leonhart, R., Linster, H. W., & Barth, J. (2010). Working alliance inventory-short revised (WAI-SR): Psychometric properties in outpatients and inpatients. *Clinical Psychology & Psychotherapy, 17*, 231–239.

National Committee for Quality Assurance. (2014). *Standards and guidelines for NCQA's patient centered medical home (PCMH)*. Retrieved from http://store.ncqa.org/index.php/2014-pcmh-standards-andguidelines-epub-single-user.html.

Patel, V., Chowdhary, N., Rahman, A., & Verdeli, H. (2011). Improving access to psychological treatment: Lessons from developing countries. *Behaviour Research and Therapy, 49*, 523–528.

Rahman, A., Hamdani, S., Awan, N., Bryant, R. A., Dawson, K. S., Khan, M. F., … van Ommeren, M. (2016). Effect of a multicomponent behavioral intervention in adults impaired by psychological distress in a conflict-affected area of Pakistan: A randomized clinical trial. *Journal of the American Medical Association, 316*(24), 2609–2617. https://doi.org/10.1001/jama.2016.17165

Ratzliff, A., Unutzer, J., Katon, W., & Stephens, K. (2016). *Integrated care: Creating effective mental and primary health care teams*. Hoboken, NJ: Wiley.

Robinson, P., & Reiter, J. (2016). *Behavioral consultation and primary care: A guide to integrating services* (2nd ed.). Geneva, Switzerland: Springer International Publishing.

Serrano, N., Cos, T. A., Daub, S., & Levkovich, N. (2017). Using standardized patients as a means of training and evaluating behavioral health consultants in primary care. *Families, Systems, & Health, 35*, 174–183.

United States Air Force (USAF). (2011). Primary behavioral health care services practice manual: Version 2. San Antonio: TX.

Wang, P. S., Simon, G. E., Avorn, J., Azocar, F., Ludman, E. J., McCulloch, J., … Kessler, R. C. (2007). Telephone screening, outreach, and care management for depressed workers and impact on clinical and work productivity outcomes: A randomized controlled trial. *Journal of the American Medical Association, 298*, 1401–1411.

Wayne, N., Perez, D., Kaplan, D., & Rivo, P. (2015). Health coaching reduces HbA1c in type 2 diabetic patients from a lower-socioeconomic status community: A randomized controlled trial. *Journal of Medical Internet Research, 17*(10), e224. https://doi.org/10.2196/jmir.4871

World Health Organization. (2008). *Task shifting: Rational redistribution of tasks among health workforce teams: Global recommendations and guidelines*. Geneva, Switzerland: World Health Organization.

World Health Organization. (2016). *Problem management plus (PM+): Individual psychological help for adults impaired by distress in communities exposed to adversity (generic field-trial version 1.0)*. Geneva, Switzerland: World Health Organization http://www.who.int/mental_health/emergencies/problem_management_plus/en/. Accessed 31 March 2017.

Zimmet, P. (2003). The burden of type 2 diabetes: Are we doing enough? *Diabetes & Metabolism, 29*(4 Pt 2), 6S9–6S18.

Chapter 5
Screening for Behavioral Health Problems in Adult Primary Care

Michelle Byrd, Casiana Warfield, Kristina Brookshire, and Lauren Ostarello

Introduction

Our nation is in the midst of what could be optimistically described as a major transformation in our healthcare system but may well be more likely to be thought of retrospectively as a significant dismantling of traditional systems of care. The Affordable Care Act (ACA), signed into law in 2010 and implemented in 2013, offered the promise of increased scope of coverage for behavioral health concerns both in primary care as well as in specialty behavioral healthcare settings. The Parity Law (signed in 2008) further required that insurers match funding for behavioral health services with that of medical/surgical costs. However, these significant legislative acts have cumulatively failed to provide consistent access to high-quality mental healthcare for the masses.

As the existing American healthcare system is being dismantled and new systems proposed and tried, clinical psychologists are likely to observe a historically unprecedented emphasis on cost-effectiveness and the necessity of embedding our clinical work within what are considered to be "core" streams of care, such as primary care clinics. Far from being purely political, the current changes call upon us as a profession to rely on our ethics code and scientific training to create sustainable models of care to protect and benefit ourselves, our clients, and our population at large. This may well prove to be the most significant challenge, and conversely, opportunity we have faced as a profession since our inception.

The obvious model that is best poised to meet the current demand for affordable and accessible mental health services is integrated care. A key building block to the viability of integrated care is the development and implementation of reliable, valid, and realistic screening protocols for behavioral health problems such as to allow for adequate detection and informed clinical decision-making. Whereas in the past this

M. Byrd (✉) · C. Warfield · K. Brookshire · L. Ostarello
Department of Psychology, Eastern Michigan University, Ypsilanti, MI, USA
e-mail: mbyrd@emich.edu

M. P. Duckworth, W. T. O'Donohue (eds.), *Behavioral Medicine and Integrated Care*,
https://doi.org/10.1007/978-3-319-93003-9_5

has been considered a model of practice or gold standard practice, in the future it will likely become absolutely essential for ethical care.

While integrated care has steadily and gradually gathered steam within the majority of health systems over the past two decades, it has still remained at the edge of clinical practice. Integrated care will likely now become *the* absolutely core behavioral healthcare modality to meet the needs of the American people. Over 80% of adults attended an outpatient primary care visit in the past year (Pleis & Lethbridge-Cejku, 2007), and it has been well-established that primary care is where the majority of psychological services are provided even in the current system (Wang et al., 2005, 2006). However, in the past this pattern of practice has occurred because of the gaps in the current system, causing primary care (PC) to become the country's "de facto mental healthcare system" (Regier et al., 1993). The integrated primary care setting is designed to not just provide a stopgap between referral and receipt of specialty mental healthcare services, but to planfully provide appropriate and adequate screening and intervention when and where care is initially sought, reserving specialty mental healthcare for situations or cases which exceed the short-term model of care in IPC either because of duration or severity of clinical presentation.

As such, there is an immediate and dire need to expedite the necessary evidence-based foundation to support a fully integrated system of care, as well as to adequately train the next generation of medical and behavioral health providers for this rapidly evolving clinical marketplace. There are several significant gaps in the current literature. First, few assessments and interventions have been developed, tested, and validated in the fast-paced PC setting for the most common problems in IPC, forcing BHCs to adapt evidence-based SMH interventions to the PC setting, yet these interventions are largely based on clinician experience rather than empiricism (Hunter et al., 2017). Also, out of necessity, what literature there is on adult primary care (e.g., Hunter et al., 2017) has been far more focused on describing treatment modalities than on establishing the psychometric properties of screening techniques. Quite simply, because patients are presenting with behavioral concerns in primary care at a high rate, clinicians have not been as motivated to screen for these concerns to increase the rate of detection as they have been to expand the repertoire of available treatments. Although both avenues of inquiry are sorely needed, treatment can never be successful at the programmatic level unless it is reaching all or at least the majority of those affected, and this cannot be accomplished without routine and valid screening. Finally, given that the empirical literatures on both screening and treatment are sparse, it follows that research on evaluation of these systems, including examining long-term quality-related outcomes and cost-benefit analyses, has not yet been conducted.

Rates of detection of mental health problems and active screening in primary care remain woefully low, despite increased rates of behavioral health integration and federal recommendations to screen for high-base rate behavioral concerns (Young, Klap, Sherbourne, & Wells, 2001). For example, while both lifetime and point prevalence rates of depression in adults are high, a recent study of over 30,000 primary care visits found that only depression screening occurred in only 4.2% of visits; however, when the screening did happen, it led to a new diagnosis of depression in 47% of cases, indicating that almost half of the cases would have gone undetected without routine screening (Akincigil & Matthews, 2017). Perhaps more concerning, this same study found that screening was less likely to occur in older adults and males, both demographic categories associated with higher rates of completed suicide (CDC, 2016). In addition, screening was found to occur at about half the rate among African-American patients as opposed to those identified as White, indicating a significant health disparity in screening procedures in a group that is already less likely to seek specialty mental healthcare services. The example of depression is useful as a model to illustrate the importance of screening, as this recent study speaks to the vast chasm between what the current system could be providing and the actuality of care received. Stated simply, if psychosocial concerns go undetected, they will remain untreated. If left untreated, they will result in higher rates of morbidity and mortality and ultimately result not only in greater decrements in individual quality of life but also higher healthcare utilization and spending in the long run.

In this chapter we aim to elucidate at a basic level a conceptual understanding of screening within primary care, along with discussion of critical clinical targets of screening, as well as specific recommendations for a battery of screens that may be implemented in primary care settings. For a more expansive and nuanced discussion of behavioral screening within primary care, we recommend the *Handbook of Psychological Assessment in Primary Care Settings* (Maruish, 2017).

The Nature and Necessity of Screening

As we have previously asserted (Byrd & Alschuler, 2009), screening must be distinguished from clinical assessment. Within medical settings, "screening is the systematic application of a test or inquiry to identify individuals at sufficient risk of a specific disorder to warrant further investigation or direct preventive action, amongst persons who have not sought medical attention on account of symptoms of that disorder" (Wald, 2001). Two aspects of this definition must be highlighted. First, screening is meant to determine which individuals are at "sufficient" risk, which is a critical distinction in behavioral health. Everyone is considered to be at some risk for the lifetime development of psychological illness given high base rates of common behavioral health problems. The key, then, is to be able to accurately and consistently determine who is at a heightened level of risk at a given moment in time.

The second critical aspect of this definition is that screening need not always occur at the population level, but may be specifically targeted to individuals with no known history of identified illness. Given that most people diagnosed with psychiatric conditions first present in primary care (deGruy, 1995) where the majority of mental health treatment actually occurs (Olfson et al., 2002), one could argue that these patients need not be screened since their level of symptomatology has already risen above the level of screening, but rather argues for these patients being systematically reevaluated at regular intervals to detect any changes in severity. Given that a common concern associated with screening is the systemic burden inherent in administering, scoring, and addressing cases that exceed clinical threshold, only screening on a more limited basis addresses this problem. However, depending on the scope of screening, patients who have previously screened positive for a particular concern, such as depression, may still need to be routinely screened for other concerns, such as substance abuse, particularly given high rates of comorbidity among psychological disorders.

It is important that all members of the multidisciplinary integrated care team view screening as a method of risk management. It is far better from a continuous quality improvement perspective to be able to document knowledge of all significant health concerns, even if they are not further assessed or treated at the current visit, rather than to perpetuate clinician ignorance and/or avoidance, which may not only hinder appropriate care of the mental health concern but also compromise related medical treatment plans. Screening provides a vehicle for establishing an understanding of the whole person in context, rather than reducing a person's current treatment plan to their primary medical driver in isolation of relevant psychosocial factors, and allowing for preventive services to be offered in advance of higher levels of need/care, consistent with the trend of patient-centered medical care. While providers may be concerned that screening opens the proverbial "Pandora's Box" of known behavioral concerns and thereby increases liability, in fact, remaining ignorant to the complete clinical landscape of intertwined physical and psychological concerns is much more likely to cloud clinical decision-making and impede progress toward health-related goals.

Given the criticality of screening for successful integrated care and the federal recommendations to do so (US Preventive Services Task Force, drug use (2008); alcohol misuse (2013); depression (2016)), why aren't clinics adopting screening procedures as standard clinical practice? While this question has not yet been answered empirically, experientially providers seem to have practical, logistic concerns that serve as significant barriers to systemic change. First, providers do not know what to screen for and what to screen with. Screening instruments are typically developed and disseminated by psychologists for use in primary care and, as such, are typically published in the *psychological* rather than the *medical* literature, where primary care coordinators are more likely to find them. As such, it is incumbent upon psychologists and other behavioral health researchers/integrated care providers to not only make an effort to publish their work in the body of literature in which it is most likely to benefit patients, but also to bridge the gap between these two silos of science for our medical colleagues in the meantime so that they will become aware and accepting of the existing screening instruments. Secondly, we must, in our efforts to continually develop and refine our screening tools, be mindful of the logistic demands of the primary care setting. Instruments that are difficult or time-consuming to administer, score, or interpret simply will never be broadly adopted in primary care. Some of this burden may be reduced by not actively screening patients who have already exceeded the bar for behavioral concern and are receiving appropriate follow-up consultation and/or treatment. At minimum, screening should be conducted with every new patient and at least once per year in patients who have not been previously identified as being at high risk for emotional or behavioral problems.

Given that many primary care practices have already moved to a completely digital model of medical record keeping, including having a HIPAA-secure patient portal for protected communication between providers and patients, ideally these instruments could be completed, scored, and reviewed prior to but close in time to the scheduled primary care visit, reducing the time pressure to complete these activities in person and potentially creating the opportunity for the initiation of meaningful intervention during the visit instead. In completing and submitting online screening tools, this clinical data would typically become part of the patient's medical record, allowing for ongoing tracking of biopsychosocial targets. A recent recommendation from Vogel et al. (2014) suggests future research to investigate optimal methods of entering screener data into the electronic health record (EHR) so they are available and visible to the whole integrated team as a means to inform treatment.

Targets of Screening

There is no consensus either in the literature or in clinical practice with regard to whether screening should be conducted at the general or the specific disorder level. While there are common sense arguments to err on the side of casting a wider net via more general screening, few measures have been developed with this aim in mind specifically for the primary care context (e.g., Alschuler, Hoodin, & Byrd, 2009). Instead, IPC practices have opted to screen for specific high-base rate/high-cost phenomena either instead of or in addition to more general markers of psychological concern, utilizing instruments that have been either developed or adapted for IPC use. In particular, based on prevalence rates, we argue that it may be optimal to screen for alcohol dependence, depression, and anxiety, in addition to more broad screening. We have provided a curated list of recommended screening instruments below for consideration for use in integrated systems. Please note that this list is not intended to be exhaustive and is specifically constructed for use in adult integrated care and cannot be generalized to either child/adolescent or older adult populations.

Recommended Screening Instruments

Most Commonly Used Instruments

Patient Health Questionnaire (PHQ). The PHQ is a brief, self-report screening instrument for prevalent psychopathology in an integrated or primary care setting (Spitzer, Kroenke, & Williams, 1999). The PHQ is not only the most commonly used instrument for this purpose but for good reason is considered the gold standard of broad and general screeners. In addition, the PHQ offers the added benefit of having additional associated diagnosis-specific screening questions. Therefore, an integrated care practice could conceivably purchase the entire PHQ package of screening devices to create a consistent and coherent screening program.

Importantly, the PHQ was specifically developed for use in the primary care setting. The PHQ was originally developed by adapting the *primary care evaluation of mental disorders (PRIME-MD)* so that it might be more efficiently administered. The PHQ assesses for the symptoms of eight disorders (major depressive disorder, panic disorder, other anxiety disorders, bulimia nervosa, other depressive disorders, alcohol use or dependence, somatization, and binge eating disorder) based upon patient self-report only. While the PRIME-MD's responses were largely dichotomous, the PHQ provides greater specificity in responses. Patients indicate the frequency with which they experience DSM-V symptoms for each disorder, from "not at all" to "nearly every day." In addition, respondents report the degree of distress associated with symptoms experienced, ranging from "not bothered" to "bothered a lot," allowing for indication of symptom severity (Spitzer et al., 1999). Although the PHQ cannot be considered a diagnostic instrument, the structure of the instrument clearly supports clinical decision-making with regard to differential diagnoses.

The PHQ has been investigated repeatedly and has underwent several revisions, resulting in helpful clinical recommendations for additional screening or assessment. For example, research has indicated that 10 is the recommended cutoff score for sensitively detecting depression in integrated care settings and different from the recommended cutoff in specialty mental health settings (Moriarty, Gilbody, McMillan, & Manea, 2015).

A major strength of the PHQ is that it is limited to three to four pages and takes under 5 min to administer, making it a streamlined tool for evaluating common symptoms of psychopathology and behavioral problems in primary care settings (Spitzer, Kroenke, & Williams, 1999). The PHQ is simple to score, with instructions provided on the measure itself. In addition, the PHQ has been validated for use in primary care settings as well as in detecting depression in specific clinical populations including prenatal women, individuals with high-risk anxiety, cancer, stroke, and ischemic attack (Muntingh et al., 2013; Prisnie et al., 2016; Randall, Voth, Burnett, Bazhenova, & Bardwell, 2013; Sidebottom, Harrison, Godecker, & Kim, 2012).

Several forms of the PHQ for more specialized screening have been developed in recent years including the PHQ-9 for depression, the PHQ-15 for somatic symptoms, and the GAD-7 for generalized anxiety (Kroenke, Spitzer, Williams, & Löwe, 2010). Of these, the PHQ-9 has been most widely adopted in integrated settings. This screener has high construct validity and has been found to be highly correlated with the gold standard measure of depression, but with the advantage of being less cumbersome (9 items vs. 21 items; Beck Depression Inventory (BDI); Beck, Ward,

Mendelson, Mock, & Erbaugh, 1961), offering an appropriate and cost-effective alternative in healthcare settings (Kung et al., 2013).

DUKE Health Profile (DUKE). The Duke Health Profile (DUKE) is a general but brief 17-item self-report measure of quality of life, specifically assessing the individual's physical, emotional, and social functioning (Parkerson, Broadhead, & Tse, 1990). The responses may be scored to capture specific constructs including perceived health, self-esteem, anxiety, depression, pain, and disability and/or summed as a general indicator of health. Patients indicate the extent to which each statement describes themselves, the frequency with which they experience the particular symptom, or the extent to which the symptom impacts their functioning.

The DUKE was derived from the Duke UNC-Health Profile (DUHP), a 63-item instrument examining a patient's physical, emotional, social functioning, as well as symptom status. The explicit goal of developing the DUKE was to provide a more concise screener appropriate for fast-paced primary care settings while maintaining the major domains of the DUHP. The DUKE takes less than 5 min to administer and is simple to score, as a template for scoring is provided at the end of the measure. Clinicians need only organize the patient's responses in the appropriate spaces on the scoring sheet to compute the previously mentioned health dimensions (Parkerson et al., 1990); however, it may be helpful to automate this aspect of the screening process as it may prove a barrier to adoption in integrated care.

A quick review of the literature suggests that the DUKE has been less frequently studied than the PHQ, with fewer citations in the literature. As such, the validity of the DUKE is less well-established, and the instrument has not yet been shown to be reliable for use in varied clinical populations as compared to the PHQ. However, the DUKE's utility in primary care settings has been established as well its comparability with other major (often lengthier) instruments empirically (Hart, Kang, Weatherby, Lee, & Brinthaupt, 2015; Parkerson et al., 1990). Notably, the DUKE was recently normed for use with international populations (Rapin et al., 2016), which offers a distinct advantage with regard to providing multiculturally competent care.

In particular, the DUKE has been shown to be an especially useful instrument in populations with known medical conditions. The DUKE has been validated as a measure of quality of life in individuals with progressive neuromuscular disorders (Baumann et al., 2011). The DUKE has been used frequently to capture quality of life in larger studies of various populations with known medical conditions or at higher risk of developing medical complications including prenatal women and new mothers, women with breast cancer, older adults, individuals with diabetes and their family members, and individuals recovering from stroke (Bonnaud-Antignac, Hardouin, Leger, Dravet, & Sebille, 2012; Kamimura et al., 2014; Perret-Guillaume et al., 2010; Tran et al., 2015; Wang, Liou, & Cheng, 2013). Therefore, the DUKE may be the screening instrument of choice for practices who serve either a more medically compromised population due to population-level stressors or a more internationally diverse catchment area.

Innovative and Less Commonly Used Instruments

While the previous measures are the most widely used and researched screeners in adult primary care, there are others that are commonly used and can also be considered. These are innovative and promising measures for use with specific populations.

General Health Questionnaire (GHQ). The General Health Questionnaire (GHQ) was originally developed by Goldberg and Hillier (1979) to be used as a screening instrument for nonpsychotic psychiatric disorders and has been since used widely to measure general psychological health (GPH) in community and nonpsychiatric clinical settings (Goldberg & Williams, 1988). The screening device was originally written as a 60-item questionnaire, and overtime it has been modified so that 30-, 28-, 20-, and 12-item versions have been created and validated to focus on specific clusters of psychological symptoms. Each item is rated on a 4-point Likert scale, from 0 to 3, ranging from "not at all" to "much more than usual."

The GHQ is included on this list in large part because of having been validated with many multicultural populations. The GHQ has been translated into 38 different languages including but not limited to Arabic, Malay, Greek, Japanese, Setswana, Italian, Iranian, and Spanish (Jackson, 2007; Garyfallos et al., 1991; Segopolo et al., 2009; El-Rufaie & Daradkeh, 1996; Fontanesi, Gobetti, Zimmerman-Tansella & Tansella, 1985; Montazeri, Vahdaninia, Ebrahimi & Jarvandi, 2003).

The 12-item version of the GHQ (Goldberg, 1992) has become a popular screening instrument to measure general psychological health in different settings and is appropriate for use in primary care due to its ease of administration and brevity (Molina, 2014; Werneke, Goldberg, Yalcin, & Üstün, 2000). This version only takes about 2 min to complete and can be scored quickly to yield an overall total score. In addition to being used as a general measure of psychological distress, factor analysis on the GHQ-12 has shown that the instrument may also be scored for more specific use to measure anxiety and depression, social dysfunction, and loss of confidence/self-esteem (Werneke et al., 2000).

Behavioral Health Questionnaire (BHQ). The Behavioral Health Questionnaire (Kopta & Lowry, 2002) is a brief instrument for assessing global mental health. The 20-item scale consists of four scales: global mental health, well-being, symptoms, and life functioning. Administration of the measure takes approximately 3 min. Each item asks how an individual has been feeling over the past 2 weeks and is rated on a 5-point Likert scale, ranging from 0 to 4 (ranging from extreme distress/poor functioning to no distress/excellent functioning). The global mental health scale is comprised of all 20 items. The well-being scale evaluates emotional distress, motivation, and life satisfaction. The symptoms scale assesses depression, anxiety, drug and alcohol abuse, and risk of harm to self and others. The life functioning scale assesses various psychosocial domains of interest including work, school, intimate relationships, nonfamily relationships, and life enjoyment.

The BHQ is distinguished by the efficiency with which it assesses mental health variables at both the general and specific levels, as well as relatively robust psychometric data. Support has been found for internal consistency, 2-week test-retest reliability, construct validity, concurrent validity, and independence of scales (Kopta & Lowry, 2002). Moreover, the BHQ has been tested and norms established with a variety of populations including a community sample of adults, undergraduate college students, and adults in outpatient psychotherapy (Kopta & Lowry, 2002). As such, the BHQ may be a particularly useful instrument for practices specializing in integrated care for younger and generally medically healthier adult populations.

Screening for Alcohol Dependence and Abuse

A recent review of the literature suggests that screening, assessment, and treatment of alcohol use disorders are viable and impactful in adult primary care (Pilowsky & Wu, 2012) given that approximately 6% of American adults meet criterion, and alcoholism is considered to be the fifth leading cause of premature death globally and attributable to 25% of premature deaths of people between the ages of 20 and 39 (Lim et al., 2012; NSDUH, 2015; World Health Organization, 2015). Simultaneously, clinicians in such settings demonstrate limited sensitivity in detecting such disorders without the use of self-report measures (Mitchell, Meader, Bird, & Rizzo, 2012).

CAGE. The CAGE is a 4-item brief screener for alcohol abuse and dependence that may be a useful addition to brief primary care batteries in settings serving potentially vulnerable populations (Ewing 1984). The CAGE is efficient and simple to score at only four items: Have you ever felt you should ***c***ut down on your drinking? Have people ***a***nnoyed you by criticizing your drinking? Have you ever felt bad or ***g***uilty about your drinking? Have you ever had a drink first thing in the morning to steady your nerves or to get rid of a hangover (***e***ye opener)? Commonly, two positive answers to any of the four questions warrant further assessment of symptoms in practice. However, research indicates that a threshold of one positive response may be of greater diagnostic utility (Aertgeerts, Buntinx, & Kester, 2004 as cited in Pilowsky & Wu, 2012). The CAGE has demonstrated adequate sensitivity and specificity in adult primary care settings, and its brevity makes it ideal for fast-paced healthcare delivery (Pilowsky & Wu, 2012). Given the relatively high prevalence of alcohol disorders, the high morbidity and mortality related to these disorders, and the potential for medical complications and or exacerbations related to alcohol use, along with the availability of a brief and psychometrically strong instrument in the CAGE, it is suggested that this screener be strongly considered for routine use in integrated primary care settings.

Summary and Future Directions

Given that screening in adult primary care is an integral piece in identifying behavioral health risks to prevent and reduce disease burden, screeners that are functional, quick, and help identify areas for intervention are critical to include in integrated care settings. Scott and Lewis (2015) discuss the importance of systematic data collection to guide long-term treatment planning, ongoing monitoring, and clinical decision-making, highlighting the critical need for screeners to accurately identify behavioral health risks prior to treatment. Vogel et al. (2014) called to attention the continued necessity of the development of better quality measures within primary care settings to capture the complexity and multidimensionality of health status and healthcare.

Future research should look to develop and validate screening tools that are both psychometrically sound and proven feasible within the primary care setting. Adequate and accurate screening tools that do not disrupt medical provider workflow are imperative in monitoring population health and determining accurate prevalence rates of common behavioral health clinical presentations within the medical setting. To this end, it would be helpful to create a standardized battery of primary care screening instruments about which data could be collected on an ongoing national basis for evaluation and revision accordingly. Given that clinical practice is outpacing academic research at a significant rate, it is critical that research on best practices become embedded in integrated care models.

Clearly it is the case that integrated models of care are the future and that the future is now. Perhaps unfortunately, the economic demands of integration have meant that clinical practice has preceded sound scientific understanding of best practices. Screening is a critical step in developing a sustainable model of integrated care such that patients who could potentially benefit from behavioral care within the setting will be rapidly and appropriately identified and addressed. By detecting and addressing behavioral health problems proactively in the context of routine medical care, rather than waiting for individuals to overcome the known barriers to treatment, the standard of healthcare in our country may be revolutionized and potentially improved for all of us, but particularly for many of the most vulnerable of us.

References

Aertgeerts, B., Buntinx, F., & Kester, A. (2004). The value of the CAGE in screening for alcohol abuse and alcohol dependence in general clinical populations: A diagnostic meta-analysis. *Journal of Clinical Epidemiology, 57*(1), 30–39.

Akincigil, A., & Matthews, E. B. (2017). National rates and patterns of depression screening in primary care: results from 2012 and 2013. *Psychiatric Services, 68*(7), 660–666.

Alschuler, K. N., Hoodin, F., & Byrd, M. R. (2009). Rapid assessment for psychopathology in a college health clinic: Utility of college student specific questions. *Journal of American College Health, 58*(2), 177–179.

Baumann, C., Erpelding, M. L., Perret-Guillaume, C., Gautier, A., Régat, S., Collin, J. F., … Briançon, S. (2011). Health-related quality of life in French adolescents and adults: Norms for the DUKE Health Profile. *BMC Public Health, 11*(1), 1–16.
Beck, A. T., Ward, C. H., Mendelson, M., Mock, J., & Erbaugh, J. (1961). An inventory for measuring depression. *Archives of General Psychiatry, 4*, 561–571.
Bonnaud-Antignac, A., Hardouin, J. B., Leger, J., Dravet, F., & Sebille, V. (2012). Quality of life and coping of women treated for breast cancer and their caregiver. What are the interactions? *Journal of Clinical Psychology in Medical Settings, 19*(3), 320–328.
Byrd, M. R., & Alschuler, K. N. (2009). Behavioral screening in adult primary care. In L. C. James & W. T. O'Donohue (Eds.), *The primary care toolkit: Practiced resources for the integrated behavioral care provider* (pp. 121–130). New York: Springer.
Centers for Disease Control and Injury Prevention (CDC). (2016). *Data & statistics fatal injury report for 2016.*
deGruy, F. (1995). Mental diagnoses in primary care: The next generation. *Archives of Family Medicine, 4*, 208–210.
El-Rufaie, O. E., & Daradkeh, T. K. (1996). Validation of the Arabic versions of the thirty-and twelve-item General Health Questionnaires in primary care patients. *The British Journal of Psychiatry, 169*(5), 662–664.
Ewing, J. A. (1984). Detecting alcoholism: the CAGE questionnaire. *JAMA, 252*(14), 1905–1907.
Fontanesi, F., Gobetti, C., Zimmermann-Tansella, C., & Tansella, M. (1985). Validity of the Italian version of the General Health Questionnaire in a general practice setting. *Psychological Medicine, 15*, 411–415.
Garyfallos, G., Karastergiou, A., Adamopoulou, A., Moutzoukis, C., Alagiozidou, E., Mala, D., & Garyfallos, A. (1991). Greek version of the General Health Questionnaire: accuracy of translation and validity. *Acta Psychiatrica Scandinavica, 84*(4), 371–378.
Goldberg, D. P., & Hillier, V. F. (1979). A scaled version of the General Health Questionnaire. *Psychological Medicine, 9*(1), 139–145.
Goldberg, D. P., & Williams, P. (1988). A User's Guide to the General Health Questionnaire: GHQ. GL assessment.
Goldberg, L. R. (1992). The development of markers for the Big-Five factor structure. *Psychological Assessment, 4*(1), 26.
Hart, P. D., Kang, M., Weatherby, N. L., Lee, Y. S., & Brinthaupt, T. M. (2015). Systematic review of health-related quality of life assessments in physical activity research. *World Journal of Preventive Medicine, 3*(2), 28–39.
Hunter, C., Goodie, J., Oordt, M., & Dobmeyer, A. (2017). Integrated behavioral health in primary care: Step-bystep guidance for assessment and intervention. In C. Hunter, J. Goodie, M. Oordt, & A. Dobmeyer (Eds.), (2nd ed.). Washington, DC: American Psychological Association.
Jackson, M. C. (2007). Systems approaches to management. Springer Science & Business Media.
Kamimura, A., Christensen, N., Myers, K., Nourian, M. M., Ashby, J., Greenwood, J. L., & Reel, J. J. (2014). Health and diabetes self-efficacy: A study of diabetic and non-diabetic free clinic patients and family members. *Journal of Community Health, 39*(4), 783–791.
Kopta, S. M., & Lowry, J. L. (2002). Psychometric evaluation of the Behavioral Health Questionnaire-20: A brief instrument for assessing global mental health and the three phases of psychotherapy outcome. *Psychotherapy Research, 12*(4), 413–426.
Kroenke, K., Spitzer, R. L., Williams, J. B., & Löwe, B. (2010). The patient health questionnaire somatic, anxiety, and depressive symptom scales: A systematic review. *General Hospital Psychiatry, 32*(4), 345–359.
Kung, S., Alarcon, R. D., Williams, M. D., Poppe, K. A., Moore, M. J., & Frye, M. A. (2013). Comparing the Beck Depression Inventory-II (BDI-II) and Patient Health Questionnaire (PHQ-9) depression measures in an integrated mood disorders practice. *Journal of Affective Disorders, 145*(3), 341–343.
Lim, S. S., Vos, T., Flaxman, A. D., Danaei, G., Shibuya, K., Adair-Rohani, H., … Memish, Z. A. (2012). A comparative risk assessment of burden of disease and injury attributable to 67 risk

factors and risk factor clusters in 21 regions, 1990–2010: A systematic analysis for the Global Burden of Disease Study 2010. *Lancet, 380*(9859), 2224–2260.
Maruish, M. E. (Ed.). (2017). *Handbook of psychological assessment in primary care settings*. Taylor & Francis.
Mitchell, A. J., Meader, N., Bird, V., & Rizzo, M. (2012). Clinical recognition and recording of alcohol disorders by clinicians in primary and secondary care: Meta-analysis. *The British Journal of Psychiatry, 201*(2), 93–100.
Molina, J.G., Rodrigo, M.F., Losilla, J.M., & Vives, J. (2014). Wording effects and the factor structure of the 12-item General Health Questionnaire. *Psychological Assessment, 26*(3):1031-7. https://doi.org/10.1037/a0036472. Epub 2014 Apr 7.
Montazeri, A., Vahdaninia, M., Ebrahimi, M., & Jarvandi, S. (2003). The Hospital Anxiety and Depression Scale (HADS): translation and validation study of the Iranian version. *Health and Quality of Life Outcomes, 1*(1), 14.
Moriarty, A. S., Gilbody, S., McMillan, D., & Manea, L. (2015). Screening and case finding for major depressive disorder using the Patient Health Questionnaire (PHQ-9): A meta-analysis. *General Hospital Psychiatry, 37*(6), 567–576.
Muntingh, A. D., De Heer, E. W., Van Marwijk, H. W., Adèr, H. J., Van Balkom, A. J., Spinhoven, P., & Van der Feltz-Cornelis, C. M. (2013). Screening high-risk patients and assisting in diagnosing anxiety in primary care: The Patient Health Questionnaire evaluated. *BMC Psychiatry, 13*(1), 192.
Olfson, M., Marcus, S. C., Druss, B., Elinson, L., Tanielian, T., & Pincus, H. A. (2002). Nataional trends in the outpatient treatment of depression. *Journal of the American Medical Association, 287*, 203–209.
Parkerson, G. R., Jr., Broadhead, W. E., & Tse, C. K. J. (1990). The Duke Health Profile: A 17-item measure of health and dysfunction. *Medical Care, 28*, 1056–1072.
Perret-Guillaume, C., Briancon, S., Guillemin, F., Wahl, D., Empereur, F., & Thi, P. N. (2010). Which generic health related quality of life questionnaire should be used in older inpatients: Comparison of the duke health profile and the MOS short-form SF-36? *The Journal of Nutrition, Health & Aging, 14*(4), 325–331.
Pilowsky, D. J., & Wu, L. T. (2012). Screening for alcohol and drug use disorders among adults in primary care: A review. *Substance Abuse and Rehabilitation, 3*(1), 25–34.
Pleis, J. R., & Lethbridge-Cejku, M. (2007). Summary health statistics for U.S. adults: National Health Interview Survey, 2006. *Vital Health Statistics. Series 10*, (235), 1–153.
Prisnie, J. C., Fiest, K. M., Coutts, S. B., Patten, S. B., Atta, C. A., Blaikie, L., … Jetté, N. (2016). Validating screening tools for depression in stroke and transient ischemic attack patients. *The International Journal of Psychiatry in Medicine, 51*(3), 262–277.
Randall, J. M., Voth, R., Burnett, E., Bazhenova, L., & Bardwell, W. A. (2013). Clinic-based depression screening in lung cancer patients using the PHQ-2 and PHQ-9 depression questionnaires: A pilot study. *Supportive Care in Cancer, 21*(5), 1503–1507.
Rapin, A., Dramé, M., Jolly, D., Novella, J., Mahmoudi, R., Toussaint-Thorin, M., & Boyer, F. C. (2016). Psychometric properties of the Duke Health Profile in a neuromuscular disease population. *European Journal of Physical and Rehabilitation Medicine, 52*(1), 57–64.
Regier, D. A., Narrow, W. E., Rae, D. S., Manderscheid, R. W., Locke, B. Z., & Goodwin, F. K. (1993). The de Facto US mental and addictive disorders service system. *Archives of General Psychiatry, 50*(2), 85. https://doi.org/10.1001/archpsyc.1993.01820140007001
Scott, K., & Lewis, C. C. (2015). Using measurement-based care to enhance any treatment. *Cognitive and Behavioral Practice, 22*(1), 49–59.
Sidebottom, A. C., Harrison, P. A., Godecker, A., & Kim, H. (2012). Validation of the Patient Health Questionnaire (PHQ)-9 for prenatal depression screening. *Archives of Women's Mental Health, 15*(5), 367–374. https://doi.org/10.1007/s00737-012-0295
Segopolo, M. T., Selemogwe, M. M., Plattner, I. E., Ketlogetswe, N., & Feinstein, A. (2009). A screening instrument for psychological distress in Botswana: validation of the Setswana ver-

sion of the 28-item General Health Questionnaire. *International Journal of Social Psychiatry, 55*(2), 149–156.

Spitzer, R. L., Kroenke, K., Williams, J. B., & Patient Health Questionnaire Primary Care Study Group. (1999). Validation and utility of a self-report version of PRIME-MD: the PHQ primary care study. *JAMA, 282*(18), 1737–1744.

Substance Abuse and Mental Health Services Administration (SAMHSA); National Survey on Drug Use and Health (NSDUH). (2015). Table 5.6B—Substance use disorder in past year among persons aged 18 or older, by Demographic Characteristics: Percentages, 2014 and 2015. Available at: https://www.samhsa.gov/data/sites/default/files/NSDUH-DetTabs-2015/NSDUH-DetTabs-2015/NSDUH-DetTabs-2015.htm#tab5-6b. Accessed 18 Jan 2017.

Tran, P. L., Blizzard, C. L., Srikanth, V., Hanh, V. T., Lien, N. T., Thang, N. H., & Gall, S. L. (2015). Health-related quality of life after stroke: Reliability and validity of the Duke Health Profile for use in Vietnam. *Quality of Life Research, 24*(11), 2807–2814.

Vogel, M. E., Malcore, S. A., Illes, R. A. C., & Kirkpatrick, H. A. (2014). Integrated primary care: Why you should care and how to get started. *Journal of Mental Health Counseling, 36*(2), 130–144.

Wald, N. (2001). The definition of screening. *Journal of Medical Screening, 8*(1), 1.

Wang, P., Liou, S. R., & Cheng, C. Y. (2013). Prediction of maternal quality of life on preterm birth and low birthweight: A longitudinal study. *BMC Pregnancy and Childbirth, 13*(1), 124.

Wang, P. S., Demler, O., Olfson, M., Pincus, H. A., Wells, K. B., & Kessler, R. C. (2006). Changing profile of service sectors used for mental health care in the U.S. *American Journal of Psychiatry, 163*(7), 1187–1198.

Wang, P. S., Lane, M., Olfson, M., Pincus, H. A., Wells, K. B., & Kessler, R. C. (2005). Twelve-month service use of mental health services in the United States. *Archives of General Psychiatry, 62*, 629–640.

Werneke, U., Goldberg, D. P., Yalcin, I., & Üstün, B. T. (2000). The stability of the factor structure of the General Health Questionnaire. *Psychological Medicine, 30*(4), 823–829.

World Health Organization (WHO). (2015). *Alcohol*. Available at: http://www.who.int/mediacentre/factsheets/fs349/en/# (link is external). Accessed 19 Sept 2016.

Young, A. S., Klap, R., Sherbourne, C. D., & Wells, K. B. (2001). The quality of care for depressive and anxiety disorders in the United States. *Archives of General Psychiatry, 58*(1), 55–61.

Chapter 6
Evidence-Based Treatments: Adapting Behavioral Medicine Change Strategies to Meet the Needs of Integrated Care with an Appreciation of Culture

Felipe González Castro, Manuel Barrera Jr, and Tara G. Bautista

Delivering Culturally Responsive Treatments in Integrated Treatment Settings

Systems Contexts for Implementing Empirically-Based Treatments

Currently many validated behavioral health treatment and prevention interventions have been developed, tested for effectiveness, and made available for dissemination and implementation within various agencies or organizational settings. The National Registry of Evidence-Based Programs and Practices (NREPP) has identified over 350 such programs that demonstrate varying levels of effectiveness in producing intended changes on targeted outcome measures. These programs have been designed to prevent or treat many behavioral health problems involving the general areas of co-occurring disorders, mental health promotion or treatment, and substance use disorder prevention or treatment (Substance Abuse and Mental Health Services Administration (SAMHSA), 2017). Despite this plethora of evidence-based programs, several systemic barriers exist that have limited the broad dissemination and implementation of these empirically-based programs.

From an ecodevelopmental systems perspective (Bronfenbrenner, 1986; Pantin, Schwartz, Sullivan, Prado, & Szapocznik, 2004; Sallis, Owen, & Fisher 2008), several systemic issues and barriers occur at *micro*-levels (the individual, families, healthcare organizations) and at *macro*-levels (communities, states, and the nation)

F. G. Castro (✉) · T. G. Bautista
College of Nursing and Health Innovation, Arizona State University, Phoenix, AZ, USA
e-mail: Felipe.Castro@asu.edu; Tara.Bautista@asu.edu

M. Barrera Jr
Department of Psychology, Arizona State University, Tempe, AZ, USA
e-mail: Manuel.Barrera@asu.edu

M. P. Duckworth, W. T. O'Donohue (eds.), *Behavioral Medicine and Integrated Care*,
https://doi.org/10.1007/978-3-319-93003-9_6

that impede the optimal implementation and the sustainability of otherwise efficacious prevention and treatment interventions (Castro et al., 2017).

This chapter presents an ecodevelopmental systems perspective for examining these barriers and their influences to help strategize and plan the cultural adaptation of an original empirically-based program, as this may counter or eliminate these barriers, while also increasing treatment relevance, engagement, fit, and effectiveness for residents from a local community.

Goal of Wide Dissemination and Implementation of Validated Treatments

In the recent past, two large fields of research and practice, *prevention* and *treatment*, have produced empirically-based and validated programs for reducing or eliminating major health, mental health, and drug abuse problems. Within these programs the capacity to produce significant changes on targeted outcome measures, that is, program *efficacy* or *effectiveness*, has been established based on empirical evidence obtained from randomized controlled trials (RCTs). Within the field of prevention research, these organized programs are described as *evidence-based interventions* (EBIs) (Castro, Barrera, & Holleran-Steiker, 2010). Similarly, in the treatment field, these programs are described as *empirically validated therapies* (EVTs) (Carroll et al., 2011). In this chapter, we will refer to each of these types of programs as *empirically-based treatments* (EBTs).

As noted, within the fields of prevention and treatment, a contemporary service delivery strategy has been that these tested-and-effective EBTs should be widely disseminated and their treatment protocol implemented with high fidelity (Carroll et al., 2011; Flay et al., 2005; Norcross, Beutler, & Levant, 2006; Spoth et al., 2013). Nonetheless, this broad dissemination and implementation with fidelity has not been fully realized (Carroll et al., 2011).

In the past, one challenge to this strategy of wide dissemination and fidelity in implementation is that many treatment providers felt constrained by an overly prescriptive, restrictive, or culturally insensitive manualized treatment protocol. These manualized treatment protocols were criticized for being unresponsive to the needs of certain groups of participants, including patients with comorbidities and for many racial/ethnic minority clients (Norcross, Beutler, & Levant, 2006; Sue & Zane, 2006). This dissatisfaction also prompted some service providers to introduce local *cultural adaptations* (Castro, Barrera, & Martinez, 2004), that is, changes in the treatment protocol to accommodate the needs and preferences of certain clients or patients for whom the manualized treatment was ineffective in addressing their needs and preferences. However, these adaptive changes were also regarded by some treatment developers as inappropriate, as such changes were believed to erode the intervention's established effectiveness (Elliott & Mihalic, 2004).

Abiding Challenges in the Application of Empirically-Based Treatments

Issues of engagement and retention In the areas of drug abuse prevention and treatment, several challenges persist involving low rates of client *engagement* and *retention* in these programs (Carroll et al., 2011). One approach to increase treatment engagement and retention among youth and families has been to reduce the total number of program sessions, e.g., from 12 to 8 sessions. However, such reductions may diminish EBT efficacy based on lower client exposures and/or less acquisition of essential treatment-related knowledge and skills (Kumpfer, Alvarado, Smith, & Bellamy, 2002; Kumpfer, Pinyuchon, de Melo, & Whiteside, 2008).

The Fidelity-Adaptation Dilemma

If a treatment lacks genuine *relevance* and *appeal* for certain clients, i.e., low *acceptability*, despite its efficacy, and if these clients discontinue the treatment, this undesirable outcome will fail to produce treatment-related benefits. This problem of limited treatment relevance and low client engagement contributed to the emergence of the *fidelity-adaptation dilemma*. This dilemma has been a prominent issue in the field of prevention science for almost two decades (US Department of Health and Human Services (DHHS), 2016). This dilemma has also emerged within the drug treatment field. Within the past two decades and after much debate and analysis, this Fidelity-Adaptation Dilemma has been and reframed. The contemporary view is that fidelity and adaptation are both important imperatives. In this reframed view, a preferred approach in intervention design is to maintain fidelity to core intervention goals, while also affording implementers the flexibility to make informed adaptations that promote community engagement and cultural responsiveness to the needs and preferences of various local consumer groups (Castro & Yasui, 2017).

About fidelity and adaptation *Fidelity* refers to the extent to which a treatment protocol is delivered as originally developed and prescribed by the creators of that treatment. Fidelity generally consists of implementation of a treatment protocol in close adherence to the manualized procedures, given that this protocol has been validated and shown to attain targeted outcomes as assessed within one or more randomized controlled trials (Flay et al., 2005; Hansen, 2014). By contrast, the *adaptation* of a model treatment protocol refers to modifications in one or more treatment components or activities to increase treatment *relevance*, client *engagement*, and perhaps *effectiveness* for a specific subcultural group of clients (Castro et al., 2004). Such modifications often focus on one or more of three major aspects of treatment: (a) informational content, (b) program activities, and (c) forms of delivery. Ideally, such adaptations will increase client engagement and the magnitude of treatment effects, i.e., *effect size*, thus ideally increasing treatment effectiveness.

Client segmentation using a more relevant unit of analysis A related issue is whether a validated EBT is *universal*, meaning that it would be efficacious across many populations and environments, or whether its effects are specific to a certain population or treatment site. Variations in an EBT's true efficacy across a diversity of clients and situations raise the need to identify sectors of the population that are so "culturally different," that they will not respond well to that EBT. This issue also prompts the need to accurately identify *subcultural groups* for which an original EBT may need to be adapted (Barrera, Castro, & Holleran-Steiker, 2011; Castro et al., 2010). This approach requires greater specificity when defining these subcultural groups, moving beyond a broad cultural concept, such as examining an EBT's efficacy among "all Latinos."

In accord with the field of social marketing, this more specific approach involves *audience segmentation* (Storey, Saffitz, & Rimon, 2008). This segmentation approach identifies more homogeneous subgroups of "consumers," those who share common beliefs, behaviors, and lifestyles. For example, some subcultural groups share a "drug culture" that involves "shared values, beliefs, customs, and traditions that evolve from substance use (Substance Abuse and Mental Health Services Administration (SAMHSA), 2014, p. 38). This more *micro-level* approach advances beyond an "ethnic gloss" (Trimble, 1995) that occurs under a more *macro-level* of analysis, e.g., focusing on an entire nation or ethnic group, where doing so "glosses over" important within-country or within-group differences. A major challenge in the adaptation of an original EBT involves reliably identifying specific subcultural groups that share common cultural characteristics and cognitive schemas, thus having similar treatment-related needs and preferences.

As a related issue, some studies have conducted post-hoc analyses with a subgroup of individuals who participated in a randomized controlled trial (RCT). Often, such subgroups have been defined by "race" or "ethnicity," to examine comparative EBT effectiveness, such as for a subgroup of Latinos enrolled in that RTC. This approach has generated limited evidence on the *comparative effectiveness* of EBT efficacy (Supplee, Kelly, MacKinnon, & Barofsky, 2013), among that sector of the study sample. Also, these analyses consist of smaller-sized samples, thus attenuating the power to detect the intervention effect and thus limiting the utility of these analyses.

Beyond this limitation, conceptually and methodologically, within the increasing diversification occurring within the USA, the use of a coarse indicator variable such as "race" or "ethnicity," to detect genuine "cultural differences," is becoming increasingly ineffective. For example, controlling for age, gender, and other person variables, a "high-acculturated Mexican heritage Latino," that is, an individual greatly engaged culturally in the "mainstream American culture," will differ considerably in lifestyle and treatment-related needs from a "low-acculturated Mexican heritage Latino," who is an individual with little engagement in the "mainstream American culture." In this case, being classified as a generic "Latino" does not operate as a critical indicator that accurately captures treatment-related cultural differences. By contrast, the variable of "acculturation status," which identifies distinct subgroups of Latinos, provides a more reliable variable for a more accurate assessment of existing cultural variation. Also, in the past, RCTs have not been explicitly conceptualized and designed to adequately sample culturally distinct subcultural groups in sufficient-sized samples to allow adequately powered tests of treatment effectiveness when conducting *comparative effectiveness analyses*.

By contrast, one recent example of a RCT designed to conduct such cultural comparisons, utilized a small well-specified sample (Supplee et al., 2013). This small RTC examined the efficacy of a behavioral activation treatment for depression (BATD) in Latinos with Spanish-speaking preference (LSSP) (Collado, Calderon, MacPherson, & Lejuez, 2016). Language preference was used as a proxy variable for "low-acculturation status." For a sample of 46 participants, when compared with supportive counseling (SC) ($n = 23$), the behavioral activation treatment for depression (BATD) ($n = 23$) was efficacious as measured by reduced symptoms of depression, increased activity levels, and higher reported environmental rewards. This study had several imitations, including a small sample size, although it provided a viable test of the BATD treatment as examined for a well-specified subcultural group of Latinos and Latinas of low-acculturation status.

Integrated Care: Toward Reducing Health Disparities in Vulnerable Populations

Within the emerging context of *integrated care*, the need exists for policy makers, treatment providers, and other professionals, to ensure high quality in service delivery to maximize the attainment of successful treatment outcomes (Rutkowski, Rawson, & Freese, 2012). In the past, the delivery of behavioral health services has been bifurcated into treatment settings that offered substance use treatment and those that offered mental health treatment. Integrative care aims to provide both substance use treatment and mental health treatment services within a single location, and as delivered by a collaborative team of health professionals.

To understand the complex interaction of biological, psychological, and sociocultural determinants of complex health conditions, a systems approach is necessary to more fully conceptualize this process as it affects the health and well-being of individuals, especially among those affected by co-occurring health problems. This systems approach is more comprehensive, offering a more complete guide for examining the integration of mental health and substance use services as delivered within a primary care setting (Collins, Hewson, Munger, & Wade, 2010).

Integrative care to improve access One approach to assessment in integrative care has described as: *screening*, *brief intervention*, and *referral to treatment* (SBIRT), which is conducted by concurrently treating substance use disorders and mental health disorders within a single primary care setting. A perspective in this approach is that integrated SPIRT services are feasible, can reach many more individuals who need treatment, promise better outcomes for patients, and can result in lower healthcare utilization costs (Rutkowski et al., 2012).

Racial/ethnic minority populations are affected by many types of health disparities and greatly need access to effective health services, although they often have limited access to these services (Agency for Healthcare Research and Quality (AHRQ), 2012). This limited access further contributes to existing low rates of service utilization. Such limited access further perpetuates existing health disparities and inequities. Furthermore, some of the worst health outcomes among racial/ethnic minority populations involve comorbidities, the presence of coexisting disorders such as a somatic health problem co-occurring a mental disorder. The National Institute of Mental Health (NIMH) (2006) reports that individuals with severe mental illness (SMI) die prematurely with a loss of 11–32 years of life when affected by a preventable and treatable health condition such as cardiovascular heart disease and type 2 diabetes that is also compounded by a mental disorder such as depression.

Cultural factors in integrated care Some racial/ethnic minority patients are sensitive to the stigma involved in seeking mental healthcare services (Snowden, 2001), as contrasted with seeking these services from a primary care physician. Thus, integrating mental health services within a primary care setting may provide a more comfortable venue that diminishes this stigma, while also providing greater access for the treatment of mental and substance use disorders.

Prior studies of stigma among Latinos have described this discomfort (Corrigan, Kuwabara, & O'Shaughnessy, 2009). Recent data from the National Epidemiologic Survey on Alcohol and Related Conditions (NES-ARC) reveals subcultural group differences within the Latino population, in their patterns of health service utilization, when examined by certain subcultural groups: (a) immigrants (typically low-acculturated) Latinos, (b) bilingual-bicultural Latinos, and (c) high-acculturated (primarily English-speaking) Latinos.

An epidemiological study conducted by Keys and collaborators (2012) revealed that "cultural factors such as ethnic identity and language/social preferences are potentially important drivers of mental healthcare among Latinos in the U.S." (Keys et al., 2012, p. 392). Among several findings these investigators also report that: (a) respondents with a stronger Spanish-language identity and Latino social preferences were less likely to utilize mental health services even after controlling for factors associated with service utilization such as insurance, income, and symptom severity and (b) Spanish-dominant (low-acculturation) patients exhibited a preference for seeing Spanish-speaking healthcare providers and that this preference was associated with lower health service utilization when these providers are not available (Keys et al., 2012). These investigators also asserted that "… continued disparities among Latinos with varying degrees of language/social preferences and ethnic identity signal the need for public health initiatives to expand access and culturally competent care for a broad range of psychiatric disorders" (Keys et al., 2012, p. 392).

Efficacy of behavioral interventions in integrated care settings The need for integrative care services is especially acute for patient populations affected by the co-occurrence of somatic disease and psychological disorders such as depression.

Such *comorbidities* are associated with a poorer quality of life, greater disability, poor disease outcomes, and higher mortality (Lemmens, Molema, Versnel, Baan, & de Bruin, 2015). Based on a *chronic disease conceptual model*, integrated care programs have been defined as those having two or more of the following components: (a) a healthcare system as a venue for the delivery of integrative services, (b) community resources that support the delivery of integrative services, (c) support for client self-management, (d) a delivery systems design that fosters the delivery of effective care, (e) decision support that includes empirically-based guidelines and technical support from experts, and (f) a clinical information system for information sharing and client reminders (Lemmens et al., 2015).

In a systematic review and meta-analysis of programs that provide *integrated care programs* when compared with *usual care programs*, integrated care was shown to be more effective in treating depression (Lemmens et al., 2015). In these comparisons, integrated care showed moderate effectiveness for the outcomes of patient satisfaction and cost-effectiveness. By contrast, there was insufficient evidence regarding the effectiveness of integrating care: (a) in the management of glycosylated hemoglobin (HbA1c) among diabetic patients, (b) in health-related quality of life, (c) in reducing mortality, and (d) in promoting adherence to prescribed medical care. However, these comparisons of integrated care programs versus usual care programs were limited by program heterogeneity across sites and by heterogeneity among the patient who attended these programs. Despite these limitations, this systematic review and meta-analysis showed that when compared with usual care, integrative care is effective on selected patient outcomes (Lemmens et al., 2015). It should be noted that this meta-analysis did not examine minority status used as a moderator variable, so this study did not examine the differential effects of integrated care for minority patients relative to White nonminority patients.

From another research and clinical perspective, to the extent that "treatment as usual" (TAU) within an integrated care setting does not address salient cultural factors for local subcultural groups, treatment limitations observed with these groups would suggest the need for modifying the current TAU. As related to Latino populations, major considerations for improving TAU include (a) recognizing the importance of language, cultural values, cultural beliefs, and barriers to healthcare access; (b) supporting public health initiatives that facilitate access to care and to culturally competent health services for a psychiatric disorders; and (c) examining the influences of contextual community factors to increase the relevance of TAU and thus to increase service utilization and quality of care for these patients (Keys et al., 2012).

A Conceptual Model to Guide Integrative Care

A four-phase model Aarons and collaborators developed a conceptual model of conditions and factors that influence the implementation of empirically-based practices within public service delivery agencies. This model consists of four sequential adaptation phases that range from initiation to the maintenance of service delivery. These implementation phases are (a) exploration, (b) adoption decisions and preparation, (c) active implementation, and (d) sustainment. Within each of these four phases, implementation is influenced by several factors that occur within each of two contexts: (a) *outer contexts*, which refers to the service environment, the inter-organization environment, and consumer support and advocacy, and (b) *inner contexts*, which refers to intraorganization characteristics and individual adaptor characteristics, such as the personal characteristics of the agency's principal administrator (Aarons, Hurlburt, & Horowitz, 2011).

This complex model has been used as a guiding framework for understanding the combination of macro-level factors (outer contexts) and micro-level factors (inner contexts) that facilitate or impede the delivery of empirically-based programs or interventions. As one example, *funding* is a major factor that exerts multiple systemic influences across phases of delivery and across contexts. The analysis of funding across phases from start-up to sustainability shows that when missing or insufficient, inadequate funding can impede the delivery of EBTs in as delivered within healthcare settings. Furthermore, when funding is available yet inflexible in adjusting to emergent organizational needs, such funding also constitutes a barrier to integrative service delivery. Similarly, across phases, *organizational characteristics* and *leadership* also emerge as core organizational factors that if weak will impede the efficacious delivery of EBTs.

An index of integrative care service delivery Within this context, an instrument has been developed to reliably assess an agency's capacity to deliver integrated health services, the Dual Diagnosis Capability in Health Care Settings (DDCHCS). This index was developed to assess the degree of integration of behavioral health, mental health, and substance use services, when delivered within conventional medical care settings. The DDCHCS assesses seven core components: (a) *program structure* (e.g., an organizational identity as it would favor integration and financial reimbursement mechanism), (b) *program milieu* (e.g., materials that address behavioral health), (c) *assessment* (e.g., integrated medical and behavioral care assessment), (d) *treatment* (e.g., having an integrated treatment plan), (e) *continuity of care* (e.g., integrated discharge planning), (f) *staffing* (e.g., on-site staff with mental health and addiction credentials), and (g) *training* (e.g., offering training regarding co-occurring disorders) (McGovern, Urada, Lambert-Harris, Sullivan, & Mazade, 2012). This instrument has effectively distinguished between clinics that offer singular care as usual, dual diagnosis capable (DDC) agencies, and dual diagnosis enhanced (DDE) agencies.

"Outer contexts" in integrative care In a study of the levels of integrative care in the provision of substance abuse and mental health services when delivered by primary care organizations in Kern County, California, *Project Care* assessed seven core components of integrative healthcare services (Padwa et al., 2016). These seven factors are: (a) on-site mental health and substance use screens for primary care patients, (b) on-site brief intervention and treatment services for patients with mild to moderate disorders, (c) referrals to specialty mental health and substance use services, (d) regular case management meetings, (e) use of electronic health records, (f) provider training regarding integrated care, and (g) reimbursement for behavioral health services delivered on the same day.

This 3-year study showed that the *Project Care* intervention was effective in increasing the level of integrative care services provided within three primary care organizations (Padwa et al., 2016). These three organizations increased their level of integrative care across a 3-year period from a "partially integrated" (PI) level toward a "fully integrated" (FI) level. This organizational-level study showed how select primary care organizations can improve their level of integrative care services by incorporating behavioral health services that include select substance abuse treatments. This study, however, did not assess health outcomes such as general health outcomes, patient satisfaction, or treatment costs for their patients. This study did highlight the importance of internal and external contextual factors, such as sufficient and flexible funding, in the delivery of integrative care. Sufficient funding along with positive staff attitudes toward the delivery of integrative care services emerged as important factors that contribute to the viability and sustainability of integrative services as provided within primary care settings.

Geographic factors and integrative care Historically, access to integrated care services has been limited within communities that contain large clusters of racial/ethnic minority residents (Guerrero & Kao, 2013). This geographically based discrepancy constitutes a barrier to the reduction of health disparities and health inequities for racial/ethnic minority and in low-income patients. Furthermore, many of these minority and low-income community residents are affected by co-occurring disorders. This co-occurrence increases problem severity and makes recovery much more difficult. This noted *geographic disparity* is a naturally occurring ecological factor that limits access to integrated mental health and substance use treatments, limiting the availability of efficacious treatments for these co-occurring disorders and perpetuating existing health disparities and inequities among certain low-income Latino patients (Guerrero & Kao, 2013).

Intervention-Related Factors in Adaptation

In principle, an EBT's activities and procedures that constitute the treatment's "core components" are based on one or more applicable theories that explain the EBT's mechanisms of effect (Rohrbach, 2014). These core components are regarded as the "active ingredients" that produce desired therapeutic outcomes. For example, a treatment that utilizes principles from social cognitive theory (Bandura, 1986) and cognitive-behavioral procedures, e.g., *contingency management*, will typically produce expected changes in human behavior, so long as this contingency is established and maintained. Although contingency management is a well-established behavior therapy technique that works well across many situations and cultural settings, differences among clients in their level of education and understanding or acceptance of specific types of contingencies can impede the implementation of this established technique. In this case, a cultural challenge involves conceptualizing how best to adapt an original EBT, to create an adapted EBT that is acceptable and engaging for individuals from an identified subcultural group of "new consumers," so that they participate actively in that adapted treatment, which also retains fidelity to the original EBT's core components.

Castro et al. (2004) outlined three major domains of EBT adaptation: (a) *cognitive information processing*, modifying the original EBT's informational characteristics to accommodate a subcultural group's language or literacy levels; (b) *affective-motivational* characteristics, modifying the original EBT to address gender, racial/ethnic identity, cultural background, religious background, socioeconomic status, and other sociocultural factors to facilitate participation in EBT activities; and (c) *environmental* characteristics, considering aspects of EBT fit when "grounded" within the institutional or ecological contexts of the local community in which the EBT is being delivered. Conceptually, the viability of developing a treatment that is well adapted for a particular setting and for a specific subcultural group of patients depends establishing a good "match" between treatment features and setting characteristics. Conversely, setting-treatment "mismatches" will likely render that treatment ineffective within that setting and/or with the identified subcultural group.

Cognitive-informational adaptation This form of treatment adaptation involves changing the program informational contents or activities which a client or patient is unable to understand or comprehend (Castro et al., 2004). Language adaptation, such as translating an EBT's curriculum from English to Spanish is the most fundamental form of cultural adaptation. A linguistic translation aims for equivalence in meaning (conceptual equivalence) and not a literal "word-for-word" translation (Geisinger, 1994; Gonzalez, Stewart, Ritter, & Lorig, 1995). Such a translation should also consider the literacy level of individuals from the identified subcultural group. Similarly, scientific or complex constructs/concepts may require a reframing to help "consumers" from a specific subcultural group to comprehend that cultural concept, particularly if it is a core factor within that EBT.

Affective-motivational adaptation This type of adaptation consists of modifications of program content or activities that can induce *cultural conflict* or that can *prompt reactance* (behavioral resistance) among individuals from the local community. As one example, a Westernized cultural approach that encourages male clients to publicly disclose their drug dependence or to discuss sexual issues in the presence of certain family members may be contraindicated within subcultural groups. This practice can be perceived as culturally inappropriate by traditional males from that subcultural group, if they feel stigmatized and resist participation, likely also dropping out of treatment. Thus, a review of these aspects of a treatment by a local Cultural Advisory Committee could reveal the need for a cultural adaptation. Recommendations from this Cultural Advisory Committee can aid in making best adaptation decisions, to resolve cultural conflicts, coupled with efforts to maintain fidelity to the scientific principles that drive the efficacy of that EBT (van der Kreeft, Jongbloet, & Van Havere, 2014).

Environmental adaptation This form of adaptation involves making ecological changes in a client's family system, in the client's home neighborhood, or within the treatment setting, to modify local environmental contexts as this can facilitate the client's recovery. Within this domain, two basic forms of adaptation consist of: (a) modifying *program contents* that conflict with the community environment and (b) modifying the *form of program delivery*. Modification of content would include *surface structure* or *deep-structure changes* in that content (Resnicow, Soler, Braithwait, Ahluwalia, & Butler, 2000). Changes in form of delivery can involve presenting the same treatment content, with changes in (a) the *characteristics of delivery personnel*, e.g., the use of lay health workers rather than health educators; (b) the *channel of delivery*, Internet delivery rather than a group session; or (c) the *location of delivery,* improving access by delivering the program within a church setting, rather than within an integrative treatment center.

Cultural Considerations in Diverse Communities in the USA

Concepts of Culture: Theory and Application

The world is very diverse place. Worldwide, large variations exist on several social and cultural factors that include language, literacy, religious and cultural belief systems, sociocultural attitudes, cultural and familial values, and social and cultural norms. Worldwide there also exists a dynamic tension between sociocultural forces that promote *modernization* and quests for change versus *traditionalism* and quests for the preservation of established beliefs, traditions, practices, and a resistance to change (Shiraev & Levy, 2010). Factors that promote *modernism*, such as international globalization, emphasize growth and standardization in currencies, consumer products, and in other factors toward homogenizing cultural practices across diverse settings. By contrast, factors that promote *traditionalism* (Ramirez, 1999) tend to diversify whole populations into distinct *subcultural groups*, by emphasizing the retention of unique subcultural identities, tribal traditions, and traditional lifeways. These broad cultural influences introduce a systemic context against which to consider the cultural adaptation of empirically-based treatments (EBTs).

Absence of cultural factors in principles of drug treatment In 1999, the National Institute on Drug Abuse published *NIDA's 13 Principles of Drug Addiction Treatment* (National Institute on Drug Abuse (NIDA), 1999). These principles are:

(a) No single treatment is appropriate for all individuals.
(b) Treatment needs to be readily available, since delays in treatment availability often result in a loss of clients.

(c) Effective treatment attends to multiple needs, not just to drug use, and this includes attention to medical, psychological, social, vocational, legal, other needs.
(d) A continuous assessment and modification of a client's treatment plan is necessary to monitor and respond to changing needs,
(e) Remaining in treatment for an adequate period of time is crucial to treatment success –typically clients should remain in treatment for at least 3 months.
(f) Counseling and behavioral therapies are crucial components of treatment, as they address treatment motivation, skill building, and problem solving.
(g) Medications are important components of treatment as these can reduce cravings, and this includes psychotropic medications for clients who need these.
(h) Integrated treatment is needed for clients with psychiatric comorbidity.
(i) Medical detox is an important first step in treatment.
(j) Treatment need not be voluntary to be effective, whereby engagement in compulsory treatment is facilitated by specific sanctions (NIDA, 1999).

It is noteworthy that at that time, none of these 13 principles directly addressed issues of "culture" in the treatment of drug-dependent clients (Castro, Nichols, & Kater, 2007). A few years earlier, the need for sensitivity to cultural and ethnic factors emerged as an important consideration for providing culturally relevant drug abuse treatments to racial/ethnic minority clients (Ja & Aoki, 1993; Terrell, 1993). Important issues for ethnic minority clients included: (a) assessing the client's immigration and acculturation experiences including *cultural stress* (Cervantes, Cardoso, & Goldbach, 2015), as factors that can erode the protective effects of a client's traditional or native culture; (b) assessing a client's experiences with *discrimination*; and (c) developing *culturally responsive* treatment interventions (Terrell, 1993). In contemporary treatments, aspects of race, ethnicity, gender, sexual orientation, and other *cultural factors* are now considered important for the delivery of a more comprehensive treatment among diverse drug-dependent clients (Castro & Hernandez-Alarcon, 2002; Castro et al., 2007).

Within Latino cultures, important cultural constructs that can be considered as cultural factors include:

(a) *Acculturation*, when defined at the individual level refers to a process of cultural change in values, beliefs, and behaviors
(b) *Ethnic pride*, positive feelings toward one's ethnic group
(c) *Familism*, a strong family orientation and family bonding
(d) *Personalismo*, a preference for personal attention in interpersonal relationships
(e) *Respeto*, the value of respect toward others with attention to the other person's social position
(f) *Simpatía*, a deferential posture toward others in efforts to avoid conflicts and to maintain harmony in interpersonal relations
(g) *Traditionalism*, a preference for old-fashioned lifeways, including conservative values and traditional beliefs about the correct way to live one's life (Castro et al., 2017)

A consideration of cultural factors is relevant to the core informational content that is presented to individuals from various racial/ethnic subcultural groups and can be important for the active engagement and retention of these patients.

From the NIDA Clinical Trials Network (Carroll et al., 2011), lessons learned from 10 years of research have yielded the following important conclusions: (a) retention remains a major problem in substance abuse treatment whereby treatment retention is critical to treatment success; (b) EBTs are not broadly implemented in practice, and when implemented they are often delivered with low fidelity; and (c) at the agency level, effort, support, and commitment are essential factors for adopting and sustaining an EBT given the costs of implementation, staff training, and supervision (Carroll et al., 2011). Cultural factors can include a local community's cultural environment, e.g., a community enclave, that offers recent immigrants cultural resources and social support (Portes & Rumbaut, 2014).

Cultural Awareness and Competency Among Healthcare Providers

The emergence of *cultural competence* in the 1990s as a core competency required of health professionals (Orlandi, Weston, & Epstein, 1992; Substance Abuse and Mental Health Services Administration (SAMHSA), 2014) emphasized the acquisition of progressive levels of cultural sensitivity, competence, and proficiency as skills for greater responsiveness to cultural issues in service delivery among people of color. Within the contemporary integrated care environment, cultural competence remains important. This includes competencies in the analysis of systemic factors that influence access and quality of care for diverse clients and patients and particularly those from vulnerable populations.

For various health providers, training in these cultural competences is important. This includes higher ranking health providers such as psychiatrists. Such training involves developing the requisite knowledge, attitudes, and skills for understanding the role of integrated care within complex healthcare systems. Such professional competencies as related to integrated care include: (a) understanding and working with the organizational dynamics of complex healthcare systems, (b) assuming various leadership roles for working collaboratively within complex healthcare systems, and (c) providing mentorship to other providers to improve quality of care (Sunderji, Waddell, Gupta, Sokaridis, & Steinberg, 2016).

Today integration in the delivery of healthcare services includes the integration of heretofore disconnected types of healthcare services, such as substance use treatment services and mental health services. Unfortunately, in the past such integrated care was lacking, especially for low-income, aging, uninsured, rural, and racial/ethnic minority clients. The delivery of truly integrated healthcare services remains as an important step toward reducing health disparities and inequities in behavioral healthcare (Davis et al., 2015).

As noted, providing culturally relevant services to people of color is facilitated by the *cultural competence* of service delivery personnel. This includes their ability to adapt evidence informed and best practices to make them more relevant for patients of color. Such adaptations can enhance client-therapist engagement and promote greater sensitivity to a minority client's cultural issues (Davis et al., 2015).

Regarding core competencies for practicing integrated care, a recent mixed methods study identified specific knowledge and skills that constitute important competencies for psychiatrists working in integrated care settings. The relevance and applicability of such competencies was related to the seniority of the psychiatrist (a senior psychiatrist versus a resident in training) and varied in its relevance to the psychiatrist's professional roles. Among several identified competencies and activities important for psychiatrists who work in integrated care settings, these competencies include: (a) understanding community contexts and patient problems within a systemic community context; (b) assisting patients in navigating the mental healthcare system; (c) forming working relationships with other providers; (d) navigating the dual roles of expert/leader and equal team member; (e) knowledge of team dynamics; (f) tolerating ambiguity, uncertainty, and complexity; and (g) tailoring patient education to the audience's existing knowledge and expertise (Sunderji et al., 2016). It is noteworthy that beyond a relevance to psychiatry, many of these skills are also relevant for providers from other professions including social work, nursing, public health, and clinical psychology.

Cultural Considerations in Delivering Empirically-Based Treatments

Culture and its related constructs such as *acculturation* are factorially complex constructs (Lopez-Class, Castro, & Ramirez, 2011; Schwartz et al., 2010). From a psychological perspective, culture consists of a *human schema*, an "explanatory model," or a "world view," which consists of symbols, attitudes, behaviors, values, and norms that are transmitted across generations. This explanatory model aids in interpreting the world and in promoting survival and well-being (Lehman, Chiu, & Schaller, 2004; Shiraev & Levy, 2010). Persons who relocate to a new cultural environment, whether between nations or within a nation, often face the challenges of acculturation and assimilation when adapting to that new cultural environment (Berry, 1980, 2005). *Acculturation* refers to a "sociocultural process in which members of one cultural group adopt the beliefs and behaviors of another group" (Lopez-Class et al., 2011, p. 1556). *Assimilation* refers to an individual's or a group's integration into a new host society as one outcome of the process of acculturation (Portes & Zhou, 1993).

One challenge in the delivery of behavioral health treatments involves implementing a scientific empirically-based treatment in a manner that will "make sense" to a client or patient. This is especially challenging in treatment delivery with persons from low-literacy and indigenous subcultures, e.g., Hmong patients, who culturally are significantly different from the White American mainstream culture in their use of language and literacy, schemas of health and illness beliefs, and their family contexts (Meschke, & Jaung, 2014). Establishing rapport with such clients is more challenging, as is communicating Westernized treatment-related information and skills and engaging them in a manner that inspires their confidence in the provider, inspires sustained treatment participation, and provides hope for recovery. Conversely, if a treatment as implemented fails to promote positive expectations for improvement, then the client may not engage in that treatment. Thus, a strategic adaptation that aids in engaging such clients would be needed (Bernal, Jimenez-Chafey, & Domenich-Rodriguez, 2009; Kumpfer et al., 2002).

Approaches to Treatment Adaptation and Relevance to Diverse Clients

Steps in the Cultural Adaptation of an Empirically-Based Treatment

The formal adaptation of an original empirically-based treatment (EBT) can be conducted under a basic five-step process (Barrera, Castro, Strycker, & Toobert, 2013). Ideally, this five-step process can include a formal randomized controlled trial, although in many treatment settings, conducting step 5 is not viable for various practical reasons. In the absence of that option, four of these five stages can be conducted using a community-based participatory research (CBPR) approach, as overseen by a well-informed Cultural Advisory Committee (CAC) (Minkler, Wallerstein, & Wilson, 2008). This would involve input from *key informants* and *stakeholders* and a review of consumer feedback, to conduct culturally sensitive and scientifically informed decisions for developing a viable cultural adaptation. The CBPR approach consists of a bidirectional process involving a collective dialogue (Donovan et al., 2011) to attain well-reasoned and planned group decisions for making best adaptations to an original EBT protocol. Based in this framework and process, these five steps are the following:

Step 1 – Information Gathering The first step is "information gathering," which involves reviewing the research literature to identify evidence of subcultural group differences in: (a) risk and protective factors, (b) intervention engagement, and (c) outcomes. Subcultural group differences suggest the need for cultural adaptation to identify the risk/protective factors that can be incorporated into modifications to an original EBT. In addition, a mixed methods methodology can be used to gather formative qualitative and quantitative data using focus groups, key informant, and/or stakeholder interviews. This formative information can include an assessment of subcultural group members' views of the original EBT's cultural fit. For adaptations designed specifically for integrated care, it would be critical to gather information from caregivers who work in the identified treatment settings. This step would include an initial assessment of whether there is a need to conduct a cultural adaptation. This can involve a review and analysis of relevant drug treatment literature as background to identify implementation problems and sources of client-treatment mismatches (Castro et al., 2004), as linked to three major domains of cultural adaptation assessment: (a) participant characteristics, (b) program delivery staff, and (c) administrative/community factors (see Castro et al., 2004).

Step 2 – Preliminary Adaptation Design When there exists sufficient justification for conducting a cultural adaptation of an original EBT, the second step, "preliminary adaptation design," involves the development of proposed modifications in the original EBT. This step would include the analysis, assessment, and integration of recommendations provided by a Cultural Adaptation Committee that can be staffed by: (a) stakeholders, (b) community experts, (c) providers from the integrated care settings, (d) developers of the EBT, and (e) former clients/patients or representatives who participated previously in the treatment (i.e., treatment insiders). Step 2 can also be conducted as a treatment quality assessment and for ongoing EBT refinement and needed modification, even if the decision is made not to conduct a cultural adaptation. In principle, core intervention components would be preserved, unless convincing evidence accrues that the intervention protocol contains one or more of these core components that are detrimental to the well-being of clients from one or more identified subcultural groups.

Step 3 – Preliminary Adaptation Tests This step examines whether adapted EBT will "work as intended." This serves as another occasion for gathering qualitative and quantitative quality control data to assess: (a) implementation problems, (b) difficulties with program content or activities, (c) client satisfaction with treatment elements, and (d) client suggestions for improvements. Accordingly, the design and pilot testing of this preliminary adapted version of the original EBT can consist of: (a) the elimination of prior implementation difficulties, (b) the emergence of problems with content or activities, (c) client satisfaction with treatment elements, and (d) suggestions for improvement.

Step 4 – Adaptation Refinement Step 4 is "adaptation refinement." Evaluative feedback from this pilot testing can inform the need for additional modifications to the adapted EBT, which can subsequently be tested in a full "cultural adaptation trial" (in Step 5).

Step 5 – A Formal Cultural Adaptation Trial A final goal is to formally assess the efficacy of this adapted EBT in a randomly controlled field trial that compares the *adapted EBT* to a treatment as usual (TAU) control group or to the *original EBT* (Castro et al., 2017). This adapted EBT's effectiveness can be assessed as it would change targeted psychological and health outcome variables, while also assessing indicators of EBT *engagement* (e.g., client involvement, client attendance, treatment completion).

Although seldom evaluated within the cultural adaptation trial stage, intervention evaluators or research investigators can assess the effects of the adapted EBT on specified mediators and moderators (MacKinnon, 2008). An example is if a culturally adapted EBT involves the addition of a module on *cultural pride*, as this added treatment component may improve one or more of the identified health outcomes. A *mediation analyses* could determine whether the intervention produced expected changes in increasing *cultural pride* and then if this cultural pride enhancement produces significant increments on the targeted outcome variables, e.g., avoiding drug relapse. Similarly, *moderator* analyses can be conducted as comparative *effectiveness analyses* to determine if the culturally adapted EBT is differentially effective: (a) for men versus for women, (b) for clients high versus low in levels of acculturation, (c) among immigrant clients versus native-born clients, or (d) for any other potential moderators of intervention effectiveness (Barrera, Toobert, Strycker, & Osuna, 2012).

The long-term use and evaluation of a cultural adaptation could reveal possible issues in its adoption and sustainability within a community setting and in a setting that provides integrated care (Barrera, Berkel, & Castro, 2016). Currently little is known about the factors that affect the *sustainability* of culturally adapted interventions. If producing a new cultural adaptation is successful in attaining a good fit with local clients and the organization's culture, this adapted EBT would appear to have a greater likelihood of being sustained within this organization's ecological environment.

Mixed Methods Approaches and Methodologies

Emergence of mixed methods research The mixed methods field has emerged within the past decade as a "third paradigm" beyond the conventional qualitative and the quantitative research paradigms (Johnson, Onwuegbuzie, & Turner, 2007). The mixed methods field offers novel methodologies for attaining more in-depth (deep structure), informative, and applicable research results (Resnicow et al., 2000; Tashakkori & Teddle, 2010). Mixed methods analyses can generate explanatory "thick description" narratives that add depth of understanding about complex and temporal aspects of treatment implementation. Mixed methods approaches can be *exploratory* in form and can complement formal quantitative methods in the analyses of program effects that utilize observational, experimental, or other types of research designs, which yield *confirmatory* result on program effects and outcomes.

The field of mixed methods research has grown considerably during the past decade. A series of mixed methods designs and methodologies have emerged for a greater integration of qualitative and quantitative evidence (Castro, Kellison, Boyd, & Kopak, 2010; Creswell, 2014), under a research approach that can yield "the best of both" methods and more informative research results. Unfortunately, in the field of prevention research, existing mixed methods studies have remained methodologically weak in their design and implementation. Major areas of weakness as identified for these prevention research studies included: (a) an unspecified mixed methods design, where information is unclear about the mixed methods design used and the purpose of the design utilized; (b) weak or unspecified "purposeful sampling" (Morgan, 2014); (c) the use of a one-group experimental design, thus limiting limited internal validity; and (d) the use of impressionistic qual-quan integration (Castro, Morera, Kellison, & Aguirre, 2014). Nonetheless, such studies can be improved with a more rigorous application of mixed methods methodologies. Several texts are now available to aid in the conceptualization, design (Creswell, 2014; Tashakkori & Teddlie, 2010), implementation, and evaluation (Bernard, Wutich, & Ryan, 2017; Curry & Nunez-Smith, 2015; Morgan, 2014) of mixed methods studies. Mixed methods methodologies can help in planning, implementing, and assessing the treatment effectiveness, as delivered within an integrative care setting. Rigor and cultural sensitivity in treatment assessment and delivery within a healthcare setting can be attained by using a well-specified research design, coupled with the well-planned implementation of a mixed methods research or program evaluation study.

Mixed methods analyses in integrated care Studies conducted within an integrative care setting that utilize mixed methods research designs can conduct in-depth interviews with well-conceptualized *purposeful sampling* of strategically selected groups of participants, for conducting an in-depth assessment of treatment outcomes and of quality in adapted EBT implementation (Castro et al., 2014; Creswell, Klassen, Plano Clark, & Smith, 2011). These approaches can also provide deep-structure analyses of client and therapist observations and detailed evidence about factors: (a) that may operate as core treatment components, (b) that become sources of problems within treatment, and (c) that work well and should be kept and (d) that clients believe to be necessary for enhancing the content and delivery of a treatment, thus for refining that adapted EBT.

Mixed methods research designs Mixed methods research designs have been used extensively in implementation research and offer considerable promise for identifying factors and conditions that can improve the dissemination, adoption, implementation, and sustainability of EBTs across diverse settings. In principle, this information can aid in eliminating implementation barriers for improved EBT implementation within integrative care settings (Palinkas et al., 2011). In their analysis of mixed methods studies as conducted within the past 5 years, Palinkas et al. (2011) identified three major elements of mixed methods research as utilized in implementation studies. These three major elements were: (a) *structure*, the study's mixed methods research design that consists either of the *concurrent* or *sequential* approaches, as well as the relative importance afforded in this design's qualitative and quantitative components (e.g., "QUAL → Quan" or "QUAL + QUAN"); (b) *function*, one of four major purposes of a mixed methods study (i.e., convergence, complementarity, expansion, development, or sampling); and (c) *process*, the manner in which the qualitative and quantitative components are integrated (i.e., merged, connected, embedded).

Thus, as conceptualized within this framework, the application of mixed method designs in implementation research can offer "the best of both" (QUAL and QUAN) methodologies, depending on the particular application of these qualitative and quantitative methodologies within a proposed mixed methods study. Well-designed mixed methods research studies offer the promise of generating more informative data to advance the field of implementation research.

The Matrix Model: Exemplar of an Efficacious EBT for Treating Drug Dependence

The Matrix Model is a manualized multicomponent model treatment that in its basic form consists of a 16-week program delivered in 3 sessions per week for a total of 48 sessions (Obert et al., 2000). The Matrix Model treatment includes: (a) 12 family therapy sessions, (b) 4 social support group sessions, (c) 4 individual treatment sessions, and (d) a weekly breath alcohol testing and urine testing protocol. This treatment is nonjudgmental and non-confrontational and includes positive reinforcement from therapists and peers that support appropriate behavior change (Hillhouse, Martinelli-Casey, Gonzales, Ang, & Rawson, 2007; Rawson et al., 1995).

The Matrix Model was developed from the integration of empirically-based interventions and "grassroots" clinical experiences (Rawson et al., 1995). This manualized treatment includes patient handouts and a patient workbook that introduce empirically-based recovery activities as developed from the integration of five theory-based treatment approaches: (a) cognitive-behavioral therapy (CBT), (b) 12-step facilitation, (c) motivational interviewing, (d) contingency management, and (e) family therapy (Obert et al., 2000).

As developed from these five treatment approaches, the formal core components of the Matrix Model consist of: (a) early recovery phase treatment activities, (b) relapse prevention training, (c) social support groups, (d) family and conjoint sessions, (e) individual sessions, (f) urine testing, (g) relapse analysis, and (h) family education groups. The Matrix Model is guided by eight treatment principles: (a) create clear and explicit structures and expectations; (b) establish positive, collaborative relationship with the client; (c) teach information and cognitive-behavioral concepts; (d) reinforce positive behavior change; (e) provide corrective feedback when necessary; (f) educate the family regarding stimulant/drug abuse recovery; (g) introduce and encourage self-participation; (h) use urinalysis to monitor drug use (Rawson et al., 1995; J. Obert, personal communication, April 2, 2013).

Indicators of effective treatment program implementation are: (a) *engagement*, staying in treatment as assessed at the 2-week and 1-month observations; (b) *retention*, sustained treatment involvement as measured by the number of weeks remaining in treatment, with a maximum of 16 weeks, and also as measured by staying in treatment for 90 days or more versus less than 90 days; (c) *abstinence*, the average number of drug-free urinalysis tests collected during treatment and the occurrence of three consecutive drug-free urine analyses during treatment; and (d) *completion*, the completion of the 16-week Matrix Model treatment with no more than 2 consecutive missed weeks of treatment versus noncompletion of this 16-week program (Hillhouse et al., 2007). Thus, having an empirically-based understanding of the structure and core components of an EBT is important for making necessary cultural adaptations that can optimize learning of knowledge and skills while also optimizing patient engagement and active involvement in that treatment, thus to produce best treatment outcomes (Mejia, Leijten, Lachman, & Parra-Cordoba, 2017). This also includes an assessment of both inner and outer contexts, which can also influence the delivery of that EBT as intended.

Cultural adaptation of the Matrix Model The cultural adaptation of the Matrix Model or any EBT begins by identifying problems in treatment implementation and by identifying sources of client-treatment mismatches (non-fit) (Castro et al., 2004). This is followed by making strategic adaptations in treatment content, activities, or forms of delivery as recommended by consumer feedback from key informants or stakeholders and as reviewed by a Cultural Advisory Committee. These adaptations would be accomplished: (a) while maintaining the identified core treatment components (essential program activities); (b) increasing the cultural relevance of the treatment for local consumers (clients and subcultural groups); (c) increasing client motivation, engagement, and treatment involvement; (d) sustaining the efficacy of the treatment effect (i.e., maintaining the effect size on targeted outcomes); and (e) ideally increasing the treatment's effect size (Castro et al., 2010), that is, increasing the magnitude of change on targeted outcome variables. Moreover, effective cultural adaptation can ideally advance "beyond the black box" (Simpson, 2004), meaning that these adaptations would directly modify the mediators of: (a) *knowledge* of how to avoid a return to illegal drug use, i.e., knowledge about relapse prevention; (b) *perceptual awareness* that involves recognizing risk events, i.e., "triggers" for relapse behavior; and (c) *personal skills* in avoiding or "walking away" from high risk situations.

Need for gender sensitivity In the past drug abuse treatments emerged primarily as treatments for drug-dependent male clients, inadvertently exhibiting insensitivity to the needs of many female drug-dependent clients (Greenfield et al., 2007). Such treatments did little to address certain critical issues that affected drug-dependent women, such as their victimization from domestic violence and abuse imposed by their partners, some of whom were also drug-dependent individuals. Thus, program adaptations involving gender, i.e., gender-sensitive programs, have been developed for implementation with drug-dependent women. These gender-sensitive treatments have shown greater efficacy in addressing certain problems that are common among substance abusing women (Greenfield et al., 2007).

Efficacy of Culturally Adapted Health and Mental Health EBTs

In integrated care, the efficacy of interventions for illness and health behaviors (e.g., diabetes, exercise) and for mental health (e.g., depression) is important, especially for reducing or eliminating the health disparities and inequities that disproportionately affect many individual racial/ethnic minority patients. Integrated care interventions and providers can offer services that are supported by evidence of treatment-related improvements on targeted health outcomes. Even when they originate from empirically-based treatments, in principle, cultural adaptations still require rigorous evaluation to assess their efficacy within a local setting.

Culturally adapted health interventions Barrera et al. (2013) observed that the efficacy of culturally adapted health interventions has been supported by meta-analyses and narrative reviews that have been conducted for treating asthma (Bailey et al., 2009), diabetes (Glazier, Bajcar, Kenne, & Wilson, 2006; Hawthorne, Robles, Cannings-John, & Edwards, 2010; Sarkisian, Brown, Norris, Wintz, & Mangione, 2003; Whittemore, 2007), and HIV/AIDS (Darbes, Crepaz, Lyles, Kennedy, & Rutherford, 2008), mammography use (Han et al., 2009), nutrition (Eyles & Mhurchu, 2009), and nutrition and exercise (Mier, Ory, & Medina, 2010). By contrast, two reviews have concluded that there is insufficient evidence regarding the efficacy or effectiveness of culturally adapted interventions (Whitt-Glover & Kumanyika, 2009; Wilson & Miller, 2003). However, those two reviews acknowledged the limitations in the studies reviewed, such as low statistical power and the development of weak cultural adaptations.

Efficacy of cultural adaptations of psychotherapies Hall, Ibaraki, Huang, Marti and Stice (2016) observed that prior to their own meta-analysis, 11 meta-analyses has been published on the efficacy of culturally adapted psychotherapies. Overall, meta-analytic reviews showed that cultural adaptations of psychotherapies produce at least moderate effect sizes (culturally adapted intervention outcomes were superior to control condition outcomes), when effect sizes were calculated under several control conditions including a no intervention condition and unadapted intervention controls.

A review by Benish, Quintana and Wampold (2011) merits special recognition because it tested a possible mechanism that would account for the effectiveness of culturally adapted psychotherapies. They proposed that an adapted intervention's ability to change clients' *explanatory models of illness* (e.g., "illness myths") served as the active psychotherapeutic mechanism. Explanatory models are rooted in culture and used by clients to understand the problems they experience, the perceived origin of these problems, and the plausibility of proposed interventions to relieve suffering. Frank and Frank (1993) argued that there are four essential features of therapeutic practice: (a) the provision of a model that explains illness and its remedy, (b) a meaningful relationship with a culturally sanctioned healer, (c) a specialized setting that contains cultural symbols of healing, and (d) a set of procedures (healing practices) for overcoming illness. Clients achieve relief from their suffering when their ineffective explanatory models are replaced by another model that mobilizes hope, healthful thinking, and effective behavior.

The meta-analyses conducted by Benish and collaborators (2011) showed that cultural adaptations had meaningful effect sizes when compared to heterogeneous control conditions ($d = 0.41$) and to other active therapies ($d = 0.32$). As noted, in a unique "mediation" analysis, Benish and collaborators (2011) demonstrated that cultural adaptations that addressed *clients' explanatory models* accounted for the beneficial effects of culturally adapted psychotherapies. The authors explained that an implication of their findings is that intervention providers should initiate treatment by assessing and then respecting clients' initial explanatory models, before attempting to change them. Next, practitioners and patients should collaborate in formulating new explanatory models that place patients in a better position to enact positive changes.

In conclusion, several literature reviews support the efficacy of culturally adapted health and psychotherapy interventions for a variety of disorders. Practitioners in integrated care settings have many options for providing empirically-based culturally adapted interventions that are directed at improving health, mental health, and drug dependence. However, in the absence of formal culturally adapted interventions, a general strategy for culturally informed practice might be for clinicians to work collaboratively with members of subcultural groups to initially understand their explanatory models and then to modify these explanatory models to promote better health outcomes.

Examples of integrated care outcome studies with ethnic minority participants The IMPACT (Improving Mood – Promoting Access to Collaborative Treatment) study is one of the most prominent studies of integrated care (Unützer et al., 2002). Patients ($N = 1801$) with chronic health conditions and depression participated in this project that included 18 primary care clinics in five states. Ethnic minority participants constituted 23% of the total sample. Depression care managers and consulting psychiatrists were added to the clinics' staffs to provide "collaborative stepped care" in which depression treatment could be modified by varying combinations of antidepressant medication and problem-solving psychotherapy when patients did not show improvement. Compared to usual care, integrated care resulted in greater reductions in depression at the 12-month assessment.

In a study directed primarily at Spanish-speaking Latino patients (about 70% of the sample), the IMPACT depression intervention was combined with a culturally relevant diabetes intervention (Project *Dulce*) to treat depression in those receiving diabetes care in three southern California community clinics (Gilmer, Walker, Johnson, Philis-Tsimikas, & Unützer, 2008). By combining the two interventions, the overall project could be described as a "co-located, co-managed" form of integrated care. Project *Dulce* consisted of a peer-led diabetes self-management intervention. IMPACT (described in the preceding paragraph) was delivered by bilingual staff and was culturally adapted by making it "more flexible for responding to cultural norms and beliefs, low literacy, socioeconomic barriers, and social stigma" (p. 1324). In this pre-post intervention evaluation, depressed diabetes patients were able to significantly lower depression scores at the 6-month assessment period (an average of 7.5 points on the PHQ-9) and significantly increase healthful nutrition.

A study of low-income medical patients also focused on depression treatment (Miranda, Azocar, Organista, Dwyer, & Areane, 2003). This was an example of *col-located integrated care* in that outpatients at San Francisco General Hospital and affiliated clinics were referred by their primary care providers to San Francisco General Hospital's Depression Clinic. Participants were 199 primary care patients, including 77 Spanish-speaking Latinos, 46 African Americans, and 18 Asians and American Indians. They were randomly assigned to receive a cognitive-behavioral therapy (CBT) group therapy intervention, or the CBT intervention combined with clinical case management designed to increase engagement (reduce dropout). CBT involved 12 group sessions based on a manualized treatment protocol. Clinical case management, which was implemented for up to 6 months, involved telephone contacts between participants and staff member that were devoted to solving problems associated with employment, housing, and relations with family and friends. Ostensibly, those problems could be barriers to treatment engagement. The investigators adapted the CBT intervention for low-income/low-education patients and for Latino patients. Spanish- and English-language manuals were written at appropriate reading levels. The pleasant activities component suggested many activities that were free of charges. Session leaders were bilingual-bicultural, and these leaders were trained to conduct sessions with interpersonal warmth consistent with the Latino cultural values of *respeto*, *personalismo*, and *simpatia*.

Findings showed that those who received group CBT plus case management attended more CBT sessions and were less likely to drop out of therapy than those who received group CBT alone. The effects of treatment condition on depression outcomes were moderated by patients' language use. For Spanish-speaking participants, those who received group CBT plus case management reported less depression at 6-month follow-up than those who received group CBT alone. For English-speaking participants, there were no differences between treatment conditions on depression at the 6-month follow-up.

Conclusions and Directions for Future Research and Practice within Integrative Health Settings

From this analysis of the cultural adaptation of EBTs, we offer five observations and recommendations.

1. *Treatment relevance and fit.* A treatment that is not designed in accord with the needs of a specific subcultural group may exhibit insensitivity to that group's cultural of other needs and preferences. For example, given that early drug abuse treatments emerged with as distinct male focus, these treatments exhibited insensitivity to the needs of many drug-dependent women. To deliver integrated health, mental health, and substance abuse treatments within healthcare settings, aspects of the local community culture can be considered for "grounding" an

EBT to operate in harmony with the environmental contexts that exist within the local healthcare system.

2. *Enhancing client engagement*. Sufficient client engagement in treatment is necessary to promote client retention and treatment completion. Currently, low rates of client engagement remain as a pervasive problem that affects treatment efficacy and the benefits that can be obtained from treatment (Carroll et al., 2011). It is thus essential that existing EBTs and any adapted versions increase their capacity for client engagement and retention.
3. *Importance of cultural factors*. Recent studies have highlighted the importance of considering various cultural factors, such as gender, racial or ethnic identity, sexual orientation, and levels of acculturation and any of several cultural constructs (Castro & Hernandez-Alarcon, 2002), important treatment-related factors that can aid in relieving the health and mental health problems that affect diverse ethnocultural clients. These treatments can be enhanced by selectively integrating cultural factors into the EBT's protocol, based on advisory feedback from a Cultural Advisory Committee (Castro et al., 2007).
4. *Enhancing cultural relevance with a culturally relevant module*. Increasing an existing EBTs cultural relevance need not involve a complete reconstruction of the original EBT. Adding relevant cultural contents or developing a specific *cultural module* may be sufficient to enhance the treatment's cultural relevance and fit for members of an identified subcultural group.
5. *Cultural adaptation as a systematic and team effort*. The effective adaptation of an EBT consists of a planned and systematic team effort as aided by input from a Cultural Advisory Committee. This effort benefits from a scientist-provider partnership that involves the developers of the treatment and other stakeholders (Donovan et al., 2011; Mejia et al., 2017). Organized agency structures are also needed and should be developed to conduct the most rigorous treatment adaptation possible within a local healthcare setting and to plan and sustain the delivery of that treatment with the requisite fidelity that is needed to produce efficacious treatment outcomes.

References

Aarons, G. A., Hurlburt, M., & Horowitz, S. M. (2011). Advancing a conceptual model of evidence-based practice implementation in public service sectors. *Administration Policy and Mental Health, 38*, 4–23.

Agency Healthcare Research and Quality (AHRQ). (2012). *National health disparities report*. Retrieved from http://www.ahrq.gov/research/findings/nhqrdr/nhdr12/2012nhdr.pdf

Bailey, E. J., Cates, C. J., Kruske, S. G., Morris, P. S., Brown, N., & Chang, A. B. (2009). Culture-specific programs for children and adults from minority groups who have asthma. *Cochrane Database System Reviews*, (2). Art. No. CD006580. https://doi.org/10.1002/14651858.CD006580.pub4

Bandura, A. (1986). *Social foundations of thought and action: A social cognitive theory*. Englewood Cliffs, NJ: Prentice Hall.

Barrera, M., Jr., Berkel, C., & Castro, F. G. (2016). Directions for the advancement of culturally adapted preventive interventions: Local adaptations, engagement, and sustainability. *Prevention Science, 18,* 640–648. https://doi.org/10.1007/s11121-016-0705-9

Barrera, M., Jr., Castro, F. G., & Holleran-Steiker, L. K. (2011). A critical analysis of approaches to the development of prevention interventions for subcultural groups. *American Journal of Community Psychology, 48,* 439–454.

Barrera, M., Jr., Castro, F. G., Strycker, L. A., & Toobert, D. J. (2013). Cultural adaptation of behavioral health interventions: A progress report. *Journal of Consulting and Clinical Psychology, 81,* 196–205. https://doi.org/10.1037/a0027085

Barrera, M., Jr., Toobert, D. J., Strycker, L. A., & Osuna, D. (2012). Effects of acculturation on a culturally-adapted diabetes intervention for Latinas. *Health Psychology, 31,* 51–54. https://doi.org/10.1037/a0025205

Berry, J. W. (1980). Acculturation as varieties of adaptation. In A. M. Padilla (Ed.), *Acculturation: Theory, models, and some new findings* (pp. 9–25). Boulder, CO: Westview Press.

Berry, J. W. (2005). Acculturation: Living successfully in two cultures. *International Journal of Intercultural Relations, 29,* 697–712.

Benish, S. G., Quintana, W., & Wampold, B. (2011). Culturally adapted psychotherapy and the legitimacy of myth: A direct comparison meta-analysis. *Journal of Counseling Psychology, 58,* 279–289. https://doi.org/10.1037/a0023626

Bernal, G., Jimenez-Chafey, M. I., & Domenech Rodriguez, M. M. (2009). Cultural adaptation of treatments: A resource for considering culture in evidence-based practice. *Professional Psychology Research and Practice, 40,* 361–368.

Bernard, H. R., Wutich, A., & Ryan, G. W. (2017). *Analyzing qualitative data: Systematic approaches* (2nd ed.). Los Angeles, CA: Sage.

Bronfenbrenner, U. (1986). Ecology of the family as a context for human development: Research perspectives. *Developmental Psychology, 22,* 723–742.

Carroll, K. M., Ball, S. A., Jackson, R., Martino, S., Petry, N. M., Stitzer, M. L., … Weiss, R. D. (2011). Ten take home lessons from the first 10 years of the CTN and 10 recommendations for the future. *The American Journal of Drug and Alcohol Abuse, 37,* 275–282.

Castro, F. G., Barrera, M., Jr., & Holleran Steiker, L. K. (2010). Issues and challenges in the design of culturally-adapted evidence-based interventions. *Annual Review of Clinical Psychology, 6,* 213–239.

Castro, F. G., Barrera, M., Jr., & Martinez, C. R. (2004). The cultural adaptation of prevention interventions: Resolving tensions between fidelity and fit. *Prevention Science, 5,* 41–45.

Castro, F. G., Bautista, T. G., Hombrados Mendieta, M. I., Ramirez, S. O., Heydarian, N. M., & Hughes, A. S. (2017). Systems contexts for designing culturally-adapted prevention interventions. In S. J. Schwartz & J. B. Unger (Eds.), *Oxford handbook of acculturation and health* (pp. 411–432). New York, NY: Oxford. Oxford University Press.

Castro, F. G., & Hernández-Alarcón, E. (2002). Integrating cultural factors into drug abuse prevention and treatment with racial/ethnic minorities. *Journal of Drug Issues, 32,* 783–810.

Castro, F. G., Kellison, J. G., Boyd, S., & Kopak, S. (2010). A methodology for conducting integrative mixed methods research and data analyses. *Journal of Mixed Methods Research, 4,* 342–360.

Castro, F. G., Morera, O. F., Kellison, J. G., & Aguirre, K. M. (2014). Mixed methods research design for prevention science: Methods, critiques, and recommendations. In Z. Sloboda & H. Petras (Eds.), *Advances in prevention science* (pp. 453–490). New York, NY: Springer.

Castro, F. G., Nichols, E., & Kater, K. (2007). Relapse prevention with Hispanic and other racial/ethnic populations: Can cultural resilience promote relapse prevention? In K. Witkiewitz & G. A. Marlatt (Eds.), *A therapist's guide to evidence-based relapse prevention* (pp. 259–292). Boston, MA: Academic Press.

Castro, F. G., & Yasui, M. (2017). Advances in EBI development for diverse populations: Towards a science of intervention adaptation. *Prevention Science, 18,* 623–629. https://doi.org/10.1007/s11121-017-0809-x

Cervantes, R. C., Cardoso, J. B., & Goldbach, J. T. (2015). Examining differences in culturally based stress among clinical and nonclinical Hispanic adolescents. *Cultural Diversity and Ethnic Minority Psychology, 21*, 458–467.

Collado, A., Calderon, M., MacPherson, L., & Lejuez, C. (2016). The efficacy of behavioral activation treatment among depressed Spanish-speaking Latinos. *Journal of Consulting and Clinical Psychology, 84*, 651–657.

Collins, C., Hewson, D. L., Munger, R., & Wade, T. (2010). *Evolving models of behavioral health integration in primary care*. New York, NY: Millbank Memorial Fund. Retrieved from: http://www.milbank.org/uploads/documents/10430EvolvingCare/10430EvolvingCare.html

Corrigan, P. W., Kuwabara, S. A., & O'Shaughnessy, J. (2009). The public stigma of mental illness and drug addiction: Findings from a stratified random sample. *Journal of Social Work, 9*, 139–147.

Creswell, J. W. (2014). *Research design: Qualitative, quantitative, and mixed methods approaches*. Los Angeles, CA: Sage.

Creswell, J. W., Klassen, A. C., Plano Clark, V. L., & Smith, K. C. (2011). *Best practices for mixed methods research in the health sciences*. Bethesda, MD: Office of Behavioral and Social Science Research (OBSSR).

Curry, L., & Nunez-Smith, M. (2015). *Mixed methods in health sciences research: A practical primer*. Los Angeles, CA: Sage.

Darbes, L., Crepaz, N., Lyles, C., Kennedy, G., & Rutherford, G. (2008). The efficacy of behavioral interventions in reducing HIV risk behaviors and incident sexually-transmitted diseases in heterosexual African Americans. *AIDS, 22*, 1177–1194. https://doi.org/10.1097/QAD.0b013e3282ff624e

Davis, T. S., Guada, J., Reno, R., Peck, A., Evans, S., Sigal, L. M., & Swenson, S. (2015). Integrated and culturally relevant care: A model to prepare social workers for primary care behavioral health practice. *Social Work in Health Care, 54*, 909–938.

Donovan, D. M., Daley, D. C., Brigham, G. S., Hodgkins, C. C., Perl, H., & Floyd, A. S. (2011). How practice and science are balanced and blended in the NIDA clinical trials network: The bidirectional process in the development of the STAGE-12 protocol as an example. *The American Journal of Drug and Alcohol Abuse, 37*, 408–416.

Elliot, D. S., & Mihalic, S. (2004). Issues in disseminating and replicating effective prevention programs. *Prevention Science, 5*, 47–53.

Eyles, H. C., & Mhurchu, C. N. (2009). Does tailoring make a difference? A systematic review of the long-term effectiveness of tailored nutrition education for adults. *Nutrition Reviews, 67*, 464–480. https://doi.org/10.1111/j.1753-4887.2009.00219.x

Flay, B., Biglan, A., Boruch, R. F., Castro, F. G., Gottfriedson, D., Kellam, E. K., … Ji, P. (2005). Standards of evidence: Criteria for efficacy, effectiveness, and dissemination. *Prevention Science, 6*(3), 151–175.

Frank, J. D., & Frank, J. B. (1993). *Persuasion and healing: A comparative study of psychotherapy* (3rd ed.). Baltimore, MD: Johns Hopkins University Press.

Geisinger, K. F. (1994). Cross-cultural normative assessment translation and adaptation issues influencing the normative interpretation of assessment instruments. *Psychological Assessment, 6*, 304–312.

Gilmer, T. P., Walker, C., Johnson, E. D., Philis-Tsimikas, A., & Unützer, J. (2008). Improving treatment of depression among Latinos with diabetes using project Dulce and IMPACT. *Diabetes Care, 31*(7), 1324–1326.

Glazier, R. H., Bajcar, J., Kenne, N. R., & Wilson, K. (2006). A systematic review of interventions to improve diabetes care in socially disadvantaged populations. *Diabetes Care, 29*, 1675–1688. https://doi.org/10.2337/dc05–1942

Gonzalez, V. M., Stewart, A., Ritter, P. L., & Lorig, K. (1995). Translation and validation of arthritis outcome measures into Spanish. *Arthritis and Rheumatism, 38*, 1429–1446.

Greenfield, S. F., Brooks, A. J., Gordon, S. M., Green, C. A., Kropp, F., McHugh, R. K., … Miele, G. M. (2007). Substance abuse treatment entry, retention, and outcome in women: A review of the literature. *Drug and Alcohol Dependence, 86*, 1–21.

Guerrero, E. G., & Kao, D. (2013). Racial/ethnic minority and low-income hotspots and their geographic proximity to integrated care providers. *Substance Abuse Treatment, Prevention, and Policy, 8*, 34–43.

Hall, G. C., Ibaraki, A. Y., Huang, E. R., Marti, C. N., & Stice, E. (2016). A meta-analysis of cultural adaptations of psychological interventions. *Behavior Therapy, 47*(6), 993–1014.

Han, H. R., Lee, J. E., Kim, J., Hedlin, H. K., Song, H., & Kim, M. T. (2009). A meta-analysis of interventions to promote mammography among ethnic minority women. *Nursing Research, 58*, 246–254. https://doi.org/10.1097/NNR.0b013e3181ac0f7f

Hansen, W. B. (2014). Measuring fidelity. In Z. Sloboda & H. Petras (Eds.), *Defining prevention science* (pp. 335–359). New York, NY: Springer.

Hawthorne, K., Robles, Y., Cannings-John, R., & Edwards, A. G. K. (2010). Culturally appropriate health education for type II diabetes in ethnic minority groups: A systematic and narrative review of randomized controlled trials. *Diabetic Medicine, 27*, 613–623. https://doi.org/10.1111/j.1464-5491.2010.02954.x

Hillhouse, M. P., Martinelli-Casey, P., Gonzales, R., Ang, A., & Rawson, R. A. (2007). Predicting in-treatment performance and post-treatment outcomes in methamphetamine users. *Addiction, 102*(Suppl 1), 84–95.

Ja, D., & Aoki, B. (1993). Substance use treatment: Cultural barriers in the Asian American community. *Journal of Psychoactive Drugs, 25*, 61–71.

Johnson, R. B., Onwuegbuzie, A. J., & Turner, L. A. (2007). Toward a definition of mixed methods research. *Journal of Mixed Methods Research, 1*, 112–133.

Keys, K. M., Martins, S. S., Hatzenbuehler, M. L., Blanco, C., Bates, L. M., & Hasin, D. S. (2012). Mental health service utilization for psychiatric disorders among Latinos living in the United States: The role of ethnic subgroup, ethnic identity, and language/social preferences. *Social Psychiatry & Psychiatric Epidemiology, 47*, 383–394.

Kumpfer, K. L., Alvarado, R., Smith, P., & Bellamy, N. (2002). Cultural sensitivity in universal family-based prevention interventions. *Prevention Science, 3*, 241–244.

Kumpfer, K. L., Pinyuchon, M., de Melo, A., & Whiteside, H. O. (2008). Cultural adaptation process for international dissemination of the strengthening families program (SFP). *Evaluation and Health Professions, 33*(2), 226–239.

Lehman, D. R., Chiu, C., & Schaller, M. (2004). Psychology and culture. *Annual Review of Psychology, 55*, 689–714.

Lemmens, L. C., Molema, C. C. M., Versnel, N., Baan, C. A., & de Bruin, S. R. (2015). Integrated care programs for patients with psychological comorbidity: A systematic review and meta-analysis. *Journal of Psychosomatic Research, 79*, 580–594.

Lopez-Class, M., Castro, F. G., & Ramirez, A. G. (2011). Conceptions of acculturation: A review and statement of critical issues. *Social Science and Medicine, 72*, 1555–1162.

MacKinnon, D. P. (2008). *Introduction to statistical mediation analysis*. New York, NY: Lawrence Erlbaum.

McGovern, M. P., Urada, D., Lambert-Harris, C., Sullivan, S. T., & Mazade, N. A. (2012). Development and initial feasibility of an organizational measure of behavioral health integration in medical care settings. *Journal of Substance Abuse Treatment, 43*, 402–409.

Mejia, A., Leijten, P., Lachman, J. M., & Parra-Cordoba, J. R. (2017). Different strokes for different folks? Contrasting approaches to cultural adaptation of parenting interventions. *Prevention Science, 18*(6), 630–639.

Meschke, L. L., & Juang, L. P. (2014). Obstacles to parent-adolescent communication in Hmong American families: Exploring pathways to adolescent mental health promotion. *Ethnicity & Health, 19*, 144–159.

Mier, N., Ory, M. G., & Medina, A. A. (2010). Anatomy of culturally sensitive interventions promoting nutrition and exercise in Hispanics: A critical examination of existing literature. *Health Promotion Practice, 11*, 541–554. https://doi.org/10.1177/1524839908328991

Miranda, J., Azocar, F., Organista, K. C., Dwyer, E., & Areane, P. (2003). Treatment of depression among impoverished primary care patients from ethnic minority groups. *Psychiatric Services, 54*, 219–225.

Minkler, M., Wallerstein, N., & Wilson, N. (2008). Improving health through community organization and community building. In K. Glanz, B. K. Rimer, & K. Viswanath (Eds.), *Health behavior and health education: Theory, research, and practice* (4th ed., pp. 287–312). San Francisco, CA: Jossey-Bass.

Morgan, D. L. (2014). *Integrating qualitative & quantitative methods: A pragmatic approach*. Los Angeles, CA: Sage.

National Institute on Drug Abuse (NIMH). (1999). *Principles of drug addiction treatment: A research-based guide. NIH publication no. 99–4180*. Rockville, MD: National Institute on Drug Abuse.

National Institute of Mental Health (NIMH). (2006). *Benefits to employers outweigh enhanced depression-care costs*. Retrieved from http://www.nimh.nih.gov/science-news/2006/benefits-to-employers-outweigh-enhanceddepression-care-costs.shtml

Norcross, J. C., Beutler, L. E., & Levant, R. F. (2006). *Evidence-based practice in mental health: Debate and dialogue on the fundamental questions*. Washington, DC: American Psychological Association.

Obert, J. L., McCann, M. J., Martinelli-Casey, P., Weiner, A., Minsky, S., … Rawson, R. (2000). The matrix model of outpatient stimulant abuse treatment: History and description. *Journal of Psychoactive Drugs, 32*, 157–164.

Orlandi, M. A., Weston, R., & Epstein, L. G. (1992). *Cultural competence for evaluators*. Rockville, MD: Office of Substance Abuse Prevention.

Padwa, H., Teruya, C., Tran, E., Livinger, K., Antonini, V. P., Overholt, C., & Urada, D. (2016). The implementation of integrated behavioral health protocols in primary care settings in *Project Care*. *Journal of Substance Abuse Treatment, 62*, 74–83.

Palinkas, L. A., Aarons, G. A., Horwitz, S., Chamberlin, P., Hurlburt, M., & Landsverk, J. (2011). Mixed methods design in implementation research. *Administration Policy and Mental Health, 38*, 44–53.

Pantin, H., Schwartz, S. J., Sullivan, S., Prado, G., & Szapocznik, J. (2004). Ecodevelopmental HIV prevention programs for Hispanic adolescents. *American Journal of Orthopsychiatry, 74*, 545–558.

Portes, A., & Rumbaut, R. A. (2014). *Immigrant America: A portrait* (4th ed.). Berkeley, CA: University of California Press.

Portes, A., & Zhou, M. (1993). The new second generation: Segmented assimilation and its variants. *Annals of the American Academy of Political and Social Science, 530*, 74–96.

Ramirez, M. (1999). Multicultural psychotherapy: *An approach to individual and cultural differences* (2nd ed.). Boston: Allyn & Bacon.

Rawson, R. A., Shoptaw, S. J., Obert, J. L., McCann, M. J., Hasson, A. L., Martinelli-Casey, P. J., … Ling, W. (1995). An intensive approach to cocaine abuse treatment. *Journal of Substance Abuse Treatment, 12*, 117–127.

Resnicow, K., Soler, R., Braithwait, R. L., Ahluwalia, J. S., & Butler, J. (2000). Cultural sensitivity in substance abuse prevention. *Journal of Community Psychology, 28*, 271–290.

Rohrbach, L. A. (2014). Design of prevention interventions. In Z. Sloboda & H. Petras (Eds.), *Defining prevention science* (pp. 275–291). New York, NY: Springer.

Rutkowski, B. A., Rawson, R. A., & Freese, T. E. (2012). Editors' introduction: The evidence for integrated care – substance use disorders, mental health, and primary care: California Substance Abuse Research Consortium (SARC) meetings, 2011. *Journal of Psychoactive Drugs, 44*, 281–241.

Sallis, J. F., Owen, N., & Fisher, E. (2008). Ecological models of health behavior. In K. Glanz, B. K. Rimer, & K. Viswanath (Eds.), *Health behavior and health education: Theory, research, and practice* (4th ed., pp. 465–485). San Francisco, CA: Jossey-Bass.

Sarkisian, C. A., Brown, A. F., Norris, K. C., Wintz, R. L., & Mangione, C. M. (2003). A systematic review of diabetes self-care interventions for older, African-American, or Latino adults. *Diabetes Educator, 29*, 467–479. https://doi.org/10.1177/014572170302900311

Schwartz, S. J., Weisskirch, R. S., Zamboanga, B. L., Castillo, L. G., Ham, L. S., Huynh, Q., … Cano, M. A. (2010). Dimensions of acculturation: Associations with high risk behaviors among college students from immigrant families. *Journal of Counseling Psychology, 20*, 1–15.

Shiraev, E. B., & Levy, D. A. (2010). *Cross-cultural psychology: Critical thinking and contemporary applications*. Boston, MA: Allyn & Bacon.
Simpson, D. D. (2004). A conceptual framework for drug treatment process and outcomes. *Journal of Substance Abuse Treatment, 27*(4), 99–121.
Snowden, L. R. (2001). Barriers to effective mental health services for African Americans. *Mental Health Services Research, 3*, 181–187. https://doi.org/10.1023/A:1013172913880
Spoth, R., Rohrbach, L. A., Greenberg, M., Leaf, P., Brown, C. H., Fagan, A., ... Society for Prevention Research Type 2 Translational Task Force Members and Contributing Authors. (2013). Addressing core challenges for the next generation of type 2 translation research and systems: The translation science to population Impact (TSci Impact) framework. *Prevention Science, 14*, 319. https://doi.org/10.1007/s11121-012-0362-6
Storey, J. D., Saffitz, G. B., & Rimon, J. G. (2008). Social marketing. In K. Glanz, B. K. Rimer, & K. Viswanath (Eds.), *Health behavior and health education: Theory, research, and practice* (4th ed., pp. 435–464). San Francisco, CA: Jossey-Bass.
Substance Abuse and Mental Health Services Administration (SAMHSA). (2014). *Improving cultural competence: Quick guide for clinician.* Treatment Improvement Protocol (TIP) Series No. 59. HHS Publication No. (SMA) 14–4849. Rockville, MD: Substance Abuse and Mental Health Services Administration. Retrieved from http://store.samhsa.gov/product/TIP-59-Improving-Cultural-Competence/SMA14-4849?sortBy=3
Substance Abuse and Mental Health Services Administration (SAMHSA). (2017, May). The National Registry of Evidence-based Programs and Practices (NREPP). Retrieved from http://www.samhsa.gov/nrepp
Sue, S., & Zane, N. (2006). Ethnic minority populations have been neglected by evidence-based practices. In J. C. Norcross, L. E. Beutler, & R. F. Levant (Eds.), *Evidence-based practices in mental health: Debate and dialogue on the fundamental question* (pp. 329–337). Washington DC: American Psychological Association.
Sunderji, N., Waddell, A., Gupta, M., Soklaridis, S., & Steinberg, R. (2016). An expert consensus on core competencies in integrated care for psychiatrists. *General Hospital Psychiatry, 41*, 45–52.
Supplee, L. H., Kelly, B. C., MacKinnon, D. M., & Barofsky, M. Y. (2013). Introduction to the special issue: Subgroup analysis in prevention and intervention research. *Prevention Science, 14*, 107–110.
Tashakkori, A., & Teddle, C. (2010). *Sage handbook of mixed methods in social and behavioral research* (2nd ed.). Los Angeles, CA: Sage.
Terrell, M. D. (1993). Ethnocultural factors and substance abuse towards culturally sensitive treatment models. *Psychology of Addictive Behaviors, 7*, 162–167.
Trimble, J. E. (1995). Toward an understanding of ethnicity and ethnic identity, and their relationship with drug abuse research. In G. J. Botvin, S. Schinke, & M. A. Orlando (Eds.), *Drug abuse prevention with multiethnic youth* (pp. 3–27). Thousand Oaks, CA: Sage.
Unützer, J., Katon, W., Callahan, C. M., Williams, J. W., Jr., Hunkeler, E., Harpole, L., ... Areán, P. A. (2002). Collaborative care management of late-life depression in the primary care setting: A randomized controlled trial. *JAMA, 288*(22), 2836–2845.
U.S. Department of Health and Human Services (DHHS). (2016). *Facing addiction in America: The surgeon general's report on alcohol, drugs, and health*. Washington, DC: HHS.
van der Kreeft, P., Jongbloet, J., & Van Havere, T. (2014). Factors affecting implementation: Cultural adaptation. In Z. Sloboda & H. Petras (Eds.), *Defining prevention science* (pp. 315–334). New York, NY: Springer.
Whittemore, R. (2007). Culturally competent interventions for Hispanic adults with type 2 diabetes: A systematic review. *Journal of Transcultural Nursing, 18*, 157–166. https://doi.org/10.1177/1043659606298615
Whitt-Glover, M. C., & Kumanyika, S. K. (2009). Systematic review of interventions to increase physical activity and physical fitness in African-Americans. *American Journal of Health Promotion, 23*, S33–S56. https://doi.org/10.4278/ajhp.070924101
Wilson, B. D. M., & Miller, R. L. (2003). Examining strategies for culturally grounded HIV prevention: A review. *AIDS Education and Prevention, 15*, 184–202. https://doi.org/10.1521/aeap.15.3.184.23838

Part III
Key Challenges to Care Integration

Chapter 7
Healthcare Transformation: The Electronic Health Record

Dana Edberg and Jeanne Wendel

Introduction

A significant part of clinical healthcare involves collecting, analyzing, and synthesizing data to create information to provide health-related advice and treatment to patients (Swinglehurst & Greenhalgh, 2015). It might be possible to view clinical healthcare providers (HCPs[1]) as incredibly sophisticated and flexible analytical systems capable of gathering and analyzing varied types of data to prescribe healthcare solutions. As the amount, type, and differing sources of data related to patient healthcare continue to grow, HCPs need the support of computer-based information technology (IT) to help store and process the data required to support effective clinical decisions.

IT is used in many industries to help people and organizations collect and analyze data more effectively (Lee, 2002). Health policy-makers in the USA hoped that more effective and ubiquitous IT could generate similar efficiencies in the healthcare industry (Blumenthal, 2009). The Office of the National Coordinator (ONC) was established in 2004 to begin developing standard definitions for core data to be stored in electronic health record (EHR) systems, technical standards for transmitting data, and standards for EHR systems.

An EHR is a digital version of the traditional patient chart, which is updated by the HCP during each patient encounter. This record serves as a consolidated source of truth about the healthcare delivered to a specific patient over time (Kohli & Tan, 2016). An EHR includes both the database (typically described as "data at rest") and

[1] We use the acronym HCP to represent both medical and behavioral healthcare providers.

D. Edberg (✉)
Department of Information Systems, University of Nevada, Reno, Reno, NV, USA
e-mail: dte@unr.edu

J. Wendel
Department of Economics, University of Nevada, Reno, Reno, NV, USA

M. P. Duckworth, W. T. O'Donohue (eds.), *Behavioral Medicine and Integrated Care*,
https://doi.org/10.1007/978-3-319-93003-9_7

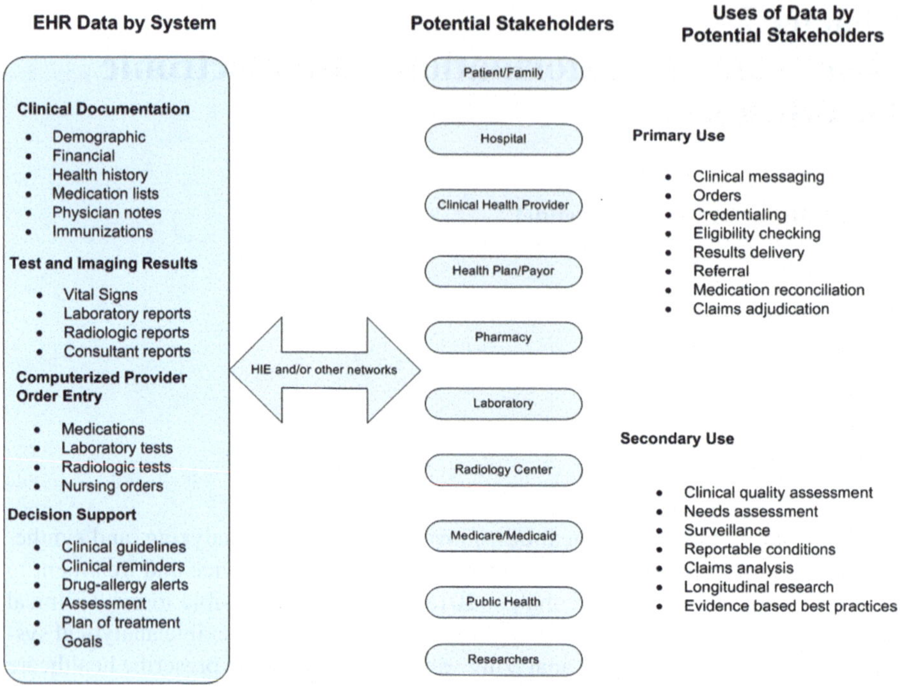

Fig. 7.1 Overview of EHR with potential stakeholders

the applications that facilitate the management of that database and communication of relevant information stored in that database.

EHRs were not intended to stand alone; they were intended to serve as key source data for a nationwide network of interconnected health data. The ONC also established standards for structured data and a common clinical data set that EHRs must meet in order to qualify as certified electronic health record technology (CEHRT) (ONC, 2016a). This certification program facilitates sharing patient data among disparate EHR systems, and it reduces buyer uncertainty about the technical qualifications of software offered by vendors.

The 2009 Health Information Technology for Economic and Clinical Health (HITECH) Act funded programs to incentivize widespread adoption of EHRs and development of state-level or area-level infrastructure to support electronic health information exchange (HIE) to facilitate data sharing (ONC, 2016b). This funding was viewed as an investment to improve healthcare quality, safety, and efficiency through the promotion of health IT.

The vision funded by HITECH included a series of HIEs that would allow healthcare providers to share data stored in individual EHRs. Figure 7.1 shows an overview of the relationship between the EHR data collected by HCPs (one of the stakeholders for EHR) and the potential uses of that data to convert it into information to support decision-making in healthcare.

This chapter explores how electronic health record systems can potentially support clinical healthcare in a HCP office. The second section of this chapter explains why EHR systems are expected to deliver the dual miracles of strengthening healthcare quality while also reducing the cost associated with delivering that care. The third section gives an overview of the data stored in an EHR system to help understand the challenges that must be addressed to use this data to support clinical decision-making. The fourth section describes potential issues as healthcare providers implement EHR systems and work to use them to support clinical decision-making. This section also highlights issues that are particularly relevant to an integrated care environment. The concluding section discusses actions required to optimize the use of an EHR system in a practice environment.

Potential Impacts of Health Information Technology

The federal government has actively supported and incentivized the use of EHR systems and the development of platforms to support HIE. A 2008 Congressional Budget Office (CBO) report (CBO, 2008) summarized evidence indicating that EHR systems can provide essential infrastructure to help healthcare providers develop systems to:

- Decrease duplicate tests, eliminate or reduce transcription costs, and reduce administrative expenditures associated with transmitting records between provider organizations
- Increase coordination of care
- Provide relevant information, at the provider's decision point, about evidence-based treatment protocols for a diagnosed patient condition, routine tests, and preventive care that should be ordered for a specific patient, and generic drugs available for specific brand-name pharmaceuticals
- Increase patient safety by using algorithms to check for potential interactions among the set of drugs prescribed for a specific patient
- Support new types of cost-effectiveness and comparative effectiveness studies, using the large datasets generated by electronic medical record systems

These anticipated benefits of HIT range from straightforward provision of relevant information to support the delivery of high-quality healthcare to significant reengineering of the healthcare delivery system. The new efficiencies are expected to occur in a range of settings. Some efficiencies may be generated within the work of one clinician. Others will streamline the interactions among clinicians, or between clinicians and payers. The technology also offers opportunities for large provider organizations and payers to strengthen population-based healthcare strategies. In addition, the Centers for Medicare & Medicaid Services (CMS) is funding pilot programs denoted as Accountable Health Communities, to explore strategies to harness this technology to strengthen coordination between healthcare providers and agencies that provide social services.

Individual healthcare providers (or provider organizations) may view an EHR system as an investment that will strengthen their ability to work efficiently, provide high-quality care, meet quality-based payment incentives, or submit accurate claims to payers (Adler-Milstein & Bates, 2010). Unlike most investment goods, EHR systems may also generate benefits for other entities (e.g., other provider organizations, payers, and public health agencies), and the systems are expected to generate databases that will support significant research activities. This array of potential beneficiaries implies that the IT personnel developing EHR software must consider a wide array of stakeholders as shown on Fig. 7.1. In addition, these systems must be designed to accomplish a broad array of tasks, including generating accurate bills, supporting day-to-day care delivery, generating data useful for measuring and reporting quality of care, supporting provider-level quality improvement activities, and facilitating communication across provider organizations (Blumenthal, 2009). In addition, policy-makers, payers, accountable care organizations, patient-centered medical homes, and managed care organizations plan to use EHR-generated data to develop new strategies for managing care.

Using Data Generated by EHRs

The anticipated new efficiencies stem from two types of uses of data: "primary uses" and "secondary uses." Activities such as using an EHR system to share patient information with care team members are categorized as *primary uses* of data (examples are provided in Fig. 7.1). In this situation, data is used to directly support delivery of care. Other examples of primary uses of data include electronic transmission of prescriptions (e-prescribing), displaying lists of medications currently prescribed for patients, displaying lists of completed vaccinations, and sharing physician notes with care team members.

Activities that require aggregating data for sets of patients are categorized as *secondary uses* of data (examples are provided in Fig. 7.1). Measuring and reporting quality of care is a common example. Computing and reporting the proportion of a physician's diabetic patients with A1c levels within the recommended range would require two steps. The EHR system would identify patients with a diagnosis of diabetes (this would be the denominator of the measure). The system could also compute the number of the physician's diabetic patients with A1c levels within the recommended range (this would be the numerator of the measure). Computing this ratio would be a time-consuming task for a practice using paper patient charts. The EHR system can compute this ratio quickly; however the HCPs would need to invest time to ensure accurate entry of relevant information, so that the EHR system can provide an accurate computation of this quality measure.

Potential EHR-generated efficiencies span the full range of the levels of problem-solving articulated in Polya's classic work on problem-solving methods

(Polya, 2014).[2] Activities such as eliminating or reducing transcription costs simply fine-tune existing processes that occur within a physician or practice office. These activities are categorized as *Level 1* efficiencies, if they streamline existing activities without generating significant changes in workflow within the office. Providing timely and relevant information to a HCP, to help that HCP avoid ordering redundant or unnecessary tests, is another example of a Level 1 solution. This information helps the physician make care delivery decisions during a patient visit, without making significant changes in the process of delivering that care.

Using an EHR system to facilitate communication within a care team could generate *Level 2* efficiencies. For example, the new types of communication could support the development of new models of team care within an office practice. In this situation, the EHR serves as a tool to support reengineering of the process for delivering care. The federal website, healthit.gov (2017), emphasizes the importance of workflow redesign for successful EHR implementation and provides resources to guide this process.

Using EHR data to develop predictive models that identify patients who are at risk for developing significant health problems could generate *Level 3* efficiencies. If the ability to identify at-risk patients supports implementation of strategies to prevent those health problems from actually occurring, the new strategies could help move the US healthcare system from its current focus on "curing" health conditions to "preventing" those conditions. This type of system redesign creates Level 3 efficiencies.

Efficiencies generated from primary and secondary uses of data can potentially occur at all three levels. Table 7.1 provides an overview of examples of Levels 1, 2, and 3 efficiencies that may be generated by primary and secondary uses of data.

Transforming Healthcare

The notion that widespread adoption of EHR systems will support innovation at all three levels is important. The implications of this idea are explored in the thoughtful and interesting book, *The Innovator's Prescription*. Christensen, Grossman, and Hwang (2009) argued that significant systems-level reengineering is needed to accomplish the goals of reducing healthcare costs and strengthening the quality of healthcare. Christensen et al. (2009) argued that it is important to recognize that "healthcare" is not a homogeneous set of activities. Instead, it is useful to think about an array of healthcare activities on a spectrum from intuitive to precision medicine.

---

[2] For a discussion of the application of these ideas in a healthcare setting, see Quality improvement: Boon or boondoggle? By Paterson, Mary A., Wendel, Jeanne, Hospital Topics, 00185868, Fall94, Vol. 72, Issue 4.

Table 7.1 Types of efficiencies potentially generated by EHR systems

Solution type	Primary use of data	Secondary use of data
Level 1	HCP uses EHR system for convenient access to information: To reduce duplicate tests, by reviewing existing test results To deliver evidence-based care by reviewing relevant guideline information prior to prescribing tests, drugs, or treatments	HCP analyzes patient data to identify issues associated with a low score on a quality performance measure and fine-tunes office procedures to address these issues ACO analyzes EHR data, to reduce inappropriate ER use by identifying locations for new clinics
Level 2	Large primary care practice uses EHR to support coordination among members of the care team	Third-party vendor uses EHR data to generate quality measures, and reports the measures to CMS to compute payment adjustments under MACRA
Level 3	EHR supports and documents protocol-based care delivered by nurse practitioner, to facilitate coordination with HCP. EHR system in primary care practice facilitates coordination between the healthcare providers and organizations that provide social service (e.g., housing assistance, food stamps, energy assistance)	HMO applies predictive modeling strategies to EHR data, to identify patients at risk for a costly medical condition ACO analyzes paid claim data to understand ambulatory care utilization and physician decisions prior to hospital admissions for ambulatory care sensitive conditions Researchers use EHR data analyze a range of issues: Demographic and health characteristics associated with inappropriate ER use Factors associated with racial differences in health outcomes (e.g., physician decision-making, patient utilization decisions, or restrictions imposed by insurers) Cost-effectiveness and comparative effectiveness analyses

Activities such as the diagnosis and treatment of strep throat are categorized as *precision medicine*. Activities in this category meet three criteria:

1. The strategy for diagnosing the condition is well-defined.
2. Once the condition is diagnosed, the strategy for treating the condition is well-defined.
3. The treatment does not require significant behavior modification or complex (or long-term) at-home management by the patient.

Diagnosis and treatment of conditions that do not meet the first two criteria are categorized as *intuitive medicine*. These activities require the healthcare provider to apply significant medical knowledge and understanding to develop a diagnosis and manage the treatment plan. Treatment of conditions that do not meet the third criteria differs from the intuitive medicine category, because these treatments also require significant patient participation.

Health information technology, including EHR systems, is expected to support the development of new types of efficiencies in areas of the healthcare that deliver precision medicine. For conditions such as strep throat, EHR systems can support protocol-driven diagnostic and treatment procedures. This innovation, by itself, generates a Level 1 efficiency when the HCP uses the EHR to provide protocol-based information. However, increased use of protocol-driven procedures for diagnosing and treating strep throat then provides additional data to the system and could support additional changes with the HCP, as information about best practices is disseminated directly through the EHR system. The HCP might decide to hire a nurse practitioner to deliver protocol-driven care to provide precision medicine for some types of patients. This would allow the physician to focus on providing care for patients with more complex issues who require intuitive medicine. In the language of workflow analysts, the physician would spend more time practicing "top of his license" rather than spending time with patients with less complex conditions (Friedberg et al., 2014). This reengineering of the office processes would generate a Level 2 efficiency.

In addition, entrepreneurs might open retail clinics in which protocol-driven care is delivered by nurse practitioners outside a HCP office. These retail clinics operate in large retail stores such as the MinuteClinics operated by CVS. They provide a defined set of precision medicine services and treatments (e.g., sports physicals, vaccinations, and treatment for strep throat). The clinic model differs from the typical HCP practice model in several ways: these clinics post the price for each service and treatment, prices are typically substantially below the rates charged by HCPs, the clinics offer extended hours, and they do not require appointments. Christensen et al. (2009) argue that competition from new types of healthcare providers is an essential component of the larger health system reengineering process.

The potential impacts of EHR support for protocol-driven diagnosis and treatment of strep throat provide a straightforward example of the range of impacts anticipated by policy-makers. Other innovations anticipated by policy-makers are more complex. These innovations include fine-tuning and redesigning processes within practices to generate Level 1 and Level 2 efficiencies that ensure consistent delivery of evidence-based care (Kellermann & Jones, 2013). Kellermann and Jones (2013) also argued that these efficiencies will be triggered by combining EHR adoption with quality-based payment incentives and that these efficiencies will focus on treatment of healthcare conditions that meet the criteria for precision medicine.

In addition, it is useful to understand that precision and intuitive medicine are not distinct binary categories. Instead, each category represents a wide spectrum of medical activities. There is a broad area between the two categories that can be supported with *empirical medicine*. This term, *empirical medicine*, refers to large-scale efforts to apply pattern recognition techniques to EHR data to identify best practices. This secondary use of data from EHRs is intended to help professionals in specific medical fields develop and follow standardized treatment protocols, to increase the degree to which healthcare is "evidence-based." These efforts can potentially expand the set of healthcare activities that can be completed by non-physician professionals such as nurse practitioners.

Use of IT systems to generate Level 2 efficiencies through process reengineering (and to trigger subsequent Level 3 efficiencies through larger systems redesign efforts) is not unique to the healthcare industries. Advocates for subsidies to boost EHR adoption and utilization, and for quality-based payment incentives to complement the EHR strategy, point to significant efficiencies generated outside the healthcare industry. Brynjolfsson and Hitt (2003) used firm-level data on 527 large US firms to estimate the impact of IT adoption on efficiency gains outside the healthcare industry during years following substantial computerization (from 1987 to 1994). These authors conclude that computerization generated first-year benefits that were approximately equal to the cost of purchasing and implementing the computer systems. Over the following 5–7 years, however, computerization generated benefits that were five times the magnitudes of the first-year benefits. These authors explain this finding as follows:

> Computers are best described as a general-purpose technology whose primary contribution is to make new production methods possible when combined with complementary investments such as new work systems, organizational redesign, and business process reengineering These changes, in turn, yield substantial productivity improvements and perhaps even structural changes in the economy over longer periods of time.
>
> … Rather than merely substituting a cheaper input (e.g., computers) for another input (e.g., labor) in the context of a fixed production process, companies can combine computers with other innovations to fundamentally change their production processes.

Applying this logic and evidence to the process of computerization in the healthcare industry suggests that the EHR system will not – by itself – generate significant net benefits. Instead, the EHR system is a tool to support process fine-tuning to generate Level 1 efficiencies, process redesign to generate Level 2 efficiencies, and system redesign to generate Level 3 efficiencies. Healthcare provider organizations (including managed care organizations, patient-centered medical homes, and accountable care organizations), public health agencies, and competing entrepreneurs (such as retail clinics) will develop these innovations. Large payers are attempting to incentivize and reward these efforts through quality-based payment systems.

Impacts on HCPs

While HCPs may applaud some of these anticipated changes and decry others (Benin et al., 2005; Friedberg et al., 2014; Hersh et al., 2013), the use of EHR is incentivized in federal law and in Medicare payment policy. The Affordable Care Act (ACA) defined a process for accountable care organizations to provide care for panels of Medicare patients, CMS announced an intention to place increasing emphasis on value-based payment (VBP), and the 2015 Medicare Access and CHIP Reauthorization Act (MACRA) detailed the legal framework for the CMS quality-based payments.

Under MACRA, physicians face quality-based payment adjustments that are scheduled to begin at 4% in 2019 and increase to 9% in 2022 (Arend, 2017; CMS, 2017a; CMS, 2017b). Exceptional performers, with quality scores in the top 25%, may earn additional bonuses up to 10% (The National Council, 2017. Healthcare providers who treat significant numbers of patients covered by Medicare will either work under the Merit-Based Incentive Payment System (MIPS) or the Advanced Alternative Payment Models (AAPM). It is expected that most psychologists will work under MIPS. MIPS includes four components:

- Performance on quality measures will have an initial weight of 60% in the payment adjustment metric, which will decrease to 30% in subsequent years. These required reporting measures are expected to be a subset of the Physician Quality Reporting System measures.
- Resource utilization will have a weight of 30% after the transition period.
- The Advancing Care Information (ACI) performance category replaces the Meaningful Use metrics that measured the intensity with which providers were using health information systems. This category will have a weight of 25%.
- Improvement activities have a weight of 15%. Providers will select a small number of measures from a list of over 90 measures. This category includes eight mental/behavioral health measures, which are listed in Table 7.2.

Behavioral healthcare providers may be impacted by these incentives in two settings. First, clinical psychologists who treat patients covered by Medicare will begin reporting quality measures in 2019 and will be impacted by payment adjustments beginning in 2021. Second, psychologists working in integrated care settings will be working to help primary care and other HCPs achieve quality goals. HCPs will begin reporting quality measures in 2017, and they will be impacted by payment adjustments beginning in 2019. EHR systems will provide essential infrastructure to support practice-level efforts to strengthen performance on the quality metrics, compute and report the quality measures, and implement ongoing quality improvement strategies.

Psychologists in Independent Practices

Behavioral psychologists working in independent practices will report metrics included in the four MIPS categories, and they will be impacted by the resulting payment adjustments. Their EHR systems will also function as important tools for computing and reporting these measures. These psychologists will also rely on electronic records to strengthen performance on the quality measures and resource measures, demonstrate performance on the ACI measures, and support performance on the measures of Improvement Activities. Larger practices may employ analysts or consultants to implement secondary uses of data, to identify gaps in the application of guideline-based care and patient utilization patterns, and to test whether quality improvement initiatives actually lead to improvements in measured quality

Table 7.2 Improvement activities (MACRA): behavioral and mental health

Activity name (weight)
1. *Implementation of co-location PCP (Primary Medical-Care Provider) and MH services (high)*
Integration facilitation and promotion of the co-location of mental health services in primary and/or non-primary clinical care settings
2. *Implementation of integrated PCBH model (high)*
Offer integrated behavioral health services to support patients with behavioral health needs, dementia, and poorly controlled chronic conditions that could include one or more of the following: Use evidence-based treatment protocols and treatment to goal where appropriate Use evidence-based screening and case finding strategies to identify individuals at risk and in need of services Ensure regular communication and coordinated workflows between eligible clinicians in primary care and behavioral health Conduct regular case reviews for at-risk or unstable patients and those who are not responding to treatment Use of a registry or certified health information technology functionality to support active care management and outreach to patients in treatment and/or integrate behavioral health and medical care plans and facilitate integration through co-location of services when feasible
3. *Depression screening (medium)*
Depression screening and follow-up plan: Regular engagement of MIPS eligible clinicians or groups in integrated prevention and treatment interventions, including depression screening and follow-up plan for patients with co-occurring conditions of behavioral or mental health conditions
4. *Diabetes screening (medium)*
Diabetes screening for people with schizophrenia or bipolar disease who are using antipsychotic medication
5. *Electronic health record enhancements for BH data capture (medium)*
Enhancements to an electronic health record to capture additional data on behavioral health (BH) populations and use that data for additional decision-making purposes (e.g., capture of additional BH data results in additional depression screening for at-risk patient not previously identified)
6. *MDD prevention and treatment interventions (medium)*
Major depressive disorder: Regular engagement of MIPS eligible clinicians or groups in integrated prevention and treatment interventions, including suicide risk assessment for mental health patients with co-occurring conditions of behavioral or mental health conditions
7. *Tobacco use (medium)*
Tobacco use: Regular engagement of MIPS eligible clinicians or groups in integrated prevention and treatment interventions, including tobacco use screening and cessation interventions for patients with co-occurring conditions of behavioral or mental health and at-risk factors for tobacco dependence
8. *Unhealthy alcohol use (medium)*
Unhealthy alcohol use: Regular engagement of MIPS eligible clinicians or groups in integrated prevention and treatment interventions, including screening and brief counseling for patients with co-occurring conditions of behavioral or mental health conditions

Source: https://qpp.cms.gov/mips/improvement-activities (CMS, 2017c)

(HealthIT.gov, 2013). Careful multivariate statistical analysis of the EHR data can help provider organizations identify opportunities for improvement, target improvement efforts to situations with high potential impact, and develop strategies for measuring impacts. Notably, McCullough, Parente, and Town (2013) concluded that health information technology did not generate a significant reduction in mortality for most hospital patients; however it did generate a significant mortality reduction for patients with complex conditions. Identifying subsets of patients that are likely to benefit from improvement processes is an essential component of efforts to generate measurable quality improvements. EHR data is needed to support this type of econometric analysis.

Psychologists Working in Integrated Care

For psychologists working in integrated care, MACRA offers an opportunity to demonstrate a clear business case and healthcare quality case for HCPs to employ or partner with psychologists. For physicians treating significant numbers of patients covered by Medicare, the difference between a potential bonus of 9% or a potential penalty of 9% could represent a significant dollar amount. Successful integrated care providers that help a HCP achieve quality goals could strengthen patient health while also contributing to the financial stability of the practice.

Achieving the dual miracles of improved healthcare quality and decreased healthcare costs requires profound and innovative transformation of healthcare work processes. IT is a tool that can help support existing work processes, but its transformative capabilities will only occur once HCPs understand its use in enough depth to create new practices that are only possible with technology. For example, WalMart could have used IT as a tool to support its existing methods of purchasing inventory for its stores, using reports to view product purchase levels, call vendors and place orders when inventory of a certain product became low. Historically, inventory management was a reactive process – organizations ordered new items when products sold out or were close to selling out. WalMart transformed the inventory management process by using IT to create a new proactive process. Instead of contacting vendors personally, the Walmart computer systems calculated the anticipated demand for products at each location, gained online access to their vendor's systems so that IT could scan vendor inventory of products and their prices, and then ordered the products in real time from vendors offering low cost and high quality, without any human intervention (Lee, 2002). This type of process transformation offers low prices to consumers, but it is not possible without IT, and it is not accomplished by simply automating existing processes or replacing inventory clerks with computers who perform the same tasks. Instead, it requires fundamental process redesign.

The next section describes in more detail the progression and evolution of EHRs, focusing on the data that is currently stored in the systems. HCPs need to understand how data is stored in order to facilitate better use of IT to transform healthcare processes.

Electronic Health Record Data

Many EHR systems grew from practice management systems that focused on billing and claims activities (AMA, 2014). The original stakeholders of practice management systems were the back-office administrative personnel whose workflow and practices are significantly different from workflows that characterize the clinical processes for delivering care (Colligan, Potts, Finn, & Sinkin, 2015). The original practice management systems served a small set of stakeholders (administrative personnel and payers) who required accurate coding to support billing. Procedure and diagnostic codes were captured in *standardized and structured formats* intended primarily for billing (Bowman, 2005). Three sets of codes were developed to capture reasons for hospital admission (diagnosis-related groups (DRGs), patient diagnoses (International Classification of Diseases (ICD-9 or ICD-10)), and medical procedures (Current Procedural Terminology (CPT)). These coding systems were originally designed to standardize the business aspects of healthcare while also allowing for some standardization of care records (Colligan et al., 2015; de Lusignan, 2005). "Standardization" in this case means that the codes identified for billing are relatively predictable and consistent across healthcare practices.

Some healthcare data, such as blood pressure or cholesterol level, is stored as structured data. Once an appropriate unit of measure is determined, this data can be analyzed within standard metrics and ranges. If it is possible to predict in advance the type of data that will be gathered (a date, set of numbers, a combination of letters and numbers), the size of the data (number of characters either exactly or within a defined size range), and the meaning of the data, then that data can be stored as *structured* data (Hoffer, Venkataraman, & Topi, 2015). Other data, such as healthcare provider notes, a picture, or a fax of a test result, are unstructured. With *unstructured* data, it may not be possible to predict in advance the type, size, or meaning of the data (Baars & Kemper, 2008).

HCPs may (or may not) depend upon DRG, ICD-10, or CPT codes for the clinical treatment of patients. Instead, they may rely on the patient chart to understand the patient's health (Petrakaki, Klecun, & Cornford, 2016; Swinglehurst & Greenhalgh, 2015). This patient chart is a text-based document which uses data in an *unstructured* format to describe the clinical treatment of a patient. For example, instead of coding a patient with coronary heart disease using a pre-defined numeric system (i.e., structured, standardized data), each HCP might use his/her own unstructured text to provide more detailed data. The HCP might note that he/she found "raised cardiac enzymes," "myocardial ischemia," "triple vessel coronary artery disease," or "myocardial infarction" rather than selecting a code number pre-defined within a coding and classification system (de Lusignan, 2005). Before EHR systems, that patient chart was written or transcribed. It could use variable terms and formats and could convey nuanced information using data about the time frame when symptoms were presented (i.e., yesterday or 6 months ago), the relative severity of symptoms, ideas about the possible etiology of the disease, and behavioral data directly related to the symptoms (lack of exercise, smoking, diet) (Bowman, 2013; Swinglehurst & Greenhalgh, 2015).

When practice management billing systems were repurposed to capture medical care-related data for healthcare rather than simply supporting billing and accounting processes, these required more precise coding of medically related data (de Lusignan, 2005). The act of coding medical data for the purpose of medical care not only changed the purpose of the EHR system but also changed the processes followed by HCPs (Swinglehurst & Greenhalgh, 2015). This meant that an uncertain diagnosis, or a set of potential diagnoses, might be treated as more certain than initially intended (Varpio et al., 2015). Creating a code and assigning it to a medical record could imply unwarranted (and unintended) assertions about diagnostic certainty (Swinglehurst & Greenhalgh, 2015).

HCPs are now documenting their diagnoses and care through structured data entered via templates in EHR systems (Swinglehurst, Greenhalgh, & Roberts, 2012). The ICD-10 codes created for billing are inadequate for the detailed granularity of data required for the clinical care of a patient (Bowman, 2005), so HCPs are also documenting their work through unstructured, non-standardized text in physician's notes and summaries of findings. The data collected in the EHR is supposed to serve as the single source of reference for patient care while also continuing to support billing and accounting (AMA, 2014). Thus, the data stored in an EHR includes both structured, standardized data that is primarily used for billing and external reporting, and unstructured, non-standardized data that is used to deliver healthcare to patients.

What Data Is Stored in an EHR?

An EHR is categorized as "basic" or "comprehensive" by the data it stores and the analysis, communication, and reporting tools offered to providers (Jha et al., 2009). The types of stored data are grouped into four broad categories as shown in Table 7.3. The first, clinical documentation, focuses on data stored in the system that will be generated by the HCP who enters the data for a patient within the EHR. The second and third sets of data, test and imaging results and computerized provider order entry, typically support communication across providers or across provider organizations. Data in the category, computerized provider-order entry, provides a history of tests and medications ordered by the HCP. These orders can be transmitted electronically to the entities that will conduct the tests or fill the prescriptions. The outcomes of these lab tests and imaging orders are stored in the category, test and imaging results. The last category, decision support, contains some data that might be generated by the initiating HCP (the HCP will likely enter information about the goals for the patient), while other data, such as alerts and reminders, will be generated by the EHR. Compared with the elements included in a basic EHR, the CEHRT-2015 standards require clinical documentation for a different set of information, they place more emphasis on CPOE and less on storage for test and imaging results, and they place more emphasis on decision support (ONC, 2016a).

Table 7.3 EHR data

Data requirement by system	Comprehensive EHR (Jha et al., 2009)	Basic EHR	CEHRT-2014	CEHRT-2015
Clinical documentation				
Patient demographics	X	X	Some data	Some data
Problem lists	X	X	X	X
Medication lists	X	X	X	X
Discharge summaries	X	X		
Advanced directives	X			
Physician notes	X			
Nursing assessments	X			
Unique device identifiers for patient's implantable device				X
Immunizations				X
Test and imaging results				
Vital signs	X	X	X	X
Laboratory reports	X	X		
Radiologic reports	X	X		
Diagnostic test results	X	X		
Radiologic images	X			
Diagnostic test images	X			
Consultant reports	X			
Computerized provider-order entry				
Medications	X	X	X	X
Laboratory tests	X		X	X
Radiologic tests	X		X	X
Consultation requests	X			X
Nursing orders	X			X
Decision support				
Clinical guidelines	X			
Clinical reminders	X			
Drug-allergy alerts	X		X	
Drug-drug interaction alerts	X			
Drug-dose support	X			
Assessment and plan of treatment				X
Goals				X
Health concerns				X

Adapted from Jha et al. (2009), ONC (2016a)

A key difference between a comprehensive and basic EHR, as well as the requirements for a certified EHR, is the storage of unstructured vs. structured data. A basic EHR stores data that can be structured, such as medication orders, into well-defined data types with pre-defined sizes and ranges of data, while the data in a comprehensive EHR will most likely include unstructured and non-standardized data, such as physician notes.

How Are Data Stored in an EHR?

The distinction between structured and unstructured data is important because the two types of data yield very different responses when trying to access, aggregate, or summarize the data. The primary reason is that it is difficult to locate specific data within stored unstructured data. For example, if you store a person's name in structured data, it is possible for a computer to search through a series of names quickly to identify the name you are seeking. If you store that same person's name in an unstructured document, like a photo of a fax, it will not be possible for a computer to quickly search through multiple pictures and identify which name matches the one you are seeking. Structured data is stored in separate rows and columns with a pre-defined data type and size in a database that can be accessed programmatically through a standard programming language such as the Structured Query Language (SQL). Unstructured data is typically stored as text or a "picture" of data that cannot be subdivided readily into its component parts. Computer science researchers are working to develop strategies to extract structured data from unstructured documents. A continuous stream of new tools are being created and patented, but it remains a difficult and inconsistent process (Felix, Pandey, & Bertini, 2017; McCallum, 2005).

By default, therefore, EHR systems encourage creating structured data out of unstructured text to facilitate better data standardization and reporting. This results in two issues related to the implementation and use of EHRs: (1) EHRs have decreased the efficiency of some HCPs providing healthcare using traditional processes; and (2) studies do not show consistent increases in quality of care after implementation of an EHR. We discuss those issues in the next section.

Issues in the Implementation and Use of EHR

The rapid implementation of EHR in the USA, and the significant level of government involvement in that implementation, has contributed to the identification of issues related to the effective use of IT to support clinical healthcare practices (Adler-Milstein, Embi, Middleton, Sarkar, & Smith, 2017; Colligan, Sinsky, Goeders, Schmidt-Bowman, & Tutty, 2016; Sinsky et al., 2016). Two of the key issues related to the general implementation and use of EHR are discussed in the next two subsections, while the third subsection discusses issues directly pertinent to HCPs working within an integrated care setting.

EHR Has Decreased the Productivity of Some HCPs

Recent research shows that the use of EHR in clinical practices has decreased the productivity and efficiency of some healthcare professionals (Colligan et al., 2016; Hill, Sears, & Melanson, 2013; Sinsky et al., 2016). One time-and-motion study of 57 US physicians found that for every 1 h of direct clinical face time with patients, the physicians spent almost 2 h of time on EHR and "desk work" after meeting with the patient (Sinsky et al., 2016). This study used direct observation of physicians rather than relying on physician reporting, so the observations are independent of participant bias. Of that almost 2 h of extra time, the physicians spent 59% of the time using an EHR. Notably, that study also reported that 37% of the physician-patient face time was spent looking at the computer screen. The researchers suggest that more documentation support through dictation or assistant services could help decrease the amount of physician time spent using the EHR (Sinsky et al., 2016).

Another study tracked the number of mouse clicks performed by 16 different HCPs to process the EHR requirements for each patient within an emergency department of one facility using a single system from one EHR vendor (Hill et al., 2013). The researchers found that 160 mouse clicks were required, on average, to process the EHR requirements for a given patient. They documented that it took 6 mouse clicks to order a 325 mg aspirin and 227 mouse clicks to document an examination of right upper quadrant abdominal pain. Of course, there was much variation among patients depending on the type of order entry required, but the researchers estimated that HCPs working a 10-h shift performed about 4000 mouse clicks (Hill et al., 2013). Other studies surveying HCPs have noted that it takes longer to enter the data (28 clicks for a Pap smear) than it does to actually perform some procedures (Colligan et al., 2016). Surveys of HCPs have identified the time it takes to enter data into an EHR as one of the major sources of dissatisfaction and stress with the job (Babbott et al., 2014; Colligan et al., 2016; Friedberg et al., 2014).

An evaluation of the issues with EHR systems conducted by the American Medical Association (AMA) indicates that much of the data entry conducted in current EHR systems is performed by physicians, which has changed the workflow and organizational practices in many healthcare groups (AMA, 2014). One qualitative study of physician notes in an emergency department examined the pre-, during, and post-EHR time required to complete the notes (Park, Lee, & Chen, 2012). They found that the division of labor among nurses, residents, and attending physicians was changed through the introduction of an EHR. With paper charts, the work load was split more evenly among the three groups of HCPs, but after introduction of an EHR system, the residents did most of the data entry work, increasing the amount of time it took to document work by three or four times for that one type of HCP. In addition, they also found that overall it took more time to use an EHR than to complete a paper-based patient record. This is consistent with survey results indicating that physicians believe that their productivity has been negatively impacted (Colligan et al., 2016). However, there are few pre- and post-studies that compare time spent on administrative work or charting prior to the implementation of an EHR system, so it is difficult to evaluate accurately the impact of the EHR on HCP productivity.

Mixed Results About the Relationship of Care Quality and Use of EHR

Studies of the relationship between healthcare quality and the use of EHR have demonstrated mixed results (Lau, Kuziemsky, Price, & Gardner, 2010). Numerous studies have attempted to understand the relationship between the quality of care and the use of EHR in a variety of healthcare environments; hence researchers have undertaken meta-analyses of these studies (Bardhan & Thouin, 2013; Campanella et al., 2015; Moja et al., 2014; Nuckols et al., 2014). The results of these meta-analyses are also mixed. Some have found no relationship, while others have found a moderate relationship between care quality and the use of EHR. It seems to depend on the type of care quality and the functionality of the EHR used for comparison. The studies performed by Campanella et al., 2015 and Nuckols et al., 2014 provided evidence that the use of EHR can improve the quality of healthcare, especially reducing medication errors and adverse drug effects, while Moja and his colleagues (Moja et al., 2014) found no impact between computerized decision support (a part of EHR systems) and mortality. However, McCullough et al. (2013) provide a caution regarding interpretation of the results of this type of study. These authors report that hospital EHR use did not significantly impact average mortality, but it did significantly reduce mortality for the subset of patients with complex health conditions.

Some of these studies are using relatively old data (Bardhan & Thouin, 2013 rely on data gathered from 2004 to 2006) without considering the potential lag between the implementation of IT and the impact of the results of IT. Most of the studies do not incorporate data that could help us understand the social or cultural context of the implementation and instead look for simple effects of one variable on another. For example, none of the studies discussed above describe whether IT helped transform or even change the processes of the organization, so we are forced to assume that most organizations simply tried to use EHRs in exactly the same way as the traditional paper charts. However, Holroyd-Leduc, Lorenzetti, Straus, Sykes, and Quan (2011) reviewed studies that estimated impact of EHR use on process measures and – separately – on outcome measures. These authors report that some studies report significant impacts of EHR on process measures such as proportions of patients completing cancer screenings.

Table 7.4 Final set of measures considered for inclusion in EHR

Measures	Sociodemographic	Psychosocial	Health Behaviors
Recommended	Residential address for geocoding Race/ethnicity Education Overall financial resource strain	Stress Depression Social connections/isolation Intimate partner violence	Physical activity Tobacco use Alcohol use
Not ready for implementation	Country of origin Food insufficiency Housing insecurity Employment	Anxiety Conscientiousness Optimism Patient engagement Self-efficacy Stress in childhood Sexual identity	Dietary pattern Health literacy Sexual behavior

Matthews et al. (2016)

Issues in the Implementation and Use of EHR for Integrated Care

With the advent of more integrated care environments, EHR systems are being modified to include behavioral health data. The next subsections describe the new behavioral health data that may be stored in the EHR, how EHR systems will change to incorporate the new behavioral health data, how workplace processes will change, and the privacy considerations of including behavioral health data in an EHR.

What Behavioral Health Data Should Be Stored in the EHR?

According to the Summary Report of Findings for the Behavioral Health Roundtable held in September 2012, "the ONC aims to coordinate the adoption and use of health IT to support the broader objectives of integrating behavioral health and primary care" (RTI International, 2013). As part of the coordination effort, the ONC is guiding the discussion with the National Academies of Medicine (formerly the Institute of Medicine) about the data related to behavioral health that should be stored in the EHR. Table 7.4 is the set of data/measures determined from phase 2 of this effort considered for inclusion in the EHR (Matthews, Adler, Forrest, & Stead, 2016).

The data that were considered "not ready for implementation" did not have enough research to support its usefulness in clinical practice, was not defined using a standard measure, or was not considered by the committee to be "actionable" in with the sense that there was no consensus on the "acceptable range" (Matthews et al., 2016).

A challenge with storing the recommended data displayed in Table 7.4 is that there are few standardized measures accepted uniformly throughout the behavioral healthcare profession (Adler & Stead, 2015). On a relatively simple level, for example, imagine a university where ethnicity and race are collected using different codes in different systems. Some of the systems record only a few ethnicity categories, so that a large number of individuals are recorded in the category of "other," while other systems at the university store information on a detailed set of ethnicity categories. In this situation, it is not feasible to consolidate that data across differing systems, without losing the detail stored in the more comprehensive systems. On a more complex level, there are many different ways to evaluate "depression" including the Center for Epidemiologic Studies Depression Scale, the Beck Depression Inventory, the Patient Health Questionnaire (PHQ-9 or PHQ-2), and the PROMIS-8 (Matthews et al., 2016). In order to record that data as part of an EHR, it would be necessary to select a preferred scale or create a way to link/crosswalk the different measures. The selection of a preferred scale is important because this decision standardizes the procedure for measuring depression, privileges the results from that measure, and affects how people are evaluated and how new HCPs are taught to work with that data and that scale (Greenhalgh, Potts, Wong, Bark, & Swinglehurst, 2009; Hall et al., 2015).

In addition to the data listed in Table 7.4, some are considering the need to include patient-generated health data to engage patients more closely in integrated care (Adler-Milstein et al., 2017). Data produced from devices such as network-connected smart weight scales, smartphones, Fitbits, and diabetic insulin pumps could all be considered "patient-generated" because these data points are derived from devices located outside of the HCP's office. This data is not typically included as part of the formal EHR, but it may be in the future, if it is found to be helpful for the full integration patient care (Adler-Milstein et al., 2017). Patient-generated health data could support more accurate measurement of some of the data recommended in Table 7.4 (such as physical activity) or the data that is "not ready for implementation" (such as dietary patterns).

This behavioral and patient-generated data is not defined by the formal standards and structured formats that are accepted across EHR systems (Matthews et al., 2016). Thus, HCPs who are adding patient-generated data into existing systems may have to change the format or content of the data in the future, to support more interoperability of systems or data collection for research and public health (Cifuentes et al., 2015).

How Should EHR Systems Change to Support Integrated Care?

Entering new behavioral data in an EHR typically requires modification of the current templates in the EHR system. Templates are used to enter data, perform error checking, and provide flags regarding HCP protocol for EHR systems (Swinglehurst et al., 2012). A study found that EHR systems generally lacked standard templates to document the additional inputs of the new behavioral data into structured fields (Cifuentes et al., 2015). This is not surprising since behavioral health and medical care differ in their "language, classifications, codes, data, reporting requirements, and regulations" (Cifuentes et al., 2015). For example, traditional mental healthcare may document HCP notes in long narrative form, focusing on telling the person's story, while integrated behavioral and primary healthcare will likely document those notes as focused on a specific problem, intervention, and follow-up plan within a relatively structured data field for physician's notes (Hall et al., 2015).

In addition to new templates for data entry and error checking, new forms of decision support tools are also necessary. Care coordination requires immediate communication with other members of the team either directly or through the data available in the EHR. Decision support tools should provide the longitudinal information necessary to support care decision-making. This information could be displayed in a patient dashboard that included important indicators of patient health over time, rather than a single point in time, as it is displayed in many current EHR systems (O'Malley, Draper, Gourevitch, Cross, & Scholle, 2015). Other suggestions for changes in the decision support features of an EHR system include (Cifuentes et al., 2015; Hall et al., 2015; O'Malley et al., 2015):

- Care plans with agreed upon goals, steps to reach those goals, as well as changes in the care plan over time
- "Huddle" sheets and pre-visit planning tools that can be populated with important patient data
- Patient registry
- Lists of patients who have related needs in order to form potential subgroups, such as patient management, grief counseling, or diabetes diet management
- Individual, customizable patient dashboard formats
- Lists of high-risk patients
- Measurement feedback systems
- Customizable aggregate/summary reports

Modifying EHR systems to support integrated care processes will require (1) more participation on the part of HCPs specializing in behavioral health, (2) a process for modifying the existing EHR systems, and (3) a willingness on the part of EHR vendors to place increasing focus on issues important to integrated care (Bruns, Hyde, Sather, Hook, & Lyon, 2016; Lyon et al., 2016). HCPs need to understand the technology, so they can change both their processes and the technology used to transform their work practices. For example, HCP input will help structure the new templates, identify variables that must be defined to support quality measurement, and specify valuable communication flows within integrated care teams.

What Organizational Changes Might Be Triggered by EHR Use in Integrated Care?

In an integrated care setting, an EHR system is expected not only to standardize the way data related to behavioral health is stored but also to contribute to enhanced communication among HCPs from a variety of different backgrounds (O'Malley et al., 2015). Some authors anticipate that using an EHR for both documentation and communication in integrated care will lead to better healthcare outcomes but will require organizational changes to achieve those improved outcomes (Bae, Hockenberry, Rask, & Becker, 2017; Matthews et al., 2016). Organizational changes may include greater standardization of documentation such as the continuity of care document (CCD) so that it can be understood by different types of HCPs to avoid double documentation and duplicate data entry (Cifuentes et al., 2015). In addition, there should be agreement among HCPs on the standard protocols used to enter data through templates to facilitate more consistency among data stored (RTI International, 2013). Since much of the data is entered as unstructured text, organizations might have to consider employing additional types of personnel such as medical scribes to accompany HCPs and enter data more quickly and accurately into the EHR (Gellert, Ramirez, & Webster, 2015). Another important organizational issue to consider is to determine who is responsible for follow-up with patients. Since patients may be seen by multiple HCPs, there should be a clear definition of who is ultimately responsible for responding to the alerts generated from the EHR (Cifuentes et al., 2015). A final change to consider is who in the practice is ultimately responsible for the accuracy of the EHR. Since data in the EHR is considered a legal document, the overall accuracy must be reviewed by a HCP (RTI International, 2013). Coordinating care among multiple people requires that HCPs determine which practitioners are reviewing the EHR for accuracy and correctly and legally signing off on each document (Cifuentes et al., 2015).

What Are the Privacy Issues Involved in Incorporating Behavioral Data in the EHR?

Incorporating behavioral-related data into the EHR elevates risk and privacy concerns for all HCPs (Hoerbst & Ammenwerth, 2010). Primary care HCPs should be educated about federal behavioral health privacy regulations. For example, the Federal Confidentiality of Alcohol and Drug Abuse Patient Records regulations specify the conditions and requirements of disclosure of patient information regarding substance abuse treatment programs. Primary care HCPs may know that these regulations require patient consent to share substance abuse treatment information, but they may not know that the regulations also prohibit re-disclosure without re-consent (RTI International, 2013). Many EHR vendors do not have a way to specify privacy settings for different types of data, making it impossible to disclose some data and not disclose other data in the database.

Patient-generated health data (PGHD) introduces additional privacy and legality concerns. If this data is entered into the EHR, then a HCP must attest to its validity as part of the EHR legal document. However, PGHD is not currently protected by HIPAA, and the incorporation of its use into medical care will require new policies and protection strategies (Adler-Milstein et al., 2017).

Conclusion

While EHR system limitations have come under increasing scrutiny from policy-makers, this technology is now an established tool in healthcare provider organizations (Leventhal, 2017). It is an essential tool for storing information, facilitating communication, and computing and reporting quality measures. However, behavioral psychologists may find that the systems that are currently available are not well-suited to supporting work processes traditionally used by many HCPs. This may be particularly true for behavioral psychologists, because this segment of HCPs does not have a history of high utilization of EHR systems. Fortunately, the process of improving these tools is underway.

Some HCPs may assume that the responsibility for improving the quality of EHR systems should and would be shouldered by IT professionals. However, it is clear that HCPs, including behavioral psychologists, can make important contributions to the process of shaping EHR systems into useful and user-friendly tools that support efficient delivery of high-quality healthcare. It is also clear that health information technology, by itself, will not deliver the twin "miracles" of strengthening quality and reducing per capita healthcare costs. Instead, this technology offers infrastructure to support efforts by providers and provider organizations to transform the US healthcare system. Much of the heavy lifting required to change the system will be undertaken by proactive and innovative healthcare providers.

References

Adler, N. E., & Stead, W. W. (2015). Patients in context—EHR capture of social and behavioral determinants of health. *Obstetrical & Gynecological Survey, 70*(6), 388–390.

Adler-Milstein, J., & Bates, D. W. (2010). Paperless Healthcare: Progress and Challenges of an IT-enabled Healthcare System. *Business Horizons, 53*(2), 119–130.

Adler-Milstein, J., Embi, P. J., Middleton, B., Sarkar, I. N., & Smith, J. (2017). Crossing the health IT chasm: Considerations and policy recommendations to overcome current challenges and enable value-based care. *Journal of the American Medical Informatics Association, 24*, 1036.

AMA. (2014). Improving care: Priorities to improve electronic health record usability. *American Medical Association*, 1–10.

Arend, E. (2017). *MACRA's quality payment project: What does it mean for your Agency's Medicare Reimbursement.* Retrieved from https://www.thenationalcouncil.org/wp-content/uploads/2016/08/MACRA-Quality-PP-web-Final.pdf

Baars, H., & Kemper, H.-G. (2008). Management support with structured and unstructured data—an integrated business intelligence framework. *Information Systems Management, 25*(2), 132–148.

Babbott, S., Manwell, L. B., Brown, R., Montague, E., Williams, E., Schwartz, M., … Linzer, M. (2014). Electronic medical records and physician stress in primary care: Results from the MEMO Study. *Journal of the American Medical Informatics Association, 21*(e1), e100–e106.

Bae, J., Hockenberry, J. M., Rask, K. J., & Becker, E. R. (2017). Evidence that electronic health records can promote physician counseling for healthy behaviors. *Health Care Management Review, 42*(3), 258–268.

Bardhan, I. R., & Thouin, M. F. (2013). Health information technology and its impact on the quality and cost of healthcare delivery. *Decision Support Systems, 55*(2), 438–449.

Benin, A. L., Vitkauskas, G., Thornquist, E., Shapiro, E. D., Concato, J., Aslan, M., & Krumholz, H. M. (2005). Validity of using an electronic medical record for assessing quality of care in an outpatient setting. *Medical Care, 43*(7), 691–698.

Blumenthal, D. (2009). Stimulating the Adoption of Health Information Technology. *New England Journal of Medicine, 360*(15), 1477–1479. https://doi.org/10.1056/NEJMp0901592

Bowman, S. (2005). *Coordination of SNOMED-CT and ICD-10: Getting the most out of electronic health record systems.* Retrieved from http://library.ahima.org/doc?oid=106578#.WWKJfIQrKUk

Bowman, S. (2013). Impact of electronic health record systems on information integrity: Quality and safety implications. *Perspectives in Health Information Management, 10*(Fall), 1c.

Bruns, E. J., Hyde, K. L., Sather, A., Hook, A. N., & Lyon, A. R. (2016). Applying user input to the design and testing of an electronic behavioral health information system for wraparound care coordination. *Administration and Policy in Mental Health and Mental Health Services Research, 43*(3), 350–368.

Brynjolfsson, E., & Hitt, L. M. (2003). Computing productivity: Firm-level evidence. *The Review of Economics and Statistics, 85*(4), 793–808.

Campanella, P., Lovato, E., Marone, C., Fallacara, L., Mancuso, A., Ricciardi, W., & Specchia, M. L. (2015). The impact of electronic health records on healthcare quality: A systematic review and meta-analysis. *The European Journal of Public Health, 26*, 60 ckv122.

CBO. (2008). *Evidence on the costs and benefits of health information technology*. (Pub. No. 2976). Washington: Congress of the United States Retrieved from http://www.cbo.gov/ftpdocs/91xx/doc9168/05-20-HealthIT.pdf.

Christensen, C. M., Grossman, J. H., & Hwang, J. (2009). *The innovator's prescription: A disruptive solution for health care*. New York, NY: McGraw-Hill.

Cifuentes, M., Davis, M., Fernald, D., Gunn, R., Dickinson, P., & Cohen, D. J. (2015). Electronic health record challenges, workarounds, and solutions observed in practices integrating behavioral health and primary care. *The Journal of the American Board of Family Medicine, 28*(Supplement 1), S63–S72.

CMS. (2017a). MACRA: Delivery system reform, medicare payment reform. Retrieved from https://www.cms.gov/Medicare/Quality-Initiatives-Patient-Assessment-Instruments/Value-Based-Programs/MACRA-MIPS-and-APMs/MACRA-MIPS-and-APMs.html

CMS. (2017b). Retrieved from https://qpp.cms.gov/

CMS. (2017c). Retrieved from https://qpp.cms.gov/mips/improvement-activities

Colligan, L., Potts, H. W., Finn, C. T., & Sinkin, R. A. (2015). Cognitive workload changes for nurses transitioning from a legacy system with paper documentation to a commercial electronic health record. *International Journal of Medical Informatics, 84*(7), 469–476.

Colligan, L., Sinsky, C., Goeders, L., Schmidt-Bowman, M., & Tutty, M. (2016). *Sources of physician satisfaction and dissatisfaction and review of administrative tasks in ambulatory practice: A qualitative analysis of physician and staff interviews*. Retrieved from https://www.ama-assn.org/sites/default/files/media-browser/public/ps2/ps2-dartmouth-study-111016.pdf

de Lusignan, S. (2005). Codes, classifications, terminologies and nomenclatures: Definition, development and application in practice. *Journal of Innovation in Health Informatics, 13*(1), 65–69.

Felix, C., Pandey, A. V., & Bertini, E. (2017). TextTile: An Interactive Visualization Tool for Seamless Exploratory Analysis of Structured Data and Unstructured Text. *IEEE Transactions on Visualization and Computer Graphics, 23*(1), 161–170.

Friedberg, M. W., Chen, P. G., Van Busum, K. R., Aunon, F., Pham, C., Caloyeras, J., … Brook, R. H. (2014). Factors affecting physician professional satisfaction and their implications for patient care, health systems, and health policy. *Rand health quarterly, 3*(4), 1.

Gellert, G. A., Ramirez, R., & Webster, S. L. (2015). The rise of the medical scribe industry: Implications for the advancement of electronic health records. *JAMA, 313*(13), 1315–1316.

Greenhalgh, T., Potts, H. W., Wong, G., Bark, P., & Swinglehurst, D. (2009). Tensions and paradoxes in electronic patient record research: A systematic literature review using the meta-narrative method. *Milbank Quarterly, 87*(4), 729–788.

Hall, J., Cohen, D. J., Davis, M., Gunn, R., Blount, A., Pollack, D. A., … Miller, B. F. (2015). Preparing the workforce for behavioral health and primary care integration. *The Journal of the American Board of Family Medicine, 28*(Supplement 1), S41–S51.

HealthIT.gov. (2013). Meaningful Use Case Studies. Retrieved from https://www.healthit.gov/providers-professionals/quality-improvement-primary-care-practice

Hersh, W. R., Weiner, M. G., Embi, P. J., Logan, J. R., Payne, P. R., Bernstam, E. V., … Cimino, J. J. (2013). Caveats for the use of operational electronic health record data in comparative effectiveness research. *Medical Care, 51*(8 0 3), S30.

Hill, R. G., Sears, L. M., & Melanson, S. W. (2013). 4000 clicks: A productivity analysis of electronic medical records in a community hospital ED. *The American Journal of Emergency Medicine, 31*(11), 1591–1594.

Hoerbst, A., & Ammenwerth, E. (2010). Electronic health records: A systematic review of quality requirements. *Methods of Information in Medicine, 49*(4), 320–336.

Hoffer, J., Ramesh, V., Topi, H. (2015) *Modern Database Management*. Upper Saddle River, New Jersey: Prentice Hall.

Holroyd-Leduc, J. M., Lorenzetti, D., Straus, S. E., Sykes, L., & Quan, H. (2011). The impact of the electronic medical record on structure, process, and outcomes within primary care: A systematic review of the evidence. *Journal of the American Medical Informatics Association, 18*(6), 732–737.

Jha, A. K., DesRoches, C. M., Campbell, E. G., Donelan, K., Rao, S. R., Ferris, T. G., … Blumenthal, D. (2009). Use of electronic health records in U.S. Hospitals. *New England Journal of Medicine, 360*(16), 1628–1638. https://doi.org/10.1056/NEJMsa0900592

Kellermann, A. L., & Jones, S. S. (2013). What it will take to achieve the as-yet-unfulfilled promises of health information technology. *Health Affairs, 32*(1), 63–68.

Kohli, R., & Tan, S. S.-L. (2016). Electronic health records: How can IS researchers contribute to transforming healthcare? *MIS Quarterly, 40*(3), 553–573.

Lau, F., Kuziemsky, C., Price, M., & Gardner, J. (2010). A review on systematic reviews of health information system studies. *Journal of the American Medical Informatics Association, 17*(6), 637–645.

Lee, H. L. (2002). Aligning supply chain strategies with product uncertainties. *California Management Review, 44*(3), 105–119.

Leventhal, R. (2017, July 11, 2017). ONC's new leadership emphasizes shifting priorities in media briefing. Retrieved from https://www.healthcare-informatics.com/article/ehr/onc-s-new-leadership-emphasizes-shifting-priorities-media-briefing

Lyon, A. R., Wasse, J. K., Ludwig, K., Zachry, M., Bruns, E. J., Unützer, J., & McCauley, E. (2016). The contextualized technology adaptation process (CTAP): Optimizing health information technology to improve mental health systems. *Administration and Policy in Mental Health and Mental Health Services Research, 43*(3), 394–409.

Matthews, K. A., Adler, N. E., Forrest, C. B., & Stead, W. W. (2016). Collecting psychosocial "vital signs" in electronic health records: Why now? What are they? What's new for psychology? *American Psychologist, 71*(6), 497.

McCallum, A. (2005). Information extraction: Distilling structured data from unstructured text. *Queue, 3*(9), 48–57.

McCullough, J. S., Parente, S., & Town, R. (2013). *Health information technology and patient outcomes: The role of organizational and informational complementarities*. (NBER working paper 18684). National Bureau of Economic Research.

Moja, L., Kwag, K. H., Lytras, T., Bertizzolo, L., Brandt, L., Pecoraro, V., … Mangia, M. (2014). Effectiveness of computerized decision support systems linked to electronic health records: A systematic review and meta-analysis. *American Journal of Public Health, 104*(12), e12–e22.

Nuckols, T. K., Smith-Spangler, C., Morton, S. C., Asch, S. M., Patel, V. M., Anderson, L. J., … Shekelle, P. G. (2014). The effectiveness of computerized order entry at reducing preventable adverse drug events and medication errors in hospital settings: A systematic review and meta-analysis. *Systematic Reviews, 3*(1), 56.

O'Malley, A. S., Draper, K., Gourevitch, R., Cross, D. A., & Scholle, S. H. (2015). Electronic health records and support for primary care teamwork. *Journal of the American Medical Informatics Association, 22*(2), 426–434.

ONC. (2016a). *Common clinical data set*. Retrieved from https://www.healthit.gov/sites/default/files/commonclinicaldataset_ml_11-4-15.pdf

ONC. (2016b). Health IT legislation and regulations. Retrieved from https://www.healthit.gov/policy-researchers-implementers/health-it-legislation-and-regulations

Park, S. Y., Lee, S. Y., & Chen, Y. (2012). The effects of EMR deployment on doctors' work practices: A qualitative study in the emergency department of a teaching hospital. *International Journal of Medical Informatics, 81*(3), 204–217.

Petrakaki, D., Klecun, E., & Cornford, T. (2016). Changes in healthcare professional work afforded by technology: The introduction of a national electronic patient record in an English hospital. *Organization, 23*(2), 206–226.

Polya, G. (2014). *How to solve it: A new aspect of mathematical method*. Princeton university press.

RTI International. (2013). *Behavioral health roundtable: Using information technology to integrate behavioral health and primary care*. Washington, D.C.: Office of Policy and Planning, Office of the National Coordinator for Health Information Technology Retrieved from https://www.healthit.gov/sites/default/files/bh-roundtable-findings-report_0.pdf.

Sinsky, C., Colligan, L., Li, L., Prgomet, M., Reynolds, S., Goeders, L., … Blike, G. (2016). Allocation of physician time in ambulatory practice: a time and motion study in 4 specialties. *Annals of Internal Medicine, 165*(11), 753–760.

Swinglehurst, D., & Greenhalgh, T. (2015). Caring for the patient, caring for the record: An ethnographic study of 'back office'work in upholding quality of care in general practice. *BMC Health Services Research, 15*(1), 177.

Swinglehurst, D., Greenhalgh, T., & Roberts, C. (2012). Computer templates in chronic disease management: Ethnographic case study in general practice. *BMJ Open, 2*(6), e001754.

The National Council. (2017). MACRA's quality payment program: What does it mean for your Agency's Medicare Reimbursement? Retrieved from https://www.thenationalcouncil.org/wp-content/uploads/2016/08/MACRA-Quality-PP-web-Final.pdf

Varpio, L., Day, K., Elliot-Miller, P., King, J. W., Kuziemsky, C., Parush, A., … Rashotte, J. (2015). The impact of adopting EHRs: How losing connectivity affects clinical reasoning. *Medical Education, 49*(5), 476–486.

Chapter 8
The Neglected Constructs of Health Literacy, Shared Decision-Making, and Patient-Centered Care in Behavioral Health: An Integrated Model

Brendan Willis and William T. O'Donohue

Introduction

Healthcare costs in the United States have continued to increase faster than the rate of inflation, with healthcare spending reaching \$3.2 trillion in 2015, which equates to about \$9990 per person (Centers for Medicare & Medicaid Services, 2015). Behavioral health costs have followed a similar trajectory, with 36.2 million Americans paying a total of \$57.5 billion in 2006 for behavioral health services (National Institute of Mental Health, 2006). Thus, behavioral health expenditures are approximately 2% of the total healthcare budget. This has led to the proposal of a number of possible solutions to reign in the escalating cost of both medical and behavioral health treatment. Among these proposals are three important, and what will be argued interrelated, concepts: behavioral health literacy, shared decision-making, and patient-centered care.

While these constructs are frequently mentioned as possible avenues to reduce healthcare costs and generally improve the quality and experience of care, the terms themselves are ill-defined, and consequently poorly measured, and inconsistently implemented. Despite the lack of agreed-upon definitions, several methods of defining and measuring these three constructs have been developed, but it raises the question about what these constructs and measures are actually capturing. If there is no consensus on what these terms mean, how can these be measured with any degree of reliability or validity? Additionally, how can the researchers and clinicians be sure that these constructs will lead to improved quality of care and reduced healthcare costs without first properly establishing exactly how these are defined and best implemented? Are these constructs being used in a rhetorical fashion—to imply positive aspects of service delivery without appropriate substance? In addition, there has been little exploration of the possible interrelationships between these three key constructs.

B. Willis (✉) · W. T. O'Donohue
Department of Psychology, University of Nevada, Reno, Reno, NV, USA
e-mail: brendanwillis@nevada.unr.edu

M. P. Duckworth, W. T. O'Donohue (eds.), *Behavioral Medicine and Integrated Care*,
https://doi.org/10.1007/978-3-319-93003-9_8

The Realm of Behavioral Healthcare

Little has been done to adapt these terms for use in the unique context of behavioral healthcare delivery. Behavioral health has focused almost exclusively on the constructs of empirically supported treatments (e.g., Chambless & Hollon, 1998), and the field has not paid sufficient attention to other key constructs related to the quality of care delivery, including these three. These terms have largely emerged in the medical literature (see Makoul & Clayman, 2006; Luxford, Safran, & Delbanco, 2011; and Zarcadoolas, Pleasant, & Greer, 2005 for the medical usage of these constructs), and for the most part, these have been applied both infrequently and haphazardly to the field of behavioral health, with little specific guidance or understanding regarding how these constructs would actually function inside of an outpatient therapist's office, an inpatient psychiatric unit, or an integrated healthcare setting. To illustrate an example of the complexities of applying these constructs, consider the concept of shared decision-making. How best is the process of shared decision-making implemented when that patient is under an emergency legal order suspending many of their rights for a period of time? By definition, such an order implies that a professional has decided the patient is unable to make reasonable decisions for themselves, often as the result of psychotic symptoms or suicidal/homicidal ideation. An even less complicated but much more common situation also illustrates the problem—suppose a person with rather routine depression presents to an outpatient therapist: What information ought the patient have to make a literate, informed decision about treatment? What exactly would a "shared" decision process look like? What attributes ought the patient's experience have in order for it to properly be experienced as "patient centered?" These and other questions illustrate the complexities of the behavioral health world and demonstrate the field cannot simply adopt these constructs without first deciding how they are to be adapted and faithfully implemented.

What follows is a critical review of the existing definitions of each construct, with the intent of developing a more useful, adequate definition for each construct. Additionally, methods of adapting each construct to behavioral health applications will be proposed. Given the limited existing literature regarding the use of these constructs in behavioral health, this review will primarily focus on how these have been defined in the medical literature. However, a conclusions section will provide a guideline of how an integrated construct comprising of the three constructs might be implemented in the behavioral health setting.

In our recommendations for applying these constructs to behavioral health settings, we argue that a definition ought to meet the following criteria in order for it to be considered adequate:

1. The definitions should be specific (i.e., lay out clear criteria that can be converted into policy and procedure, and provide clear avenues for further research such as psychometric evaluation) and clearly applied to the context of delivering behavioral health services.

2. The definitions should include dimensions that can be measured. As will be discussed below, many of the definitions for these constructs are so vague that these do not lend themselves to measurement. As a result, attempts at measuring these constructs must often begin by redefining the constructs, leading to further inconsistency across definitions. To remedy this, an adequate definition must include specific, measurable factors. This of course is important for accountability.
3. The construct definitions should also present clear applications/implementation for both providers and patients. It is vital to understand that these constructs are not simply things that are "done" to the patient. These constructs represent changing how behavioral health services are delivered in general and require training programs and guidelines to help providers become more proficient in their use. One of the clearest examples of this is behavioral health literacy. Providers must understand behavioral health problems, treatment options, and other related concerns before they are able to help educate their patients.

Behavioral Health Literacy

Behavioral health literacy has a somewhat more established definition than the other two constructs, having been first coined in 1997 by Jorm and colleagues. Its original definition was "knowledge and beliefs about mental disorders which aid their recognition, management or prevention" (Jorm et al., 1997, p. 182). Since then, this definition has become the de facto standard definition for the behavioral health field. However, key questions still remain regarding if this definition is sufficient or if it is lacking in essential components. The clearest evidence of this comes from the similar medical construct, health literacy. Health literacy also has a variety of definitions without a single unanimously accepted one, with many of the components and dimensions of health literacy still under debate (Sørensen et al., 2012). An examination of the various definitions of health literacy in the medical literature should prove useful in identifying how the construct of behavioral health literacy can be expanded and improved.

Current Definitions

Health literacy as a construct was introduced by Simonds (1974), and in 2012, Sorensen and colleagues completed a systematic review of the various definitions. The researchers concluded that there were 17 separate ways the construct has been defined. Their findings are summarized in Table 8.1.

As can be seen in Table 8.1, these definitions vary in scope and content, making it difficult to build a coherent, consensual construct. Further complicating the issue is some indecision regarding if health literacy itself is a "community" construct or an "individual" construct. That is, does the construct apply to the overall ability of

Table 8.1 Definitions of health literacy found by Sørensen et al. (2012)

1	WHO (Kickbusch & Nutbeam, 1998)	Skills (both cognitive and social) that determine motivation and ability of individuals to access, understand, and use information to promote and maintain good health
2	American Medical Association (AMA) (1999)	Constellation of skills, including basic reading and numeral tasks, needed to function in a healthcare setting
3	Nutbeam (2000)	The personal, cognitive, and social skills that determine a person's ability to gain access to,understand, and use information for the promotion and maintenance of good health
4	Institute of Medicine (Nielsen-Bohlman, Panzer, Hamlin, & Kindig, 2004)	Capacity to obtain, process, and understand basic health information and services needed to make health decisions
5	Kickbusch, Wait, Maag, and Banks (2006)	Ability to make sound health decisions in the context of everyday life. Represents a critical empowerment strategy to increase the consumer's control and responsibility over their health as well as access to health information
6	Zarcadoolas, Pleasant, and Greer (2003, 2005, 2009)	Range of skills and competencies developed to find, understand, evaluate, and use health information to make informed choices, reduce health risks, and increase quality of life
7	Paasche-Orlow and Wolf (2007)	The possession of needed skills for making health-related decisions. Health literacy must always be viewed in the context of the specific task to be accomplished
8	European Union (European Commission, 2007)	Ability to read, filter, and understand health-related information and use to make sound judgments
9	Pavlekovic (2008)	Capacity to obtain, understand, interpret, and use health information and services to enhance health
10	Rootman and Gordon-El-Bihbety (2008)	Ability to access, understand, evaluate, and communicate information in ways to promote, maintain, and improve health in a variety of contexts across the life span
11	Ishikawa and Yano (2008)	Knowledge, abilities, and skills pertaining to interactions with the healthcare system
12	Mancuso (2008)	An evolving process that encompasses the life span and involves capacity, comprehension, and communication. The attributes of health literacy are integrated in the skills, strategies, and abilities embedded in the competencies required to attain literacy in health matters
13	Australian Bureau of Statistics (2008)	Knowledge and skills needed to use and understand health-related information and issues, such as substance abuse, disease treatment and prevention, as well as accident prevention, first aid, and staying healthy
14	Yost et al. (2009)	Degree of capacity to read and comprehend health-related printed material, identify, and interpret information presented in graphical forms and ability to perform arithmetic operations in order to make healthcare decisions

(continued)

Table 8.1 (continued)

15	Adams et al. (2009)	Ability to understand and interpret health information in written, spoken, or digital forms how this motivates people to follow or ignore health-related actions
16	Adkins and Corus (2009)	Ability to derive meaning from different modes of communication through the use of a variety of skills in order to accomplish health-related goals
17	Freedman et al. (2009)	Degree that individuals and groups can obtain, understand, process, evaluate, and use information needed to make public health choices that benefit the community

From Sørensen et al. (2012), p. 4

some community to understand health information, or does it rather deal with how individuals themselves have knowledge and skills to properly navigate the healthcare system? Should an intervention be targeted at improving how an entire neighborhood, town, city, family, or specific population possesses and uses health information? Or should it be taken on a more individualistic patient-by-patient basis? Even then, is it important that individuals in the patient's support network (however large this may be) also be literate?

Of the 17 different definitions identified by Sorensen and colleagues, the following have been selected as being sufficiently unique and useful from the other definitions particularly to the behavioral health domain. All definitions share a central concept of being able to utilize and understand health-related information, but they differ in scope and other vital details.

World Health Organization (Kickbusch & Nutbeam, 1998) The needed social and cognitive skills that determine motivation and ability of individuals to access, understand, and use information to promote and maintain good health.

This definition incorporates "cognitive and social skills" as well as "motivation," in the definition, both of which would be important in an overall definition of behavioral health literacy, although making measurement more complex. Interacting with the healthcare system requires a level of social competency, being able to call and set appointments, appropriately assert needs, and interact competently with a variety of healthcare personnel. Additionally, a level of cognitive skill is needed to be able to understand the information that is received during interactions with the healthcare system. In addition, skills may be needed to see information as incomplete or contradictory and to seek additional information. However, this definition does not specify how much of each factor is needed to be able to be considered "health literate." For cognitive skills, is there a certain IQ at which health literacy is not possible or at least very difficult? Or do certain behavioral health disorders that impact social skills such as unassertiveness or social phobia prevent someone from becoming health literate? Or does this also include the skill of the healthcare provider to adapt the information to the cognitive and social skill of the patient so that understanding is achieved? This definition also emphasizes health as opposed to curing illness, which some see as more comprehensive and holistic.

American Medical Association (AMA) (1999) "The constellation of skills, including the ability to perform basic reading and numeral tasks required to function in the healthcare environment" (p. 553).

The American Medical Association definition illustrates that health literacy is a combination of various skills. The definition also includes what some of those skills are, namely, basic reading and numeral tasks. Reading and numeral skills are not frequently part of the definition of health literacy, but these are still vitally important. If an individual is unable to read, or read in the language used in the healthcare system, they will be at a severe disadvantage. Additionally, part of dealing with the healthcare system in the United States often involves insurance plans, and basic arithmetic and numerical skills are needed to understand rates per session, deductibles, out-of-pocket maximums, in-network vs out-of-network rates, and so on. However, it is unclear if basic literacy and numeracy are sufficient to fully comprehend, appraise, and formulate reasonable action plans relevant to this information. However, the definition states that there are other skills included in the constellation, but does not define what these are. Furthermore, it states that these skills are needed to function in the healthcare environment, but no cutoff is provided for exactly what constitutes "functioning." One can also imagine that there are many other skills relevant to this functioning—e.g., being assertive, handling stress, finding a job to pay medical bills, tolerating side effects, etc. Is solely utilizing emergency services as one's primary form of interacting with the healthcare system considered functional? Or should functioning also include other basic behaviors, such as being able to call and set up an appointment with a primary care doctor and thus avoid the expense of an emergency department visit? This has further implications for behavioral health, given the complexities and difficulty in navigating the behavioral health system. How much knowledge is needed to be considered functional? Does a person need to just know the basic mental health resources in their area and how to contact them, or should they also understand how so-called behavioral health "carve-outs" work on their insurance policy?

Institute of Medicine (Nielsen-Bohlman et al., 2004) "The individual's capacity to obtain, process, and understand basic health information and services needed to make appropriate health decisions" (p. 32).

The Institute of Medicine's definition of health literacy is typical of many definitions, highlighting the importance of understanding and using health information in order to make decisions regarding healthcare. However, this definition is still quite vague. For example, just what is meant by "basic health information?" Is there some general health information that all need to have (e.g., regarding vaccines, diet), and then what constitutes basic health information concerning a particular diagnosis such as autism? Furthermore, what is meant by "appropriate health decisions?" Who decides whether the decision was appropriate—or by what criteria? This is especially salient in behavioral health where a particular issue can be treated with a variety of therapeutic modalities and more basically a variety of diagnostic practices. What may be an appropriate treatment for one may not be for someone with a similar presenting problem but different overall context.

Zarcadoolas, Pleasant, and Geer (2009) "The wide range of skills and competencies that people develop to seek out, comprehend, evaluate and use health information and concepts to make informed choices, reduce health risks and increase quality of life" (p. 5).

Zarcadoolas, Pleasant, and Geer (2009) emphasized that health literacy is a combination of a wide variety of skills, highlighting the complexity of the term itself. In this sense, it gives much more detail and appropriately indicates that it is a much more involved cognitive task than the WHO definition. Unfortunately, this definition does not explain exactly what these skills and competencies are. For example, evaluating information is a very complex skill and can occur at a variety of different levels of sophistication—what level is sufficient to satisfy this definition? The definition does add the concept of using health information to make informed choices, reduce risks, and increase quality of life. These are more specific outcomes than many of the other definitions, especially with the focus on risk reduction and increasing quality of life. This has a great deal of relevance to behavioral health, as the selection of treatment modality can have a huge impact on how long a person struggles with a particular disorder based on their individual circumstances. Additionally, the idea of risk management can be extended to behavioral health as well. Patients will need to know what treatment options will help them minimize the risk of worsening symptoms, or family members will need to know what they can do to minimize the risk of self-injurious behavior or suicide. Finally, risk management in behavioral health situations is a concept that all clinicians should be familiar with and includes understanding warning signs that a patient could have a worsening condition or might imminently try to harm themselves or someone else. Thus, behavioral health literacy is not just a concept to be applied to the patient but to the provider as well. This definition also assumes that knowledge is sufficient for healthy behavior. However, knowledge alone is not sufficient for individuals to engage in healthy behaviors. Individuals may know that certain things are bad for them but do not have other psychological factors (such as motivation) or the skills to desist from engaging in these behaviors, which may range from safe sex to exercise and healthy eating.

Paasche-Orlow and Wolf (2007) "An individual's possession of requisite skills for making health-related decisions, which means that health literacy must always be examined in the context of the specific tasks that need to be accomplished. The importance of a contextual appreciation of health literacy must be underscored" (p. 20).

Paasche-Orlow and Wolf emphasized context as an important part of health literacy, although "context" itself is a very vague term. One is always, in some larger setting, leading to the important question of what are the boundaries of "context." The context of behavioral health differs substantially from other medical care settings in a number of ways, as there are often different rules about insurance, often different locations from where the person usually seeks medical attention, different diagnostic tests and procedures, and an entire unique language that is both esoteric and confusing. These differences underscore an important point of behavioral health literacy, namely, that a person can be more literate in one area and less literate in another. Individuals, through necessity, may have become literate in working with the primary care system or dealing with a specialty care system, but that does not automatically indicate that the person will be literate in all healthcare situations. In terms of applicability to behavioral health, it is important to remember a person can be extremely competent at dental care, primary healthcare, and other forms of medical care but struggle in trying to understand how the behavioral health system works. Therefore, it is the responsibility of behavioral health providers to help acclimate individuals to the unique behavioral health context. This definition is also vague in that what "needs" to be done might be vague or poorly understood—what do you need to do today for your health?

Australian Bureau of Statistics (2008) Knowledge and skills needed to use and understand health-related information and issues, such as substance abuse, disease treatment and prevention, as well as accident prevention, first aid, and staying healthy.

The Australian Bureau of Statistics definition of health literacy closely resembles the Jorm et al. (1997) definition of behavioral health literacy in that it includes knowledge and skills needed to navigate health issues including the prevention of diseases and accidents. Knowing the signs that a disease is developing or getting worse is an important part of health literacy as well as behavioral health literacy. Additionally, the Australian Bureau of Statistics definition is one of the only current definitions that attempts to specify the major factors that fall under the behavioral health banner, namely, drug and alcohol problems, indicating the applicability of the construct to behavioral health. Furthermore, this definition also includes helping individuals understand the appropriate level of care for their specific situation, whether they need emergency care, first aid, or help in avoiding those entirely through disease prevention and treatment. Helping individuals understand where to go and what level of service to seek help for their mental health issues is a vital component of behavioral health literacy. However, the definition is still incomplete, as it is vague on what individuals should do with the information and skills they have acquired about health issues. The definition simply states "use" the information, but what is the information being used for and how is it known that individuals are using the information correctly? Furthermore, there is no indication of where this information is supposed to come from. Calabretta (2002) stated that more and more individuals are relying on Internet-based sources for information about healthcare issues. In fact, in the year 2000 alone, 60% of individuals surveyed indicated that they had visited a health or medical website. But there are serious questions regarding the quality of the information available to the public. Good health literacy, and by extension good behavioral health literacy, must include getting accurate information into the hands of consumers.

Freedman et al. (2009) "The degree to which individuals and groups can obtain, process, understand, evaluate, and act upon information needed to make public health decisions that benefit the community."

This definition is particularly interesting in that it is squarely in the camp of health literacy focusing more on the community than the individual. Here, individuals are only considered literate in health matters if they make public health decisions that will benefit the community as a whole. But what about choices with no direct impact on the community, only on the individual? Does the choice of preferred therapy modality actually impact the good of the community? And if a person is forced to make a choice that is not of benefit to the community due to insurance issues, does that automatically make the person health illiterate?

Building a New Behavioral Health Literacy Definition

As can be seen by the preceding examples, there are a wide variety of definitions of health literacy, many of which go beyond the original definition of behavioral health literacy proposed by Jorm et al. (1997). Even that definition was expanded upon, with Jorm (2012) stating that behavioral health literacy has a number of components, including knowledge of how to prevent mental disorders, recognition that a disorder is developing, knowledge of help-seeking options and treatments available, knowledge of effective self-help strategies for milder problems, and first aid skills to support others who are developing a mental disorder or who are in some sort of behavioral health crisis. Taking these components as well as the aforementioned definitions, it is possible to fashion a more complete definition of behavioral health literacy.

Sørensen et al. (2012) laid the foundation for such a definition by creating an integrated definition of overall health literacy. To Sorenson and colleagues, health literacy is defined as a process requiring four competencies: the ability to obtain health information, the ability to comprehend health information that is accessed, the ability to evaluate the obtained information, and the ability to communicate and use that information to make decisions that will improve or maintain health.

Applying the Sørensen et al. (2012) definition to behavioral health as well as incorporating elements from the previous medical definitions and Jorm (2012) yields the following definition of behavioral health literacy[1]:

Behavioral health literacy can be defined as a series of competencies specific to the domain of behavioral health problems. These competencies can be defined as:

1. The ability to obtain valid and relevant behavioral health information, often with consultation with healthcare professionals.
2. The ability to evaluate and synthesize the obtained behavioral health information.
3. The ability to use that information to make sound behavioral healthcare decisions relating to both wellness and the treatment of illness. This includes an understanding of important treatment factors such as duration, safety, possible side effects, and costs.
4. The ability to understand the factors that contribute to prevention of psychological disorders and the promotion of overall wellness.

[1] It should be noted that this definition applies to the provider as well as the patient. Specifically, the provider should have access to the necessary information to help their patients become literate in behavioral health concerns or know where to find said information.

Some key domains of literacy include:

1. Being able to recognize when a disorder is beginning or worsening
2. How to prevent behavioral health disorders
3. Knowledge of effective and safe treatment options
4. An understanding of stepped care in behavioral health, including effective self-help strategies for managing behavioral health issues and knowing when to seek higher levels of care
5. How to successfully access the treatment options, including where those options are located, who are competent providers, and how services can be obtained (insurance vs self-pay vs free clinics, etc.)

Based on the wide variety of health literacy definitions, it is not expected that there will be total agreement on this proposed definition. However, in combining elements from the various proffered conceptualizations, this definition should serve as a base from which future research can build to refine and hone the definition into a construct that is both more comprehensive and relevant to improving healthcare delivery.

Measuring Behavioral Health Literacy

Several scales have been developed to measure various aspects of health literacy, and some have focused more on generic literacy (i.e., basic reading skills) of the patient, while others have focused more on the patients' understanding of health-related material. Jorm et al. (1997) developed one of the more frequently used behavioral health literacy measures, the Mental Health Literacy Questionnaire. The questionnaire presents respondents with a vignette of an individual suffering from a diagnosable mental illness and then asks the respondent to identify what, if anything, is wrong with the individual and what could be done to help them in the best way. This measure has been used in research but has limitations in terms of clinical application. The vignettes only present an individual suffering with either schizophrenia or depression and therefore are applicable to research settings but may fail to capture the variety of behavioral health problems that an individual may be suffering from in a clinical setting. Unfortunately, psychometrics on the Mental Health Literacy Questionnaire is not readily available, further complicating attempts at using it in both research and clinical settings. Issues remain regarding its utility across different cultures as well as its ability to adapt to the new diagnostic requirements of the latest addition of the *Diagnostic and Statistical Manual of Mental Disorders*. Further research is needed to develop a valid and reliable behavioral health literacy measure for clinical applications.

Ideally, a psychometrically sound measurement of behavioral health literacy for clinical applications should focus on the general class of behavioral problems the patient is presenting with, allowing clinicians to gauge how much the individual understands about their particular presenting problem and how much they need to be educated on this information. This measure could be administered after a diagnosis has been made initially and then given at time of termination to gauge how much the patient has learned as well as for quality improvement purposes. This would allow healthcare systems to identify what patients with what type of behavioral health problems are not being sufficiently educated. Furthermore, such a measure should also assess the desire of the patient to know more about their particular diagnosis. Not all patients will want to have the same level of information given to them. Some will be satisfied with a basic understanding of the problem and possible treatments, while others will desire a near-expert level understanding. This is important information to understand at the beginning of treatment so that efforts to educate the patient match how much they are willing to learn.

Shared Decision-Making

Shared decision-making is perhaps the most ill-defined of the three concepts under review here, being vaguely described as a verb and a process by which practitioners and clients somehow work together (Drake, Deegan, & Rapp, 2010). Shared decision-making is supposed to be able to help clients feel more empowered by allowing them a voice in processes of making choices regarding various treatment details, such as what treatments will be used or how long they will last. As a result, shared decision-making is supposed to improve client motivation, engagement, and compliance. The possibility exists that it could also improve health literacy, as part of this sharing ought to be the sharing of relevant information from the healthcare professional. However, there has been little research detailing how shared decision-making should actually be implemented in the behavioral health domain, especially given the unique challenges faced by mental health professionals in situations where a client's ability to choose may be impacted by a metal health problem or temporarily suspended for their own safety.

Current Definitions of Shared Decision-Making

As before, an examination of the medical literature will prove useful in establishing a more precise definition of shared decision-making and aid in applying it to behavioral health situations.

President's Commission for the Study of Ethical Problems in Medicine (President's Commission, 1982) Shared decision-making consists of "discussions between professional and patient that bring the knowledge, concerns, and perspectives of each to the process of seeking agreement on a course of treatment. Simply put, this means that the physician or other health professional invites the patient to participate in a dialogue in which the professional seeks to help the patient understand the medical situation and course of action and the patient conveys his or her concerns and wishes" (p. 44).

Interestingly, this definition tends to be clearer and more precise than many of the attempts that would follow. Specifically, the President's Commission (1982) indicates shared decision-making is a collaboration between a healthcare professional and a patient, with the end goal of meeting the needs of the patient by presenting various options and reaching a decision together. Though this is an excellent foundation, it still is lacking critical detail. The definition lacks any mention of how much the decision needs to be shared between physician and patient. In fact, a more basic question is what parties are involved in the decision-making—which healthcare providers (e.g., should primary care physician be involved)—should family members; should payors (payors often are involved whether wanted or not). Additionally, is the decision made equally by all parties (if so equal, on what dimensions and how will it be measured)? What information ought each party have before a decision can be properly reached (relevant to health literacy above)? Or does one party have more influence than the other, at least in some situations? What about situations in which a patient prefers to abdicate any decision-making role and prefers to let the healthcare provider make the decision for them? What happens if there is any disagreement between physician and patient? How ought pragmatic issues like cost and geographical distance play into such decisions? Are there cultural variables which affect how "shared" is defined—perhaps some allegedly collectivist cultures may differ from more individualistic ones? Additionally, some research has indicated that, depending on the kind of medical issue being dealt with, some patients may prefer more information about their condition but do not want to have an increased role in making decisions. This was demonstrated in Hamann, Cohen, Leucht, Busch, and Kissling's (2005) work with shared decision-making in population of patient suffering from schizophrenia. They found that their participants' desire for information was considerably higher than their desire for participation in the actual decision-making process. Any definition of shared decision-making must then include assessing the degree to which a patient would like to be included in the decision-making process as well as ensuring that the information about treatment options has been conveyed, as described in behavioral health literacy. This also raises a key question of whether the patient's desire to share in decision-making itself ought to be a treatment target.

Charles, Gafni, and Whelan (1997) Shared decision-making involves at least two participants, the professional and the patient. Both parties take steps to participate in the process of making decisions about treatment, beginning with the sharing of information. Treatment decisions are made when both parties agree to the course of action.

One of the most frequently cited definitions of shared decision-making (Makoul & Clayman, 2006) builds upon the President's Commission by adding that decisions need to be made only after both the professional and the patient agree on the course of action as well as the importance of sharing information at the beginning in order for the patient to be aware of the various options available. One can see how health literacy seems to be a key component of shared decision-making, as "sharing of information" is mentioned in the definition. Here though the gaining and processing of this information seem to be more of an explicitly shared task rather than a solitary one. Again however, this definition does nothing to address how "shared" the decision needs to be. Does every decision in healthcare need to be shared? Are there circumstances in which one side or the other needs to have more control over the decision-making process? Finally, what if a consensus cannot be reached between physician and patient, then what? Is no treatment attempted—is the treatment provider obligated to attempt to find a healthcare professional who might provide the patient's preference? And thus does one side—particularly the healthcare professional—need to acquiesce to the demands of the other? Certainly, the case of an inappropriate opioid-seeking patient would be a counterexample to this, where the patient's reported need for opiate medication is overridden by good clinical judgment and concerns for the patient's safety. In terms of behavioral health, these questions are especially salient. In selecting a course of treatment for a particular disorder, a behavioral health provider will need to be objective in presenting the details about various treatment options, especially if those options belong to therapy modalities that are different from the provider's.

Charles et al. (1997) also identified that decision-making exists on a spectrum, with the physician as agent, or paternalistic, model on one extreme and informed decision-making on the other. The physician as agent model is defined as the physician having total control over the decision-making process, while the informed decision-making model has the patient in complete control over their decisions, with only marginal input from the physician to communicate information. Charles et al. (1997) saw shared decision-making as existing between these two extremes, allowing the physician to explain options and make recommendations while at the same time being sensitive to the patient's needs and goals. This view is especially applicable in behavioral health, where many disorders have multiple potential avenues of treatment, including watchful waiting, various face-to-face therapeutic strategies (e.g., group or individual), bibliotherapy, and psychopharmacology options. Any definition of shared decision-making for behavioral health needs to include a detailed explanation of all treatment options so the client can be well informed before making a decision. However, since decision-making is between both the provider and patient, the provider should also give their recommendations about which option is best for dealing with the client's specific issue.

Adams, Drake, and Wolford (2007) "Shared decision making denotes the process of enabling clients to participate actively and meaningfully in their treatment by providing them with accessible information and choices" (p. 1219).

Here, Adams et al. (2007) again demonstrate the relevance of health literacy to shared decision-making. Shared decision-making is about ensuring that the client is participating actively and has actual informed choices about the treatment options. This places a greater burden on the provider to make sure that the client is involved in a meaningful way during the decision-making process. However, a number of important questions remain, such as what exactly is a meaningful choice. Do meaningful choices extend to what kind of medication a patient should be taking, even if the patient has little understanding of pharmacology? What about in the behavioral health setting when patients are placed in emergency involuntary commitment orders? How are they supposed to be able to make meaningful choices when their right to make many decisions has been temporarily suspended for their own safety?

In terms of applicability to the behavioral health context, this definition does remind providers of the vital importance of behavioral health literacy. If a patient does not know what options are available, along with the pros and cons of each choice, they cannot participate effectively in the shared decision-making process. Additionally, it emphasizes that the information should be presented in an accessible way. Behavioral health as a whole has its own unique jargon and language, one that can be difficult to understand to the layperson. When beginning the process of shared decision-making, explanations need to be simple while still being accurate and avoid as much jargon as possible. Drake et al. (2010) further suggest that decision aids, such as diagrams, charts, or handouts, be used to enhance the provider's ability to explain treatment options.

Makoul and Clayman (2006) Makoul and Clayman (2006) conducted a literature review of shared decision-making and crafted a more integrated definition, taking into account the previous attempts at defining it. Specifically, they stated that shared decision-making begins with patients and providers defining and explaining the problem to be addressed. At this point, the provider should review any options that do exist as well as their risks and benefits. The process also involves a discussion of the patient's sense of self-efficacy and their ability to follow through with the plan, in order to identify potential roadblocks to compliance. During the process, both sides should periodically check for understanding of the facts and perspectives, providing clarification as needed. Finally, consistent follow-up is needed to gauge the outcome of the decision that has been made and make any needed adjustments.

This more integrated model is more psychological sophisticated as it sees the psychological complexities of the patient involved in shared decision-making. It also has the advantage of combining elements of a number of different definitions while also addressing several of the weaknesses. The model even makes mention that there are times where no choices exist for the patient and a certain course of action must be followed, such as during emergency hospitalization. Of additional importance, this definition also conforms to rational or strategic problem-solving, as outlined by Nezu, Nezu, and D'Zurilla (2012), in which a problem is defined, alternative solutions are generated, a decision is made, the solution is implemented, and finally verification is done to ensure that the solution had the desired effect.

Towel and Godolphin (1999) Towel and Godolphin developed a series of eight specific competencies that they used as their definition of shared decision-making. The competencies are as follows:

1. Develop a partnership with the patient.
2. Establish or review the patient's preferences for information (such as amount or format).
3. Establish or review the patient's preferences for role in decision-making (such as risk-taking and degree of involvement of self and others) and the existence and nature of any uncertainty about the course of action to take.

4. Ascertain and respond to patient's ideas, concerns, and expectations (such as about disease management options).
5. Identify choices (including ideas and information that the patient may have), and evaluate the research evidence in relation to the individual patient.
6. Present (or direct patient to) evidence, taking into account competencies 2 and 3, framing effects (how presentation of the information may influence decision-making), etc. Help patient to reflect on, and assess the impact of alternative decisions with regard to his or her values and lifestyle.
7. Make or negotiate a decision in partnership with the patient and resolve conflict.
8. Agree an action plan and complete arrangements for follow-up.

Towle and Godolphin (1999) offer one of the more concrete and specific definitions of shared decision-making. It has a number of important advantages including providing detailed steps for implementation. After developing a partnership with the patient or, as behavioral health providers would say, "establishing rapport," the provider proceeds to determine how much influence over the decisions the patient would like to have. Equally critical, the provider seeks to resolve any misgivings or misunderstandings the patient may be harboring, reducing the likelihood that the patient will simply agree with the provider despite their concerns or fears. Additionally, this definition makes clear mention of the importance of follow-up to see if the agreed-upon course of action has been followed. If it has not, then the provider can restart the shared decision-making process to determine what went wrong. However, some clarification is still needed in this definition. Competency 7 states that conflicts need to be resolved but states little to help understand how that resolution should take place. Are the patient's desires and wishes always more important than the provider's opinion, or are there instances where the provider must override the decision of the patient? There are clear examples of this in behavioral health, as mentioned before, so the question remains how to best carry out shared decision-making in cases where a person's right to choose has been temporarily limited.

Building a Shared Decision-Making Definition

Using Towle and Godolphin (1999) as a base, it is possible to further refine it into a definition of shared decision-making for behavioral healthcare.

1. Establish the necessary rapport between clinician and patient.
2. Establish or review the patient's preferences for information (such as amount and format).
3. Establish or review the patient's preferences for role in decision-making (such as risk-taking and degree of involvement of self and others) and the existence and nature of any uncertainty about the course of action to take. This should include resolving any uncertainty about how much the patient wishes to be involved in the decision-making.

4. Ascertain and respond to patient's ideas, concerns, and expectations about their current situation and possible treatment (such as about disease management options).
5. The provider should provide information about available evidence-based treatments as well as any options the patient brings to the table, along with an honest and as unbiased as possible discussion of the risks and benefits of each option. The clinician should provide or direct the patient to sources of additional information and evidence about each option, taking into account the preferred formats from competencies 2 and 3. The clinician should help the patient assess the impact of alternative decisions with regard to his or her own individual values, beliefs, and lifestyle. The provider should also endeavor to correct misconceptions the patient may have about their disorder or treatment options. The provider should supply information about pragmatics such as costs, waits, side effects, and availability of services.
6. The patient and provider should then mutually select a course of action, depending on how much shared decision-making was decided upon at the outset. Any conflicts should be identified and resolved. By mutual, we mean that the course of action should be decided by both patient and provider who are actively participating in the decision-making process. The patient is actively participating at the desired level established in step 3, and the provider is respecting the previously agreed-upon level of participation. Critically, the provider must verify throughout the treatment process that the patient is indeed participating in the decision-making at the desired level. It is not enough to assume that they are, as patients may become agreeable to whatever the provider wants due to the power difference inherent in a provider-patient relationship.
7. Mutually agree to an action plan. Afterward, the provider will verify to see how well the decision was implemented and address any problems or concerns. If the patient has failed to follow through on the agreed-upon decision, the provider can return to the beginning of the shared decision-making process to uncover the causes of the noncompliance and address them with the patient.

In terms of the special circumstances discussed previously of involuntary commitment, Hamann et al. (2005) found that even in a sample of participants suffering with schizophrenia scored on average scored 46 on the autonomy preference index, a measure of the patient's wish to be participate in making medical decisions. The scale ranges from 0 to 100, with an average of 48 indicating a strong desire to work together with behavioral health specialists in making treatment decisions. The patients did not want to let the doctors make all the decisions, but they also do not want to make the decisions completely by themselves. Of note, an average of 46 on the API is also slightly higher than those who reported solely for primary care concerns (33–42), meaning that even those suffering from serious mental illness still wished to be involved in the decision-making process. Hamann and colleagues also addressed the issue of involuntary commitment and shared decision-making, by stating that there will be times in which shared decision-making will not be feasible. However, they recommend that shared decision-making be used as soon as is appropriate with involuntary patients. This can be done even while still under an order of commitment by finding treatment options that the patient can participate in, such as where or when a therapy session might be held. Such less critical treatment decisions can be used, while the person is working to leave the involuntary commitment order.

Measuring Shared Decision-Making

Some attempt has been made to create measures assessing patient involvement in the decision-making process (see Elwyn et al. (2001) for a review of a number of observation-based assessments of shared decision-making), but there has been limited development of measures for clinical use. Most of the measures that have been developed are subscales within broader assessments or have been designed to be used by a researcher or supervisor watching the interaction between provider and patient. While useful for training and research purposes, a more applicable clinical measure of shared decision-making should first begin during the initial appointment and assess the degree to which the patient wishes to be involved. A scale, such as the aforementioned autonomy preference index (Ende, Kazis, Ash, & Moskowitz, 1989), could be used as a base to develop such a measure of desired shared decision-making. The scale is divided into two subscales, assessing decision-making and information seeking. The scales had a test-retest reliability of 0.84 for decision-making and 0.83 for the information-seeking scale. Both scales achieved a Cronbach's alpha of 0.82, indicating a good degree of internal consistency and reliability. Additional testing should be done to ensure the cross-cultural applicability of the measure, as it was originally tested on a sample of Caucasian and African-American participants, with a small number of participants identifying as Hispanic or Others (Ende et al., 1989). At termination of treatment, the patient should be assessed to determine how involved they felt they were in the decision-making process and if it was in accordance with their desired level of involvement. This way, healthcare systems can verify if their providers utilize appropriate levels of shared decision-making and make adjustments if needed.

One final note, there do appear to be some possible racial and ethnic differences, as well as some gender differences in the level of desired shared decision-making. Levinson, Kao, Kuby, and Thisted (2005), using the US General Social Survey, found that women tended to prefer a more active role in decision-making compared to men. Also, when compared to the Caucasian respondents, African-American and Hispanic respondents were more likely to prefer physician-directed interactions, though the cause for this is unknown and could potentially be related to differential treatment based on race. Overall however, the survey revealed that 96% of respondents preferred to be offered choices during their medical consultations, indicating a strong desire to at the very least be aware of treatment options.

Patient-Centered Care

Patient-centered care is also a construct that has been around for quite some time, but similar to the other terms, it has been vaguely defined and poorly measured. Some work has been done on attempting to define the construct; however, similar to the previous terms, these attempts have largely neglected applying patient-centered care to behavioral health settings. Refining the definition and application of patient-centered care is especially important in the search for methods to decrease health-care costs and increase quality of healthcare delivery. Despite the lack of a unified definition, research conducted on patient-centered care has linked it with decreased healthcare utilization, often in the form of decreased referrals and decreased number of diagnostic tests (Bertakis & Azari, 2011).

Current Definitions of Patient-Centered Care

As with the previous terms, the following are all attempts at defining patient-centered care, drawn primarily from the medical literature.

Epstein and Street (2011) Epstein and Street (2011) pointed out the tendency of patient-centered healthcare to be confused with efforts that are quite superficial. Due to the lack of a clear definition of what patient-centered care is, often hospitals and other facilities will make changes in an attempt to enhance the patient experience, such as adding greenery, greeters, and coffee shops, but these changes are not necessarily core to the construct of patient-centered care. Even the deployment of electronic health record systems is not necessarily patient centered unless the system actually helps patients understand more about their own health or enhances their experience of care in some other way.

Thus, Epstein and Street defined patient-centered care as an approach to care that respects patient preferences. Similar to shared decision-making, patient-centered care seeks to help patients be more active in their care and avoid the centuries-old tradition of physician-dominated interactions. Additionally, patient-centered care involves training providers to be more mindful of patient preferences, informative, and empathic.

While a good beginning, this definition still relies is vague and does not clearly define what patient-centered care actually is. Furthermore, like the other constructs discussed, there is no clear indication of how patient-centered care should be applied in the behavioral health setting. Many of the skills described in the definition are applicable to behavioral health, such as empathic listening and respect for preferences. However, this construct appears to be more "meta" and is concerned with the overall nature of care as opposed to just being felt understood at some point in time in therapy. As mentioned earlier, there are instances where providers are unable to respect a client's preferences, such as when they are making homicidal or suicidal threats. How to keep patient-centered care in mind while dealing with such a situation has not been discussed.

Stewart et al. (2000) Stewart and colleagues attempted to bring some clarity to the construct by identifying six interactive components of patient-centered care. These components are as follows:

1. The clinician's exploration of the client's presenting problem and the experience of the illness itself
2. The clinician's understanding of the whole person
3. The clinician and client working together to build a consensus regarding the management of the illness
4. The clinician incorporating prevention and health promotion into their visits with the client
5. The enhancement of the clinician-client relationship
6. Ensuring that the patient-centered practice be realistic

However, this model lacks specifics and clear definitions of what each of the components means. Exploration of the presenting problem and understanding the whole person are unclear. Additionally, there are no specifics on what "realistic" in the last component actually implies. Despite these problems, there are some ideas that are of use to a behavioral health definition of patient-centered care. Patient-centered behavioral healthcare should emphasize the context that a person is living in and not solely focus on the disorder itself. This means that relevant aspects of a client's life should be considered while rendering behavioral health treatment. Is the client not exercising? Are they smoking or engaging in other unhealthy lifestyles? By examining the whole context in which person lives, clinicians can identify targets for change that may assist in treating the presenting problem and improve overall quality of life.

US Veterans Administration (Dobscha, Cromer, Crain, & Denneson, 2016) As a massive provider of medical and behavioral health services in the United States, the VA has a vested interest in methods of improving quality and lowering healthcare costs. The VA developed their own, more succinct definition of patient-centered care, namely, that patient-centered care involves placing the veteran at the center of the healthcare experience and healthcare practice, with healing environments, healing relationships, a focus on proactive health and well-being, and personalized healthcare plans (Dobscha et al., 2016).

The VA definition has the advantage of being slightly more specific than the previous definitions; however it still leaves many questions to be answered. For example, what is meant by "healing environments" or "healing relationships?" What exactly does it mean that the veteran is at the center of the healthcare practice? However, of most use to behavioral health applications is the metaphor of placing the patient at the center of the behavioral health practice. While ill-defined in the VA conceptualization, this can be taken to mean changing the practice to be more convenient and pleasing for the patient instead of the provider. Patients would appropriately be seen as consumers needing to be satisfied rather than individuals who have few other choices and who ought simply to be satisfied with the way things currently are structured. Therefore, accommodations should be made if patients prefer extended evening hours, or if patients can only meet on the weekends, or if patients want to be able to check and pay their bill online through a simple online portal.

Another crucial aspect of patient-centered care that has not been discussed in the previous definitions is the idea of marketing. In the United States, service industries such as healthcare have surpassed manufacturing industries in terms of size and importance to the country's economy. However, despite this, the healthcare industry has been slow to even acknowledge the importance of marketing principles in informing, attracting, and retaining patients (Corbin, Kelley, & Schwartz, 2001). Traditionally, the healthcare industry has been slow to seek out the benefits of improved customer satisfaction and retention efforts. Recent changes in insurance premiums and other factors are pushing hospital systems to investigate and apply marketing and customer satisfaction techniques in an effort to reduce costs, increase quality of service delivery, and secure the loyalty of returning patients. Marketing itself is focused on understanding and providing the consumer (in our case the patient) with features that they want, which makes it inexorably tied to patient-centered care. However, marketing also involves the development and implementations of features that the consumer may not be aware that they want. An example is online patient portals, where patients can log in to view their bills, communicate with providers, respond to quality improvement requests, and set appointments, among other functions. These online portals were inconceivable in the early 1990s but are now becoming common place. Other examples may include using newly improved biometric security devices to facilitate secure and speedy access to medical records, increasing the availability of telehealth and telecrisis services, or implementing a mental health crisis line that can respond to both text messages and phone calls. Therefore, an important component of building a patient-centered practice is the continual research into and development of features that will improve the patient experience but that the patients themselves are not aware that they want.

Building a Patient-Centered Care Definition

In terms of a patient-centered care definition specific to behavioral health, the VA definition can be used as a starting point. While most of the healthcare in the VA would be free of charge, another aspect of patient-centered care is providing high value for the dollar and specifically attempting to drive down cost. Patient-centered care can be defined by the following concepts:

1. Patient-centered behavioral healthcare involves making behavioral healthcare as easy to access and use as possible and pleasing and providing good value for the dollar.
2. Examples include the aforementioned changes in schedule, including multilingual signs and materials in the office that might be useful, ensuring that clinics and offices are accessible by disabled persons, and providing staff on hand who can explain the complexities of behavioral health insurance to patients.
3. Patient-centered care also extends to ensuring good listening skills and empathetic communication on the part of staff members, but it cannot end there.

4. Patient-centered care should not be thought of as a dichotomous variable but rather as a continuous one. A practice is not either patient centered or non-patient centered. Instead, it should be viewed as a spectrum, running from less patient centered to more patient centered. The more features present to help patients learn more about their health and access and utilize the behavioral health services, the more patient centered the practice is.
5. A critical aspect of patient-centered care is the development, implementation, and assessment for quality improvement of both features patients have stated that they want as well as features they are unaware they want. Quality improvement efforts should be both bottom up—asking patients what they like and dislike about the totality of their care as well as suggestions for improvement—and a search for innovation from other sources such as innovative industries such as retailing and the computer industries. Especially with the development of new features, continual QI is needed to ensure that the features are having the desired effect and to identify and solve problems quickly.

Discussions regarding this construct often stop at good listening skills (Stewart et al., 2000). This is much too narrow of a focus. In true patient-centered care, what is lost is a delivery system driven by the convenience of the provider or the healthcare industry. Currently, many providers structure their practices around their own convenience, including location, pricing, hours, insurances accepted, therapies offered, and referrals made. In essence, the care is not centered on the needs and requirements of the patient, but rather the provider, making it provider-centered care. Patient-centered care has the possibility of increasing patient involvement in and follow through with treatment, but it also carries the cost of making it much less convenient for the provider. Longer hours, weekend shifts, hiring of extra staff, and adding additional insurance panels are all examples of improvements that can make a practice more patient centered while adding additional cost or work for the provider. In other words, patient care needs to transition from provider centered to patient or consumer centered.

Measuring Patient-Centered Care

In terms of measurement, measuring patient-centered care should be focused more on the organizational level rather than the level of individual practitioners. Any measure of the construct should assess what features are present in the system and patients' reactions to these as well as suggestions for improvement. A systematic quality improvement system would be most conducive to gaining this information—as it would be perpetual and require iterative attempts at reform. This system is vital to a patient-centered organization, as constant attempts at quality improvement allow the organization to detect problems that need to be solved, evaluate the effectiveness of new interventions, and identify programs that are working and should be expanded. Further research is also needed to determine the respective weight that different patient-centered care features should have. For example, is having multilingual materials and signs available in the practice more important than extended hours on the weekends? Such a measure should also take into account the differing needs of the population to be served, as not all populations will need the same set of features to make the practice patient centered.

From the literature that has been reviewed, it is apparent that none of these constructs can be defined independently. These each depend on each other in order to be described properly and to be implemented properly. The interconnectedness of these constructs implies an integrated definition and model incorporating all three in order to better understand how each construct relates to the others. A proposed integrated model is listed in Fig. 8.1. At the core of the model is behavioral health literacy. This construct is essential, as without it the other two will not be able to be properly defined. Individuals cannot participate in the decision-making process if they do not understand the available options, along with their risks and benefits. Furthermore, providers will be hard-pressed to provide adequate shared decision-making encounters for their clients if the providers and the patients do not know the available resources and options for their particular situation. Additionally, providers will be unable to focus care on the patient's needs if they are unable to recognize and accurately diagnose behavioral health disorders or do not know to whom they can refer the patient if they suspect such

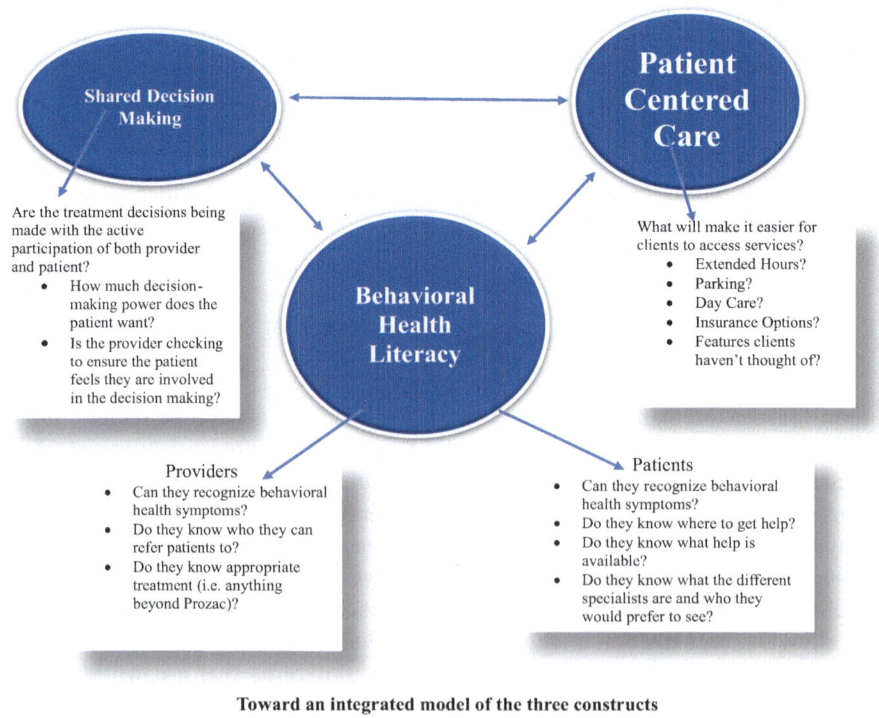

Fig. 8.1 Proposed integrated model

a problem exists and further assessment is needed. Therefore, providers must be literate in behavioral health matters as well in order to implement care that is both collaborative and patient centered.

Shared decision-making, in turn, has an impact on both behavioral health literacy and patient-centered care. In terms of behavioral health literacy, shared decision-making serves as a motivating force for providers to become more literate in behavioral health issues and treatments themselves. The need to provide patients with all accurate and complete information about available evidence-based options for their specific difficulties also motivates clinicians to make connections with other providers who offer specialized services, become more knowledgeable about insurance matters, and potentially seek additional training in therapeutic protocols in order to better serve their patient population. Shared decision-making also helps to improve patient-centered care, as patients when informed about stepped care options may decide to utilize self-help strategies rather than engage in full psychotherapy. A patient-centered practice would have accurate and easy-to-access self-help materials on hand in order to facilitate such a patient decision. Likewise, patient-centered care influences shared decision-making by providing the clinician with the needed interpersonal skills to help empower the client to share in the decision-making process as well as effectively educating patients to facilitate behavioral health literacy. If a client does not feel comfortable in sharing in the decision process, a clinician should be able to identify and work to alleviate these feelings. Patient-centered care also helps to remind the provider that if a patient prefers that the provider takes a lead in decisions, that is, in itself, a decision and should be respected.

Patient-centered care should begin with effective training of the staff so they can interact and communicate with patients in a clear and understandable manner. Providers need to be trained to listen completely to their clients as well as check for understanding when decisions are being made. Therefore, through training the providers in the tenants of good patient-centered care, shared decision-making can be facilitated and enhanced. Furthermore, shared decision-making and behavioral health literacy cannot be implemented if there are no patients coming to the clinic or practice. Because patient-centered care is concerned with factors that help make the patient's access and use of services easier, it in turn permits behavioral health literacy and shared decision-making to function.

A Systems Perspective of Health Literacy, Shared Decision-Making, and Patient-Centered Care

Understanding that these three constructs are interconnected is not sufficient however. Frequently, shared decision-making, patient-centered care, and behavioral health literacy are seen as nothing more than a specific set of clinical skills to be developed by individual clinicians. In essence, these can be seen as a "bottom-up" approach to improving healthcare that by improving a specific set of skills of clinicians in each of these areas, healthcare costs will be lowered and quality of service will be increased. However, it can be argued that such an approach is not the most efficient method of implementing these constructs nor a sufficient method. Instead of viewing them as mere clinical skills, these should instead be conceptualized as a system of care. Therefore, the best place to deploy a delivery system deploying these constructs is at the organizational level, not solely at the level of individual clinicians. Accessibility, extended hours, and multilingual support are all improvements that an organization, rather than isolated providers, is best able to implement. Trainings in how to best utilize shared decision-making are most efficiently delivered to groups of providers, where progress can be measured and issues resolved, rather than allowing each clinician to apply or not apply the shared decision-making principles at their own discretion. Finally, behavioral health literacy interventions can be enhanced through the availability and use of Internet databases, provider directories, and community partnerships to help patients understand more about their particular condition, what treatment options are available, and where to find them. These types of programs are best created and maintained by organizations who can keep them current and easily accessible for providers and patients alike.

It would be useful to craft an integrated definition that combines these three terms into a working delivery system, demonstrating the shared dependencies that are necessary for these three constructs to work. The following is a proposed integration of the three constructs:

Behavioral health literacy, shared decision-making, and patient-centered care do not operate independently of one another but rather together in a coordinated system of healthcare delivery. This system can be defined by the following:

1. A system that educates patients on behavioral health diagnoses and treatments.
2. This information and education enable shared decision-making to arrive at a mutually agreed-upon course of action.
3. Both are facilitated by making the patient the center of clinical and practice organization decisions, which should result in making it as easy as possible for a client to access, understand, and use the services provided.

A hypothetical case example should help to illustrate potentially how such a system of behavioral health literacy, patient-centered care, and shared decision-making might function. Before even arriving at a provider's office, a patient should be able to access a well-designed website with clear cost information and a provider schedule that allows them easy access to the services. A patient then presents to their primary care physician complaining of symptoms of anxiety. The primary care doctor, having been educated in the basics of anxiety disorders as well as where to make referrals, can give the preestablished materials about the disorder as well as where to find additional, reliable information. These materials should be designed to address the basic information regarding the disorder to help educate the patient as well as helping to guide the patient in selecting treatment options, such as watchful waiting, self-help, or deciding to engage in psychotherapy. If psychotherapy is needed, then the patient is referred to the organization's behavioral health provider, who begins by ascertaining how much information the patient desires to know about the disorder and how much they want to be involved in the treatment process. Using the information gathered, the behavioral health provider crafts a treatment plan with the desired participation of the patient, making sure to inform the patient of all possible evidence-based treatment options, so they can make an informed decision regarding their care. Before a decision is made, the patient should be clearly informed of the cost of treatment (i.e., explaining how the patient's insurance may or may not pay for the treatment) as well as educated on the different levels of treatment available so that the appropriate level (watchful waiting vs self-help vs outpatient or inpatient treatment) can be selected. Once a course of action has been decided upon, the treatment will be implemented with the behavioral health provider checking in routinely to see if the intervention is working and if it is still something the patient wishes to continue. If the patient at any time decides they no longer wish to seek treatment, the behavioral health provider should attempt to educate the patient on self-care strategies and other methods of managing their anxiety until they wish to seek treatment again. This entire process will be facilitated by ensuring that the clinic itself has therapy appointments available when the patient has time, has reading materials in the patient's language, and offers child care, so the patient can still attend when they are unable to find someone to watch their children, while they are in session. Other factors, such as a well-designed and comfortable waiting room and convenient parking, will also serve to further enhance the patient's experience and improve the quality of care they are receiving. Lastly, should the patient decide to pursue treatment with another provider in the future, an effective and efficient records management program will be vital to ensure timely and accurate transmission of information for the purposes of coordinating care.

An additional consequence of such a system is the need for additional specialists in the field of psychology. Traditionally, the clinical psychologist tended to be a jack-of-all-trades, often attempting to perform most if not all the duties required in running a clinical practice, including billing, patient education, and taking the trash out. However, for this proposed system to function most efficiently, other specialists should be trained to reduce the burden on the behavioral health providers. An example of such a specialist can be found in the field of diabetes treatment, where diabetes educators train patients in the skills and knowledge needed to modify their behavior and successfully self-manage their disease (Duncan et al., 2011). Diabetes educators have been shown to significantly reduce the cost of diabetes treatment, for example, reducing it from $1012.66 for participants with no diabetes education to $887.44 for those receiving training with a diabetes educator. A similar career path could be adapted to the behavioral health world, with master's level professionals serving as behavioral health educators. These educators could take over the responsibility of educating patients on different treatment modalities, self-care strategies, and techniques for maintaining the improvements made in therapy. Such professionals would fill a vital role in helping patient who may need less intensive care, thus reducing the workload of other clinicians, as well as helping to educate other patients to become more literate in regard to their behavioral health. In turn, this will allow patients to participate more effectively in their treatment.

A Question of Measurement

As previously illustrated, there is a need for further measure development in assessing these constructs. This also applies to the proposed integrated definition, and methods will need to be developed to reliably and validly measure a patient's experience of behavioral health literacy, shared decision-making, and patient-centered care. One possible form such a measure could take is a short survey conducted at the termination of treatment. Building off of the quality improvement aspect of patient-centered care, such a measure should include questions asking patients if they felt that they participated in their treatment at the level that they desired, if they were more knowledgeable about their disorder now than at the beginning of treatment, and if there were any barriers in the clinic itself that made it more difficult for them to obtain services. This measure could be administered in either paper or electronic form, depending on the available resources. More importantly, the measure should be delivered during the patient's last appointment or mailed out to patients who drop out of treatment. Utilizing this type of quality improvement measure at the end of treatment will allow clinics and practices to assess their success in implementing interventions based around the proposed integrated definition.

Conclusions

In summary, behavioral health literacy, shared decision-making, and patient-centered care define a consumer-centered perspective, one that emphasizes the needs and experience of the patient. It is a perspective that goes beyond clinical skills and extends to the entire interaction between a patient and a behavioral health service delivery system. These constructs define a system that makes it easier for a patient to find services, understand what those services are, access services, participate in the decision-making process, and interact with behavioral health professionals in order to get their needs met.

This chapter has presented potential integrated definitions for three of the common methods of reducing healthcare costs and their application to behavioral health. Behavioral health literacy, shared decision-making, and patient-centered care have been lacking unified definitions for years, which has hampered research and quality improvement measures alike. It is our goal that the definitions presented here will form a base of integrated definitions that empirical research can expand and refine, making them more useable as the field searches for methods of reducing healthcare costs while at the same time delivering high-quality behavioral health treatments.

References

Ad Hoc Committee on Health Literacy for the Council on Scientific Affairs AMA. (1999). Health literacy: Report of the council on scientific affairs. *Journal of the American Medical Association*, 552–557.

Adams, J. R., Drake, R. E., & Wolford, G. L. (2007). Shared decision-making preferences of people with severe mental illness. *Psychiatric Services, 58*(9), 1219–1221.

Adams, R. J., Stocks, N. P., Wilson, D. H., Hill, C. L., Gravier, S., Kickbusch, I., & Beilby, J. J. (2009). Health literacy: A new concept for general practice? *Australian Family Physician, 38*(3), 144.

Adkins, N. R., & Corus, C. (2009). Health literacy for improved health outcomes: Effective capital in the marketplace. *Journal of Consumer Affairs, 43*(2), 199–222.

Australian Board of Statistics. (2008). *Adult literacy and life skills survey: Summary results*. Canberra, Australia: Australian Bureau of Statistics.

Bertakis, K. D., & Azari, R. (2011). Patient-centered care is associated with decreased health care utilization. *The Journal of the American Board of Family Medicine, 24*(3), 229–239.

Calabretta, N. (2002). Consumer-driven, patient-centered health care in the age of electronic information. *Journal of the Medical Library Association, 90*(1), 32.

Centers for Medicare & Medicaid Services. (2015). *Highlights*. Retrieved from Centers for Medicare & Medicaid Services: https://www.cms.gov/Research-Statistics-Data-and-Systems/Statistics-Trends-and-Reports/NationalHealthExpendData/downloads/highlights.pdf

Chambless, D. L., & Hollon, S. D. (1998). Defining empirically supported therapies. *Journal of Consulting Psychology, 66*, 7–18.

Charles, C., Gafni, A., & Whelan, T. (1997). Shared decision-making in the medical encounter: What does it mean? (or it takes at least two to tango). *Social Science & Medicine, 44*(5), 681–692.

Corbin, C. L., Kelley, S. W., & Schwartz, R. W. (2001). Concepts in service marketing for healthcare professionals. *The American Journal of Surgery, 181*(1), 1–7.

Dobscha, S. K., Cromer, R., Crain, A., & Denneson, L. M. (2016). Qualitative analysis of US Department of veterans affairs mental health clinician perspectives on patient-centered care. *International Journal for Quality in Health Care, 28*(3), 355–362.

Drake, R. E., Deegan, P. E., & Rapp, C. (2010). The promise of shared decision making in mental health. *Psychiatric Rehabilitation Journal, 34*, 7–13.

Duncan, I., Ahmed, T., Li, Q., Stetson, B., Ruggiero, L., Burton, K., … Fitzner, K. (2011). Assessing the value of the diabetes educator. *The Diabetes Educator, 37*(5), 638–657.

Elwyn, G., Edwards, A., Mowle, S., Wensing, M., Wilkinson, C., Kinnersley, P., & Grol, R. (2001). Measuring the involvement of patients in shared decision-making: a systematic review of instruments. *Patient Education and Counseling, 43*(1), 5–22.

Ende, J., Kazis, L., Ash, A., & Moskowitz, M. A. (1989). Measuring patients' desire for autonomy. *Journal of General Internal Medicine, 4*(1), 23–30.

Epstein, R. M., & Street, R. L. (2011). The values and value of patient-centered care. *Annals of Family Medicine, 9*(2), 100–103 https://doi.org/10.1370/afm.1239

European Commission. (2007). Together for health: A strategic approach for the EU Commission of the European Communities: Brussels 2008–2013.

Freedman, D. A., Bess, K. D., Tucker, H. A., Boyd, D. L., Tuchman, A. M., & Wallston, K. A. (2009). Public health literacy defined. *American Journal of Preventive Medicine, 36*(5), 446–451.

Hamann, J., Cohen, R., Leucht, S., Busch, R., & Kissling, W. (2005). Do patients with schizophrenia wish to be involved in decisions about their medical treatment. *American Journal of Psychiatry, 162*, 2382–2384.

Ishikawa, H., & Yano, E. (2008). Patient health literacy and participation in the health-care process. *Health Expectations, 11*(2), 113–122.

Jorm, A. F. (2012). Mental health literacy: empowering the community to take action for better mental health. *American Psychologist, 67*(3), 231.

Jorm, A. F., Jacomb, P., Jacomb, P. A., Christensen, H., Rodgers, B., & Pollitt, P. (1997). "Mental health literacy": A survey of the public's ability to recognise mental disorders and their beliefs about the effectiveness of treatment. *Medical Journal of Australia, 166*, 182–186.

Kickbusch, I., & Nutbeam, D. (1998). *Health promotion glossary*. Geneva, Switzerland: World Health Organization.

Kickbusch, I., Wait, S., Maag, D., & Banks, I. (2006). *Navigating health: The role of health literacy*. London, UK: Alliance for Health and the Future, International Longevity Centre.

Levinson, W., Kao, A., Kuby, A., & Thisted, R. A. (2005). Not all patients want to participate in decision making. *Journal of General Internal Medicine, 20*(6), 531–535.

Luxford, K., Safran, D. G., & Delbanco, T. (2011). Promoting patient-centered care: A qualitative study of facilitators and barriers in healthcare organizations with a reputation for improving the patient experience. *International Journal for Quality in Health Care, 23*, 510–515.

Makoul, G., & Clayman, M. L. (2006). An integrative model of shared decision making in medical encounters. *Patient Education and Counseling, 60*, 301–312.

Mancuso, J. M. (2008). Health literacy: A concept/dimensional analysis. *Nursing & Health Sciences, 10*(3), 248–255.

National Institute of Mental Health. (2006). *Mental healthcare cost data for all Americans (2006)*. Retrieved from National Institute of Menal Health. https://www.nimh.nih.gov/health/statistics/cost/mental-healthcare-cost-data-for-all-americans-2006.shtml

Nezu, A. M., Nezu, C. M., & D'Zurilla, T. (2012). *Problem-solving therapy: A treatment manual*. New York, NY: Springer Publishing Company.

Nielsen-Bohlman, L. T., Panzer, A. M., Hamlin, B., & Kindig, D. A. (2004). Institute of Medicine. *Health literacy: A prescription to end confusion*. Committee on Health Literacy, Board on Neuroscience and Behavioral Health.

Nutbeam, D. (2000). Health literacy asa public health goal: A challenge for contemporary health education and communication strategies into the 21st century. *Health Promotion International, 15*, 259–267.

Paasche-Orlow, M. K., & Wolf, M. S. (2007). The causal pathways linking health literacy to health outcomes. *American Journal of Health Behavior, 31*(1), S19–S26.

Pavlekovic (Ed.). (2008). *Health literacy: Programmes for training on reseach in public health for south eastern eurpoe* (Vol. IV). Health Promotion and Disease Prevention.

President's Commission for the Study of Ethical Problems in Medicine, Biomedical, & Behavioral Research (US). (1982). *Making Health Care Decisions* (Vol. 1). President's Commission for the study of ethical problems in medicine and biomedical and behavioral research.

Rootman, I., & Gordon-El-Bihbety, D. (2008). *A vision for a health literate Canada*. Ottawa, ON: Canadian Public Health Association.

Simonds S.K. (1974). Health education as social policy. *Health Education Monograph, 2*, 1–25.

Sørensen, K., Van den Broucke, S., Fullam, J., Doyle, G., Pelikan, J., Slonska, Z., & Brand, H. (2012). Health literacy and public health: A systematic review and integration of definitions and models. *BMC Public Health, 12*(1), 80.

Stewart, M., Brown, J. B., Donner, A., McWhinney, I. R., Oates, J., Weston, W., & Jordan, J. (2000). The impact of patient-centered care on outcomes. *The Journal of Family Practice, 49*(9), 1–13.

Towle, A., & Godolphin, W. (1999). Framework for teaching and learning informed shared decision making. *BMJ: British Medical Journal, 319*(7212), 766.

Yost, K. J., Webster, K., Baker, D. W., Choi, S. W., Bode, R. K., & Hahn, E. A. (2009). Bilingual health literacy assessment using the Talking Touchscreen/la Pantalla Parlanchina: Development and pilot testing. *Patient Education and Counseling, 75*(3), 295–301.

Zarcadoolas, C., Pleasant, A., & Greer, D. S. (2003). Elaborating a definition of health literacy: A commentary. *Journal of Health Communication, 8*(S1), 119–120.

Zarcadoolas, C., Pleasant, A., & Greer, D. S. (2005). Understanding health literacy: An expanded model. *Health Promotion International, 20*(2), 195–203.

Zarcadoolas, C., Pleasant, A., & Greer, D. S. (2009). *Advancing health literacy: A framework for understanding and action* (Vol. 45). San Fransisco: Wiley.

Part IV
Health Risk and Care Delivery Factors That Are Key to Healthcare Cost Containment

Chapter 9
Behavioral Health and Diabetes: Increasing Treatment Adherence

Rebecca Crochiere and Amy Hughes Lansing

Diabetes is a chronic illness in which the body struggles to produce or process insulin correctly. Insulin is a hormone created by the pancreas that allows glucose (blood sugar) from the food humans consume to enter the body's cells and be used for energy. When insulin is absent or not working effectively in the body, glucose accumulates in the bloodstream, depriving the body's cells of energy in the short term and producing dire health consequences over the long term, such as kidney failure, heart disease, blindness, and serious infections requiring amputation. Thus, to measure the severity of diabetes, providers collect blood samples to assess average glucose levels in the bloodstream, called the glycated hemoglobin percentage (HbA1c). Upwards of 29.1 million people in the United States or approximately 1 in every 11 Americans lives with diabetes (Centers for Disease Control and Prevention, 2014). In this chapter, we focus on the two most prevalent types of diabetes: type 1 and type 2.

Type 1 diabetes (sometimes referred to as juvenile diabetes) is a chronic disease in which the immune system attacks the cells within the pancreas that create insulin. Since the pancreas becomes unable to produce insulin for people with type 1 diabetes, those with the disease must dose insulin daily to survive. While the etiology of type 1 diabetes is complex, individuals are genetically predisposed to develop the disease, and most of those with type 1 diabetes are diagnosed between childhood and young adulthood. Within the United States, type 1 diabetes disproportionately affects non-Hispanic white individuals compared to individuals of other races or ethnicities (Centers for Disease Control and Prevention, 2015). Approximately 5% of all people with diabetes have type 1 diabetes (Centers for Disease Control and Prevention, 2014).

R. Crochiere
Department of Psychology, Drexel University, Philadelphia, PA, USA
e-mail: rjc356@drexel.edu

A. H. Lansing (✉)
Department of Psychology, University of Nevada, Reno, Reno, NV, USA
e-mail: alansing@unr.edu

M. P. Duckworth, W. T. O'Donohue (eds.), *Behavioral Medicine and Integrated Care*,
https://doi.org/10.1007/978-3-319-93003-9_9

Type 2 diabetes is much more common, making up 90–95% of all diabetes diagnoses. In most instances of type 2 diabetes, the pancreas still produces insulin, but the body's cells and tissues no longer use the insulin properly—a condition termed insulin resistance. Insulin resistance develops gradually and may initially result in prediabetes—or elevated blood glucose levels that do not quite reach the threshold for a diabetes diagnosis—which afflicts more than a third of (86 million) Americans and significantly increases one's chances of developing diabetes in the future (Centers for Disease Control and Prevention, 2014). Both genetic and lifestyle factors heighten risk of developing type 2 diabetes, including family history of diabetes, ethnicity (with African Americans, American Indians, Asian Americans, Pacific Islanders, and Hispanic Americans/Latinos experiencing higher risk), sedentariness, being overweight, and having high blood pressure, among others (Centers for Disease Control and Prevention, 2011; The National Institute of Diabetes and Digestive and Kidney Diseases, 2016). Physicians recommend weight loss, exercise, and often medications that lower blood glucose levels to prevent type 2 diabetes for those at risk, as well as to treat the disease post-diagnosis. Some individuals with type 2 diabetes eventually will require insulin treatments, as prolonged insulin resistance can lead to the death of the cells in the pancreas that produce insulin. The age of onset for type 2 diabetes is usually mid to late adulthood, but type 2 diabetes is increasing in youth and young adults.

Diabetes management, whether for type 1 or type 2 diabetes, requires a complex regimen of multiple daily adherence behaviors, including, but not limited to, self-monitoring of blood glucose, dosing accurate amounts of insulin or taking other diabetes-related medication, and maintaining a low-fat, high-fiber diet. Regular physical activity also helps the body use insulin more effectively (American Diabetes Association, 2015). The merits of exercise and related behavioral medicine approaches are extensively examined in another chapter, so we have limited our discussion of physical activity. Rather, this chapter focuses on behavioral medicine practices for three main components of diabetes management: blood glucose monitoring, medication adherence, and eating behavior/lifestyle changes.

Adherence to the diabetes medical regimen is critical to improving glycemic control and health outcomes, including reductions in microvascular and neurologic complications—major culprits of increased mortality among those with diabetes (Diabetes Control and Complications Trial Research Group, 1993). In the United States, approximately half or fewer of individuals with diabetes meet the suggested level of glycemic control set forth by the American Diabetes Association (Nyenwe, Jerkins, Umpierrez, & Kitabchi, 2011; Wood et al., 2013). In a meta-analysis ranking adherence to 17 different disease and condition regimens using data gathered from 569 studies, diabetes emerged as the second worst in terms of adherence (Dimatteo, 2004). These high rates of nonadherence are particularly alarming because nonadherence to the diabetes regimen not only is associated with worse glycemic control (Feldman et al., 2014; Hood, Peterson, Rohan, & Drotar, 2009) but also increased risk of all-cause hospitalization and mortality (Currie et al., 2012; Ho et al., 2006).

Proper management of diabetes and optimal adherence requires the completion of multiple, daily health behaviors. First, increased self-monitoring of blood glucose (SMBG) levels has been shown to be a strong, objective indicator of adherence to the diabetes regimen, and increased SMBG is associated with improved glycemic control (Diabetes Control and Complications Trial Research Group, 1993; Miller et al., 2013). Nevertheless, only two-thirds of people engaging in SMBG self-report meeting the daily SMBG clinical recommendation (Centers for Disease Control and Prevention, 2015). Second, consistent and timely medication adherence (e.g., insulin doses or metformin—an oral diabetic medicine that helps control blood glucose levels) also positively impacts glycemic control (Diabetes Control and Complications Trial Research Group, 1993; Morris et al., 1997). However, recent data showed that about two-thirds of insulin-pump-wearing individuals with type 1 diabetes miss one or more meal-specific insulin doses weekly, and missing just two of these insulin doses weekly can significantly detriment glycemic control, raising HbA1c levels by 0.5% on average (Datye, Moore, Russell, & Jaser, 2015). Individuals with type 2 diabetes have shown similarly poor adherence to insulin dose regimens and oral antidiabetic drugs, with most studies reporting well below 80% of individuals are adherent (Krass, Schieback, & Dhippayom, 2015).

Third, adherence to nutrition therapy—an individualized meal plan that aims for a healthy macronutrient distribution, monitors carbohydrate consumption, and accounts for the influence of food on glucose levels—has been associated with reduced HbA1c (Delahanty & Halford, 1993); nonetheless, fewer than 10% of patients with established diabetes have visited a nutritionist (Robbins, Thatcher, Webb, & Valdmanis, 2008). In addition, individuals with diabetes have self-reported less adherence to dietary recommendations than to insulin prescriptions and oral agents—adhering only one-third of the time to a strict diet targeting sugar, fat, and calorie consumption to achieve weight loss and improve health (Vijan et al., 2005).

Barriers to Adherence and Diabetes Management

There are a multitude of barriers that can hinder progress toward adherence goals for individuals with diabetes. Peyrot et al. (2005) conducted interviews with healthcare providers and patients with diabetes residing in 13 countries around the world, finding low levels of adherence to diabetes-related clinical recommendations. These researchers also found that patients experienced high rates of diabetes-specific distress and low psychological well-being; patients and providers held significantly different opinions on patients' degree of adherence; and providers felt they lacked the resources to adequately tackle the psychosocial factors inhibiting their patients' progress toward better health (Peyrot et al., 2005). Thus, to comprehensively understand why a patient struggles to meet medical recommendations, barriers to care must be evaluated from a personal (e.g., psychopathology), social (e.g., ineffective communication with caregivers), and societal level (e.g., high cost of diabetes supplies) (Naranjo, Mulvaney, McGrath, Garnero, & Hood, 2014).

Mental health. Rates of depression are significantly higher in youth and adults with diabetes than in those without diabetes (Ali, Stone, Peters, Davies, & Khunti, 2006; Hood et al., 2006). Several studies and meta-analyses suggest that depression or depressive symptoms are significantly associated with decreased adherence (Gonzalez et al., 2008; Hood et al., 2006; Lin et al., 2004). More specifically, some research has found that major depression is linked with lower adherence to medications, reduced exercise, and unhealthy eating habits (Lin et al., 2004) and that individuals with diabetes and depression are three times less likely to adhere to specific aspects of the diabetes regimen than are their non-depressed counterparts (Dimatteo, Lepper, & Croghan, 2000). Further, depressive symptoms negatively impact glycemic control through suboptimal adherence to the diabetes regimen (McGrady, 2009; McGrady & Hood, 2010), and depressive symptoms are negatively associated with glycemic control across ages (Grey, Whittemore, & Tamborlane, 2002; Lustman & Clouse, 2005).

However, researchers also have challenged the notion that depression diagnoses are as prevalent and uniformly linked to the diabetes disease process as the abovementioned research would suggest (Fisher, Gonzalez, & Polonsky, 2014). Researchers provide evidence to imply that depressive symptoms below the threshold of a depression diagnosis are more strongly linked to certain nonadherence behaviors such as diet, exercise, and medication adherence than is major depression (Gonzalez et al., 2007). In addition, their data imply that the depressive symptomology found in individuals with diabetes may be less closely related to major depression than it is to diabetes distress or unique emotional distress stemming from the burden, worry, and burnout that coincide with managing a chronic illness (Fisher et al., 2010; Polonsky et al., 2005). Diabetes distress is highly common, occurring in approximately 30% of individuals with diabetes in one study; in fact, there is evidence to suggest that diabetes distress is more prevalent than is major depression in this population (Fisher et al., 2008). Diabetes distress reflects the chronic strain this disease can exert on one's emotional functioning, relationships, physical health, and ability to lead a normal life (Nicolucci et al., 2013)—for example, diabetes self-management can take up to 2 h per day even among individuals well-practiced in adherence behaviors (Russell, Suh, & Safford, 2005). Diabetes distress has been linked with worse adherence to the diabetes regimen (Fisher et al., 2014) and more strongly linked with poor glycemic control than has depression (Fisher et al., 2010). Thus, when considering how the burden of diabetes is intricately linked with the well-being, adherence, and glycemic control of individuals living with diabetes, it may be critical to differentiate whether depression or diabetes distress plays a stronger mechanistic role, and use that information to guide intervention.

In addition, because successful adherence to the diabetes regimen can require daily completion of several painful behaviors (e.g., pricking your finger to ascertain blood glucose level or dosing insulin through needle injections), anxiety, phobias, and aversions related to these painful adherence behaviors have been shown to influence diabetes management (Nyomba, Berard, & Murphy, 2002; Zambanini, Newson, Maisey, & Feher, 1999). For example, evidence suggests some patients with diabetes avoid self-monitoring of their blood glucose levels because it is too painful (Nyomba et al., 2002). Other research has examined how general and injection-specific anxiety influences adherence and glycemic control in diabetic patients treated with insulin, finding that 14% of patients avoided injections because of anxiety, 42% were troubled by the prospect of needing more frequent injections, and both avoidance of injections and worry of increased injections were associated with greater general anxiety.

Cognitive and behavioral factors. Various cognitive and behavioral factors also can hinder implementation of the major lifestyle changes needed to achieve optimal adherence to the diabetes regimen, such as self-regulation, self-efficacy, illness representations, and disease management knowledge. Self-regulation—one's ability to regulate cognitions, emotions, and behaviors toward a long-term goal—is an overarching construct encompassing many facets of cognitive and behavioral control that have been associated with diabetes adherence, such as self-control (Lansing et al., 2017; Lansing & Berg, 2014) forgetfulness (Vietri, Wlodarczyk, Lorenzo, & Rajpathak, 2016), lack of motivation (Koponen, Simonsen, & Suominen, 2018), as well as perceived inconvenience and valuation of adherence behaviors (Nyomba, Berard, & Murphy, 2004). Relatedly, executive function skills, such as the ability to plan, inhibit impulses, and initiate activity, have been linked with nonadherence to the diabetes regimen in a variety of studies (Duke & Harris, 2014; Feil, Zhu, & Sultzer, 2012). These findings suggest that problems with self-regulation or executive function impairments may put individuals at risk for nonadherence to the diabetes regimen and, consequently, poor glycemic control.

Additionally, individuals' thoughts about how well they can manage diabetes (Iannotti et al., 2006; Nouwen, Urquhart Law, Hussain, McGovern, & Napier, 2009) and the effectiveness of their medical regimen (Farmer, Kinmonth, & Sutton, 2006; Hampson, Glasgow, & Foster, 1995) have been linked to adherence and glycemic control (Griva, Myers, & Newman, 2000). Many of these beliefs and cognitions may be influenced by illness representation, or the patient's schema of an illness, which is theorized to shape disease-related self-regulation and decision making (Leventhal, Meyer, & Nerenz, 1980; Howard Leventhal, Brissette, & Leventhal, 2003). For example, researchers have found that components of the illness representation model, such as illness-specific self-efficacy and perception of treatment effectiveness, were directly linked to diabetes distress and adherence (Nouwen et al., 2009) and glycemic control (Griva et al., 2000).

In youth with type 1 diabetes, beliefs that an individual can carry out diabetes-specific self-management behaviors appropriately and effectively (i.e., self-efficacy) are associated with better adherence (Iannotti et al., 2006). In addition, greater confidence in the effectiveness of treatment has been associated with improved adherence (Hampson et al., 1995).

Finally, a sufficient knowledge base in diabetes self-management is critical to making informed decisions about adherence to the diabetes regimen (Funnell et al., 2009). Despite this, some research shows less than 7% of adults with type 2 diabetes on private insurance attend self-management education training within 12 months of being diagnosed (Li et al., 2014). In fact, attending just one diabetes education session has been associated with significant reductions in hospitalizations (approximately 9 fewer hospitalizations per 100 person years) and hospital costs (savings of over $11,000 per person; Robbins et al., 2008). In addition, meta-analyses have indicated that diabetes self-management training or education improves self-monitoring of blood glucose, adherence to dietary recommendations, and glycemic control (Cooke et al., 2013; McGowan, 2011). Thus, people's cognitive abilities, cognitions, and knowledge—what they believe and know about diabetes as well as their self-regulatory capacity—play a significant role in their ability to manage diabetes successfully.

Social factors. Nevertheless, it is important not only to consider an individual's capacity for managing diabetes but also the capacity of family members involved in the individual's diabetes care (Anderson & Laffel, 1997; Lansing, Crochiere, Cueto, Wiebe, & Berg, 2017). In both youth and adults with diabetes, family involvement, support, and shared responsibility in managing this disease are highly encouraged by healthcare providers and are considered to be a critical component of optimal diabetes management (Chiang, Kirkman, Laffel, & Peters, 2014; Nicolucci et al., 2013). For example, in a large sample of adults with diabetes living in 17 different countries, 85% reported experiencing support and help with self-management from family members (Nicolucci et al., 2013). Higher levels of perceived social support are also positively associated with better adherence (Kouris, Wahlqvist, & Worsley, 1988). Further, among adolescents, active parental monitoring of diabetes adherence behaviors (Berg, Wiebe, & Butner, 2011; Palmer et al., 2011), low diabetes-related family conflict or stress (Anderson et al., 2009; Berlin, Rabideau, & Hains, 2012), and a clear understanding of who—parent or youth—is responsible for specific diabetes adherence behaviors (Anderson et al., 2009; Lewin et al., 2006) have been associated with improved adherence and glycemic control.

In addition to relationships between individuals with diabetes and family members, relationship quality between patient and provider also may influence adherence to medical recommendations. For example, in a study examining barriers to care in 780 youth with type 1 diabetes, Valenzuela et al. (2014) found that almost half of the participants identified receipt of information from providers or communication with providers as impediments to adequate self-care. Even when diabetes providers and patients share the same language and nation of origin, providers' explanations of the disease and self-management are incompatible with the patients' understanding (Weller, Baer, Garcia de Alba Garcia, & Salcedo Rocha, 2012). The use of provider communication techniques that enhance patient comprehension of diabetes self-management, such as evaluation of patient's recall, increases the likelihood that a patient will have better glycemic control (Schillinger et al., 2003). Patient-provider dyads with a dismissing attachment style and poor communication have been linked with worse adherence and glycemic control (Ciechanowski, Katon, Russo, & Walker, 2001).

Systemic factors. Research suggests that individuals with diabetes coming from low-income, less-educated, or socially disadvantaged backgrounds disproportionately experience problems related to access and quality of care, which are associated with worse glycemic control and increased risk of health complications (Naranjo, Hessler, Deol, & Chesla, 2012; Valenzuela et al., 2014). Relatedly, the cost of proper diabetes self-management is considered one of the most pervasive and challenging barriers to care (Daly et al., 2009; Valenzuela et al., 2014), and an inability to meet the costs of care have been associated with worse adherence and less engagement in preventative measures (Karter et al., 2003; Roblin et al., 2005). In one study, approximately one-third of participants reported monitoring their blood glucose levels less frequently than is recommended because of the high cost of testing strips, and simply providing testing strips free of cost predicted increased self-monitoring of blood glucose and improved glycemic control (Nyomba et al., 2002). It is critical while considering individual and social barriers to adherence to also acknowledge and work toward ameliorating systemic inequities associated with worse adherence and disease outcomes.

Screening Tools to Assess Barriers to Adherence and Diabetes Self-management

Mental Health. Some screening tools that assess psychosocial barriers to diabetes self-management were initially developed for more general populations but have shown efficacy in diabetes-specific populations. For example, the patient health questionnaire-9 (PHQ-9; Kroenke, Spitzer, & Williams, 2001) and patient health questionnaire-2 (PHQ-2; Kroenke, Spitzer, & Williams, 2003) serve as sound, validated depression screening tools in diabetes patients (van Steenbergen-Weijenburg et al., 2010). By using the PHQ-2 as a first-line screener and only employing the PHQ-9 for individuals that screen positive on the PHQ-2 (i.e., at least one item positive), burden on patients can be limited. Similarly, the general anxiety disorder screener-7 has been validated in diabetes patients (GAD-7; Spitzer, Kroenke, Williams, & Löwe, 2006). Since these screeners have only a few items, they represent efficient tools that provide a reliable measure of depressive or anxiety symptoms and take considerably less time to implement than the gold standard, a structured clinical interview (Esbitt, Tanenbaum, & Gonzalez, 2013).

The Diabetes Distress Scale-17 (DDS-17; Polonsky et al., 2005) and the Diabetes Distress Scale-2 (DDS-2; Fisher, Glasgow, Mullan, Skaff, & Polonsky, 2008) are two measures shown to be sensitive indicators of diabetes-related distress. Additionally, the diabetes-related emotional problem domain on the 20-item Problem Areas in Diabetes Scale (PAID; Polonsky et al., 1995) has been used to capture diabetes-specific distress, and briefer versions of this scale, notably the PAID-5 and the PAID-1 (McGuire et al., 2010), also have shown good reliability, sensitivity, and specificity. Again, these measures allow for a brief first-line screening tool to assess diabetes distress while limiting patient burden related to completing screening forms.

Cognitive, Behavioral, and Social Factors. Moreover, several measures were designed to evaluate multiple psychosocial barriers to the diabetes regimen, a "one-stop shop" tool for providers seeking to determine which psychosocial factors may be influencing suboptimal adherence in any given patient. For example, the

Diabetes Care Profile (DCP; Fitzgerald et al., 1996) indexes diabetes-specific attitudes, self-control, self-efficacy, knowledge, and social support in people with type 1 or type 2. Other measures, such as the 9-item Risk Index for Poor Glycemic Control (RI-PGC; Schwartz, Axelrad, & Anderson, 2013) and the 21-item Barriers to Diabetes Adherence (BDA; Mulvaney et al., 2011), were developed to ascertain psychosocial risk of nonadherence in youth with type 1 diabetes. The PedsQL Diabetes Module, although described as a quality of life scale, also represents a reliable and valid measure of diabetes-specific barriers to treatment, including worries and communication issues. The Psychosocial Assessment Tool (PAT; Kazak et al., 2001) also is commonly used to assess psychosocial risk in youth with chronic illnesses more generally. Finally, the Psychosocial Risk Screening Measure (PRiSM; Schwartz, Cline, Hansen, Axelrad, & Anderson, 2010) is a semi-structured interview that may be used to further assess for risk of nonadherence by evaluating socioeconomic, mental health, and family risk factors in youth with type 1 diabetes. Employing a combination of these screening tools can help providers quickly identify barriers to adherence, facilitate brief behavioral medicine interventions, and determine appropriate referrals to additional services.

Brief Intervention to Improve Adherence

Because patients often experience combinations of the abovementioned barriers to care, the gold standard method to promote adherence is a multicomponent intervention that addresses the numerous psychosocial barriers impeding proper self-management. Generally, such an approach is not feasible in the time-constricted space of brief behavioral medicine interventions. Thus, a critical purpose of the screening assessment tools is to identify the most high-need area (or two) to address in a brief intervention. Education, behavioral problem-solving, and motivational interviewing approaches have been supported as important for improving diabetes adherence, and there is a growing role for the use of technology in extending the reach of brief behavioral medicine interventions to promote diabetes management. Employing these methods during primary and specialty care visits for diabetes may increase adherence and promote health, while preserving limited outpatient psychological services for patients with complex presentations of psychosocial problems that are not responsive to time-limited interventions.

Diabetes self-management education (DSME) is essential to optimal adherence but, on its own, may not be sufficient to significantly improve adherence to the diabetes regimen. Especially in youth, interventions aimed at promoting diabetes self-management via DSME have shown little effectiveness or efficacy in achieving better glycemic control (Murphy, Rayman, & Skinner, 2006). In adult populations, DSME interventions have led to modest improvements in disease severity (Gary, Genkinger, Guallar, Peyrot, & Brancati, 2003), with interventions that employ in-person instruction, physical activity content, and cognitive reframing approaches being more likely to change glycemic control (Ellis et al., 2004). Other research corroborates that short educational programs may moderately ameliorate diabetes outcomes, such as one randomized controlled trial finding that a single 6-h educational session resulted in greater weight loss and smoking cessation in individuals with newly diagnosed type 2 diabetes (Davies et al., 2008). Thus, while DSME alone may not drastically boost adherence, it is necessary, and referrals to DSME should be made when knowledge is interfering with optimal adherence.

Interventions that target behavior modification via problem-solving, behavioral skills, and coping have been more effective in achieving improved adherence than has DSME (Padgett, Mumford, Hynes, & Carter, 1988). Interventions promoting goal-setting and problem-solving skills, self-monitoring behavior, and positive reinforcement have led to improvements in diabetes-related health outcomes, including weight loss maintenance (Wing, Tate, Gorin, Raynor, & Fava, 2006) and dietary behavior (Glasgow, Toobert, & Hampson, 1996). Further, Glasgow et al. (1996) achieved these improvements using just a single session office-based intervention, supporting the notion that these types of interventions can effectively be delivered in brief formats. Other researchers have found that simply adding self-regulation content—e.g., highlighting problem-solving techniques like goal identification—to an information session focused on increased fruit and vegetable consumption led to greater fruit and vegetable intake even 2 years post-intervention (Stadler, Oettingen, & Gollwitzer, 2010). Another promising model for providing this type of brief intervention is that of collaborative care, in which nurses meet with patients 1–2 times a month and use problem-solving and goal-setting techniques to help patients manage diabetes and depression. Research has shown this type of model to be effective at improving diabetes and mental health outcomes, requiring only weekly supervision from a provider, psychologist, and psychiatrist (Katon et al., 2010).

This behavioral problem-solving approach also has shown to be effective in the context of family functioning surrounding diabetes management, most commonly for youth with type 1 diabetes. Researchers have been able to incorporate programs targeting diabetes-related family functioning into clinic settings. For example, researchers developed a family-focused intervention occurring after regularly scheduled diabetes visits that targeted responsibility-sharing and problem-solving within the family system; this ambulatory intervention boosted family involvement in diabetes and buffered against the worsening of glycemic control (Laffel et al., 2003). These examples suggest that promoting problem-solving and behavioral skills at both the patient and family level can be beneficial in improving diabetes adherence and health.

Motivational interviewing, a client-focused, therapeutic approach to behavioral change, is another evidence-based approach that can be easily incorporated into regular medical visits and may help patients adopt healthy behaviors required for optimal adherence (Rollnick & Miller, 1995). This approach emphasizes a communication style that help healthcare providers to come alongside patients by asking open questions, affirming, reflecting, and summarizing when discussing behavior change. Several randomized trials have found that motivational interviewing interventions improve adherence to the diabetes regimen and glycemic control in adults (Chen, Creedy, Lin, & Wollin, 2012; West, DiLillo, Bursac, Gore, & Greene, 2007) and youth (Channon et al., 2007). For example, Channon et al. (2007) implemented a motivational interviewing program for youth in which two trained nurses worked with youth on awareness building, considering alternatives, and goal setting in the context of diabetes management. The motivational interviewing sessions lasted 20–60 min and were scheduled as needed, with participants engaging in four sessions on average across 12 months. Motivational interviewing compared to a nondirective support program led to significantly lower HbA1c at end of treatment. West et al. (2007) found that five 45-min sessions of motivational interviewing that focused on promoting change talk and the alignment of values with behavioral change for overweight women with type 2 diabetes resulted in greater weight loss over 18 months compared to the control group. Other common features of these programs included a focus on free choice in making behavior changes, use of readiness rulers to discuss importance of and confidence in specific behavior change, and how to respond to failures in behavior change (relapse prevention).

Moreover, training providers and other healthcare personnel to employ motivational interviewing techniques may prove beneficial for patient diabetes outcomes. For example, researchers have randomized general practitioners to engage in a 1 1/2-day training program on motivational interviewing, during which they were coached by a trained instructor on the primary components of motivational interviewing, as well as two half-day follow-up trainings within the year. The results indicated that training providers in motivational interviewing led their patients to experience enhanced autonomy, motivation to adhere, and perceived importance of preventative behaviors and glycemic control (Rubak, Sandbaek, Lauritzen, Borch-Johnsen, & Christensen, 2009). Also, dieticians randomly assigned to a 2-day motivational interviewing training plus a 1-day follow-up workshop exhibited more empathy and reflection when interacting with patients than did the control group, and these interactions spurred by motivational interviewing were linked with improved dietary adherence (Brug et al., 2007). Thus, primary and specialty diabetes care settings could benefit from training patient-facing staff in motivational interviewing as well as having expert behavioral health providers available for brief motivational interviewing sessions in the context of more problematic health behaviors.

In addition, the recent advent of technological tools designed to improve health, such as mHealth apps that facilitate self-monitoring and engagement in health-related behaviors or a web-based, diabetes-specific Coping with Depression course (van Bastelaar, Pouwer, Cuijpers, Riper, & Snoek, 2011), may allow providers to "prescribe" patients a mobile or computer-based solution to address barriers to adherence. For example, the diabetes-specific Coping with Depression course offers eight weekly online lessons that require minimal involvement from providers (i.e., limited to providing concise, standardized feedback on homework assignments). The course was adapted from an existing online depression module by adding diabetes content focused on training coping skills for the management of problematic cognitions and emotions related to poor test results, fluctuations in blood glucose, and other diabetes-related worries as well as social skills for communicating with healthcare professionals and talking to others about diabetes. This course has been shown to reduce depressive symptoms and diabetes-related distress in a randomized controlled trial of over 250 adults with diabetes (van Bastelaar et al., 2011). Recent meta-analyses also suggest that mHealth interventions can significantly improve health outcomes and management of chronic illness in adults (Liang et al., 2010) and youth, and involvement of caregivers in mHealth interventions may produce greater improvements in youth chronic illness management (Fedele et al., 2017). Further, due to the universality of mobile devices and ease of inputting and integrating diabetes-related data (e.g., blood glucose levels or carbohydrates) into mobile apps, mHealth programs may boost providers' ability to access, monitor, and synthesize patient data and offer support in real time (Naranjo et al., 2014). While these advances represent exciting and efficient tools for healthcare systems already overstretched to provide adequate care, these mHealth interventions must undergo stringent clinical trials to ensure they are effective and efficacious.

Finally, interventions on the healthcare system itself also may help mitigate some of the psychosocial barriers to optimal diabetes adherence. For example, healthcare systems could adopt a case management approach, with personnel like nurses serving as team leaders, which has shown to be effective in improving patient adherence (Welch, Garb, Zagarins, Lendel, & Gabbay, 2010). In fact, simply enhancing the involvement of nurses providing diabetes care has been associated with improvements in patient health outcomes (Renders, Valk, & Griffin, 2001). Additionally, diabetes care provided by physicians may be enhanced longitudinally via easy-to-implement tools that offer performance improvement feedback (Ziemer et al., 2006). To this end, a study found that encouraging provider screening of diabetic complications, goal setting with patients, and continuing education courses reduced complications and HbA1c over 6 years (Olivarius et al., 2001). Thus, the ways in which medical professionals frame and organize healthcare may ease the burden of adherence on patients and lead to better health outcomes.

Summary

Diabetes management requires a complex regimen of multiple daily adherence behaviors, and many individuals with diabetes struggle to achieve optimal adherence and glycemic control. Various psychosocial issues may be inhibiting individuals' ability to engage in proper diabetes self-management, including mental health problems, cognitive, behavioral, and social factors, and systemic obstacles. Several well-established screening tools can be implemented in clinical settings to detect these psychosocial barriers to adherence and inform potential brief behavioral medicine intervention approaches. While DSME may be critical to attain excellent adherence, it may not be sufficient to enact behavioral health change. Other approaches, such as those employing problem-solving, behavioral skills, and coping techniques as well as those utilizing motivational interviewing in brief intervention formats, have shown greater effectiveness in improving diabetes outcomes. Advances in technology and the advent of mHealth tools may help to disseminate these intervention approaches at a low cost, and research suggests mHealth interventions can be effective in bolstering chronic illness management. Last, some simple steps can be taken to redesign our healthcare systems so that providers and healthcare teams can better support individuals struggling to manage diabetes.

References

Ali, S., Stone, M., Peters, J., Davies, M., & Khunti, K. (2006). The prevalence of co-morbid depression in adults with type 2 diabetes: A systematic review and meta-analysis. *Diabetic Medicine, 23*, 1165–1173.

American Diabetes Association. (2015). *Food and fitness: What we recommend*. Retrieved May 18, 2017, from http://www.diabetes.org/food-and-fitness/fitness/types-of-activity/what-we-recommend.html

Anderson, B., Holmbeck, G., Iannotti, R., Mckay, S., Lochrie, A., Volkening, L., & Laffel, L. (2009). Dyadic measures of the parent–child relationship during the transition to adolescence and glycemic control in children with type 1 diabetes. *Families, Systems, & Health, 27*, 141–152.

Anderson, B., & Laffel, L. M. (1997). Behavioral and psychosocial research with school-aged children with type 1 diabetes. *Diabetes Spectrum, 10*, 227–284.

Berg, C. A., Wiebe, D. J., & Butner, J. (2011). Affect covariation in marital couples dealing with stressors surrounding prostate cancer. *Gerontology, 57*, 167–172.

Berlin, K. S., Rabideau, E. M., & Hains, A. A. (2012). Empirically derived patterns of perceived stress among youth with type 1 diabetes and relationships to metabolic control. *Journal of Pediatric Psychology, 37*, 990–998.

Brug, J., Spikmans, F., Aartsen, C., Breedveld, B., Bes, R., & Fereira, I. (2007). Training dietitians in basic motivational interviewing skills results in changes in their counseling style and in lower saturated fat intakes in their patients. *Journal of Nutrition Education and Behavior, 39*, 8–12.

Centers for Disease Control and Prevention. (2011). National Diabetes Fact Sheet, 2011.

Centers for Disease Control and Prevention. (2014). *National diabetes statistics report: Estimates of diabetes and its burden in the United States*. Atlanta, GA: U.S. Department of Health and Human Services.

Centers for Disease Control and Prevention. (2015). Diabetes Report Card, 2014.

Channon, S. J., Huws-Thomas, M. V., Rollnick, S., Hood, K., Cannings-John, R. L., Rogers, C., & Gregory, J. W. (2007). A multicenter randomized controlled trial of motivational interviewing in teenagers with diabetes. *Diabetes Care, 30*, 1390–1395.

Chen, S. M., Creedy, D., Lin, H. S., & Wollin, J. (2012). Effects of motivational interviewing intervention on self-management, psychological and glycemic outcomes in type 2 diabetes: A randomized controlled trial. *International Journal of Nursing Studies, 49*, 637–644.

Chiang, J., Kirkman, M., Laffel, L., & Peters, A. (2014). Type 1 diabetes through the life span: A position statement of the American Diabetes Association. *Diabetes Care, 37*, 2034–2054.

Ciechanowski, P. S., Katon, W. J., Russo, J. E., & Walker, E. A. (2001). The patient-provider relationship: Attachment theory and adherence to treatment in diabetes. *American Journal of Psychiatry, 158*, 29–35.

Cooke, D., Bond, R., Lawton, J., Rankin, D., Heller, S., Clark, M., & Speight, J. (2013). Structured type 1 diabetes education delivered within routine care: Impact on glycemic control and diabetes-specific quality of life. *Diabetes Care, 36*, 270–272.

Currie, C. J., Peyrot, M., Morgan, C. L., Poole, C. D., Jenkins-Jones, S., Rubin, R. R., … Evans, M. (2012). The impact of treatment noncompliance on mortality in people with type 2 diabetes. *Diabetes Care, 35*, 1279–1284.

Daly, J. M., Hartz, A. J., Xu, Y., Levy, B. T., James, P. A., Merchant, M. L., & Garrett, R. E. (2009). An assessment of attitudes, behaviors, and outcomes of patients with type 2 diabetes. *The Journal of the American Board of Family Medicine, 22*, 280–290.

Datye, K. a., Moore, D. J., Russell, W. E., & Jaser, S. S. (2015). A review of adolescent adherence in type 1 diabetes and the untapped potential of diabetes providers to improve outcomes. *Current Diabetes Reports, 15*, 621.

Davies, M. J., Heller, S., Skinner, T. C., Campbell, M. J., Carey, M. E., Cradock, S., … Khunti, K. (2008). Effectiveness of the diabetes education and self management for ongoing and newly diagnosed (DESMOND) programme for people with newly diagnosed type 2 diabetes: Cluster randomised controlled trial. *BMJ, 336*, 491–495.

Delahanty, L. M., & Halford, B. N. (1993). The role of diet behaviors in achieving improved glycemic control in intensively treated patients in the Diabetes Control and Complications Trial. *Diabetes Care, 16*, 1453–1458.
Diabetes Control and Complications Trial Research Group. (1993). The effect of intensive treatment of diabetes on the development and progression of long-term complications in insulin-dependent diabetes mellitus: Diabetes Control and Complications Trial. *New England Journal of Medicine, 329*, 977–986.
Dimatteo, M. R. (2004). Social support and patient adherence to medical treatment: A meta-analysis. *Health Psychology, 23*, 207–218.
Dimatteo, M. R., Lepper, H. S., & Croghan, T. W. (2000). Depression is a risk factor for non-compliance with medical treatment meta-analysis of the effects of anxiety and depression on patient adherence. *Archives of Internal Medicine, 160*, 2101–2107.
Duke, D. C., & Harris, M. A. (2014). Executive function, adherence, and glycemic control in adolescents with type 1 diabetes: A literature review. *Current Diabetes Reports, 14*, 532.
Ellis, S., Speroff, T., Dittus, R., Brown, A., Pichert, J., & Elasy, T. (2004). Diabetes patient education: A meta-analysis and meta-regression. *Patient Education and Counseling, 52*, 97–105.
Esbitt, S., Tanenbaum, M., & Gonzalez, J. S. (2013). Disentangling clinical depression from diabetes-specific distress: Making sense of the mess we've made. In *Screening for depression and other psychological problems in diabetes. A practical guide* (pp. 27–46), New York, NY: Springer.
Farmer, A., Kinmonth, A., & Sutton, S. (2006). Measuring beliefs about taking hypoglycaemic medication among people with Type 2 diabetes. *Diabetic Medicine, 23*, 265–270.
Fedele, D. A., Cushing, C. C., Fritz, A., Amaro, C. M., & Ortega, A. (2017). Mobile health interventions for improving health outcomes in youth. *JAMA Pediatrics, 41*, 835–848.
Feil, D. G., Zhu, C. W., & Sultzer, D. L. (2012). The relationship between cognitive impairment and diabetes self-management in a population-based community sample of older adults with Type 2 diabetes. *Journal of Behavioral Medicine, 35*, 190–199.
Feldman, B. S., Cohen-Stavi, C. J., Leibowitz, M., Hoshen, M. B., Singer, S. R., Bitterman, H., … Balicer, R. D. (2014). Defining the role of medication adherence in poor glycemic control among a general adult population with diabetes. *PLoS One, 9*, e108145. https://doi.org/10.1371/journal.pone.0108145
Fisher, L., Glasgow, R. E., Mullan, J. T., Skaff, M. M., & Polonsky, W. H. (2008). Development of a brief diabetes distress screening instrument. *Annals of Family Medicine, 6*, 246–252.
Fisher, L., Mullan, J., Arean, P., Glasgow, R., Hessler, D., & Masharani, U. (2010). Diabetes distress but not clinical depression or depressive symptoms is associated with glycemic control in both cross-sectional and longitudinal analyses. *Diabetes Care, 33*, 23–28.
Fisher, L., Skaff, M. M., Mullan, J. T., Arean, P., Glasgow, R., & Masharani, U. (2008). A longitudinal study of affective and anxiety disorders, depressive affect and diabetes distress in adults with type 2 diabetes. *Diabetic Medicine, 25*, 1096–1101.
Fisher, L., Gonzalez, J. S., & Polonsky, W. H. (2014). The confusing tale of depression and distress in patients with diabetes: A call for greater clarity and precision. *Diabetic Medicine, 31*, 764–772.
Fitzgerald, J. T., Davis, W. K., Connell, C. M., Hess, G. E., Funnell, M. M., & Hiss, R. G. (1996). Development and validation of the diabetes care profile. *Evaluation & the Health Professions, 19*, 208–230.
Funnell, M., Brown, T., Childs, B., Haas, L., Hosey, G., Jensen, B., … Weiss, M. (2009). National standards for diabetes self-management education. *Diabetes Care, 32*, S87–S94.
Gary, T. L., Genkinger, J. M., Guallar, E., Peyrot, M., & Brancati, F. L. (2003). Meta-analysis of randomized educational and behavioral interventions in type 2 diabetes. *The Diabetes Educator, 29*, 488–501.
Glasgow, R. E., Toobert, D. J., & Hampson, S. E. (1996). Effects of a brief office-based intervention to facilitate diabetes dietary self-management. *Diabetes Care, 19*, 835–842.

Gonzalez, J. S., Peyrot, M., McCarl, L. A., Collins, E. M., Serpa, L., Mimiaga, M. J., & Safren, S. A. (2008). Depression and diabetes treatment nonadherence: A meta-analysis. *Diabetes Care, 31*, 2398–2403.

Gonzalez, J. S., Safren, S. A., Cagliero, E., Wexler, D. J., Delahanty, L. M., Wittenberg, E., … Grant, R. W. (2007). Depression, self-care, and medication adherence in type 2 diabetes. *Diabetes Care, 30*, 2222–2227.

Grey, M., Whittemore, R., & Tamborlane, W. (2002). Depression in type 1 diabetes in children: Natural history and correlates. *Journal of Psychosomatic Research, 53*, 907–911.

Griva, K., Myers, L. B., & Newman, S. (2000). Illness perceptions and self efficacy beliefs in adolescents and young adults with insulin dependent diabetes mellitus. *Psychology & Health, 15*, 733–750.

Hampson, S., Glasgow, R., & Foster, L. (1995). Personal models of diabetes among older adults: Relationship to self-management and other variables. *The Diabetes Educator, 21*, 300–307.

Ho, P. M., Rumsfeld, J. S., Masoudi, F. A., McClure, D. L., Plomondon, M. E., Steiner, J. F., & Magid, D. J. (2006). Effect of medication nonadherence on hospitalization and mortality among patients with diabetes mellitus. *Archives of Internal Medicine, 166*, 1836–1841.

Hood, K., Huestis, S., Maher, A., Butler, D., Volkening, L., & Laffel, L. M. (2006). Depressive symptoms in children and adolescents with type 1 diabetes: Association with diabetes-specific characteristics. *Diabetes Care, 29*, 1389–1391.

Hood, K., Peterson, C., Rohan, J., & Drotar, D. (2009). Association between adherence and glycemic control in pediatric type 1 diabetes: A meta-analysis. *Pediatrics, 124*, e1171–e1179.

Iannotti, R., Schneider, S., Nansel, T., Haynie, D., Plotnick, L., Clark, L., … Simons-Morton, B. (2006). Self-efficacy, outcome expectations, and diabetes self-management in adolescents with type 1 diabetes. *Journal of Developmental & Behavioral Pediatrics, 27*, 98–105.

Karter, A. J., Stevens, M. R., Herman, W. H., Ettner, S., Marrero, D. G., Safford, M. M., … Brown, A. F. (2003). Out-of-pocket costs and diabetes preventive services: The Translating Research Into Action for Diabetes (TRIAD) study. *Diabetes Care, 26*, 2294–2299.

Katon, W. J., Lin, E. H. B., Von Korff, M., Ciechanowski, P., Ludman, E. J., Young, B., … McCulloch, D. (2010). Collaborative care for patients with depression and chronic illnesses. *The New England Journal of Medicine, 363*, 2611–2620.

Kazak, A., Prusak, A., McSherry, M., Simms, S., Beele, D., Rourke, M., … Lange, B. (2001). The Psychosocial Assessment Tool (PAT)©: Pilot data on a brief screening instrument for identifying high risk families in pediatric oncology. *Families, Systems, & Health, 19*, 303–317.

Koponen, A. M., Simonsen, N., & Suominen, S. B. (2018). Success in weight management among patients with type 2 diabetes: Do perceived autonomy support, autonomous motivation, and self-care competence play a role? *Behavioral Medicine, 44*, 151–159.

Kouris, A., Wahlqvist, M. L., & Worsley, A. (1988). Characteristics that enhance adherence to high-carbohydrate/high-fiber diets by persons with diabetes. *Journal of the American Dietetic Association, 88*, 1422–1425.

Krass, I., Schieback, P., & Dhippayom, T. (2015). Adherence to diabetes medication: A systematic review. *Diabetic Medicine, 32*, 725.

Kroenke, K., Spitzer, R. L., & Williams, J. B. W. (2001). The PHQ-9: Validity of a brief depression severity measure. *Journal of General Internal Medicine, 16*, 606–613.

Kroenke, K., Spitzer, R. L., & Williams, J. B. W. (2003). The Patient Health Questionnaire-2: Validity of a two-item depression screener. *Medical Care, 41*, 1284–1292.

Laffel, L., Vangsness, L., Connell, A., Goebel-Fabbri, A., Butler, D., & Anderson, B. (2003). Impact of ambulatory, family-focused teamwork intervention on glycemic control in youth with type 1 diabetes. *The Journal of Pediatrics, 142*, 409–416.

Lansing, A. H., & Berg, C. A. (2014). Adoelscent self-regulation as a foundation for chronic illness self-management. *Journal of Pediatric Psychology, 39*, 1091–1096.

Lansing, A. H., Crochiere, R., Cueto, C., Wiebe, D. J., & Berg, C. A. (2017). Mother, father, and adolescent self-control and adherence in adolescents with type 1 diabetes. *Journal of Family Psychology, 31*, 495–503. https://doi.org/10.1037/fam0000292

Lansing, A. H., Turner, S. L., Osborn, P. G., Winnick, J. B., Taheri, K., Murray, M., ... Berg, C. A. (2017). Academic achievement and metabolic control in adolescents with type 1 diabetes. *Children's Health Care, 47*, 16–33.

Leventhal, H., Brissette, I., & Leventhal, E. (2003). The common-sense model of self-regulation of health and illness. In *The Self-Regulation of Health and Illness Behaviour* (pp. 42–65), New York, NY: Routledge.

Leventhal, H., Meyer, D., & Nerenz, D. (1980). The common sense representation of illness danger. In: S. Rachman, Ed., *Contributions to Medical Psychology (*17–30*)*, New York, NY: Pergamon Press.

Lewin, A. B., Heidgerken, A. D., Geffken, G. R., Williams, L. B., Storch, E. A., Gelfand, K. M., & Silverstein, J. H. (2006). The relation between family factors and metabolic control: The role of diabetes adherence. *Journal of Pediatric Psychology, 31*, 174–183.

Li, R., Shrestha, S. S., Lipman, R., Burrows, N. R., Kolb, L. E., Rutledge, S., & Centers for Disease Control and Prevention (CDC). (2014). Diabetes self-management education and training among privately insured persons with newly diagnosed diabetes--United States, 2011-2012. *Morbidity and Mortality Weekly Report, 63*, 1045–1049.

Liang, X. H., Wang, Q. Q., Yang, X. L., Cao, J., Chen, J. C., Mo, X. B., ... Gu, D. F. (2010). Effect of mobile phone intervention for diabetes self-management support on glycemic control: A meta-analysis. *Cardiology, 117*, 120.

Lin, E. H. B., Katon, W., Von Korff, M., Rutter, C., Simon, G. E., Oliver, M., ... Young, B. (2004). Relationship of depression and diabetes self-care, medication adherence, and preventive care. *Diabetes Care, 27*, 2154–2160.

Lustman, P. J., & Clouse, R. E. (2005). Depression in diabetic patients: The relationship between mood and glycemic control. *Journal of Diabetes and Its Complications, 19*(2), 113–122.

McGowan, P. (2011). The efficacy of diabetes patient education and self-management education in type 2 diabetes. *Canadian Journal of Diabetes, 35*, 46–53.

McGrady, M. (2009). Depressive symptoms and glycemic control in adolescents with type 1 diabetes mediational role of blood glucose monitoring. *Diabetes Care*, 1–11.

McGrady, M. E., & Hood, K. K. (2010). Depressive symptoms in adolescents with type 1 diabetes: Associations with longitudinal outcomes. *Diabetes Research and Clinical Practice, 88*, e35. https://doi.org/10.1016/j.diabres.2010.03.025

McGuire, B. E., Morrison, T. G., Hermanns, N., Skovlund, S., Eldrup, E., Gagliardino, J., ... Snoek, F. J. (2010). Short-form measures of diabetes-related emotional distress: The Problem Areas in Diabetes Scale (PAID)-5 and PAID-1. *Diabetologia, 53*, 66–69.

Miller, K. M., Beck, R. W., Bergenstal, R. M., Goland, R. S., Haller, M. J., McGill, J. B., ... Hirsch, I. B. (2013). Evidence of a strong association between frequency of self-monitoring of blood glucose and hemoglobin A1c levels in T1D exchange clinic registry participants. *Diabetes Care, 36*, 2009–2014.

Morris, A. D., Boyle, D. I. R., McMahon, A. D., Greene, S. A., MacDonald, T. M., & Newton, R. W. (1997). Adherence to insulin treatment, glycaemic control, and ketoacidosis in insulin-dependent diabetes mellitus. *Lancet, 350*, 1505–1510.

Mulvaney, S. A., Hood, K. K., Schlundt, D. G., Osborn, C. Y., Johnson, K. B., Rothman, R. L., & Wallston, K. A. (2011). Development and initial validation of the barriers to diabetes adherence measure for adolescents. *Diabetes Research and Clinical Practice, 94*, 77–83.

Murphy, H. R., Rayman, G., & Skinner, T. C. (2006). Psycho-educational interventions for children and young people with type 1 diabetes. *Diabetic Medicine., 23*, 935.

Naranjo, D., Hessler, D., Deol, R., & Chesla, C. (2012). Health and psychosocial outcomes in U.S. adult patients with diabetes from diverse ethnicities. *Current Diabetes Reports, 12*(6), 729–738.

Naranjo, D., Mulvaney, S., McGrath, M., Garnero, T., & Hood, K. (2014). Predictors of self-management in pediatric type 1 diabetes: Individual, family, systemic, and technologic influences. *Current Diabetes Reports, 14*, 1–8.

Nicolucci, A., Kovacs Burns, K., Holt, R., Comaschi, M., Hermanns, N., Ishii, H., ... DAWN2 Study Group. (2013). Diabetes Attitudes, Wishes and Needs second study (DAWN2TM):

Cross-national benchmarking of diabetes-related psychosocial outcomes for people with diabetes. *Diabetic Medicine, 30*, 767–777.

Nouwen, A., Urquhart Law, G., Hussain, S., McGovern, S., & Napier, H. (2009). Comparison of the role of self-efficacy and illness representations in relation to dietary self-care and diabetes distress in adolescents with type 1 diabetes. *Psychology & Health, 24*, 1071–1084.

Nyenwe, E. A., Jerkins, T. W., Umpierrez, G. E., & Kitabchi, A. E. (2011). *Management of type 2 diabetes: Evolving strategies for the treatment of patients with type 2 diabetes*. Metabolism: Clinical and Experimental.

Nyomba, B., Berard, L., & Murphy, L. (2002). The cost of self-monitoring of blood glucose is an important factor limiting glycemic control in diabetic patients. *Diabetes Care, 25*, 1244–1245.

Nyomba, B. L., Berard, L., & Murphy, L. J. (2004). Facilitating access to glucometer reagents increases blood glucose self-monitoring frequency and improves glycaemic control: A prospective study in insulin-treated diabetic patients. *Diabetic Medicine, 21*, 129–135.

Olivarius, N. D. F., Beck-Nielsen, H., Andreasen, A. H., Hørder, M., Pedersen, P. A., Horder, M., & Pedersen, P. A. (2001). Randomised controlled trial of structured personal care of type 2 diabetes mellitus. *BMJ, 323*, 970–970.

Padgett, D., Mumford, E., Hynes, M., & Carter, R. (1988). Meta-analysis of the effects of educational and psychosocial interventions on management of diabetes mellitus. *Journal of Clinical Epidemiology, 41*, 1007–1030.

Palmer, D. L., Osborn, P., King, P. S., Berg, C., Butler, J., Butner, J., … Wiebe, D. (2011). The structure of parental involvment and relations to disease managment for youth with type 1 diabetes. *Journal of Pediatric Psychology, 36*, 596–605.

Peyrot, M., Rubin, R. R., Lauritzen, T., Snoek, F. J., Matthews, D. R., Skovlund, S. E., … Delamater, A. (2005). Psychosocial problems and barriers to improved diabetes management: Results of the Cross-National Diabetes Attitudes, Wishes and Needs (DAWN) Study. *Diabetic Medicine, 22*, 1379–1385.

Polonsky, W., Anderson, B., Lohrer, P., Welch, G., Jacobson, A., Aponte, J., & Schwartz, C. (1995). Assessment of diabetes-related distress. *Diabetes Care, 18*, 754–760.

Polonsky, W., Fisher, L., Earles, J., Dudl, R., Lees, J., Mullan, J., & Jackson, R. (2005). Assessing psychosocial distress in diabetes: Development of the Diabetes Distress Scale. *Diabetes Care, 28*, 626–631.

Renders, C., Valk, G., & Griffin, S. (2001). Interventions to improve the management of diabetes in primary care, outpatient, and community settings a systematic review. *Diabetes Care, 24*, 1821–1833.

Robbins, J. M., Thatcher, G. E., Webb, D. A., & Valdmanis, V. G. (2008). Nutritionist visits, diabetes classes, and hospitalization rates and charges. *Diabetes Care, 31*, 655–660.

Roblin, D. W., Platt, R., Goodman, M. J., Hsu, J., Nelson, W. W., Smith, D. H., … Soumerai, S. B. (2005). Effect of increased cost-sharing on oral hypoglycemic use in five managed care organizations: How much is too much? *Medical Care, 43*, 951–959.

Rollnick, S., & Miller, W. R. (1995). What is motivational interviewing? *Behavioural and Cognitive Psychotherapy, 23*, 325–334.

Rubak, S., Sandbaek, A., Lauritzen, T., Borch-Johnsen, K., & Christensen, B. (2009). General practitioners trained in motivational interviewing can positively affect the attitude to behaviour change in people with type 2 diabetes. One year follow-up of an RCT, ADDITION Denmark. *Scandinavian Journal of Primary Health Care, 27*, 172–179.

Russell, L. B., Suh, D., & Safford, M. M. (2005). Time requirements for diabetes self-management: Too much for many? *Journal of Family Practice, 54*, 52–56.

Schillinger, D., Piette, J., Grumbach, K., Wang, F., Wilson, C., Daher, C., … Bindman, A. B. (2003). Closing the loop: Physician communication with diabetic patients who have low health literacy. *Archives of Internal Medicine, 163*, 83–90.

Schwartz, D., Axelrad, M., & Anderson, B. (2013). Psychosocial risk screening of children newly diagnosed with type 1 diabetes: A training toolkit for healthcare professionals. *MedEdPORTAL, 9*, 9643. https://doi.org/10.15766/mep_2374-8265.9643.

Schwartz, D. D., Cline, V. D., Hansen, J. A., Axelrad, M. E., & Anderson, B. J. (2010). Early risk factors for nonadherence in pediatric type 1 diabetes: A review of the recent literature. *Current Diabetes Reviews, 6*, 167–183.

Spitzer, R., Kroenke, K., Williams, J., & Löwe, B. (2006). A brief measure for assessing generalized anxiety disorder: The GAD-7. *Archives of Internal Medicine, 166*, 1092–1097.

Stadler, G., Oettingen, G., & Gollwitzer, P. (2010). Intervention effects of information and self-regulation on eating fruits and vegetables over two years. *Health Psychology, 29*, 274–283.

The National Institute of Diabetes and Digestive and Kidney Diseases. (2016). *Risk factors for type 2 diabetes*. Retrieved May 18, 2017, from https://www.niddk.nih.gov/health-information/diabetes/overview/risk-factors-type-2-diabetes

Valenzuela, J. M., Seid, M., Waitzfelder, B., Anderson, A. M., Beavers, D. P., Dabelea, D. M., … Mayer-Davis, E. J. (2014). Prevalence of and disparities in barriers to care experienced by youth with type 1 diabetes. *Journal of Pediatrics, 164*, 1369–1375.

van Bastelaar, K. M. P., Pouwer, F., Cuijpers, P., Riper, H., & Snoek, F. J. (2011). Web-based depression treatment for type 1 and type 2 diabetic patients a randomized, controlled trial. *Diabetes Care, 34*, 320–325.

van Steenbergen-Weijenburg, K. M., de Vroege, L., Ploeger, R. R., Brals, J. W., Vloedbeld, M. G., Veneman, T. F., … van der Feltz-Cornelis, C. M. (2010). Validation of the PHQ-9 as a screening instrument for depression in diabetes patients in specialized outpatient clinics. *BMC Health Services Research, 10*, 235.

Vietri, J. T., Wlodarczyk, C. S., Lorenzo, R., & Rajpathak, S. (2016). Missed doses of oral antihyperglycemic medications in US adults with type 2 diabetes mellitus: Prevalence and self-reported reasons. *Current Medical Research and Opinion, 32*, 1519–1527.

Vijan, S., Stuart, N. S., Fitzgerald, J. T., Ronis, D. L., Hayward, R. A., Slater, S., & Hofer, T. P. (2005). Barriers to following dietary recommendations in Type 2 diabetes. *Diabetic Medicine, 22*, 32–38.

Welch, G., Garb, J., Zagarins, S., Lendel, I., & Gabbay, R. A. (2010). Nurse diabetes case management interventions and blood glucose control: Results of a meta-analysis. *Diabetes Research and Clinical Practice, 88*, 1.

Weller, S. C., Baer, R. D., Garcia de Alba Garcia, J., & Salcedo Rocha, A. L. (2012). Explanatory models of diabetes in the U.S. and Mexico: The patient-provider gap and cultural competence. *Social Science and Medicine, 75*, 1088–1096.

West, D., DiLillo, V., Bursac, Z., Gore, S., & Greene, P. (2007). Motivational interviewing improves weight loss in women with type 2 diabetes. *Diabetes Care, 30*, 1081–1087.

Wing, R., Tate, D., Gorin, A., Raynor, H., & Fava, J. (2006). A self-regulation program for maintenance of weight loss. *New England Journal of Medicine, 355*, 1563–1571.

Wood, J. R., Miller, K. M., Maahs, D. M., Beck, R. W., Dimeglio, L. A., Libman, I. M., … Woerner, S. E. (2013). Most youth with type 1 diabetes in the T1D exchange clinic registry do not meet American diabetes association or international society for pediatric and adolescent diabetes clinical guidelines. *Diabetes Care, 36*, 2035–2037.

Zambanini, A., Newson, R. B., Maisey, M., & Feher, M. D. (1999). Injection related anxiety in insulin-treated diabetes. *Diabetes Research and Clinical Practice, 46*, 239–246.

Ziemer, D. C., Doyle, J. P., Barnes, C. S., Branch, W. T., Cook, C. B., El-Kebbi, I. M., … Phillips, L. S. (2006). An intervention to overcome clinical inertia and improve diabetes mellitus control in a primary care setting: Improving Primary Care of African Americans with Diabetes (IPCAAD) 8. *Archives of Internal Medicine, 166*, 507–513.

Chapter 10
Meeting the Care Needs of Patients with Multiple Chronic Conditions

Melanie P. Duckworth, Tony Iezzi, and Gwendolyn C. Carlson

Primary care facilities and hospitals have long been aware of the significant burden borne by patients who present with chronic medical conditions. Current estimates suggest that nearly 50% of American adults have at least one chronic medical condition (Ward, Schiller, & Goodman, 2014; Wu & Green, 2000). Patients commonly present to the primary care setting for management of symptoms and functional impairments associated with hypertension, high cholesterol, diabetes, skin conditions, or arthritic conditions. Patients with chronic medical conditions often experience marked changes in overall quality of life, with varying degrees of compromise experienced across work, household, recreational, social, interpersonal, and familial domains of function. These changes in overall quality of life, in conjunction with the stress of diagnosis and the demands of disease management, often result in psychological distress that would be deemed clinically significant and require intervention. Primary care physicians are among the first healthcare providers tasked with managing these chronic medical conditions and the associated physical and psychological compromise. For patients with chronic medical conditions that require extensive intervention by medical providers or involve complex self-management regimens, patient care needs are much more likely to be assessed and managed through any number of general and specialty care clinics.

In 2010, the most prevalent chronic physical and psychological conditions experienced by American adults were hypertension (27%), hyperlipidemia (22%), allergies, sinusitis, and upper respiratory conditions (14%), arthritis (13%), depression and bipolar disorder (11%), diabetes (10%), and anxiety disorders (7%; Gerteis et al., 2014). The Centers for Medicare and Medicaid Services (2016) noted that, among Medicare and Medicaid recipients, the most

M. P. Duckworth (✉) · G. C. Carlson
Department of Psychology, University of Nevada, Reno, Reno, NV, USA
e-mail: melanied@unr.edu

T. Iezzi
Behavioral Medicine Service, London Health Sciences Center, London, ON, Canada

M. P. Duckworth, W. T. O'Donohue (eds.), *Behavioral Medicine and Integrated Care*,
https://doi.org/10.1007/978-3-319-93003-9_10

common chronic medical conditions include arthritis, asthma, atrial fibrillation, cancer, chronic kidney disease, chronic obstructive pulmonary disease, diabetes, heart failure, hepatitis (chronic viral B and C), human immunodeficiency virus (HIV)/acquired immunodeficiency syndrome (AIDS), hyperlipidemia, hypertension, ischemic heart disease, osteoporosis, and stroke. Also numbered among commonly experienced chronic conditions are psychological disorders such as depression. The increasing prevalence of such chronic physical and psychological conditions is likely due to improvements in the effectiveness of medical interventions and the associated decrease in disease-related mortality, all of which translates to fewer people dying due to disease and more people living longer with chronic medical conditions.

One of the more pressing concerns for all parties involved in healthcare provision is the marked increase in the number of patients who present with multiple, concurrent, chronic medical conditions. It has been estimated that 32% of the American adult population are experiencing and attempting to manage two or more chronic medical conditions (Gerteis et al., 2014). When compared to patients diagnosed with a single chronic medical condition, patients with two or more chronic medical conditions present with greater disruptions in function and quality of life as well as increased mortality (Anderson, 2010; Boyd & Fortin, 2010; Lee et al., 2007). In 2010, the US Department of Health and Human Services (HHS) Agency for Healthcare Research and Quality convened a workgroup aimed at creating system-wide strategies to identify and focus clinical and research attention on patients with two or more chronic medical conditions. This workgroup eventually supported the use of the term multiple chronic conditions (MCC) to refer to such patients and put forward a strategic framework for disseminating data and improving the psychometric properties of measures used to capture MCC (Anderson, 2010). For the purposes of this chapter, the term MCC will be used to refer to patients with two or more chronic medical conditions, with terms such as comorbidity and multimorbidity used only when these terms have been used by other researchers to define patient groups.

Because MCC are associated with greater healthcare utilization and costs, and because patients with MCC often experience functional impairment and disability and clinically significant psychological distress, the MCC context serves as an ideal context for the integration of behavioral health interventions and medical interventions aimed at managing multiple, co-occurring chronic medical conditions and reducing the impact of such conditions on patient quality of life and overall well-being. The current chapter describes the scope and significance of MCC, functional impairment and disability experienced consequent to MCC, risk factors that contribute to the onset of MCC, traditional disease self-management approaches used in the context of MCC, and a newly proposed treatment program aimed at applying empirically supported cognitive-behavioral interventions to the problem of MCC. In this discussion of MCC, information pertaining to adults with MCC is emphasized; however, information relevant to MCC in children and older adult populations is also presented.

Scope and Significance of MCC

Prevalence

Although prevalence estimates for MCC vary depending on the population targeted, the setting in which the survey is completed, and the survey method employed, it can be generally agreed that the number of persons with MCC is staggering. It has been estimated that some 75 million Americans have two or more medical conditions (Anderson 2010), and by the year 2020, 81 million Americans will likely experience two or more chronic medical conditions (Anderson & Horvath, 2004).

The presence of MCC is associated with elevated rates of healthcare utilization. Using data from the 2009 National Ambulatory Medical Care Survey, Ashman and Beresovsky (2013) found that, of the 326 million physician office visits made by adults 18 years of age or older, nearly 123 million of these visits were made by patients with two or more chronic medical conditions. More than 67 million office visits were made by patients with at least three chronic medical conditions. Using data from the Nationwide Inpatient Sample, the largest all-payer inpatient database, Steiner and Friedman (2013) determined that, of approximately 28 million adult patients discharged from American hospitals in 2009, 39% had two to three chronic medical conditions and 33% had four or more chronic medical conditions. Ward et al. (2014) used data from the 2010 National Health Interview Survey to estimate the prevalence of multiple chronic conditions among US adults. The data revealed that, of the 117 million US adults determined to have at least one chronic medical condition, more than 32 million of these US adults had two chronic medical conditions, and nearly 28 million had at least three chronic medical conditions. Findings from these three studies suggest that an increasingly large portion of the nation's healthcare resources are being used to manage the care needs of patients with MCC.

Data also suggest that the likelihood of experiencing MCC increases as individuals get older. Machlin and Soni (2013) used data from the 2009 Medical Expenditure Panel Survey to estimate the prevalence of MCC across two age cohorts: adults aged 45–64 years and adults aged 65 years or older. These researchers examined the rates of occurrence of a wide array of chronic medical and psychiatric conditions, including arthritis, asthma, autism spectrum disorder, cancer, cardiac arrhythmias, chronic kidney disease, chronic obstructive pulmonary disease, congestive heart failure, coronary artery disease, dementia, depression, diabetes, hepatitis, HIV infection, hyperlipidemia, hypertension, osteoporosis, schizophrenia, stroke, and substance abuse disorders. It was estimated that 25% of all adults surveyed had been treated for at least two chronic medical conditions. This estimated rate of MCC increased to 31% for adults aged 45–64 and to 67% for adults aged 65 years or older. Among adults 65 years or older, nearly 25% had been treated for four or more chronic conditions.

While research findings suggest that MCC can be considered a near normative experience among older adults, it must be acknowledged that, for a significant number of adults with MCC, their experience of MCC likely began in childhood or adolescence. It is estimated that 12% of young persons in the US have been diagnosed with MCC (Clark et al., 2015; Zhong et al., 2015). Although these findings suggest that MCC are common among young persons, no longitudinal examinations of the trajectory of MCC from childhood into adulthood were identified in the literature.

In addition to investigating the relation of MCC to advancing age, researchers have sought to determine the relation of MCC to other sociodemographic variables, including gender, race and ethnicity, and the interaction of these variables. Freid, Bernstein, and Bush (2012) used data collected from the National Health Interview Survey to examine the changing prevalence of MCC among US adults aged 45 years and older by gender, racial and ethnic group, and income. Survey participants were characterized as experiencing MCC based on the presence of two or more of the following medical conditions: diabetes, cancer, chronic bronchitis, current asthma, emphysema, heart disease, hypertension, kidney disease, and stroke. To determine the changing prevalence of MCC, survey data obtained from participants evaluated in the year 1999–2000 were compared to data obtained from participants evaluated in the year 2009–2010. Results revealed that, among adults aged 45–64 years and among adults aged 65 years and above, MCC increased for both men and women, for members of all racial and ethnic groups, and for most income groups.

Cost

Patients with MCC are high healthcare utilizers and the cost of managing the care needs of persons with co-occurring conditions contributes significantly to the financial burden borne by society. Chronic conditions cost the US government billions of dollars each year as a function of direct medical costs and costs related to reduced work productivity. It is estimated that 71% of all healthcare expenditures in the US are spent on patients with MCC and over a third of all healthcare expenditures are spent on patients with five or more health conditions (Gerteis et al., 2014). In 2010, average annual healthcare spending was estimated to be $4,731 for two chronic conditions, $6,751 for three chronic conditions, $9,162 for four chronic conditions, and $15,954 for five or more conditions (Gerteis et al., 2014).

Using data from the 2009 Medical Expenditure Panel Survey, it was determined that the average annual medical care expenditure for adults with two to three chronic conditions was $8,478 and that the average medical care expenditure for adults with four or more chronic conditions was $16,257 (Machlin & Soni, 2013). These care expenditures are in stark contrast to the average medical expenditure of $2,367 that is spent to manage the health needs of adults who do not require treatment for MCC.

Due to the fact that the Medicare program was designed to support the healthcare needs of persons aged 65 years and older as well as persons under age 65 with permanent disabilities, Medicare patients are recognized as being high healthcare utilizers and as contributing significantly to healthcare costs. Schneider, O'Donnell, and Dean (2009) examined Medicare expenditures associated with MCC across adults aged 65 years and older. Results revealed that the annual Medicare payment for beneficiaries with one condition was $7,172, the annual payment for beneficiaries with two conditions was $14,931, and the annual payment for beneficiaries with three or more conditions was $32,498.

In an older but influential study, Wolff, Starfield, and Anderson (2002) examined data from a random sample of approximately 1.2 million Medicare beneficiaries who were 65 years of age and older and found that 67% of those sampled experienced MCC. Beneficiaries with MCC accounted for 95% of Medicare costs. After controlling for the effects of age and gender, individuals with four or more chronic medical conditions were almost 100 times more likely to undergo hospitalization for a medical circumstance that could have been managed with a primary care intervention. While the average annual cost for Medicare beneficiaries with no chronic condition was $211, the average annual cost for Medicare beneficiaries with four or more chronic conditions was $13,973. The investigators concluded that improvements in primary care access and interventions could lead to a reduction in hospitalization rates and costs, especially for those beneficiaries with MCC.

As part of a finer analysis of healthcare expenditures associated with multiple chronic conditions, Skinner, Coffey, Jones, Heslin, and Moy (2016) examined the ambulatory care costs and hospitalization costs incurred by persons with chronic medical conditions. Using the 2012 State Inpatient Databases (SID), databases developed as part of the Agency for Healthcare Research and Quality Healthcare Cost and Utilization Project, Skinner and colleagues reviewed 1.43 million claims to determine the number of chronic medical conditions experienced by claimants. Findings revealed that approximately 38% of claimants had two or three chronic conditions, 30% had four or five chronic conditions, and 10% had six or more chronic conditions. Using claimants with zero or one chronic condition as the comparison group, claims data revealed that ambulatory care costs were 19% higher for claimants with two or three conditions, 32% higher for those with four or five conditions, and 31% higher for those with six or more conditions. When hospital stays involved management of acute conditions (i.e., dehydration, bacterial pneumonia, and urinary tract infections), results revealed that hospital stays were 11% longer for claimants with two or three conditions, 21% longer for those with four or five conditions, and 27% longer for those with six or more conditions. When hospital stays were required to manage chronic conditions (e.g., diabetes, chronic obstructive pulmonary disease, and congestive heart failure), the relation of increasing numbers of chronic conditions to lengthier hospital stays was again observed. Finally, it was determined that the relation of increasing chronic conditions to increasing care costs was largely a function of lengthier hospital stays experienced by persons with MCC rather than higher per day care costs.

The SID databases used by Skinner et al. (2016) include hospital discharge data from US community hospitals. Zulman and colleagues undertook the study of MCC as found among US Veterans and as managed within the Veterans Administration healthcare system (Zulman et al., 2015). To determine the economic impact of high utilization patients on the VA healthcare system, these researchers reviewed the files of 5.2 million patients who received VA healthcare services in the year 2010. The researchers found that 50% of the total VA healthcare expenditures for 2010 were made as part of managing the healthcare needs of the 5% of patients ($N = 261{,}699$) with the highest rates of care utilization. Approximately two-thirds of those patients had chronic conditions that affected three or more organ systems.

Lehnert et al. (2011) completed a systematic review of 35 studies that examined healthcare outcomes (i.e., physician use, hospital use, and medication use) and healthcare costs (i.e., medication costs, out-of-pocket costs, and total healthcare costs) among elderly persons with MCC. The authors noted that, although the synthesis of studies was limited by the variability in definitions of MCC used and the different outcomes measures employed across studies, it can be concluded that the relation of MCC to healthcare use and healthcare cost is positive, with each additional chronic condition associated with an increase in healthcare utilization and an exponential increase in the cost of that healthcare. The authors noted that there are few care models that properly attend to the needs of elderly persons with MCC. They recommended that a comprehensive care management approach be taken in treating such patients, one that would accommodate the different diseases, treatment settings, care providers, and treatment locations that are part of usual care for persons with MCC.

Using an integrated healthcare model, Bayliss and colleagues sought to demonstrate the utility of continuity of care in reducing healthcare utilization among elderly persons with MCC (Bayliss et al., 2015). This study was conducted in response to findings from earlier studies that characterized older MCC populations as more vulnerable to fragmented healthcare and indicated low continuity of care as associated with inappropriate medication use, more emergency room visits and hospitalizations, and higher mortality rates. Using the electronic records of 12,200 members of Kaiser Permanente in Colorado, a not-for-profit integrated healthcare delivery system, the researchers examined the relation between patients' perceptions of care continuity and their utilization of healthcare services. Participating patients were 65 years or older, and continuity of care was assessed using Bice and Boxerman's (1977) Continuity of Care Index. The results indicated that after controlling for demographics and clinical covariates, greater primary and specialty care continuity was associated with fewer inpatient admissions and fewer emergency room visits. Of note, analyses performed on the subgroup of patients who attended three or more primary care visits and three or more specialty care visits revealed that specialty care continuity contributed to a decrease in hospital admissions and primary care continuity contributed to a decrease in emergency room visits.

Studies examining the cost of MCC in the young are limited. In one of best available studies examining chronic conditions among young persons and the associated healthcare costs, Zhong et al. (2015) performed a retrospective cohort study of all dependents ($N = 14{,}727$) of Mayo Clinic employees over the 4-year period between 2004 and 2007. The researchers determined that, for children with no chronic condition, average annual medical costs totaled \$1,483; for children with four or five chronic conditions, average annual medical costs ranged from \$12,524 to \$33,782. Children's experiences of MCC also were determined to persist over time and to be associated with consistently high medical costs. Those children with MCC that placed them in the top 10th percentile of healthcare expenditures during the first year of the study were more likely to incur similarly high healthcare costs 3 years later.

Impairment and Disability

When a medical condition is experienced as a chronic and disabling circumstance, the effect of that condition on function tends to follow a familiar and predictable progression from disease diagnosis to functional impairment to partial or total disability (Duckworth & Iezzi, 2010; Duckworth, Iezzi, & Shearer, 2012). For patients with MCC, this progression from disease diagnosis to disability is often accelerated and associated with even greater burden. Impairment is defined as "a loss, loss of use, or derangement of any body part, organ system, or organ function," while disability is defined as "an alteration of an individual's capacity to meet personal, social or occupational demands because of an impairment" (Cocchiarelli & Andersson, 2001, p. 3). For persons with MCC, physical impairments may include the reduced ability to sit, stand, walk, lift, carry, bend, etc. Physical impairments then lead to reduced involvement in routine activities. For patients who are less than 65 years of age, the ability to work is often affected, which can lead to financial losses that interfere with MCC patients' ability to maintain basic necessities of living, including food, shelter, clothing, and healthcare. Regardless of age, the presence of MCC is associated with a marked decrease in housekeeping and home maintenance tasks, recreational activities, social interactions, familial and marital activities, and physical and nonphysical intimacy. Physical impairments can sometimes be so extreme that they render MCC patients unable to engage in basic activities of daily living (ADLs) such as eating, bathing, dressing, toileting, and sleeping. The more changes in ADLs and overall quality of life that persons with MCC experience, the more likely it is that they will experience emotional distress. The emotional distress can reach such an intensity that it can be disabling.

With the goal of identifying promising avenues for health promotion and disease prevention among older adults, Barile and his colleagues (2013) used baseline and 2-year follow-up data from 27,334 respondents to the Medicare Health Outcomes Survey to examine associations among MCC, ADLs, and quality of life. Activities of daily living were assessed using a six-item measure (Katz, Ford, Moskowitz, Jackson, & Jaffe, 1963), and health-related quality of life was assessed using two items from the CDC's Healthy Days Measures (Moriarty, Zack, & Kobau, 2003). Findings indicated that MCC, when present at baseline and as a circumstance that developed over the 2-year sampling period, were associated with reduced engagement in ADLs and poorer quality of life. The authors concluded that any effective intervention for patients with MCC would have significant effects on clinical outcomes and healthcare costs. They also emphasized the need for broad-based interventions designed to impact different aspects of MCC (i.e., increase patient engagement in health-promoting behaviors [e.g., exercise, good nutrition, and stress management] and decrease patient engagement in disease-promoting behaviors [e.g., overeating, smoking, and substance use]).

Salive (2013) examined the administrative claims of over 31 million Medicare beneficiaries for the presence of 15 prevalent medical conditions, and he reviewed 17 studies examining MCC among community samples of older adults. It was determined that 67% of the Medicare beneficiaries experienced multimorbidity, with multimorbidity present in 50% of beneficiaries younger than 65 years of age, 62% of those aged 65 to 74 years, and 82% of those aged 85 years and older. Based on his review of the 17 community studies, Salive concluded that multimorbidity was associated with adverse drug events, poor functional status, poor quality of life, increased disability, and elevated risk of death. He noted that these conclusions were consistent with two other systematic literature reviews of this literature (Fortin et al., 2004; Gijsen et al., 2001).

Gully, Rasch, and Chan (2011) used data from the Medical Expenditure Panel Survey (2002–2004) to examine the relations among MCC, disability, and healthcare utilization. Among those persons reporting limitations in any basic or instrumental ADLs, 35% experienced four or more medical conditions. The investigators also noted that limitations of any kind consistently predicted more emergency department visits and hospitalizations and greater problems with healthcare access.

In an attempt to develop models that would allow for the prediction of functional outcomes experienced by persons with MCC, Alonso-Moran, Nuno-Solinis, Onder, and Tonnara (2015) conducted a review of studies published between 1994 and 2014 that examined persons with MCC and documented the outcomes experienced by such patients. From a total of 3,674 citations, the researchers identified 29 articles that met criteria for inclusion in the review. Different measures of multimorbidity were employed across studies, with the Charlson Comorbidity Index (Charlson, Pompei, Ales, & MacKenzie, 1987) being the most frequently used measure (used in 12 of the 29 studies). Clinical and administrative data were used to establish rates of hospital admission and readmission. The diseases identified as contributing most significantly to the prediction of negative health and functional outcomes were chronic obstructive pulmonary disease, cardiac heart failure, cerebrovascular disease, and diabetes. As a multidimensional construct, ADLs served as an important predictor of functional impairment and disability.

Research has been undertaken to determine whether different patterns of multimorbidity are associated with different patterns of functional impairment and disability (Jackson et al. 2015; Quinones, Markwardt, & Botoseneanu, 2016). For their study of multimorbidity and functional impairment, Jackson and colleagues surveyed a total of 7,270 older women (aged between 76 and 81 years) who participated in the Australian Longitudinal Study on Women's Health. Survey data were collected every 3 years over the 9-year period between 2002 and 2011. Functional ability and functional decline were assessed using eight basic ADLs (grooming, eating, bathing, dressing upper body, dressing lower body, getting up from chair, walking, and toileting) and eight instrumental ADLs (doing housework, managing finances, preparing meals, taking medications, using the telephone, shopping, doing laundry, and managing transportation). Data pertaining to 31 self-identified chronic conditions were submitted to factor analysis, and three patterns of multimorbidity were revealed: (1) musculoskeletal/somatic (representing conditions such as back pain, arthritis, and headache), (2) neurological/mental health (representing conditions such as dementia, depression, anxiety, and stroke), and (3) cardiovascular (representing conditions such as hypertension, heart attack, and angina). When applied to data collected during the initial project year, persons who evidenced higher factor scores across the three patterns of multimorbidity evidenced higher levels of functional impairment (as measured by basic and instrumental ADLs [IADLs]) than did a reference group of persons who obtained lower factor scores. Findings revealed that, during the 7-year period between 2005 and 2011, women in the cardiovascular group experienced the greatest decline in basic ADLs, while women in the neuromuscular/mental group experienced the greatest decline in IADLs. The authors concluded that different multimorbidity patterns were associated with different patterns of functional decline and disability and that such findings would have implications for both the management and prevention of MCC.

A large-scale study of older Americans revealed findings similar to those obtained by Jackson et al. (2015) in their study of older Australian women. Using data from the Health and Retirement Study and employing a prospective cohort design, Quinones et al. (2016) examined 8,782 participants, aged 65 years and older, to identify combinations of chronic conditions and to determine the manner in which different combinations of chronic conditions contribute to functional impairment and disability. Unlike the Jackson et al. study, depressive symptoms were included as one of the chronic conditions evaluated in this study. The three most prevalent combinations of chronic conditions were (1) hypertension and arthritis; (2) hypertension, arthritis, and cardiovascular disease; and (3) hypertension, arthritis, and diabetes. Only one of the 14 identified multimorbidity combinations included depressive symptoms. Compared to persons with any other single chronic condition or combination of chronic conditions, persons who reported the combination of arthritis, hypertension, and depressive symptoms evidenced the highest level of disability across both basic ADLs and IADLs. This finding held even after the influence of age, gender, education, race/ethnicity, and body mass index was controlled. The authors indicated that, when added to other chronic conditions, depressive illness might confer a level of burden greater than that associated with adding another chronic medical condition (e.g., asthma).

The importance of disability to the health and survival of persons with chronic medical conditions was made even more salient by Marengoni, von Strauss, Rizzuto, Winblad, and Fratiglioni's (2009) examination of data from the Kungsholmen Project (1987–2000), a Swedish, community-based, prospective study of aging and dementia. Data from 2,368 persons, aged 75 years and older, were used to determine the independent and combined contributions of MCC and disability to function and survival outcomes at three-year follow-up. At baseline assessment, 52% of participants were diagnosed with MCC and 12% experienced partial or total disability, with partial disability defined as need for assistance with two to four basic ADLs and total disability defined as the need for assistance with five to six basic ADLs. At 3-year follow-up, the health status of 85 participants had worsened and 365 participants had died. The number of diagnosed conditions was positively and significantly associated with risk of functional decline but was not significantly associated with risk of mortality. Interestingly, baseline disability had the highest effect on survival independent of the number of MCC. The authors concluded that, among elderly persons, disability is a stronger predictor of function and survival than is multimorbidity.

Disability of any kind (physical or psychological) represents a significant complicating aspect of the MCC experience. Each additional chronic condition increases functional impairment and decreases quality of life (Jindai, Nielson, Vorderstrasse, & Quinones, 2016). In fact, the amount and kind of disability may play a more important role in the MCC experience than an actual count of chronic conditions. Additional research examining the contribution of disability to MCC-related morbidity and mortality is warranted.

MCC and Psychological Distress

It has been long recognized that patients with chronic medical conditions experience co-occurring psychological conditions, most commonly depressive disorders, anxiety disorders, and substance use disorders. However, the process by which these medical conditions and psychological conditions co-occur is not always understood. Psychological factors are known to play a significant role in the development, maintenance, and exacerbation of chronic medical conditions, and chronic medical conditions are known to precipitate psychological distress reactions, even in patients who do not have any psychiatric history prior to medical diagnosis. It is also clear that some psychological disorders constitute a significant burden for the individual sufferer and for the healthcare system. Given all that is known about the interacting influences of medical and psychological conditions and the burden these conditions present in isolation and in combination, it is important to recognize that few studies have examined the relation between medical and psychological conditions in the context of MCC.

Cabassa et al. (2013) used the data from National Epidemiologic Survey on Alcohol and Related Conditions to determine the risk of MCC conferred by the presence of a psychiatric disorder as well as the risk conferred by ethnic/racial identity (African American, Hispanic, and non-Hispanic White). Data collected from 33,107 survey participants were submitted to multinomial logistic regression analyses. Findings revealed that participants diagnosed with psychiatric disorders experienced a higher likelihood of MCC than participants with no psychiatric diagnosis. It was determined that, after controlling for the effect of covariates (i.e., other sociodemographic variables, body mass index, psychiatric disorders, and quality of life), African American participants experienced the highest odds of MCC and Hispanic participants the lowest likelihood of MCC.

Byles et al. (2014) used data from 236,508 participants in the New South Wales 45 and Up Study, an ongoing study of healthy aging among Australian adults, to examine the associations among self-reported physical conditions, psychological distress (as measured by the Kessler Psychological Distress Scale; Kessler et al.,

2002), and disability (as measured by the SF-36 Physical Function subscale; Ware, Kosinski, & Keller, 1994). The investigators focused on heart attack/angina, other heart disease, stroke, and diabetes as singular physical conditions and as co-occurring physical conditions. As singular conditions, all medical conditions were associated with higher risk of high to very high psychological distress; the significance of the relation of individual medical conditions to psychological distress was maintained even after comorbidity, disability, and sociodemographic factors were added to the prediction model. When compared to participants reporting no need for assistance with daily life tasks, women who reported needing assistance with daily life tasks were seven times more likely to experience marked psychological distress, and men who reported needing assistance with daily life tasks were nine times more likely to experience marked psychological distress. Participants who were unable to work due to illness or disability had the highest rates of psychological distress.

Finally, Banhato et al. (2016) examined depressive symptoms in a sample of 1,558 Brazilian patients with MCC, all of whom attended a center that treated patients with hypertension, diabetes, and chronic kidney disease and underwent semi-structured interview over the 3-month study period. Results revealed that 33% of the study sample had depressive symptoms. After controlling for age and education, the presence of depressive symptoms was predicted by being female, being a smoker, and having diabetes. Although study findings regarding the prevalence of depressive symptoms are interesting, depressive symptoms were measured using only two items from a patient history form. These findings need to be replicated using brief but psychometrically sound measures of depression and other psychological disorders that are common among persons with chronic medical conditions.

Although clinically significant psychological distress occurs in relation to MCC, healthcare providers sometimes fail to recognize symptoms of psychological distress and/or appreciate the influence of distress symptoms on the health and treatment outcomes experienced by patients with MCC. Also key to the healthcare provider's effective evaluation and treatment of such patients is knowledge of the coping strategies, both adaptive and maladaptive, that patients routinely employ to managing their medical conditions and the associated changes in function. Early and ongoing assessment and management of the psychological symptoms serve to improve patients' overall health and well-being and need to become a routine component of care provision for patients with MCC.

Biological and Environmental Risk Factors Associated with MCC

Biological and environmental risk factors for a single medical condition such as cardiovascular disease, diabetes, stroke, arthritis, renal disease, respiratory disease, or cancer have been long recognized; however, the relation of these risk factors to

MCC has not been well established. There are a handful of studies that actually examine biological and lifestyle risk factors that contribute to the etiology of MCC. Overall, the evidence seems to provide stronger support for the contribution of environmental factors to MCC.

Gijsen et al. (2001) reviewed 82 studies that examined the causes and consequences of medical comorbidity. Only four of the reviewed studies revealed support for genetic susceptibility and familial risk as causes of comorbidity, and the support for these biological variables relations was considered weak. On the other hand, evidence for the relation of comorbidity to healthcare utilization, quality of life, and mortality was stronger. In a more recent review, Salive (2013) identified 16 studies that examined the prevalence of multimorbidity in elderly community samples. He noted that body mass index was one biological risk factor associated with multimorbidity. He also indicated that there was more evidence for the role of childhood financial hardship, lifetime earnings, lower education, tobacco use, poor dietary habits, alcohol consumption, and physical inactivity as contributants to multimorbidity.

Using data from a sample of 1,594 adults with long-term physical disability due to muscular dystrophy, post-polio syndrome, or spinal cord injury, Smith, Molton, and Jensen (2016) examined the incidence, prevalence, age at onset, as predictors of five chronic conditions: arthritis, cancer, coronary heart disease, diabetes, and hypertension. During the 3.5-year study period, the most commonly reported new-onset conditions were arthritis (14%), hypertension (9%), and cancer (7%). The report of new conditions occurred most frequently among participants between the ages of 56 and 65 years, and the strongest risk factors included greater body mass index and waist circumference and the presence of another comorbid condition at baseline. Research examining whether changes in modifiable factors (e.g., exercise) at midlife or earlier can help to prevent or delay onset of comorbid conditions was recommended by the authors.

More evidence is beginning to accumulate supporting the significance of the relation of adverse childhood events (ACE) to long-term health and overall well-being (Ben-Shlomo & Kuh, 2002; McCrory, Dooley, Laytr, & Kenny, 2015; Raposa, Hammen, Brennan, O'Callaghan, & Najman, 2014). ACE include family dysfunction, parental illness, neglect, and abuse of all types. The exact manner in which ACE influence the development of physical disease later in life has yet to be empirically proven; however, McCrory et al. (2015) proposed three approaches that might be taken in modeling the contribution of ACE to disease in later adulthood. For one set of explanatory models, the authors propose that ACE be viewed as distal factors that act on proximal factors (e.g., low education leading to lower occupational position and income), which then specify environmental conditions in adulthood (e.g., substandard housing, poor nutrition, and poor health behavior) and contribute to the onset of chronic conditions. As a second approach, aspects of the early psychosocial environment would be viewed as instrumental in going from ACE to disease. For example, children who grow up in risky social environments may be more likely to develop maladaptive coping styles, emotional dysregulation, and social cognitions that increase their exposure to stress and affect their responses to stress later in life (Repetti, Taylor, & Seeman, 2002). As a third approach, these authors recommend that emphasis be placed on neurophysiological pathways (e.g., endocrine and immunologic systems) in determining children's responses to stress. These models would emphasize the chronic activation of the sympathetic nervous system and activation of the hypothalamic-pituitary-adrenal axis that characterize responses to stress. Chronic activation of these systems can lead to chronic homeostatic dysregulation, which can exhaust physiological systems and increase the risk for disease.

In one of the few empirical examinations of the relation of ACE to disease, McCrory et al. (2015) used data from 6,912 participants in the initial wave of the Irish Longitudinal Study on Aging to examine the influence of ACE on disease risk, disease onset, and disease comorbidity. A four-item measure was used to document participants' experiences of ACE, and the risk, onset, and comorbidity related to nine chronic disease types were established by doctor diagnosis. Results indicated that ACE were associated with increased risk of cardiovascular disease, lung disease, and emotional, nervous, or psychiatric disorders. The relation of ACE to disease conformed to a dose-response pattern, with increased numbers of ACE translating to increased disease risk later in life. ACE were also associated with earlier onset for any physical disease or psychological disorder. The authors concluded that childhood may be a sensitive period for the development of medical conditions and highlighted the import of using a lifespan approach to studying chronic conditions.

Another study examined the relation between self-reported ACE and multimorbidity and the contribution of other social, behavioral, and psychological factors to that relation (Sinnott, McHugh, Fitzgerald, Bradley, & Kearney, 2015). Data were collected from 2,047 participants recruited from a large primary care center as part of the Mitchelstown cohort phase of the Cork and Kerry Diabetes and Heart Disease Study. The number of ACE experienced was documented using the Center for Disease Control ACE measure. Multimorbidity status was defined as 0 chronic diseases, 1 chronic disease, or 2 or more chronic diseases. ACE were reported by 28% of participants in the multimorbidity group, 21% of participants in the single-disease group, and 16% of participants with no chronic diseases. Results of ordinal logistic regression analyses revealed that, after adjusting for education, health coverage, smoking, exercise, diet, body mass index, and anxiety/depression scores, a positive history of ACE conferred a 1.4 increased risk for multimorbidity.

Medical Management of MCC

The medical management of a chronic medical condition is usually dictated by well-established, condition-specific guidelines for use of pharmacotherapy as well as condition-specific recommendations around exercise, nutrition, and other lifestyle behaviors. For example, the management of cardiovascular disease can initially include a host of medications (e.g., antihypertensive, statin, beta-blocker, angiotensin-converting enzyme, aspirin, antidepressant, and anxiolytic), which then might be followed by physical rehabilitation and psychological management when indicated.

Medical management of MCC consists of similar approach but requires an appreciation for the complexity of managing several serious medical conditions at the same time. Although there are a number of different medical models of care, the most influential model is the Chronic Care Model (CCM; Wagner, Austin, & Von Korff, 1996; Wagner et al., 2001). The CCM has become the standard in guiding the assessment and management of MCC. It was largely developed out of a recognition that chronically ill patients are often dealing with co-occurring physical, psychological, and cognitive sequelae and require an integration of care systems to meet their needs. The CCM is a collaborative, patient-centered, and goal-oriented model of care and dictates that healthcare providers and patients collaboratively generate the care plan and set goals for accomplishing that plan, that healthcare providers train and support patients in their self-management efforts, and that follow-up care be provided to alter and redefine the care plan as needed.

Wagner et al. (1996) also noted that, regardless of research design employed to study the treatment of chronic illness, components of high-quality care were characterized by the following: (1) using clearly defined plans and protocols; (2) changing the organization of practice to provide more time, variety of resources, and closer monitoring to be more able to meet the needs of patients (e.g., when appointments are scheduled); (3) providing systematic attention to the information and attending to behavioral change in patients (e.g., self-management); (4) relying on quick access to specialty services (e.g., expert consultation); and (5) providing information that is supportive (e.g., reminders or feedback). Development of the CCM also led to the development of stepped care protocols (Von Korff, 2000). Stepped care interventions are clinical guidelines that go from least costly and demanding to most costly and demanding and are assigned to patients based on observable outcomes. Stepped care for individuals requires higher levels of coordination among service providers (e.g., PCPs, specialist care providers, providers repesenting other allied care disciplines, or case managers).

Bleich et al. (2015) conducted a systematic review of programs treating patients with high-need and high-cost MCC. Their review yielded 27 treatment studies, with 12 of the 27 studies being randomized control trials (RCTs) that covered 5 models of care (care or case management, chronic disease self-management, disease management, nursing home care, and transitional care). With the exception of the transitional care model, all models of care yielded some positive clinical outcomes, but most studies did not show these models of care to be associated with marked improvements in clinical outcomes, patient satisfaction, or healthcare utilization and spending. The care or case management and disease management models were the only two models of care associated with improvements across all three outcome categories, with the care or case management model having its greatest effect on healthcare utilization and spending and the disease management model having its greatest effect on clinical outcomes. The authors did add the caveat that model processes and applications varied considerably across studies and these variations may explain the different model effects observed within and across outcome categories.

Smith, Wallace, O'Dowd, and Fortin (2016) completed a systematic review of interventions for patients with multimorbidity in primary care and community settings.

Eighteen RCTs were identified, with nine studies focusing on more commonly experienced comorbid conditions and the remaining nine studies focusing on multimorbidity among older adults. In 12 studies, the organization of care served as the target for intervention (i.e., changing the care context from standard care to case management or a multidisciplinary team approach). In six studies, interventions were delivered directly to patients, with emphasis placed on education and self-management. Overall, the results were mixed, with no clear improvements observed across clinical outcomes or healthcare utilization and only small to moderate improvements observed across measures of mental health, patient-reported functional outcomes, medication compliance, and patient-related health behaviors. The authors concluded that it is difficult to improve clinical and associated outcomes among patients with multimorbidity.

Brady et al. (2013) conducted a meta-analysis of 23 studies evaluating the physical and psychological benefit of the Chronic Disease Self-Management Model (Lorig et al., 1999), a 6-week community-based intervention aimed at improving self-management of chronic conditions by increasing self-efficacy skills. Results indicated moderate improvements in self-efficacy and small to modest improvements in psychological health and health behaviors 12 months posttreatment. However, improvements across physical health outcomes were less consistent.

Integrating Empirically Supported Cognitive-Behavioral Strategies for the Management of MCC

Rehabilitation strategies that can be used across different medical conditions are required to manage the physical and psychological sequelae of MCC. Interventions that serve to improve coping strategies used in relation to a single chronic condition are likely to be beneficial to persons experiencing MCC. Treatment programs for MCC should be guided by a philosophy that dictates that the complexity and challenge of living with MCC be fully appreciated and that every effort be made to maintain as much function as possible across as many life domains as possible. The following sections present an array of empirically supported strategies that we have found useful in our efforts to help patients identify and manage their chronic conditions and the functional limitations and psychosocial challenges that are often associated with MCC.

Goal Setting

While patients will have to accept physical limitations associated with MCC, patients will still want to optimize their functioning and make improvements across life domains in which change is possible. Goal setting is characterized by the identification of a specific behavioral goal. Rather than immediately implementing a behavior change, patients can benefit from the progressive change that occurs through goal setting. Goal setting involves the creation of an action plan and a timeframe for the completion of each goal-directed action. To enhance the objectivity of goals and action plans, goals should be specific, measurable, achievable, realistic/relevant, and timed (SMART; Doran, 1981; Bovend'Eerdt, Botell, & Wade, 2009). Patients may have a difficult time identifying clear and realistic goals and physicians and psychologists should assist patients in the identification of patient-specific SMART goals. Appropriate SMART goals in the context of MCC management may include increasing compliance with treatment recommendations and decreasing treatment interfering behaviors.

Adherence to the action plan is critical to achieving an identified goal. Pacing is a strategy that can optimize the likelihood of both action plan adherence and goal achievement. Pacing involves increasing an infrequent behavior in a controlled manner. The goals of pacing are to increase patients' consistent engagement in desired behaviors and decrease the influence mood has on patients' engagement in the desired behaviors (Nielson, Jensen, Karsdorp, & Vlaeyen, 2013). There is a strong association between mood and engagement in goal-directed behaviors, with negative mood predicting less behavioral engagement and positive mood predicting more behavioral engagement (Andrews, Strong, & Meredith, 2012). While patients with MCC may understand the way in which negative mood and underactivity can hinder treatment, patients may not intuitively understand the way in which overactivity can also hinder treatment. Overactivity refers to a level of behavior that exceeds the level specified within a patient's action plan. Patients should be oriented to the risk of exhaustion and burnout associated with overactivity and the cyclical nature of overexertion and underactivity. To increase the likelihood of achieving treatment goals, patients with MCC should adhere to their action plans, neither over nor under engaging in goal-oriented behaviors.

Therapeutic Writing and the Psychological Benefits of the Medical Narrative

Therapeutic writing is a strategy that patients can use to monitor their medical conditions; the physical, psychological, and functional changes they experience consequent to their medical conditions; and the interaction of these experiences throughout the treatment and management of their medical conditions. Therapeutic writing is also referred to as expressive writing or journaling in the psychological intervention literature. Therapeutic writing involves personal reflection and/or emotional disclosure through writing on multiple occasions over a period of time (Cummings, Hayes, Saint, & Park, 2014). In their review examining the health benefits of therapeutic writing, Baikie and Wilhelm (2005) found that therapeutic writing was associated with improvements in the following health-related outcomes: blood pressure, immune system function, lung function, mood/affect, and self-reported psychological well-being. Baikie and Wilhelm also found that therapeutic writing was associated with fewer days in the hospital, fewer stress-related visits to the doctor, and fewer posttraumatic stress and avoidance systems. The results of other reviews have suggested that the effects of therapeutic writing may be more modest than previously thought (Frisina, Borod, & Lepore, 2004; Zachariae & O'Toole, 2015). Despite small effect sizes, Zachariae and O'Toole conclude that therapeutic writing may still be clinically relevant due to the inexpensive and easily disseminable nature of writing interventions.

Although the general effectiveness of therapeutic writing as a psychological intervention has been demonstrated, there are number of implementation strategies that psychologists and other behavioral health specialists can utilize to optimize the effectiveness of therapeutic writing. The benefits of therapeutic writing will be further enhanced when delivered in the context of a multicomponent intervention that incorporates empirically supported and complimentary therapeutic strategies. Miller (2014) outlined several strategies for the use of therapeutic writing in psychotherapy including interactive journaling, structured writing prompts for patients pertaining to treatment-relevant information, and encouraging patients to integrate the information they learn into their journal entries. Miller also suggested that interactive journaling may promote behavior change. Cummings et al. (2014) recommended that psychologists and other behavioral health specialists monitor patient's engagement in writing and consider incorporating designated writing time into sessions. Patients should be encouraged to monitor the relation of skills learned in treatment to the experience of psychological distress. Psychologists and other behavioral health specialists should consider therapeutic writing as a tool to help patients gain insight regarding effective and ineffective coping strategies. Therapeutic writing can help patients to track the changes they make in treatment and promote continued change.

A medical narrative is important in addressing the psychological distress that often accompanies MCC. A medical narrative is a written, first-person account of all that the patient has experienced as a consequence of the medical condition. Outside of the medical context, narratives have been incorporated into the treatment of posttraumatic stress reactions (Monson et al., 2006; Resick & Schnicke, 1993) as well as the treatment of stress responses, more broadly. To construct a narrative, individuals are asked to write about their stressful experience and their interpretation about the event and their role in the event. Given the stress and life-changing consequences associated with medical conditions, narratives are highly applicable to patients with MCC. The narrative analysis centers on the way a patient tells his/her narrative. The psychologist or behavioral health specialist assesses the amount of narrative details provided, narrative coherence, amnesia for or gaps in the chronology of the event, the affect that accompanies the telling (e.g., shame), and the interpretations that are made (e.g., lack of agency). Consistent with cognitive-behavioral therapy and cognitive processing therapy, psychologists and other behavioral health specialists help patients to identify inaccurate and unhelpful interpretations within the narrative and adopt more adaptive interpretations of their experience (Hofmann, Asnaani, Vonk, Sawyer, & Fang, 2012; Monson et al., 2006). It is assumed that more objective interpretations of their medical condition and their current life circumstances will lead to more positive affect and more adaptive behavioral responses to the unique challenges associated with having MCC. Beyond objective interpretation, there is evidence that increased integration of stressful life experiences into the macronarrative of one's life is predictive of decreased psychological distress (Holland, Currier, Coleman, & Neimeyer, 2010; Lancaster & Carlson, 2015). The use of medical narratives can influence the way in which medical conditions are placed within a patient's larger life context and the meaning a patient makes of their medical conditions. Medical narratives can aid the integrated care team members in identifying those person-specific interpretations and reactions to medical conditions that most influence recovery and quality of life and guide interventions related to the patient's acquisition and use of the most effective coping strategies.

Therapeutic Reading and the Psychological Benefits of Reading

Bibliotherapy is one form of self-help that has been developed based on empirically supported psychological treatments and has been shown to be effective at reducing psychological distress and pain and improving quality of life across a variety of clinical populations (Högdahl, Birgegård, & Björck, 2013; Johnston, Foster, Shennan, Starkey, & Johnson, 2010; Thorsell et al., 2011). Muschalla, Glatz, and Linden (2013) found bibliotherapy to improve health-related knowledge among patients with cardiovascular disease. It appears that reading about illness may help to familiarize patients with treatment options and the healthcare system in which they are being treated. Bibliotherapy is also a convenient self-help resource for patients with MCC, particularly if constraints associated with their medical conditions impact patients' physical functioning and mobility. Patients can access treatment within their home and complete treatment at a pace that corresponds to their individual level of strength and stamina. The empirical basis and practical nature of bibliotherapy make it an appropriate treatment option for patients with MCC.

While the first aim of bibliotherapy is to reduce psychological distress, bibliotherapy and therapeutic reading can result in other positive effects. Therapeutic reading refers to patients' use of literature as a resource for understanding, expressing, and managing challenges specific to their medical problems as well as other difficult life circumstances. The use of books can also help patients to gain insight into personal challenges and promote positive identification with others who are experiencing similar challenges (Heath, Sheen, Leavy, Young, & Money, 2005). Information about chronic illnesses and their associated consequences are often presented to patients in a formal manner. To supplement the formal presentation of medical information, Kaptein, Meulenberg, and Smyth (2015) suggested that patients may benefit from exposure to art forms that depict illness, including novels. Kaptein and colleagues proposed that informal representations of illness may help to humanize medical conditions and medical care. In summary, therapeutic reading has obvious implications for the treatment of psychological distress as well as the potential to increase health-related knowledge and patients' emotional understanding of their condition-specific experiences.

Self-Advocacy and Effective Management of System Issues

Navigating the healthcare system can be challenging, particularly when patients are managing MCC and frequently interacting with multiple healthcare providers. The ability to obtain, understand, process, and communicate health-related information is referred to as health literacy (Institute of Medicine, 2004). Following the onset of medical conditions, efforts to minimize the condition symptoms (secondary prevention) and to minimize the functional impairments that are associated with the condition symptoms (tertiary prevention) are necessarily complex (Hayes, Barlow, & Nelson-Gray, 1999). The success of such efforts depends on person-level variables, including prior history of chronic disease, prior history of coping with medical conditions, availability and ability to access support within their own social network, availability and ability to access healthcare, ability to negotiate compensation systems (e.g., the worker's compensation system, insurance companies, and the legal system), as well as system-level variables, including healthcare initiatives and mass media campaigns designed to increase awareness of resources both to prevent health-related adverse events and to limit the negative consequences of medical conditions. Patients with MCC need to educate themselves about their medical conditions, the roles of their various healthcare providers, and the larger healthcare system.

While understanding the healthcare system is an important skill, patients are also expected to take an active part in their treatment. Medical self-advocacy refers to a patient's assertiveness regarding his/her healthcare needs, willingness to challenge healthcare providers, and active participation in treatment decision-making (Brashers, Haas, & Neidig, 1999). Martin et al. (2011) examined the relation of literacy skills to patients' self-advocacy, which was measured by responses to a vignette that described barriers to scheduling a medical appointment. Responses were coded as counterproductive, passive, somewhat proactive, becoming proactive, and proactive, with level of proactivity equated with level of self-advocacy. Results revealed that literacy skills were associated with more proactive responses to the vignette.

Closely related to medical self-advocacy is patient activation. Patient activation refers to the skills and confidence that allow patients to actively engage in their healthcare (Hibbard & Greene, 2013). Hibbard, Greene, Shi, Mittler, and Scanlon (2015) examined the influence of patient activation on health-related outcomes at a 4-year follow-up assessment among patients with chronic conditions. Results revealed that higher activation at baseline was associated with greater self-management and functioning and less costly healthcare utilization at the 4-year follow-up assessment. Most recently, Hibbard, Mahoney, and Sonet (2017) examined the impact of patient activation on health-related outcomes among cancer patients. Findings demonstrated that patients who were actively involved in their treatment were more likely to perceive their treatment plan as consistent with their values, cope with treatment side effects effectively, and initiate healthier diets in comparison to less activated patients. It appears that patients who actively engage in treatment are more likely to experience positive outcomes than patients who take a less active role in their treatment.

In addition to engagement in treatment, patient activation skills include interpersonal effectiveness skills. Interpersonal effectiveness skills are used to optimize the likelihood that patients will successfully manage the complex healthcare system and experience improved health outcomes. In the context of medical consultation, patients should first acknowledge the effort healthcare providers are putting into their treatment and the components of treatment the patient finds to be helpful. Second, patients should indicate the components of treatment that have not been found to be helpful and about and/or request alternative treatment options in an assertive manner. Third, patients should explain why honoring their request or exploring the proposed alternatives would benefit the healthcare provider (e.g., greater patient treatment compliance or patient gratitude). The patient should highlight their shared goal with the healthcare provider, improving the patient's health. These components are consistent with the components of dialectical behavior therapy (DBT) interpersonal effectiveness skills (Linehan, 2014). The goals of DBT interpersonal effectiveness skills include: obtaining the objective goal; maintaining self-respect; and maintaining relationships. Because the goal of medical self-advocacy is to optimize desired health outcomes, interpersonal effectiveness skills can help patients to effectively convey their requests and maintain a working relationship with their healthcare providers. Positive relationships between patients and healthcare providers can further increase the likelihood of patients experiencing improved health outcomes.

Acceptance and Life Purpose

While there are multiple skills patients can learn that can improve their current situation, there are circumstances in which improvements are limited. This is particularly true for a patient with MCC and the impact medical conditions can have on a patient's level of functioning. Acceptance and the re-creation of life purpose are a model of coping often referred to within the chronic pain literature (McCracken & Vowles, 2014). Acceptance is not a passive resignation aimed at tolerating illness and functional impairment. Acceptance of pain is characterized not only by the absence of attempts to control or avoid pain but by the pursuit of personal goals and engagement in valued actions regardless of pain experiences (McCracken, 1998). Valued actions can be conceptualized as activities that give life meaning. For patients with MCC, acceptance and engagement in valued action involve the identification and implementation of functional and lifestyle adjustments that are necessary for patients to have the most satisfying and normal lives possible.

Acceptance has also been discussed in the context of chronic illness. Acceptance of illness is associated with quality of life among heart failure patients, with greater illness acceptance predicting greater quality of life (Obiegło, Uchmanowicz, Wleklik, Jankowska-Polańska, & Kuśmierz, 2016). In the broader context of chronic disease, Karademas, Tsagaraki, and Lambrou (2009) examined the impact of illness acceptance among a sample of hospitalized patients with histories of cancer, chronic coronary artery disease, and chronic renal disease. Findings revealed that illness acceptance was positively associated with self-reported health and negatively associated with psychological distress. It appears that acceptance of illness may be a protective factor and a goal of treatment should be to increase acceptance among patients with MCC.

Acceptance and commitment therapy (ACT) is an empirically supported treatment that emphasizes the importance of acceptance and valued actions as mechanisms of change in the treatment of psychological distress (Hayes, Luoma, Bond, Masuda, & Lillis, 2006). ACT has been shown to improve self-reported physical functioning and distress among patients managing chronic pain (Hann & McCracken, 2014). ACT has also been shown to improve quality of life and decrease distress among cancer patients (Feros, Lane, Ciarrochi, & Blackledge, 2013). Through the lens of cognitive-behavioral therapy, acceptance can be viewed as an adaptive response for patients with MCC when efforts to reverse or limit the progression of medical conditions are no longer adaptive. Behavioral health specialists can help patients with MCC to reallocate their efforts toward developing new coping skills, rather than attempting to change fixed medical circumstances.

While accepting the changes that occur in the context of MCC is important, purpose in life has also been shown to improve health outcomes. Zilioli, Slatcher, Ong, and Gruenewald (2015) examined the impact of perceived life purpose on allostatic load and self-health locus of control at a 10-year follow-up assessment. Allostatic load consisted of measures of physiological dysregulation across the following areas: cardiovascular, lipid, glucose metabolism, inflammation, sympathetic nervous system reactivity, parasympathetic nervous system reactivity, and hypothalamic-pituitary-adrenal axis reactivity. Results revealed that greater life purpose predicted greater self-health locus of control and lower levels of allostatic load. Kim, Sun, Park, Kubzansky, and Peterson (2013) examined the relation of life purpose to health outcomes among patients with coronary heart disease and found that greater life purpose at baseline was associated with a decreased likelihood of experiencing a myocardial infarction at a 2-year follow-up assessment. In addition to cardiovascular events, Cohen, Bavishi, and Rozanski (2016) conducted a meta-analysis and found that greater life purpose predicted reduced risk for all-cause mortality. Life purpose appears to be a protective factor against morbidity and mortality, and helping patients develop a greater sense of life purpose should be a high treatment priority in the management of MCC.

Relaxation Techniques and Meditation

Similar to the relation of mood to behavior, the negative influence of stress on physical health outcomes is well documented (Thoits, 2010). Due to the stress associated with chronic medical conditions, relaxation training should be an integral part of treatment for patients with MCC. Relaxation and meditation can be performed in a number of ways, including progressive muscular relaxation, mindfulness meditation, meditative relaxation, transcendental meditation, guided imagery, and breathing retraining. Based on their 2005 review, Schneider et al. concluded that across cardiovascular disease risk factors including blood pressure, cholesterol, and smoking, transcendental meditation was found to be an effective risk reduction strategy. Across cardiovascular events and endpoints including myocardial ischemia, left-ventricular mass, and atherosclerosis, transcendental meditation effectively increased exercise tolerance and maximum work load. Across physiological neuroendocrine mechanisms that contribute to cardiovascular compromise, including baseline levels of respiration and heart rate, spontaneous skin resistance, heart rate reactivity, sympathetic adrenergic receptor sensitivity, and basal and average cortisol levels, transcendental meditation effectively reduced stress and increased relaxation. In a more recent meta-analysis examining the impact of transcendental meditation on cardiovascular health, Schneider and Carr (2014) found transcendental meditation was associated with decreased cardiovascular disease risk factors including hypertension, psychosocial stress, and smoking as well as cardiovascular events.

In addition to the physical benefits, relaxation and meditation can also help patients with MCC manage psychological distress. In their systematic review and meta-analysis examining the physiological and psychological effects of meditation, Goyal et al. (2014) found that meditation was associated with significant decreases in anxiety, depression, and pain. Galante, Galante, Bekkers, and Gallacher (2014) conducted a meta-analysis examining the influence of kindness-based meditation on psychological health outcomes. The results revealed that kindness-based meditation was associated with significant decreases in depression and significant increases in mindfulness and self-compassion. Given the comorbidity of chronic conditions and psychiatric conditions, these collective findings suggest that relaxation and meditation should be included as treatment components in the management of MCC.

Communication and Assertiveness Skills

Effective communication is characterized by a balanced exchange between two or more individuals, with each individual presenting information effectively and listening to the information being presented. Effective communication between patients and healthcare providers is essential in the treatment of MCC.

Communication skills can be sorted into two broad categories: information seeking and information verification (McGee & Cegala, 1998). In the medical context, information seeking is characterized by question asked by both the patient and members of the integrated care team. Information verification is characterized by one individual (e.g., patient or healthcare provider) requesting another individual (e.g., patient or healthcare provider) repeat previously presented information. Information verification also includes one individual (e.g., patient or healthcare provider) summarizing information that has been presented by another individual (e.g., patient or healthcare provider). It is vital that information related to the following be sought and verified: symptoms, diagnosis, prognosis, treatment, procedures/tests, physical examination, procedural information (i.e., insurance plans and paper work), follow-up appointments and referral information, and medical history (Cegala, McClure, Marinelli, & Post, 2000). Information seeking and information verification are particularly relevant to patients with MCC because their health is dependent on their ability to understand and present information about their co-occurring and interacting medical conditions.

Patients and healthcare providers comprise a communication dyad; however, the majority of research has focused on the implementation of communication skills training among healthcare providers as a means to improve patient outcomes (Boissy et al., 2016; Fujimori et al., 2014; Rao, Anderson, Inui, & Frankel, 2007; Uitterhoeve, Bensing, Grol, Demulder, & Achterberg, 2010). While training healthcare providers to communicate effectively is important, providing patients with communication skills training may provide a more direct pathway to improving patient outcomes. McGee and Cegala (1998) conducted a communication skills training among patients. During the communication skills training, participants were asked questions to encourage articulation of medical history, provided assistance with the wording and writing of questions to gather desired information, and encouraged to verify their understanding of information presented to them. Results revealed that communication skills training increased information-seeking and information-verifying behaviors, the amount of information gathered, and the amount of information recalled among patients. This finding suggests that communication skills training may increase patients' knowledge of their medical conditions.

The communication skills training protocol used by McGee and Cegala (1998) guided the content included in subsequent patient communication skills trainings. Cegala et al. (2000) also conducted communication skills training among patients. Results revealed that patients who underwent training gathered information more effectively, provided more information, and made more verifying summary statements during medical interviews than patients who did not receive communication skills training. Harrington, Noble, and Newman (2004) conducted a systematic review of studies aimed at increasing participants' communication in medical consultations. Results revealed that communication skills training increased patients' adherence to treatment recommendations, level of participation in medical consultations, perceptions of control over health, attendance of appointments, and clinical outcomes. The collective findings support the assumption that outcomes for patients with MCC are optimized when patients have medical-related knowledge and are able to share this knowledge with healthcare providers.

Given their frequent interactions with numerous healthcare providers, assertive behavior is a specific communication skill that can greatly benefit patients with MCC. Assertive behavior is characterized by making a request of others and refusing requests made by others that an individual deems to be overly burdensome or unreasonable (Duckworth & Mercer, 2006). Assertive behavior can be contrasted with aggressive and passive behavior. Aggressive behavior is characterized by an imposition of one's own requests or opinions on others, and passive behavior is characterized by an overconcern for the needs and opinions of others at the expense of one's own needs or opinions (Duckworth, 2008). Duckworth discussed the implications of aggressive and passive behavior when communicating with healthcare providers, both of which can result in patients with MCC not having their healthcare needs met. Aggressive behavior may be perceived as threatening to healthcare providers, and providers may refuse healthcare-related requests that are made in an aggressive manner. Passive behavior may lead to the non-articulation of healthcare needs. Assertive behavior optimizes the likelihood of patients getting their healthcare needs met.

Despite the potential for assertiveness skills to increase the likelihood of patients getting their health needs met, little research has examined the effects of assertiveness training among medical patients. Studies have shown assertiveness skills training to improve communication skills and satisfaction outcomes among a variety of populations including psychiatric patients, students, and healthcare providers (Lin et al., 2004, 2008; Tavakoli, Lumley, Hijazi, Slavin-Spenny, & Parris, 2009). The lack of assertiveness skill training among patients is surprising given the evidence that passive and aggressive manifestations of anger have been shown to positively relate to certain types of cancer (Penedo et al., 2006; White et al., 2007), cardiovascular disease (Kop et al., 2008; Mostofsky, Penner, & Mittleman, 2014), and chronic pain (Bruehl, Chung, & Burns, 2006; Burns et al., 2015). It appears that assertiveness skills training may serve patients with MCC in two ways: increasing the likelihood that health needs are met and decreasing the negative physical health effects associated with aggressive and passive behavior.

Duckworth (2008) provided an outline for assertiveness skills training protocols. Patients should be oriented to the rational for assertiveness skills training as well as the definitions of assertive, aggressive, and passive behavior. Targets of assertiveness skills training include nonverbal forms of communication, giving and receiving compliments and criticisms, and making and refusing requests. These skills should be learned and practiced in a variety of ways, with therapists modeling assertive verbal communication for patients, patients role-playing assertive communication with others, patients practicing assertive communication within sessions, and patients practicing assertive behavior between sessions through homework assignments. In the context of MCC, this would include practicing assertive behavior with healthcare providers. In addition to practicing skills through role-plays and real-life homework assignments, effective assertiveness skills training is characterized by providing patients with reinforcement and corrective feedback. These proposed protocol components are consistent with the protocol components (i.e., modeling, role-playing, feedback, and application) included in effective assertiveness skills trainings (Tavakoli et al., 2009). Through practice of assertiveness skills, therapists can assess patients' understanding of skills, reinforce assertive behavior, and correct aggressive and passive behavior. Assertiveness skills can decrease communication barriers that prevent patients from getting their healthcare needs met and facilitate the working alliance between patients and healthcare providers.

Social Support and Intimacy

While it is important for patients to use communication skills to strengthen their relationships with healthcare providers, it is also important that patients develop and maintain personal relationships. Social support has been proposed to contribute to improve health through two pathways. The first pathway suggests that social relationships reduce the effects of stressors by providing informational, emotional, and/or tangible resources (Cohen, Gottlieb, & Underwood, 2001). Through this pathway, relationships are conceptualized as social support that buffers the negative impact of stressors on a patient's health (Holt-Lunstad, Smith, & Layton, 2010). The second pathway suggests that the effects of social relationships on health are direct, with the biological, behavioral, cognitive, and emotional factors present within social relationships having a positive effect on patient health. Social relationship partners can model health protective behaviors and provide greater purpose in life for patients (Cohen, 2004; Cohen et al., 2001). In summary, pathways of social relationships to health outcomes are highly relevant to interventions for patients with MCC.

Regardless of the pathways through which the effects occur, the positive impact of social relationships is well documented. In their meta-analytic review, Holt-Lunstad et al. (2010) found that stronger social relationships were associated with a 50% reduced mortality risk. Within the chronic disease literature, Barth, Schneider, and von Känel (2010) examined the influence of social support on the development of coronary heart disease. Results revealed that lower functional support positively predicted all-cause mortality including cardiac-related mortality. These findings are consistent with findings from a review by Compare et al. (2013) that determined that a lack of social support (i.e., being unmarried) and the presence of depression symptoms significantly predicted poorer cardiac disease prognosis. Pinquart and Duberstein (2010) examined the impact of social support on cancer mortality. Findings demonstrated that perceived social support was associated with a 25% decrease in mortality risk, social network size was associated with a 20% decrease in mortality risk, and being married was associated with a 12% decrease in mortality risk. These findings suggest that the quantity of social support and the types of relationships that a patient possesses are predictive of disease trajectory.

Intimate relationships have been proposed to be a type of relationship that is relevant to health outcomes among patients with chronic disease (Pietromonaco,

Uchino, & Schetter, 2013; Reis & Franks, 1994). Intimacy refers to close and familiar relationships. Intimacy can take many forms including cognitive intimacy (i.e., sharing thoughts or ideas), experimental intimacy (i.e., engaging in activities together), emotional intimacy, and physical or sexual intimacy (Tolstedt & Stokes, 1983). Changes in intimacy as a result of medical conditions can happen in a number of ways, including but not limited to the following: poor physical health, physical limitations, pain, hormonal changes, medication side effects and substance use, depression, anxiety, stress, body image changes, weight gain/loss, scars, poor sleep, and chronic fatigue. Many individuals report significant changes in sexual well-being after diagnosis and treatment for medical conditions (Gandaglia et al., 2014; Schover et al., 2014). In the aftermath of medical conditions and treatment, couples will be well served by receiving psychoeducation about sexual dysfunction, sexual intimacy, and other forms of intimacy. Couples should be oriented to the fact that the social relationships a patient possesses, including intimate relationships, contribute to quality of life among patients and the partners of patients with medical conditions (Leung, Pachana, & McLaughlin, 2014; Kim, Duberstein, Sörensen, & Larson, 2005). Similar to the process of accepting limitations and redefining life purpose following the onset of chronic disease, patients and their partners should consider broadening their definition of intimacy to include forms of intimacy other than sexual intimacy. Given the protective effect social relationships and intimacy have on health outcomes, patients with MCC should be encouraged to interact with and strengthen their existing social relationships.

Future Directions

The challenge of managing MCC cannot be overstated, and the individual burden and individual and societal costs of MCC are significant. While there are established guidelines that dictate the management of single conditions, there are few empirical tests of the relative effectiveness of any condition-specific treatment when implemented in the context of multiple, comorbid medical and psychiatric conditions. Studies that have evaluated the impact of different models of care on clinical and functional outcomes experienced by patients with MCC suggest some modest benefit from care delivered in accord with a care or case management model or a disease management model. While these care models are gaining traction, it is still the case that most patients with MCC receive care that involves multiple providers across multiple care settings. It is far too often the case that patients with MCC receive medical care that is not comprehensive, not coordinated, and not co-located. It is also far too often the case that the psychosocial needs of patients with MCC are not evaluated or treated.

Given the increasing rates of MCC, and given the current realities of the healthcare system, there is great need for an integrated approach to advancing healthcare service provision and research around MCC. In 2008, the US Department of Health and Human Services undertook development of a strategic framework that would guide the conceptualization and evaluation of MCC (U.S. Department of Health and Human Services, 2010). The strategic framework identifies four overarching goals, each goal having multiple objectives that would serve to mitigate the effects of MCC:

1. Foster healthcare and public health system changes to improve the health of individuals with MCC.
2. Maximize the use of proven self-care management and other services by individuals with MCC.
3. Provide better tools and information to healthcare, public health, and social services workers who deliver care to individuals with MCC.
4. Facilitate research to fill knowledge gaps about, and interventions and systems to benefit, individuals with MCC (p. 6).

Also critical to prevention and management of MCC is research establishing the independent and interactive contributions of those biological (e.g., age, body mass, and genetics/family history of disease) and environmental (e.g., ACE) factors considered to heighten an individual's risk for MCC. Such research would go far in shaping general and targeted prevention efforts. There is also a great need for research addressing the behavioral, cognitive, emotional, interpersonal, and social factors that contribute to patients' willingness and ability to monitor their disease status; adhere to multiple, complex treatment regimens; and advocate effectively with care providers and other healthcare system representatives to receive the least intrusive, most effective, and least costly care their conditions warrant. The rehabilitation model is a care model that we think holds promise for managing the physical, functional, and psychosocial limitations that result from MCC. As part of such an approach, patients with MCC would develop and practice skills relevant to (1) medical regimen adherence; (2) goal setting aimed at increasing healthy lifestyle behaviors and reducing risky lifestyle behaviors as well as goal setting aimed at achieving maximal function across all relevant life domains; (3) assertive communication and effective self-advocacy around issues of healthcare and around issues that impact overall quality of life and well-being; (4) managing physiological arousal, emotional distress, and interpersonal discord; and (5) accepting that treatment gains have been maximized and defining a new life purpose that permits a sense of personal fulfillment.

References

Alonso-Moran, E., Nuno-Solinis, R., Onder, G., & Tonnara, G. (2015). Multimorbidity in risk stratification tools to predict negative outcomes in adult population. *European Journal of Internal Medicine, 26*, 182–189.

Anderson, G., & Horvath, J. (2004). The growing burden of chronic disease in America. *Public Health Reports, 119*, 263–270.

Anderson, G. (2010). *Chronic care: Making the case for ongoing care*. Princeton: Robert Wood Johnson Foundation.

Andrews, N. E., Strong, J., & Meredith, P. J. (2012). Activity pacing, avoidance, endurance, and associations with patient functioning in chronic pain: A systematic review and meta-analysis. *Archives of Physical Medicine and Rehabilitation, 93*(11), 2109–2121.

Ashman, J., & Beresovsky, V. (2013). Multiple chronic conditions among US adults who visited physician offices: Data from the National Ambulatory Medical Care Survey, 2009. *Preventing Chronic Disease, 10*, E64.

Banhato, E. F. C., Galil, A. G. D., Campos, T. D. S., Colugnati, F. A. D., Richter, K. P., Bastos, M. G., & Cupertino, A. P. (2016). Depression symptoms among patients with multiple chronic conditions. *Journal of Depression and Anxiety, 5*(3). https://doi.org/10.4172/2167-1044.1000230

Baikie, K. A., & Wilhelm, K. (2005). Emotional and physical health benefits of expressive writing. *Advances in Psychiatric Treatment, 11*(5), 338–346.

Barile, J. P., Thompson, W. W., Zack, M. M., Krahn, G. L., Horner-Johnson, W., & Bowen, S. E. (2013). Multiple chronic conditions and health-related quality of life in older adults, 2004-2006. *Preventing Chronic Diseases, 10*, E162.

Barth, J., Schneider, S., & von Känel, R. (2010). Lack of social support in the etiology and the prognosis of coronary heart disease: A systematic review and meta-analysis. *Psychosomatic Medicine, 72*(3), 229–238.

Bayliss, E. A., Ellis, J. L., Shoup, J., Zeng, C., McQuillan, D. B., & Steiner, J. F. (2015). Effect of continuity of care on hospital utilization for seniors with multiple medical conditions in an integrated health care system. *Annals of Family Medicine, 13*, 123–129.

Ben-Shlomo, Y., & Kuh, D. (2002). A life course approach to chronic disease epidemiology: Conceptual models, empirical challenges and interdisciplinary perspectives. *International Journal of Epidemiology, 31*, 285–293.

Bice, T. W., & Boxerman, S. B. (1977). A quantitative measure of continuity of care. *Medical Care, 15*, 347–349.

Bleich, S. N., Sherrod, C., Chaing, A., Boyd, C., Wolff, J., DuGoff, E., … Anderson, G. (2015). Systematic review of programs treating high-need and high-cost people with multiple chronic diseases or disabilities in the United States, 2008-2014. *Preventing Chronic Disease, 12*, E197.

Boissy, A., Windover, A. K., Bokar, D., Karafa, M., Neuendorf, K., Frankel, R. M., … Rothberg, M. B. (2016). Communication skills training for physicians improves patient satisfaction. *Journal of General Internal Medicine, 31*(7), 755–761.

Bovend'Eerdt, T. J., Botell, R. E., & Wade, D. T. (2009). Writing SMART rehabilitation goals and achieving goal attainment scaling: A practical guide. *Clinical Rehabilitation, 23*(4), 352–361.

Boyd, C. M., & Fortin, M. (2010). Future of multimorbidity research: How should understanding of multimorbidity inform health system design? *Public, Health Reviews, 32*, 451–474.

Brady, T. J., Murphy, L., O'Colmain, B., Beauchesne, D., Daniels, B., Greenberg, M., … Chevrin, M. (2013). A meta-analysis of health status, health behaviors, and health care utilization outcomes of the chronic disease self-management program. *Preventing Chronic Disease, 10*, 120112.

Brashers, D. E., Haas, S. M., & Neidig, J. L. (1999). The patient self-advocacy scale: Measuring patient involvement in health care decision-making interactions. *Health Communication, 11*(2), 97–121.

Bruehl, S., Chung, O. Y., & Burns, J. W. (2006). Anger expression and pain: An overview of findings and possible mechanisms. *Journal of Behavioral Medicine, 29*(6), 593–606.

Burns, J. W., Gerhart, J. I., Bruehl, S., Peterson, K. M., Smith, D. A., Porter, L. S., … Keefe, F. J. (2015). Anger arousal and behavioral anger regulation in everyday life among patients with chronic low back pain: Relationships to patient pain and function. *Health Psychology, 34*(5), 547–555.

Byles, J. E., Robinson, I., Banks, E., Gibson, R., Leigh, L., Rodgers, B., … Jorm, L. (2014). Psychological distress and comorbid physical conditions: Disease or disability. *Depression and Anxiety, 31*, 524–532.

Cabassa, L. J., Humensky, J., Druss, B., Lewis-Fernandez, R., Gomes, A. P., Wang, S., & Blanco, C. (2013). Do race, ethnicity, and psychiatric diagnoses matter in the prevalence of multiple chronic medical conditions. *Medical Care, 51*, 540–547.

Cegala, D. J., McClure, L., Marinelli, T. M., & Post, D. M. (2000). The effects of communication skills training on patients' participation during medical interviews. *Patient Education and Counseling, 41*, 209–222.

Centers for Medicare and Medicaid. (2016). *Chronic conditions*. Retrieved from https://www.cms.gov/Research-Statistics-Data-and-Systems/Statistics-Trends-and-Reports/Chronic-Conditions/CC_Main.html.

Charlson, M. E., Pompei, P., Ales, K. L., & MacKenzie, C. R. (1987). A new method of classifying prognostic comorbidity in longitudinal studies: Development and validation. *Journal of Chronic Diseases, 40*, 373–383.

Clark, N. M., Lachance, L., Benedict, M. B., Little, R., Leo, H., Awad, D., & Wilkin, M. K. (2015). The extent and patterns of multiple chronic conditions in low-income children. *Clinical Pediatrics, 54*, 515–524.

Cocchiarelli, L., & Andersson, G. B. J. (2001). *American Medical Association: Guides to the evaluation of permanent impairment* (4th ed.). Chicago, IL: Author.

Cohen, R., Bavishi, C., & Rozanski, A. (2016). Purpose in life and its relationship to all-cause mortality and cardiovascular events: A meta-analysis. *Psychosomatic Medicine, 78*(2), 122–133.

Cohen, S. (2004). Social relationships and health. *American Psychologist, 59*(8), 676–684.

Cohen, S., Gottlieb, B. H., & Underwood, L. G. (2001). Social relationships and health: Challenges for measurement and intervention. *Advances in Mind-Body Medicine, 17*(2), 129–141.

Compare, A., Zarbo, C., Manzoni, G. M., Castelnuovo, G., Baldassari, E., Bonardi, A., … Romagnoni, C. (2013). Social support, depression, and heart disease: A ten year literature review. *Frontiers in Psychology, 4*, 384–391.

Cummings, J. A., Hayes, A. M., Saint, D. S., & Park, J. (2014). Expressive writing in psychotherapy: A tool to promote and track therapeutic change. *Professional Psychology: Research and Practice, 45*(5), 378–386.

Doran, G. T. (1981). There's a SMART way to write management's goals and objectives. *Management Review, 70*(11), 35–36.

Duckworth, M. P. (2008). Assertiveness skills and the management of related factors. In J. E. Fisher & W. O'Donohue (Eds.), *Cognitive behavior therapy: Applying empirically supported techniques in your practice* (2nd ed., pp. 26–34). New York, NY: Springer.

Duckworth, M. P., & Iezzi, T. (2010). Physical injuries, pain, and psychological trauma: Pathways to disability. *Psychological Injury and Law, 3*, 241–253.

Duckworth, M. P., Iezzi, T., & Shearer, E. (2012). Retraumatization associated with disabling physical injuries. In M. P. Duckworth & V. Follette (Eds.), *Retraumatization: Assessment, treatment, and prevention* (pp. 377–421). New York, NY: Routledge Press.

Duckworth, M. P., & Mercer, V. (2006). Assertiveness training. In J. E. Fisher & W. O'Donohue (Eds.), *Practice guidelines for evidence based psychotherapy* (pp. 80–92). New York, NY: Springer Publishing Company.

Feros, D. L., Lane, L., Ciarrochi, J., & Blackledge, J. T. (2013). Acceptance and commitment therapy (ACT) for improving the lives of cancer patients: A preliminary study. *Psycho-Oncology, 22*(2), 459–464.

Fortin, M., Lapointe, L., Hudon, C., Vanasses, A., Ntetu, A. L., & Maltais, D. (2004). Multimorbidity and quality of life in primary care: A systematic review. *Health and Quality of Life Outcomes, 2*, 51.

Freid, V. M., Bernstein, A. B., & Bush, M. A. (2012). Multiple chronic conditions among adults aged 45 and over: Trends over the past 10 years. *NCHS Data Brief, 100*, 1–8.

Frisina, P. G., Borod, J. C., & Lepore, S. J. (2004). A meta-analysis of the effects of written emotional disclosure on the health outcomes of clinical populations. *The Journal of Nervous and Mental Disease, 192*(9), 629–634.

Fujimori, M., Shirai, Y., Asai, M., Kubota, K., Katsumata, N., & Uchitomi, Y. (2014). Effect of communication skills training program for oncologists based on patient preferences for communication when receiving bad news: A randomized controlled trial. *Journal of Clinical Oncology, 32*(20), 2166–2172.

Galante, J., Galante, I., Bekkers, M. J., & Gallacher, J. (2014). Effect of kindness-based meditation on health and Well-being: A systematic review and meta-analysis. *Journal of Consulting and Clinical Psychology, 82*(6), 1101–1114.

Gandaglia, G., Briganti, A., Jackson, G., Kloner, R. A., Montorsi, F., Montorsi, P., & Vlachopoulos, C. (2014). A systematic review of the association between erectile dysfunction and cardiovascular disease. *European Urology, 65*(5), 968–978.

Gerteis, J., Izrael, D., Deitz, D., LeRoy, L., Ricciardi, R., Miller, T., & Basu, J. (2014). *Multiple chronic conditions chartbook*. Rockville, MD: Agency for Healthcare Research and Quality Publications.

Gijsen, R., Hoeymans, N., Schellevis, F. G., Ruwaard, D., Satariano, W. A., & van den Bos, G. A. M. (2001). Causes and consequences of comorbidity: A review. *Journal of Clinical Epidemiology, 54*, 661–674.

Goyal, M., Singh, S., Sibinga, E. M., Gould, N. F., Rowland-Seymour, A., Sharma, R., … Ranasinghe, P. D. (2014). Meditation programs for psychological stress and Well-being: A systematic review and meta-analysis. *JAMA Internal Medicine, 174*(3), 357–368.

Gully, S. P., Rasch, E. K., & Chan, L. (2011). The complex web of health: Relationships among chronic conditions, and health services. *Public Health Reports, 126*, 495–507.

Hann, K. E., & McCracken, L. M. (2014). A systematic review of randomized controlled trials of acceptance and commitment therapy for adults with chronic pain: Outcome domains, design quality, and efficacy. *Journal of Contextual Behavioral Science, 3*(4), 217–227.

Harrington, J., Noble, L. M., & Newman, S. P. (2004). Improving patients' communication with doctors: A systematic review of intervention studies. *Patient Education and Counseling, 52*(1), 7–16.

Hayes, S. C., Barlow, D. H., & Nelson-Gray, R. O. (1999). *The scientist practitioner: Research and accountability in the age of managed care* (2nd ed.). Boston, MA: Allyn & Bacon.

Hayes, S. C., Luoma, J. B., Bond, F. W., Masuda, A., & Lillis, J. (2006). Acceptance and commitment therapy: Model, processes and outcomes. *Behaviour Research and Therapy, 44*(1), 1–25.

Heath, M. A., Sheen, D., Leavy, D., Young, E., & Money, K. (2005). Bibliotherapy: A resource to facilitate emotional healing and growth. *School Psychology International, 26*(5), 563–580.

Hibbard, J. H., & Greene, J. (2013). What the evidence shows about patient activation: Better health outcomes and care experiences; fewer data on costs. *Health Affairs, 32*(2), 207–214.

Hibbard, J. H., Greene, J., Shi, Y., Mittler, J., & Scanlon, D. (2015). Taking the long view: How well do patient activation scores predict outcomes four years later? *Medical Care Research and Review, 72*(3), 324–337.

Hibbard, J. H., Mahoney, E., & Sonet, E. (2017). Does patient activation level affect the cancer patient journey? *Patient Education and Counseling, 100*(7), 1276–1279.

Hofmann, S. G., Asnaani, A., Vonk, I. J., Sawyer, A. T., & Fang, A. (2012). The efficacy of cognitive behavioral therapy: A review of meta-analyses. *Cognitive Therapy and Research, 36*(5), 427–440.

Högdahl, L., Birgegård, A., & Björck, C. (2013). How effective is bibliotherapy-based self-help cognitive behavioral therapy with internet support in clinical settings? Results from a pilot study. *Eating and Weight Disorders-Studies on Anorexia, Bulimia and Obesity, 18*(1), 37–44.

Holland, J. M., Currier, J. M., Coleman, R. A., & Neimeyer, R. A. (2010). The integration of stressful life experiences scale (ISLES): Development and initial validation of a new measure. *International Journal of Stress Management, 17*(4), 325–352.

Holt-Lunstad, J., Smith, T. B., & Layton, J. B. (2010). Social relationships and mortality risk: A meta-analytic review. *PLoS Medicine, 7*(7), e1000316.

Institute of Medicine. (2004). *Health literacy: A prescription to end confusion*. Washington, DC: National Academic Press.

Jackson, C. A., Jones, M., Tooth, L., Mishra, G. D., Byles, J., & Dobson, A. (2015). Multimorbidity patterns are differentially associated with functional ability and decline in a longitudinal cohort of older women. *Age and Ageing, 44*, 810–816.

Jindai, K., Nielson, C. M., Vorderstrasse, B. A., & Quinones, A. R. (2016). Multimorbidity and functional limitations among adults 65 or older, NHANES 2005-2012. *Preventing Chronic Disease, 13*, 160174.

Johnston, M., Foster, M., Shennan, J., Starkey, N. J., & Johnson, A. (2010). The effectiveness of an acceptance and commitment therapy self-help intervention for chronic pain. *The Clinical Journal of Pain, 26*(5), 393–402.

Kaptein, A. A., Meulenberg, F., & Smyth, J. M. (2015). A breath of fresh air: Images of respiratory illness in novels, poems, films, music, and paintings. *Journal of Health Psychology, 20*(3), 246–258.

Karademas, E. C., Tsagaraki, A., & Lambrou, N. (2009). Illness acceptance, hospitalization stress and subjective health in a sample of chronic patients admitted to hospital. *Journal of Health Psychology, 14*(8), 1243–1250.

Katz, S., Ford, A. B., Moskowitz, Jackson, & Jaffe, M. W. (1963). Studies of illness in the aged-The Index of ADL: A standardized measure of biological and psychosocial function. *Journal of the American Medical Association, 185*, 914–919.

Kessler, R., Andrews, G., Colpe, L., Hirpi, E., Mroczek, D. K., Normand, S. L., … Zaslavsky, A. M. (2002). Shortscreen scales to monitor population prevalences and trends in non-specific psychological distress. *Psychological Medicine, 32*, 959–976.

Kim, E. S., Sun, J. K., Park, N., Kubzansky, L. D., & Peterson, C. (2013). Purpose in life and reduced risk of myocardial infarction among older US adults with coronary heart disease: A two-year follow-up. *Journal of Behavioral Medicine, 36*(2), 124–133.

Kim, Y., Duberstein, P. R., & Sörensen, S., & Larson, M. R. (2005). Levels of depressive symptoms in spouses of people with lung cancer: Effects of personality, social support, and caregiving burden. *Psychosomatics, 46*(2), 123–130.

Kop, W. J., Weissman, N. J., Zhu, J., Bonsall, R. W., Doyle, M., Stretch, M. R., … Tracy, R. P. (2008). Effects of acute mental stress and exercise on inflammatory markers in patients with coronary artery disease and healthy controls. *American Journal of Cardiology, 101*(6), 767–773.

Lancaster, S. L., & Carlson, G. C. (2015). Meaning made, distress, and growth: An examination of the integration of stressful life experiences scale. *International Journal of Stress Management, 22*(1), 92–110.

Lee, T. A., Shields, A. E., Vogeli, C., Gibson, T. B., Woong-Sohn, M., Marder, W. D., … Weiss, K. B. (2007). Mortality rate in veterans with multiple chronic conditions. *Journal of General Internal Medicine, 22*(Supple. 3), 403–407.

Lehnert, T., Heider, D., Leicht, H., Heinrich, S., Corrieri, S., Luppa, M., … Konig, H. (2011). Health care utilization and costs with elderly persons with multiple chronic conditions. *Medical Care Research and Review, 68*, 387–420.

Leung, J., Pachana, N. A., & McLaughlin, D. (2014). Social support and health-related quality of life in women with breast cancer: A longitudinal study. *Psycho-Oncology, 23*(9), 1014–1020.

Lin, Y. R., Shiah, I. S., Chang, Y. C., Lai, T. J., Wang, K. Y., & Chou, K. R. (2004). Evaluation of an assertiveness training program on nursing and medical students' assertiveness, self-esteem, and interpersonal communication satisfaction. *Nurse Education Today, 24*(8), 656–665.

Lin, Y. R., Wu, M. H., Yang, C. I., Chen, T. H., Hsu, C. C., Chang, Y. C., … Chou, K. R. (2008). Evaluation of assertiveness training for psychiatric patients. *Journal of Clinical Nursing, 17*(21), 2875–2883.

Linehan, M. (2014). *DBT® skills training manual*. New York, NY: Guilford Publications.

Lorig, K. R., Sobel, D. S., Stewart, A. L., Brown, B. W., Bandura, A., Ritter, P., … Holman, H. R. (1999). Evidence suggesting that a chronic disease self-management program can improve health status while reducing hospitalization: A randomized trial. *Medical Care, 37*, 5–14.

Machlin, S. R., & Soni, A. (2013). Health care expenditures for adults with multiple treated chronic conditions: Estimates from the medical expenditure panel survey, 2009. *Preventing Chronic Disease, 10*, E63–E71.

Marengoni, A., von Strauss, E., Rizzuto, D., Winblad, B., & Fratiglioni, L. (2009). The impact of chronic multimorbidity and disability on functional decline and survival in elderly person: A community-based, longitudinal study. *Journal of Internal Medicine, 265*, 288–295.

Martin, L. T., Schonlau, M., Haas, A., Derose, K. P., Rudd, R., Loucks, E. B., … Buka, S. L. (2011). Literacy skills and calculated 10-year risk of coronary heart disease. *Journal of General Internal Medicine, 26*(1), 45–50.

McCracken, L. M. (1998). Learning to live with the pain: Acceptance of pain predicts adjustment in persons with chronic pain. *Pain, 74*(1), 21–27.

McCracken, L. M., & Vowles, K. E. (2014). Acceptance and commitment therapy and mindfulness for chronic pain: Model, process, and progress. *American Psychologist, 69*(2), 178–187.

McCrory, C., Dooley, C., Laytr, R., & Kenny, R. A. (2015). The lasting legacy of childhood adversity for disease risk in later life. *Health Psychology, 34*, 687–696.

McGee, D. S., & Cegala, D. J. (1998). Patient communication skills training for improved communication competence in the primary care medical consultation. *Journal of Applied Communication Research, 26*, 412–430.

Miller, W. (2014). Interactive journaling as a clinical tool. *Journal of Mental Health Counseling, 36*(1), 31–42.

Monson, C. M., Schnurr, P. P., Resick, P. A., Friedman, M. J., Young-Xu, Y., & Stevens, S. P. (2006). Cognitive processing therapy for veterans with military-related posttraumatic stress disorder. *Journal of Consulting and Clinical Psychology, 74*(5), 898–907.

Moriarty, D. G., Zack, M. M., & Kobau, R. (2003). The Centers for Disease Control and Prevention's health days measure-population tracking and perceived physical and mental health over time. *Health and Quality of Life Outcomes, 1*, 37.

Mostofsky, E., Penner, E. A., & Mittleman, M. A. (2014). Outbursts of anger as a trigger of acute cardiovascular events: A systematic review and meta-analysis. *European Heart Journal, 35*(21), 1404–1410.

Muschalla, B., Glatz, J., & Linden, M. (2013). Bibliotherapy on coping with illness improves health literacy but not heart-related anxiety of patients in cardiological rehabilitation. *Psychotherapy and Psychosomatics, 82*(5), 349–350.

Nielson, W. R., Jensen, M. P., Karsdorp, P. A., & Vlaeyen, J. W. (2013). Activity pacing in chronic pain: Concepts, evidence, and future directions. *The Clinical Journal of Pain, 29*(5), 461–468.

Obiegło, M., Uchmanowicz, I., Wleklik, M., Jankowska-Polańska, B., & Kuśmierz, M. (2016). The effect of acceptance of illness on the quality of life in patients with chronic heart failure. *European Journal of Cardiovascular Nursing, 15*(4), 241–247.

Penedo, F. J., Dahn, J. R., Kinsinger, D., Antoni, M. H., Molton, I., Gonzalez, J. S., … Schneiderman, N. (2006). Anger suppression mediates the relationship between optimism and natural killer cell cytotoxicity in men treated for localized prostate cancer. *Journal of Psychosomatic Research, 60*(4), 423–427.

Pietromonaco, P. R., Uchino, B., & Schetter, C. D. (2013). Close relationship processes and health: Implications of attachment theory for health and disease. *Health Psychology, 32*(5), 499–513.

Pinquart, M., & Duberstein, P. R. (2010). Depression and cancer mortality: A meta-analysis. *Psychological Medicine, 40*(11), 1797–1810.

Quinones, A. R., Markwardt, S., & Botoseneanu, A. (2016). Multimorbidity combinations and disability in older adults. *Journal of Gerontology: Medical Sciences, 71*, 823–830.

Rao, J. K., Anderson, L. A., Inui, T. S., & Frankel, R. M. (2007). Communication interventions make a difference in conversations between physicians and patients: A systematic review of the evidence. *Medical Care, 45*(4), 340–349.

Raposa, E. B., Hammen, C. L., Brennan, P. A., O'Callaghan, F., & Najman, J. M. (2014). Early adversity and health outcomes in young adulthood: The role of ongoing stress. *Health Psychology, 33*, 410–418.

Reis, H. T., & Franks, P. (1994). The role of intimacy and social support in health outcomes: Two processes or one? *Personal Relationships, 1*(2), 185–197.

Repetti, R. L., Taylor, S. E., & Seeman, T. E. (2002). Risky families: Family social environments and the mental and physical health of offspring. *Psychological Bulletin, 128*, 330–366.

Resick, P. A., & Schnicke, M. (1993). *Cognitive processing therapy for rape victims: A treatment manual*. Newbury Park, CA: Sage Publications.

Salive, M. E. (2013). Multimorbidity in older adults. *Epidemiologic Reviews, 35*, 75–83.

Schneider, K. M., O'Donnell, B. E., & Dean, D. (2009). Prevalence of multiple chronic conditions in the United States' Medicare population. *Health and Quality of Life Outcomes, 7*, 1–11.

Schneider, R. H., & Carr, T. (2014). Transcendental meditation in the prevention and treatment of cardiovascular disease and pathophysiological mechanisms: An evidence-based review. *Advances in Integrative Medicine, 1*(3), 107–112.

Schover, L. R., van der Kaaij, M., van Dorst, E., Creutzberg, C., Huyghe, E., & Kiserud, C. E. (2014). Sexual dysfunction and infertility as late effects of cancer treatment. *European Journal of Cancer Supplements, 12*(1), 41–53.

Sinnott, C., McHugh, S., Fitzgerald, A. P., Bradley, C. P., & Kearney, P. K. (2015). Psychosocial complexity in multimorbidity: The legacy of adverse childhood experiences. *Family Practice, 32*, 269–275.

Skinner, H. G., Coffey, R., Jones, J., Heslin, K. C., & Moy, E. (2016). The effects of multiple chronic conditions on hospitalization costs and utilization for ambulatory care sensitive conditions in the United States: A nationally representative cross-sectional study. *BMC Health Services Research, 16*, 77.

Smith, A. E., Molton, I. R., & Jensen, M. P. (2016). Self-reported incidence and age of chronic comorbid medical conditions in adults aging with long-term physical disability. *Disability and Health Journal, 9*, 533–538.

Smith, S. M., Wallace, E., O'Dowd, T., & Fortin, M. (2016). Interventions for improving outcomes in patients with multimorbidity in primary care and community settings. *Cochrane Database of Systematic Reviews, 3*, CD006560.

Steiner, C. A., & Friedman, B. (2013). Hospital utilization, costs, and mortality for adults with multiple chronic conditions, Nationwide inpatient sample, 2009. *Preventing Chronic Disease, 10*, E62.

Tavakoli, S., Lumley, M. A., Hijazi, A. M., Slavin-Spenny, O. M., & Parris, G. P. (2009). Effects of assertiveness training and expressive writing on acculturative stress in international students: A randomized trial. *Journal of Counseling Psychology, 56*(4), 590–596.

Thoits, P. A. (2010). Stress and health: Major findings and policy implications. *Journal of Health and Social Behavior, 51*(Supple. 1), S41–S53.

Thorsell, J., Finnes, A., Dahl, J., Lundgren, T., Gybrant, M., Gordh, T., & Buhrman, M. (2011). A comparative study of 2 manual-based self-help interventions, acceptance and commitment therapy and applied relaxation, for persons with chronic pain. *The Clinical Journal of Pain, 27*(8), 716–723.

Tolstedt, B. E., & Stokes, J. P. (1983). Relation of verbal, affective, and physical intimacy to marital satisfaction. *Journal of Counseling Psychology, 30*(4), 573–580.

U.S. Department of Health and Human Services. (2010). *Multiple chronic conditions—A strategic framework: Optimum health and quality of life for individuals with multiple chronic conditions*. Washington, DC: Author.

Uitterhoeve, R. J., Bensing, J. M., Grol, R. P., Demulder, P. H. M., & van Achterberg, T. (2010). The effect of communication skills training on patient outcomes in cancer care: A systematic review of the literature. *European Journal of Cancer Care, 19*(4), 442–457.

Von Korff, M. (2000). Individualized stepped care of chronic illness. *Western Medical Journal, 172*, 133–137.

Wagner, E. H., Austin, B. T., Davis, C., Hindmarsh, M., Schaefer, J., & Bonomi, A. (2001). Improving chronic illness care: Translating evidence into action. *Health Affairs, 20*, 64–78.

Wagner, E. H., Austin, B. T., & Von Korff, M. (1996). Organizing care for patients with chronic illness. *The Millbank Quarterly, 74*, 511–544.

Ward, B. W., Schiller, J. S., & Goodman, R. A. (2014). Multiple chronic conditions among US adults: A 2012 update. *Preventing Chronic Disease, 11*, E62–E66.
Ware, J. E., Kosinski, M., & Keller, S. K. (1994). *SF-36 physical and mental health summary scales: A user's manual*. Boston, MA: The Health Institute.
White, V. M., English, D. R., Coates, H., Lagerlund, M., Borland, R., & Giles, G. G. (2007). Is cancer risk associated with anger control and negative affect? Findings from a prospective cohort study. *Psychosomatic Medicine, 69*(7), 667–674.
Wolff, J. L., Starfield, B., & Anderson, G. (2002). Prevalence, expenditures, and complications of multiple chronic conditions in the elderly. *Archives of Internal Medicine, 162*(20), 2269–2276.
Wu, S. Y., & Green, A. (2000). *Projection of chronic illness prevalence and cost inflation*. Washington, D.C.: RAND Health.
Zachariae, R., & O'Toole, M. S. (2015). The effect of expressive writing intervention on psychological and physical health outcomes in cancer patients—A systematic review and meta-analysis. *Psycho-Oncology, 24*(11), 1349–1359.
Zhong, W., Finnie, D. M., Shah, N. D., Wagie, A. E., Sauver, J. L., Jacobson, D. J., & Nassens, J. M. (2015). Effect of multiple chronic diseases on the health care expenditures in childhood. *Journal of Primary Care & Community Health, 6*, 2–9.
Zilioli, S., Slatcher, R. B., Ong, A. D., & Gruenewald, T. L. (2015). Purpose in life predicts allostatic load ten years later. *Journal of Psychosomatic Research, 79*(5), 451–457.
Zulman, D. M., Chee, C. P., Wagner, T. H., Yoon, J., Cohen, D. M., Holmes, T. H., … Asch, S. M. (2015). Multimorbidity and healthcare utilization among high-cost patients in the US veterans affairs health care system. *BMJ Open, 5, e007771.*

Chapter 11
Increasing Healthy Exercise in the Primary Care Setting

Terry L. Oroszi, Jacob Shoenleben, and Larry C. James

The primary care hospital and clinic settings offer many rewards to practitioners and challenges alike. One major challenge that health care professionals may often identify in the primary care setting is the sedentary lifestyle of their patients. Needless to say, the lack of healthy exercise can be a leading cause of obesity, type II diabetes, essential hypertension, as well as obesity. In this chapter we will discuss outcome research that has been shown to increase patient participation in healthy exercise and decrease the symptoms associated with the diseases (such as type II diabetes, obesity, and essential hypertension) that can be effectively treated with behavioral health interventions directly within the primary care clinics.

Exercise and weight loss industries combined are estimated to annually yield approximately $60 billion dollars in revenue, and 67% of Americans will never use the membership purchased at either a healthy club or gym (ABCNews.Com, 2012; Williams, 2013). Needless to say, the exercise industry is robust, yet Americans are described as more overweight and sedentary today than ever before (ABCNews.Com, 2012; Williams, 2013). Researchers as well as healthcare professionals have known for decades (Annesi & Tennant, 2013; Bean, Vora, & Frontera, 2004; Epstein et al., 1995) that healthy and regular exercise results in many health and psychological benefits.

In general, consumption of foods that are high in fat in combination with an increasingly sedentary lifestyle has caused an imbalance between calories consumed and calories expended (WHO, 2015). How we eat as a culture, or the norms around eating, has negatively impacted our ability to estimate the number of food-related decisions we make a day and the quality of the food consumed (Wansink & Sobal, 2007).

T. L. Oroszi
Department of Pharmacology & Toxicology, Boonshoft School of Medicine, Wright State University, Dayton, OH, USA

J. Shoenleben · L. C. James (✉)
School of Professional Psychology, Wright State University, Dayton, OH, USA
e-mail: Larry.James@wright.edu

M. P. Duckworth, W. T. O'Donohue (eds.), *Behavioral Medicine and Integrated Care*,
https://doi.org/10.1007/978-3-319-93003-9_11

Wansink and Sobal (2007) in their study regarding individual's awareness of their food-related decision making and their belief that these decisions are influenced by their environment found that the average participant made an estimated number of 226.7 decisions regarding food a day. This was statistically significant when compared to the baseline average estimate of the participant, which were approximately 14 food-related decisions a day (Wansink & Sobal, 2007). This research suggested that not only do individuals intrinsically influence their choice of foods but that also the environment can influence an individual's decision of what and how much to eat. Moreover, the World Health Organization (2015) reported that elements of social, cultural, political, physical, and structural environmental factors could affect weight status. As a result, in treating individuals struggling with type II diabetes, essential hypertension, high cholesterol, and obesity, it is vital that practitioners utilize empirically validated healthy lifestyle treatments that include low-intensity healthy exercise in addressing these facets of the individual and their environment both at the micro- and macro-levels (Wansink & Sobal, 2007).

Diet and/or exercise are the most common strategies reported in the treatment of obesity of adults (Miller, 2001). Additionally, healthy exercise is a commonly reported treatment for obesity (Miller, 2001; Wing, 2008). Exercise has been repeatedly shown to increase weight loss success influencing physiological, emotional, and behavioral aspects in addition to decreasing total fat composition (Colvin & Olson, 1984; Jeffery et al., 1984; Kayman, Stern, & Burvold, 1990). Less commonly identified techniques in the treatment of weight loss by laypersons incorporate basic methods of the behavioral and cognitive-behavioral theories. Such techniques include self-monitoring (keeping food and exercise logs), goal setting, stimulus control/problem solving (identifying situations likely to cause unhealthy eating), and cognitive restructuring (recognizing and deterring individuals from rationalizing with themselves to eat unhealthy foods after stressful events) (Wing, 2008).

Given the abundance of treatment modalities and techniques, what causes individuals to dropout of exercise and weight loss programs, regain weight after a weight loss or structured exercise program, and continue to live an unhealthy lifestyle with impending disastrous health effects? Why do some individuals successfully continue on the correct path to healthy exercise and along the way lose weight, report better mood, and maintain their weight loss and exercise regime? James et al. (1997) emphasized that it may be perhaps due to how the exercise paradigm is presented to program participants.

James, Folen, and Noce (1998), James et al. (1999) and James and Linton (2008) believed that most overweight persons eventually discontinue their exercise program because the person has unrealistic goals that are oftentimes suggested by the healthcare professionals.

Let us explain this phenomenon. The average sedentary and/or overweight patients come to the doctor (the expert) seeking guidance and direction and ask their doctor the question, "Doctor, how do I start my exercise program?" Of course the doctor or nurse usually says with a smile, "I want you to exercise at least 3 times a week for 30 min each session." This does appear ideal and technically correct, but the problem is that the doctor offering this advice has just, unknowingly, set this patient up for failure. Why? As James and his colleagues (1998, 1999) have asserted, the vast majority of these patients are sedentary and overweight, and they have never been a seasoned and disciplined athlete.

James et al. (1999) postulated that this is how most patients with type II diabetes, essential hypertension, high cholesterol, and/or obesity have arrived at the current unhealthy state. Asking patients who have never been disciplined with exercise and healthy eating to adopt to a regime, which requires discipline, is setting patients up for failure.

Other authors have demonstrated findings suggesting that diet and exercise alone are not sufficient in the long-term maintenance of weight loss or regular exercise (American Dietetic Association, 1997; Hill, Thompson, & Wyatt, 2005; Mann et al., 2007; Miller, 1999, 2001; James et al., 1997). The American Dietetic Association (1997) reported that food- and weight-related behaviors alone are likely to be counterproductive rather than therapeutic at times becoming detrimental to the health and well-being of the individual. Cooper et al. (2010) reported that even highly advanced treatments consisting of cognitive-behavioral methods demonstrated similar weight loss maintenance difficulties.

A proposed mechanism by which obese individuals are thought to have unsuccessfully maintained their weight loss is that many diets and exercise routines fail to address the environmental, psychological, and social factors of maintaining weight loss beyond the first few weeks to months of attempting weight loss (Annesi, 2012; Caldwell, Baime, & Wolever, 2012; James et al., 1998, 1999). Given these findings, psychologists must address diseases such essential hypertension, type II diabetes, and obesity treatments by boosting techniques to enhance treatment outcomes.

James et al. (1998) developed the Healthy Lifestyle LE^{3}AN Program to address the treatment concerns of obese minority men. The program consisted of 25 minority and male military service members; all had been medically diagnosed as obese, had a BMI of at least 30, and were diagnosed with type II diabetes and essential hypertension (James et al., 1998). The researchers employed a cognitive-behavioral consistent treatment program that included a 2-week inpatient hospitalization followed by a 1-week day-treatment regimen and 1 year of weekly outpatient follow-up. It was found that the patients maintained weight loss for 1 year (James et al., 1998). At 12 months post-initiation of treatment, the patients maintained a 10 percent weight loss.

This finding is significant as maintenance of weight loss after 1 year is not consistently found within the research as previously stated. At a 2-year follow-up study (James et al., 1999), information on 91 active duty officers and enlisted personnel, including males and females, demonstrated that at 12 and 18 months follow-up, statistically significant weight loss and maintenance had been achieved. Furthermore, an encouraging aspect of this treatment program was that the study did not generate adverse side effects sometimes seen in other treatment programs (James et al., 1999). From this study, the authors identified several areas that psychologists should apply to current type II diabetes, essential hypertension, and obesity treatments to enhance treatment outcomes including nutrition, exercise, healthy lifestyles, emotions, expectations, and attitudes; these areas coupled with the policy recommendations provide a foundation for developing enhanced treatment programs that go beyond the typical nutritional, behavioral, and exercise suggestions that ultimately lead to failed weight loss attempts.

A way in which James et al. (1999) enhanced their nutritional portion of the *Healthy Lifestyle* LE^3AN Program was to instill within the patients the belief that they have the ability to make healthy choices in combination with the knowledge of healthier nutritional choices. Furthermore, aspects of cognitive-behavioral therapy seen in this philosophy include mastery and self-efficacy, both working in tandem to provide the individual with the confidence in their ability and the actual ability to control their thoughts and bodies as they relate to nutrition and healthy lifestyles.

The World Health Organization (2000) promotes a diet that is low in fat and high in complex carbohydrates and contains large amounts of fruit and vegetables to combat obesity. Moreover, although individuals are ultimately the ones to choose what to eat, environmental factors should be addressed at the individual, familial, societal, and community level to encourage proper nutrition (WHO, 2000). James et al. (1998), consistent with other authors, recommend utilizing food diaries as a way to self-monitor and record actual eating habits. This is an important aspect of obesity treatment as Wansink and Sobal (2007) demonstrated that individuals are not well equipped to estimate their daily food-related decisions. To enhance the nutritional aspect of obesity treatment, individuals should be encouraged to engage in self-monitoring while practitioners foster their sense of self-efficacy and mastery.

Healthy low-intensity exercise has been consistently shown to influence weight loss and maintenance (Colvin & Olson, 1984; Jeffery et al., 1984; Kayman et al., 1990; Miller, 2001; Wing, 2008). However, diets and exercise have also been shown to typically only produce short-term success (American Dietetic Association, 1997; Hill et al., 2005; James et al., 1997; Mann et al., 2007; Miller, 1999, 2001).

To enhance an already research supported technique, practitioners should implement short bouts of activity as James et al. (1998) reported; this approach improves exercise compliance while reducing the likelihood of injury. Jakicic, Robertson, Butler, and Wing (1995) reported three benefits to short bouts of exercise (20-min periods):

- Less likelihood of injury.
- Low-intensity short-bout exercise is less painful.
- Two periods of 20 min is more manageable than a daunting long session of painful exercise.

Miller (2001) reported that even when philosophical positions of the treatment program change exercise, it is critical to the successful to successful maintenance of weight loss, emotions, and healthful behaviors. Additionally, the type and intensity of exercise should be highly individualized with a focus on encouraging repeated and regular exercise that is enjoyable (Miller, 2001). Furthermore, instilling in individuals the ability to decrease sedentary activity, such as decreasing TV watching and increasing physical activity, is effective in promoting weight loss (Epstein et al., 1995).

Resistance training may also provide additional benefits to individuals by strengthening key areas of the body that may have been neglected as a result of years of obesity, thereby improving quality of life in the future (Nicklas et al., 2015). In sum, short-bouts of enjoyable, low-intensity exercise are more beneficial, despite common conception, in promoting weight loss and maintenance.

In an effort to offer practitioners with example on increasing outcome efficacy, James et al. (1998) recommend that the provider include easily, obtainable exercise and weight loss goals (0.5–1 lb. per week). These authors asserted that this would foster a sense of accomplishment and definitive progress toward their exercise and weight loss goals. Field trips and real-life scenarios should be practiced with obese individuals during treatment as to exercise their ability to control unhealthy behaviors and continue to build their sense of self-efficacy (James et al., 1998). These recommendations related to physical and mental exercise are likely to enhance treatment outcomes by addressing long-term needs in addition to short-term effective weight loss practices.

In offering a long-term aftercare program, James et al. (1998) provided a foundation for the participants to maintain their weight loss by having weekly check-ins to encourage lifestyle changes that had been made during treatment. James et al. (1998) also included the family in the treatment program as inclusion of this factor will further encourage the participant to change their environments to reflect their weight loss needs. Encouraging lifestyle changes including reducing the availability of unhealthy food items, increasing the availability of healthy food items, having regular check-ins or discussions about progress or lapses, and setting reasonable weight loss goals will do justice in maintaining weight loss as these techniques are likely to induce positive lifestyle changes.

In addition to the commonly accepted practices of enacting weight loss and maintenance of this weight loss, coupled with low-intensity healthy exercise, James et al. (1998) recommended practitioners to address the emotions related to stress, unreasonable exercise, and weight loss expectations and attitudes of their program that impeded the participants' long-term health and success. These areas are likely to influence the success or failure of the program and have almost certainly been disregarded in previous efforts.

In addressing these areas, participants will likely sustain the lifestyle changes that have been fostered through the enhancement of typical obesity treatments. Specifically, the *Healthy Lifestyle* LE^{3}AN Program contained regular psychological visits to address the relationships between the participant's "food, social environment, body image, and emotions" (James et al., 1998).

Other researchers have also included a psychological piece to address body image with success in their treatment programs (Miller, 1999). Wing (2008) recommended utilizing cognitive restructuring when cues of overeating and underexercising become prevalent in work with obese individuals. Annesi and Tennant (2013) found that increasing self-regulation and focusing on improving mood and self-efficacy are advantageous in the treatment of obesity which we can draw associations to health exercise. As a result of the cited literature, treatment outcomes can be enhanced by addressing the expectations, emotions, and attitudes of obese individuals early and often in treatment.

Case Examples of Increasing Healthy Exercise

Case 1: Moses Moses was a 30-year-old, married, Native Hawaiian who worked as a supply supervisor. He was 5′8″ and weighed 278 pounds. Moses had many successful weight loss attempts coupled with many "embarrassing moments" at fitness centers and "work-out clubs" where he "wasted hundreds of dollars every other year." Moses was depressed and felt as though he was lost. Each time he enrolled in a "program," Moses actually gained more weight and felt worse. A program was designed so that Moses could be successful. First, Moses was encouraged to exercise in small pieces every day. It was explained to Moses that he needed to build exercise into his daily life as part of his "normal" routine rather than cope with the disruption and failure of a three times a week failure. He was encouraged to walk for 5–10 min each day. Moses was able to acquire success with this brief model of exercise and over time was able to increase his walks to 40 min each day. Within 14 months, Moses' weight slowly decreased to 220 pounds, coupled with a clinically significant decrease in his total cholesterol and blood pressure.

Case 2: Julie Julie was 39 years of age and at 5′3″ she weighed 275 pounds. She felt ashamed and perceived herself as "a loser." She cried every day, felt more alone, and knew that she needed to exercise in order to lose weight, but she would be in severe pain after all of the 1 h aerobic classes she attended. She just wanted "to give up." We designed a program to increase the likelihood that Julie would achieve exercise success. First, she was offered the advice that "pain is her enemy." And, Julie was also told to find a support system of close neighbors, relatives, co-workers, and/or friends who would be willing to exercise with her. We identified a supervised, water aerobic program at a nearby YWCA that was convenient for Julie to attend. Julie began to attend the program each morning prior to work with her sister with great success. Eventually, two of her office co-workers and an aunt began to attend the water aerobics program with Julie. Over time she began to lose weight and would walk with her husband in the evening without experiencing any leg pain.

Case 3: Cliff Cliff was a 43-year-old African-American male who was married and had three teenage boys. Cliff had had two open heart surgeries in 5 years, and he needed to lose weight as well. Cliff simply hated exercise because he disliked running due to the residual chest pain he would experience while running. Due to the time demands of his job, he lacked the time to "go for a five-mile run" two to three times a week. Cliff argued with his wife constantly about him "giving up on exercise." Cliff believed that "if it didn't involve either running, pain, or sweat, it wasn't exercise." We implemented a "short bout" of exercise for Cliff. He was encouraged to purchase a stationary bike for his home and spend just 10–15 min on the bike in the morning and 10–15 min in the evening riding the bike at a very comfortable MPH. He was asked to encourage his sons and wife to participate, and his request was welcomed with enthusiasm.

Case 4: Donnie Donnie was a 51-year-old, married white male who was 5′6″ tall and weighed 296 pounds. Donnie's blood pressure was 198/120, and his total cholesterol was 320. He reported to being tired and fatigued "all the time" and was disappointed in himself because of his appearance, and he struggled to perform sexually with his wife of 30 years. Donnie decided to compete in the US Air Force Marathon in Dayton, Ohio, in September of 2015. Regardless of the advice from his physician "to take it slow," Donnie registered for the Marathon and had a goal of jogging seven to ten miles per day from January of 2015 leading up to the Marathon in September of 2015. On January 2nd of 2015, Donnie ran 5.5 miles and collapsed on the side walk, one block from his home. Within a matter of days, Donnie required emergency surgery and had undergone a quadruple "bypass" heart surgery to save his life. Upon completion of his cardiac rehabilitation program, Donnie was referred to our office. We assisted Donnie in designing a daily, low-intensity, healthy lifestyle program that included his wife and children. One year later Donnie was continuing to walk every day with his wife for approximately 40 min at a rate of 3.2 miles per hour. We incorporated into his regimen a consultation with a registered dietitian for healthy meal planning, and after 12 months Donnie had lost 75 pounds.

What Were the Common Variables to Success in the Cases?

1. *Pain is the enemy!* In particular, for patients who have never participated in organized high school or college sports, most will lack both the discipline and exercise knowledge to be successful with exercise. Most patients will assume that in order for exercise to work, it must hurt and be painful.
2. *Group support is essential.* Attempting to lose weight, continuing an exercise program, stopping smoking or drinking without a support system are very, very difficult. The more the healthcare professional can integrate in a family member or a friend or have the patient participate in an organized exercise program, the success rate will be greatly increased.
3. *The importance of time and convenience.* Americans have full and busy lives. Each time a healthcare professional asks a patient to just add in another activity that willrequire daily 60–90 min of time, the doctor is asking the patient to fail. Usually the compliant patient will initiate the exercise activity. But he or she will usually succumb to the business of their lives. Work, family duties and responsibilities, the house, the cars, etc. will soon overcome the patient's good intentions for the exercise program. To increase the successfulness of a healthy exercise regime, assist the patient in incorporating exercise into the home or work and require shorter time periods of exercise rather than longer ones.
4. *Exercise costs are important.* Keep the costs associated with exercise down. Exercise does not need to be expensive in order for it to be successful. The important point to be mindful of is that most patients believe that they must pur-

chase an expensive membership or equipment "to work out." Thus, one should provide patients with exercise alternatives that are inexpensive alternatives such as walking in the neighborhood or joining the nearby YMCA or YWCA.

5. *Reasonable exercise goals*. Many patients who have never jogged a mile may, on their own, set running a marathon or other demanding, arduous athletic events as their goal. However, early on, goals as such are usually a recipe for failure and will set the patient up for discontinuing exercise altogether. We encourage that patients be assisted in developing smaller or more reachable goals. This will lead to patients continued excitement and increase the likelihood that the person will continue to exercise.
6. *Reasonable expectations*. Often, at the beginning of treatment that will involve exercise, many patients may have expectations that are unrealistic such as increasing exercise from 10 min a day to 60 min after only 2 days of exercise. The psychologist will need to cognitively frame expectations so that these are easily attainable and healthy.
7. *Early morning exercise*. Exercising early in the morning provides a greater sense of well-being according to Zhaoyang, Matire, and Sliwinski (2017). Moreover, in order to decrease the likelihood that the burdens and requirements of one's daily schedule will interfere with exercise, we also strongly recommend to our patients that exercising at the beginning of the day will increase the possibility of their continued success with exercise.
8. *Connect exercise with weight loss*. Connecting healthy exercise with weigh loss is common, and it will provide a concrete measure and illustrate daily, weekly, and/or monthly progress.
9. *Cognitively define and frame what exercise is and is not*. Many patients struggle to lose weight as part of a new exercise program. Yet, often these new aspirations are met with failure. Why are some many patients unsuccessful with an exercise program and weight loss? The vast majority of patients who were never a part of an organized sports team lack the true understanding of exercise versus being active. At the onset of treatment, most of our patients view walking the dog or vacuuming the house as the same as being on a tread mill for 30 min (walking at a rate of 3.0–4.5 mph). The vast majority of our patients have little (if any) understanding of "target heart rate" or how to determine if an activity is actually an exercise. Thus, the practitioner should assist patients in identifying and defining exercises that will actually assist them in their weight loss efforts.
10. *Employ fitness trackers*. Most patients miscalculate the quality and quantity of what they eat and their exercise by at least 50%. Most Americans will assume they have walked for two miles when in fact he or she walked for nine blocks. The now commonly used wrist band fitness trackers will greatly assist patients in being mindful of their "steps" per day or miles walked or jogged. Moreover, the fitness trackers are ideal to provide our patients with some assessment of their heart rate.
11. *Deliver healthy exercise and behavioral health services directly in the primary setting*. Several researchers (Hunter, Goodie, Oordt, & Dobmeyer, 2009; James

& Folen, 2005; James & O'Donohue, 2008; O'Donohue, Byrd, Cummings, & Anderson, 2005; O'Donohue, Cummings, Cucciare, Runyan, & Cummings, 2006) have posited research that clearly demonstrated that behavioral health interventions offered directly within the primary care clinics can improve patient access, increase the continuity of care, reduce mental health stigma, and increase treatment compliance.

We have found that family medicine providers are very welcoming of psychologists and other mental health professionals delivering services in the primary care setting. It is suggested that behavioral health provider collaborate with family medicine providers and offer these interventions in the family medicine clinics.

An example would be partnering clinical psychology interns and clinical health psychology postdoctoral fellows with primary care and family medicine residents to jointly offer low-intensity healthy exercise programs with the primary care clinics. In addition, programs such as tobacco cessation and weight loss group-based interventions can be delivered directly in the primary care setting.

12. *Offer web-based and social media exercise applications for laptops and cell phones.* There are many free web-based, online, applications available that will assist patients with developing a successful outcome with healthy exercise. For example, the "Top 10 Interval Training Mobile Apps to Download Right Now" can be found at https://greatist.com/fitness/10-interval-training-mobile-apps-download-right-now.

    In addition, a guide to free "fitness apps" can be found at http://www.businessinsider.com/one-free-fitness-app-has-made-a-huge-difference-for-me-and-researchers-say-it-works-too-2015-8/#-1.

More recently in 2017, the Health Psychology published published a special section of it's journal on healthy exercise. In this special edition, Bernstein and McNally (2017) provided their findings on a study that employed "acute aerobic exercise to hasten emotional recovery from a subsequent stressor." In their study with 95 participants, the researchers found that cycling may facilitate subjective emotional recovery.

An innovative study conducted by Zhaoyang et al. (2017) sought to examine the variable exercise has on self-efficacy in patients diagnosed with knee osteoarthritis. These researchers found that in 135 older adults, "morning self-efficacy" was a predictor in not only exercise outcome but morning exercise also produced a greater sense of well-being. The participants who exercised in the morning rather than in the evening or afternoon reported "emotionally feeling better."

Conclusions

Increasing healthy exercise for our patients in the primary care setting can be challenging and involve many complex variables. Often, even though patients may have good intention to exercise, all too often, time, family challenges, the financial costs of exercise, and having unrealistic goals can unintentionally place failure and a lack of success in our patient's path. Depression, chronic pain, feelings of worthlessness, and poor health are the common results of many failed attempts at exercise. Research by many primary care scholars and researchers have shown the benefits of offering healthy exercise within the primary care setting (James et al., 1998, 1999; James & Folen, 2005).

As discussed in this chapter, reasonable goals and expectations, coupled with exercise routines that are without physical pain, conveniently increase patient exercise success. Likewise, incorporating the support of family, friends, and co-workers will enhance exercise success and reduce the possibility of relapse. We also discussed that incorporating early morning exercise will increase the clinical and emotional well-being effects of healthy exercise.

References

ABCNews.Com. (2012). Weight loss by the numbers. Abcnews.go.com/Health/100-million-dieters-20billion-weight-loss-industry/story?id=16297197

American Dietetic Association. (1997). Position of the American dietetic association: Weight management. *Journal of the American Dietetic Association, 97*, 71–74.

Annesi, J. J. (2012). Supported exercise improves controlled eating and weight through its effects on psychosocial factors: Extending a systematic research program toward treatment development. *The Permanente Journal, 16*(1), 7–18.

Annesi, J. J., & Tennant, G. A. (2013). Mediation of social cognitive theory variables in the relationship of exercise and improved eating in sedentary adults with severe obesity. *Psychology, Health & Medicine, 18*(6), 714–724. https://doi.org/10.1080/13548506.2013.766354

Bean, J. F., Vora, A., & Frontera, W. R. (2004). Benefits of exercise. *Archives of Physical Medicine & Rehabilitation, 85*(Suppl 3), S31–S42.

Bernstein, E., & McNally, R. (2017). Acute aerobic exercise hastens emotional recovery from a subsequent stressor. *Health Psychology, 36*(6), 560567.

Caldwell, K. L., Baime, M. J., & Wolever, R. Q. (2012). Mindfulness based approaches to obesity and weight loss maintenance. *Journal of Mental Health Counseling, 34*(3), 269–282.

Colvin, R. H., & Olson, S. B. (1984). Winners revisited: An 18-month follow-up of our successful weight losers. *Addictive Behaviors, 9*(3), 305–306.

Cooper, Z., Doll, H. A., Hawker, D. M., Byrne, S., Bonner, G., Eeley, E., … Fairburn, C. G. (2010). Testing a new cognitive behavioral treatment for obesity: A randomized controlled trial with three-year follow-up. *Behavior Research and Therapy, 48*, 706–713. https://doi.org/10.1016/j.brat.2010.03.008

Epstein, L. H., Valoski, A. M., Vara, L. S., McCurley, J., Wisniewski, L., Kalarchian, M. A., … Shrager, L. R. (1995). Effects of decreasing sedentary behavior and increasing activity on weight change in obese children. *Health Psychology, 14*(2), 109–115. https://doi.org/10.1037/0278-6133.14.2.109

Hill, J. O., Thompson, H., & Wyatt, H. (2005). Research: Weight maintenance: What's missing? *Journal of The American Dietetic Association, 105*(*Supplement*), 63–66. https://doi.org/10.1016/j.jada.2005.02.016

Hunter, C., Goodie, J., Oordt, M., & Dobmeyer, A. (2009). *Integrated behavioral health care: Step-by-step guidance for assessment & intervention*. Washington, DC: American Psychological Association Press.

Jakicic, J., Robertson, R., Butler, B., & Wing, R. (1995). Prescribing exercise in multiple short bouts versus one continuous bout: Effects on adherence, cardiorespiratory fitness, and weight loss in overweight women. *International Journal of Obesity, 19*(12), 893–901.

James, L. C., & Folen, R. A. (2005). *The primary care consultant*. Washington, DC: American Psychological Association Press.

James, L.C., Folen, R.A., Noce, M., Pederson, D. & Page, H. (1997). Preliminary findings of a healthy lifestyle program for the treatment of obesity & hyperlipidemia in minority men. Proceedings of the National Medical Association. August 2–7. Honolulu, Hawaii.

James, L. C., Folen, R. A., & Noce, M. A. (1998). A healthy lifestyle program for the treatment of obesity in minority men. *Journal of Clinical Psychology in Medical Settings, 5*(3), 259–273. https://doi.org/10.1023/A:1026250019031

James, L. C., Folen, R. A., Page, H., Noce, M., Brown, J., & Britton, C. (1999). The Tripler LE^{3}AN program: A two-year follow-up report. *Military Medicine, 164*(6), 389–395.

James, L. C., & O'Donohue, W. (2008). *The primary care tool kit*. New York, NY: Springer.

James, L.C. & Linton, J. (2008). *Treating obseity across the lifespan*. New York: Springer Press.

Jeffery, R. W., Bjornson-Benson, W. M., Rosenthal, B. S., Lindquist, R. A., Kurth, C. L., & Johnson, S. L. (1984). Correlates of weight loss and its maintenance over two years of follow-up among middle-aged men. *Preventive Medicine, 13*(2), 155–168.

Kayman, S., Stern, J., & Bruvold, W. (1990). Maintenance and relapse after weight loss in women: Behavioral aspects. *American Journal of Clinical Nutrition, 52*(5), 800–807.

Mann, T., Tomiyama, A. J., Westling, E., Lew, A., Samuels, B., & Chatman, J. (2007). Medicare's search for effective obesity treatments: Diets are not the answer. *American Psychologist, 62*(3), 220–233.

Miller, W. (2001). Effective diet and exercise treatments for overweight and recommendations for intervention. *Sports Medicine, 31*(10), 717–724. 0112-1642/01/0010-0717.

Miller, W. C. (1999). Fitness and fatness in relation to health: Implications for a paradigm shift. *Journal of Social Issues, 55*(2), 207–219.

Nicklas, B. J., Chmelo, E., Delbono, O., Carr, J. e., Lyles, M. F., & Marsh, A. P. (2015). Effects of resistance training with and without caloric restriction on physical function and mobility in overweight and obese older adults: A randomized controlled trial. *American Journal of Clinical Nutrition, 101*(5), 991–999. https://doi.org/10.3945/ajcn.114.105270

O'Donohue, W., Byrd, M., Cummings, N., & Anderson, D. (2005). *Behavioral integrative care: Treatments that work in primary care*. New York, NY: Brunner-Routledge.

O'Donohue, W., Cummings, N., Cucciare, N., Runyan, C., & Cummings, J. (2006). *Integrated behavioral health care: A guide to effective intervention*. New York, NY: Humanity Books.

Wansink, B., & Sobal, J. (2007). Mindless eating: The 200 daily food decisions we overlook. *Environment and Behavior, 39*(1), 106–123. https://doi.org/10.1177/0013916506295573

Williams, G. (2013, January 3). *The heavy price of losing weight*. USNews&World Report. https://money.usnews.com/money/personal-finance/articles/2013/01/02/the-heavy-price-of-losing-weight

Wing, R. R. (2008). Behavioral approaches to the treatment of obesity. In G. A. Bray & C. Bouchard (Eds.), *Handbook of obesity: Clinical applications* (pp. 227–248). New York, NY: Informal Healthcare.

World Health Organization (WHO). Obesity and overweight. World Health Organization. (2015). Fact sheet No 311. Retrieved from http://www.who.int/mediacentre/factsheets/fs311/en/

World Health Organization (WHO). (2000). *Obesity: Preventing and managing the global epidemic: Report of a WHO consultation*. Geneva, Switzerland: World Health Organization.

Zhaoyang, R., Matire, L., & Sliwinski, M. (2017). Morning self-efficacy predicts physical activity throughout the day in knee osteoarthritis. *Health Psychology, 369*(6), 568–576.

Chapter 12
Smoking Cessation in the Context of Integrated Care

Brandon T. Sanford

Prevalence and Impact

According to the US Department of Health and Human Services, 15 out of every 100 (15.1%) US adults smoke cigarettes (2014). At the time of this writing, that equates to approximately 36.8 million Americans. Of course, the prevalence of smoking is not evenly distributed across gender, geographic location, ethnicity, and socioeconomic status. Cigarette smoking is more prevalent among males (16.7%) as compared to females (13.7%; Jamal, 2016), as well as those living in the south and midwestern areas of the USA (Dwyer-Lindgren et al., 2014). Smoking prevalence and tobacco consumption rates are also significantly higher among those lower in socioeconomic status (Casetta et al., 2016; Nagelhout et al., 2012), a trend that is unfortunately widening over time, particularly for females. With regard to ethnicity, those who identify as American Indian/Alaska Native are significantly more likely to smoke (21.9%), compared to those identifying as non-Hispanic white (16.6%), non-Hispanic black (16.7%), or Hispanic (10.1%; Jamal, 2016). US military veterans are also significantly more likely to smoke (Brown, 2010).

Unsurprisingly, those working in medical settings are especially likely to come into contact with smokers. Approximately 28% of acute medical admissions are smokers (Harrison, Preston, Bucur, & Fletcher, 2012). Those diagnosed with chronic obstructive pulmonary disease (COPD) have been consistently shown to be 1.5 times more likely to smoke (Vozoris & Stanbrook, 2011). This has been found to be as high as 2.5 times more likely for women diagnosed with COPD. Approximately 1 in 4 women in their first month of pregnancy is recently an active smoker, and while this rate declines during pregnancy, up to 11% of women continue to smoke at 9 months (Alshaarawy & Anthony, 2015). It is also important to note that women are more likely to conceal current smoking status during

B. T. Sanford (✉)
Department of Psychology, University of Nevada, Reno, Reno, NV, USA

M. P. Duckworth, W. T. O'Donohue (eds.), *Behavioral Medicine and Integrated Care*,
https://doi.org/10.1007/978-3-319-93003-9_12

pregnancy (Shipton et al., 2009; Cnattingius, S. (2004)). Those with diagnosed mental health or substance use disorders are also especially likely to smoke (Catchpole, McLeod, Brownlie, Allison, & Grewal, 2016) with nearly 50% of all cigarettes consumed in North America being smoked by this group (Ziedonis, Williams, & Smelson, 2003). Furthermore, while national smoking prevalence is slowly declining over time, this is not true for those with poor mental health (Steinberg, Williams, & Li, 2015).

These prevalence estimates become especially important in examining the effects of smoking on mortality, morbidity, and financial burden. The 2004 Surgeon General's report reports that smoking negatively impacts nearly every organ in the body (USD-HHS, 2004). An updated report published 10 years later causally links smoking to 12 types of cancer and over 20 chronic diseases (USD-HHS, 2014) resulting in a smoking-attributable mortality rate of 480,000 Americans per year. The relative risk of death from all causes among current smokers as compared to never smokers is 2.8 times higher for men and 2.76 times higher for women (Thun et al., 2013). Smoking is responsible for over 30% of all cancer deaths and nearly 80% of deaths from COPD and early cardiovascular disease (CDC, 2008). Those who smoke are 25 times more likely to die from both lung cancer and COPD than never smokers (Thun et al., 2013). Interestingly, approximately 17% of the excess mortality for smokers is attributed to causes not formally linked to smoking, which speaks to its globally deleterious effects on the body (Carter et al., 2015). In addition to increased mortality rates, smoking greatly impacts morbidity. Among smokers approximately 47.5% of females and 44.9% of males over the age of 65 report having been diagnosed with at least 1 smoking-related condition, with 16.9% of men and 14.3% of women reporting multiple conditions (Rostron, Chang, & Pechacek, 2014). This includes increased odds of being diagnosed with COPD, diabetes mellitus, heart attack, cancer, and stroke. Cigarette smoking not only increases the risk of developing diabetes mellitus by 50% (Eliasson, 2003) but contributes to poorer glycemic control, macrovascular complications (e.g., coronary artery disease and stroke), and microvascular complications (e.g., nephropathy and retinopathy; Tonstad, 2009). Smoking is also associated with delayed conception and infertility, ectopic pregnancy, spontaneous abortions, placental complications, fetal growth restriction, preterm birth, stillbirth, neonatal mortality, and behavioral and psychiatric disorders in childhood (Cnattingius, 2004). Smoking also represents a significant financial burden with between 6% and 18% of all healthcare spending directly attributed to tobacco use which is approximately 1% of the US GDP (Ekpu & Brown, 2015). This equals roughly $193 billion annually in health-related costs and loss of productivity. More than 60% of these costs are paid by public programs such as Medicare, Medicaid, or other federally sponsored programs (Xu, Bishop, Kennedy, Simpson, & Pechacek, 2015).

Fortunately, cessation of smoking significantly ameliorates these negative impacts. Quitting earlier in life results in the best health outcomes, with those who quit between the ages of 25 and 34 having nearly identical mortality curves to those of never smokers (Jha et al., 2013). This represents an increased life expectancy of 10 years compared to those who continue to smoke. Those who quit between ages

35 and 44 gain 9 years of life expectancy and reduce their excess risk of death from any cause by 90%. Those who quit between ages 45 and 54 and 55 and 64 gain 6 and 4 years of life expectancy, respectively, and approximately a 66% reduced excess risk of death. Compared to current smokers, each 10-year period since quitting smoking is associated with a 16% decrease in the global risk of hospitalization (Tran, Falster, Douglas, Blyth, & Jorm, 2015). In addition to direct health benefits, smoking cessation has positive impacts on communities. Community-level adult smoking rates are associated with rates of smoking in adolescents and increase the impact of perceived friends' smoking behavior on individual smoking behavior (Thrul, Lipperman-Kreda, Grube, & Friend, 2014). Similarly, children's odds of smoking are reduced by nearly 40% for those whose parents successfully quit smoking as compared to those who continue (Bricker, Leroux, Andersen, Rajan, & Peterson, 2005). Parental smoking cessation is also associated with the future smoking cessation of their adolescent children (Bricker, Otten, Liu, & Peterson, 2009). Thus, smoking cessation interventions in adults may meaningfully be contributing to the prevention of smoking in younger generations.

Evidence-based Treatments for Tobacco Use

The state of the evidence makes a compelling case for the importance of widespread effective tobacco cessation interventions. Integrated care settings represent a unique opportunity to interface with patients who smoke and deliver brief targeted treatments. Large systematic reviews of the literature have found individual and group counseling to be effective for smoking cessation as compared to minimum contact controls (Chen & Wu, 2015; Hartmann-Boyce, Stead, Cahill, & Lancaster, 2014). This effect is particularly pronounced for those with a history of depression and for women who are pregnant (Gierisch, Bastian, Calhoun, McDuffie, & Williams, 2012). The National Guidelines for Treating Tobacco Use and Dependence issue ten specific recommendations to healthcare providers which broadly encourage the identification of smokers and administration of evidence-based treatments (Fiore et al., 2008). This includes behavioral interventions (e.g., motivational interviewing, cognitive behavioral therapy, acceptance and commitment therapy, mindfulness-based treatments), stepped-care interventions (e.g., quit lines, smartphone applications), and pharmacotherapy.

Stepped-Care Interventions

Quit Lines In a meta-analysis of ten trials evaluating the efficacy of smoking cessation quit lines, patients who engaged in call-back counseling were 41% more likely to be abstinent at a 6–12-month follow-up (Stead, Perera, & Lancaster, 2007). Lichtenstein, Zhu, and Tedeschi (2010) point out that quit-line counseling has the advantages of being (1) convenient for patients, as they do need to make travel arrangements; (2) fast-moving, as the semi-anonymous nature allows for more candid discussion; (3) proactive, as the counselor can call patients which reduces attrition; and (4) structured, as the telephone format is ideal for delivering and monitoring protocol-based treatment. Behavioral care providers (BCPs) should be aware of local, state, and federal quit lines. It is also worth noting that some state quit lines can be helpful in assisting patients in obtaining free or low-cost nicotine replacement treatments.

Text Messaging and Smartphone Applications As the ubiquity of smartphones continues to increase, it opens up an additional avenue for delivering real-time health-based interventions. Over 64% of American adults are smartphone owners, and in the past year, over half of all smartphone owners have used the device to look up a health condition (Smith, 2015). Smartphone ownership remains near 50% even in the lowest income brackets meaning smoking cessation applications are useful even in settings treating underserved populations. In a Cochrane review of 12 trials encompassing nearly 12,000 patients, those who received smartphone interventions were nearly 70% more likely to be abstinent at follow-up (Whittaker, McRobbie, Bullen, Rodgers, & Gu, 2016). The majority of these trials were SMS text message based. Of the commercially available smartphone apps, the majority consist of simple trackers (i.e., money saved, days since quitting) and often exhibit a dearth of tailoring and assistance in quitting (Hoeppner et al., 2015). Of the top 50 smartphone applications recommended by app store marketplaces, only 4% have any scientific support (Haskins, Lesperance, Gibbons, & Boudreaux, 2017). One notable exception is that of the SmartQuit application, which boasts interactivity and tailoring in developing a quit plan, tracking smoking and urges successfully passed, social community features, location tracking, protocolized exercises, and achievement badges (Heffner, Vilardaga, Mercer, Kientz, & Bricker, 2015). When compared to the National Cancer Institute's QuitGuide, patients engaged with SmartQuit significantly more often and had an 88% increased rate of abstinence at 2-month follow-up (13% to 8%; Bricker et al., 2014). An updated version of the application demonstrated similar quit rates while improving patient satisfaction and usability ratings (Bricker et al., 2017). A limitation of this app is its cost ($50 as of this writing) as compared to most free or low-cost options popular in the marketplace; however, institutions and wellness programs may purchase bulk licenses for patients.

Behavioral Interventions

Motivational Interviewing A recent review found that while smoking interventions are equally effective for young adults as compared to older adults, they are less likely to engage in evidence-based treatment (Suls et al., 2012). This speaks to the importance of increasing motivation to engage in treatment. Often patients will display ambivalence about their smoking citing that they know it is unhealthy, but that now is not the time to quit or that they could not cope without the habit. In these cases, motivational interviewing (MI; Miller & Rollnick, 2012) is useful in fostering willingness to engage in change. MI is not intended to be a stand-alone treatment per se (Miller, 2012) but a therapeutic stance and set of techniques which seeks to "clarify [a patient's] strengths and aspirations, evoke their own motivations for change, and promote autonomy of decision making" (Rollnick, Butler, Kinnersley, Gregory, & Mash, 2010). Techniques used within MI include asking open-ended questions, asking about pros and cons of change, providing information, and reflective listening (Croston, 2010). A key component in this approach is evoking change talk (i.e., statements from a patient about why they want to change or how they might go about accomplishing that end), for example, asking a patient "How important is it for you to quit smoking?" or "How confident do you feel about quitting?" is likely to occasion a change response. An MI stance also encourages clinicians to roll with resistance where it is encountered by reflecting concerns and reframing to encourage future change talk. If a patient were to say they were "about a 4" when asked how confident they were in executing their change plan on a scale of 1 to 10, you may then respond "so a 4, why not a 3 or a 1?" which then occasions a response from the patient consistent with the relative importance to change. Two large meta-analyses which each reviews a total of 31 trials demonstrate a consistent advantage for MI as compared to control group, which equates to 45% improved chance of abstinence at follow-up (Heckman, Egleston, & Hofmann, 2010; Hettema & Hendricks, 2010). A more recent review of trials, utilizing primary care physicians (PCPs), hospital clinicians, nurses, and counselors, found a more modest but still significant effect for MI compared to treatment as usual (26% increased likelihood of abstinence at follow-up; Lindson-Hawley, Thompson, & Begh, 2015). Those looking for more information or training in MI should visit http://www.motivationalinterviewing.org/ to find an extensive selection of theoretical and empirical articles, example exercises and techniques, and list of upcoming trainings.

Cognitive Behavioral Therapy Cognitive behavioral therapy (CBT; Hofmann, Asnaani, Vonk, Sawyer, & Fang, 2012) for smoking cessation focuses on changing maladaptive thinking patterns and the negative behavior patterns associated with them. CBT for smoking cessation is mediated by increases in a patient's self-efficacy with respect to quitting (Hendricks, Delucchi, & Hall, 2010). CBT has been found to be effective when compared to treatment as usual or health information controls (Webb, de Ybarra, Baker, Reis, & Carey, 2010; Zelman, Brandon, Jorenby, & Baker, 1992). Some studies have found CBT outcomes are best when delivered for an extended length of time (i.e., up to 52 weeks; Hall et al., 2002, 2009; Hall, Humfleet, Reus, Muñoz, & Cullen, 2004); however, a recent large trial (n = 219) found no advantage to treatment beyond week 26 (Laude et al., 2017). Note that most CBT trials are conducted in conjunction with nicotine replacement treatment. As mentioned earlier, there may be particular benefits in administering CBT for smokers who have a history of depression, which is important in light of findings that an increasing number of treatment-seeking smokers exhibit symptoms of depression (Leyro et al., 2016). Treatments lasting 26 weeks may be a poor fit to be performed in integrated care settings, which typically focus on assessment, triage, delivery of stepped-care and brief interventions, and referrals to specialty evidence-based mental healthcare. In those cases, referral out to specialty care settings is advised.

Acceptance and Mindfulness-based Treatments There is a well-documented link between stress and both increased frequency of smoking and the increased likelihood of relapse (Carey, Kalra, Carey, Halperin, & Richards, 1993; Cohen & Lichtenstein, 1990; Kassel, Stroud, & Paronis, 2003). Anecdotally, it is not hard to recount numerous examples of patients who report quit attempts which end in lapse following a stressful event such as a family member being sent to the hospital, the breakup of a relationship, or an unexpected relocation. Acceptance and mindfulness-based interventions such as acceptance and commitment therapy (ACT; Hayes, Strosahl, & Wilson, 1999) and mindfulness-based addiction treatment (MBAT; Vidrine et al., 2016) are designed to increase an individual's willingness to experience urges without attempting to escape them via smoking and directly target the link between stress, cravings to smoke, and smoking behavior. Mindfulness has the specific aims of helping a patient:

(a) Become more aware of thoughts, feelings, and sensations from moment to moment.
(b) Develop a different way of relating to thoughts, feelings, and sensations.
(c) Increase the ability to disengage attention and choose skillful responses to any thoughts, feelings, or situations that arise.

(Vidrine et al., 2016)

Exercises are also used to connect a person with personal values associated with quitting such as health, family, or mobility, in order to enhance motivation for continued abstinence. Increased awareness of the present moment as practiced in mindfulness is useful in self-detection of relapse and return to non-smoking.

Those prone to early relapse (within 24 hours) subsequent to quit attempts perform significantly worse on distress tolerance/acceptance tasks than do those who relapse later (after 3 months; Brown, Lejuez, Kahler, & Strong, 2002; Brown et al., 2008). Poorer distress tolerance/acceptance mediates the impact of stress on smoking and relapse (Garey, Farris, Schmidt, & Zvolensky, 2016). Conversely, increases in willingness to experience cravings have been demonstrated to mediate the efficacy of quit-line treatment (Schuck, Otten, Kleinjan, Bricker, & Engels, 2014). Mindfulness training has been shown to moderate the relationship between cravings to smoke and cigarette use, such that those who engaged in mindfulness practice were less likely to smoke independent of their level of cravings (Elwafi, Witkiewitz, Mallik, Thornhill, & Brewer, 2013). Those higher in dispositional mindfulness are more likely to both achieve and maintain abstinence and to recover abstinence after an early lapse (Heppner et al., 2016).

An 11-minute mindfulness-based "urge surfing" exercise was shown to significantly reduce cigarette smoking in college students over a 7-week period as compared to a coping as usual condition (Bowen & Marlatt, 2009). A 4-week, 8-session, mindfulness training intervention was compared to a federally funded treatment as usual and demonstrated significantly higher abstinence rates at 17 weeks follow-up (31% to 6%; Brewer et al., 2011). However, a larger replication of this trial using seven weekly encounters plus a 6.5-h retreat compared to a time-matched version of the federally funded control program for low-SES smokers found no difference at 4 weeks post-treatment and a numerical, though nonsignificant, trend toward the mindfulness condition at 24 weeks. MBAT was developed in part to address the concerns raised in this previously reported trial and incorporates elements of CBT plus relapse prevention. When compared to a CBT condition and treatment as usual control, no significant differences were found between groups in prolonged abstinence; however, those in the MBAT group who lapsed were significantly more likely to regain abstinence (Vidrine et al., 2016). Thus, mindfulness training may be particularly useful as a skill trained in maintenance in order to encourage recovery from lapse.

ACT as a treatment package incorporates mindfulness training with acceptance and values elements targeting distress tolerance. When 14 sessions of ACT (7 individuals, 7 groups, over 7 weeks) were compared to nicotine replacement therapy, nonsignificantly different quit rates were found at post (35% to 33%) and 6 months follow-up (23% to 11%); however, significant differences were observed at 12 months follow-up (35% to 15%) in favor of the ACT condition (Gifford et al., 2004). The aforementioned SmartQuit intervention is also based on an ACT approach. A meta-analysis evaluating ACT for substance abuse found the subset of five trials examining smoking cessation to have a small to medium significant effect size favoring ACT compared to control ($g = 0.42$; Lee, An, Levin, & Twohig, 2015). Based on current evidence, acceptance-based interventions are effective for smoking cessation and may be particularly useful for those prone to immediate relapse or those who cite coping with stress as their primary reason for continued smoking.

Pharmacotherapy

Nicotine Replacement Therapy Nicotine replacement therapy (NRT) works by directly replacing the nicotine in tobacco products with gum, patches, lozenges, inhalers, or nasal sprays. Aggregating across all forms of NRT, individuals have an 84% increased rate of smoking cessation compared to placebo (Cahill, Stevens, Perera, & Lancaster, 2013; Hartmann-Boyce et al., 2014). These outcomes are further improved when paired with behavioral interventions. Potential adverse effects include a significant increase in cardiovascular events as compared to placebo (Samet, 2013). This effect is sustained well after NRT is discontinued and cannot be readily explained based on an understanding of nicotine's pharmacological effects. However, the benefits for cardiovascular health of sustained abstinence still outweigh the relative increase attributed to NRT such that using NRT successfully represents a net benefit.

Medications Bupropion (Zyban, Aplenzin, Wellbutrin, Forfivo) is an antidepressant that works by mitigating the symptoms of withdrawal from nicotine. It has been shown to have similar efficacy to NRT (82%; Hartmann-Boyce et al., 2014; Cahill, Stevens, Perera, & Lancaster, 2013). Varenicline (Chantix) facilitates smoking cessation by functioning as a partial nicotine agonist. It has been shown to be significantly more effective than either NRT or bupropion with a cessation rate of 127% higher than placebo. This equates to approximately 60% improved odds compared to NRT and bupropion. While roughly 13% of individuals taking varenicline will report abnormal dreams or sleep disturbance, across 13 trials there is no evidence for increased chance of suicide or attempted suicide, suicidal ideation, depression, irritability, aggression, or death (Thomas, Martin, Knipe, Higgins, & Gunnell, 2015). It should also be noted that there is no substantial advantage to using smoking cessation medication in conjunction with NRT.

Treatments to Avoid

There are several approaches to smoking cessation that either lack sufficient evidence to be employed or have accrued sufficient evidence to be avoided. Buspirone, a medication prescribed to treat anxiety, has demonstrated an inverse relationship with smoking cessation within the limited trials it has been tested in and should be avoided (Hartmann-Boyce et al., 2014). Naltrexone, an opiate agonist, selective serotonin reuptake inhibitors, and St. John's wort have all failed to demonstrate an advantage over placebo. Occasionally, patients may ask about hypnosis as a treatment for nicotine dependence. According to the most recent review on the subject, the authors conclude "We have not shown that hypnotherapy has a greater effect on six-month quit rates than other interventions or no treatment" (Barnes et al., 2010). Given the current state of the evidence, patients should be advised to pursue a combination of pharmacotherapy and intensive behavioral treatments if they have been unsuccessful using other approaches in the past.

Program Development

The review of the literature on smoking cessation up until this point should give the BCP a sufficient orientation to evidence-based treatments and for their substantial need. Virtually every behavioral approach covered here was tested exclusively, or at least primarily, in the context of specialty mental healthcare. Sustainable programs must merge unobstructively with medical professional's workflow, and thus these interventions may require adaptation. One way of accomplishing this is by the use of real-time hallway handoffs, where BCPs are able to see patients during the same encounter period they are seen by PCPs. This allows the PCP to accomplish other tasks while the smoking cessation intervention is performed and be quickly updated afterward. In order to establish such a system, we must review the medical framework for addressing smoking cessation while highlighting opportunities for behavioral providers to integrate into and improve it.

5As Approach

The 5As (Ask, Advise, Assess, Assist, Arrange) approach has been widely recommended within the medical literature as a useful way of addressing the National Guidelines for Treating Tobacco Use and Dependence (Fiore et al., 2008; Goldstein, Whitlock, & DePue, 2004; Whitlock, Orleans, Pender, & Allan, 2002). Combining findings from over 26 studies, the Advise stage alone accounts for a 76% increased rate of smoking cessation compared to no advice/treatment as usual (Hartmann-Boyce et al., 2014). Arranging follow-up increases odds of quitting by 46% when compared to no follow-up (Park et al., 2015). Clinics which institute a system change consistent with a 5As approach resulted in a 40% increase in self-reported abstinence among patients compared to patients in clinics who continued practice as usual (13.6% to 9.7%; Land et al., 2012). Additionally, there was a significant reduction (4.3%) in smoking-related office visits for those identified as smokers at sites which achieved system change. Clinics which targeted pregnant smokers showed a 16% increase in smoking abstinence after instituting a 5As approach (Olaiya et al., 2015). Yet, documented rates of successfully completing all 5As in the literature are low: Ask (87–60%), Advise (76–49%), Assess (63–42%), Assist (56–50%), and Arrange (17–3%; Lawson, Flocke, & Casucci, 2009; Park et al., 2015; King, Dube, Babb, & McAfee, 2013).

Improving 5As adherence requires adequate training for the entire staff. Training itself is associated with a 60% increase in patient cessation success (Hartmann-Boyce et al., 2014). A 3.5-h training for medical staff at 10 facilities ($n = 488$) consisting of didactics and interactive modules has been shown to increase 5As adherence at 6-month follow-up (Payne et al., 2014). Results of a meta-analysis compiling trials which examined programs designed to increase 5A utilization revealed that multicomponent approaches are significantly more efficacious than training alone (Papadakis et al., 2010). The most common components included training, screeners, desktop resources, performance feedback, checklists, electronic prompts, adjunct counseling, and cost-free NRT. At minimum the BCP should be able to offer training and adjunct counseling as needed; other elements should be implemented as available. For example, brief one-page checklists have been found to be effective in increasing the rate of documented 5As adherence. Electronic prompts inside electronic medical records have also been found to increase 5As adherence. Performance feedback can be accomplished by regularly reviewing charts to ensure 5As are properly documented. Training should address how to address patients who appear to be disinterested, how to implement each of the 5As and do so in a reasonable amount of time, and, if applicable, how to address pregnant patients and the applicability of tobacco cessation medications (Agaku et al., 2015).

As a trainer your goal is to instill confidence in the staff's ability to carry out the 5As and establish the perception that helping smokers quit is a priority of their facility. It is also important to remind the staff that tobacco dependence often requires repeated intervention and multiple attempts to quit (Fiore et al., 2008). A recent study estimates that it takes an average of 30 attempts before an individual is successful in quitting for over 1 year (Chaiton et al., 2016) with an estimated one quit attempt per year (Borland, Partos, Yong, Cummings, & Hyland, 2012). It should also be noted that between 40% and 52% of former smokers quit the first time they made a serious attempt (cf Chaiton et al., 2016), but the overarching point is that repetition is key.

Taken together, an example integrated care smoking cessation program based on a 5As approach would look like the following:

1. PCP reviews patient chart making note of smoking status.
2. *Ask*: PCP asks patient about their current smoking status.
3. *Advise*: PCP gives clear, specific, and personalized behavior change advice, including information about personal health harms from smoking and benefits of cessation (Whitlock et al., 2002).
4. PCP informs patient that a member of the behavior health staff will be in to discuss smoking and continues the medical encounter.
5. PCP or a member of medical staff informs BCP that a hallway handoff is needed and provides patient information.
6. *Assess*: BCP uses MI to assess willingness to engage in a quit attempt, explore ambivalence about quitting, and encourage change.
7. *Assist*: BCP provides evidence-based stepped-care interventions such as self-help materials and information about quit lines and smartphone applications. BCP also provides information about NRT and smoking cessation medications.
8. *Arrange*: BCP arranges follow-up either for more intensive smoking cessation counseling, telephone follow-up, or follow-up at the patient's next medical encounter.
9. BCP follows up with PCP regarding the encounter and asks about the appropriateness of NRT or medication if the patient is interested in trying them.

Quality Improvement

Continued success of a program such as this requires regular quality improvement including data collection, evaluation, and iterative change (O'Donohue & Maragakis, 2016). Perhaps the most important metric is prevalence of 5A delivery at the clinic. Low instance rates of Ask, Advise, and involve BCP would signal the need for either additional training or individual feedback depending on variance in completion. Provider satisfaction is also key, as it allows BCPs to ensure the program is not putting undue burden onto PCPs. For example, low satisfaction scores indicating that providers are getting too behind with their schedules signal that steps 6–8 need to either be completed quicker or need to be completed after the medical encounter is over and in a different room. Finally, data should be taken on patient outcomes including current smoking status, quit attempt status, current amount of smoking, and patient satisfaction. In sum, the quality improvement process becomes iterative in itself as more creative and advanced metrics are applicable and inform more nuanced programmatic improvement.

Conclusion

Smoking represents a high-prevalence, high-impact problem well suited for integrated care programs. Fortunately, BCPs have a variety of evidence-based options for treatment that can be easily scaled to fit the low-scope high-volume style of treatment often implemented in integrated care settings. The 5As approach establishes a common language in developing programs alongside medical professionals and also provides a convenient system to interject BCP intervention. In order to ensure systematic change, multicomponent implementation should be undertaken including training which addresses key concerns, checklists and/or electronic prompts, and regular feedback. The goal is to establish smoking as a principal issue within the organization and promote adherence to 5A delivery. With a program in place, BCPs work closely with medical staff completing real-time hallways handoff interventions and delivering immediate feedback on outcome. Finally, quality improvement is continuously being undertaken collecting satisfaction and outcome data which inform further improvement of the program.

References

Agaku, I. T., Olaiya, O., Quinn, C., Tong, V. T., Kuiper, N. M., Conrey, E. J., … Dee, D. (2015). A Mixed-Methods Assessment of a Brief Smoking Cessation Intervention Implemented in Ohio Public Health Clinics, 2013. *Maternal and Child Health Journal, 19*(12), 2654–2662.

Alshaarawy, O., & Anthony, J. C. (2015). Month-wise estimates of tobacco smoking during pregnancy for the United States, 2002–2009. *Maternal and Child Health Journal, 19*(5), 1010–1015.

Barnes, J., Dong, C. Y., McRobbie, H., Walker, N., Mehta, M., & Stead, L. F. (2010) Hypnotherapy for smoking cessation. *Cochrane Database of Systematic Reviews*: Reviews 2010(10). John Wiley & Sons, Ltd: Chichester, UK, 2010.

Borland, R., Partos, T. R., Yong, H. H., Cummings, K. M., & Hyland, A. (2012). How much unsuccessful quitting activity is going on among adult smokers? Data from the International Tobacco Control Four Country cohort survey. *Addiction, 107*(3), 673–682.

Bowen, S., & Marlatt, A. (2009). Surfing the urge: Brief mindfulness-based intervention for college student smokers. *Psychology of Addictive Behaviors, 23*(4), 666.

Brewer, J. A., Mallik, S., Babuscio, T. A., Nich, C., Johnson, H. E., Deleone, C. M., … Carroll, K. M. (2011). Mindfulness training for smoking cessation: Results from a randomized controlled trial. *Drug and Alcohol Dependence, 119*(1), 72–80.

Bricker, J. B., Copeland, W., Mull, K. E., Zeng, E. Y., Watson, N. L., Akioka, K. J., & Heffner, J. L. (2017). Single-arm trial of the second version of an acceptance & commitment therapy smartphone application for smoking cessation. *Drug and Alcohol Dependence, 170*, 37–42.

Bricker, J. B., Leroux, B. G., Andersen, M. R., Rajan, K. B., & Peterson, A. V. (2005). Parental smoking cessation and children's smoking: Mediation by antismoking actions. *Nicotine & Tobacco Research, 7*(4), 501–509.

Bricker, J. B., Otten, R., Liu, J. L., & Peterson, A. V., Jr. (2009). Parents who quit smoking and their adult children's smoking cessation: A 20-year follow-up study. *Addiction, 104*(6), 1036–1042.

Bricker, J. B., Mull, K. E., Kientz, J. A., Vilardaga, R., Mercer, L. D., Akioka, K. J., & Heffner, J. L. (2014). Randomized, controlled pilot trial of a smartphone app for smoking cessation using acceptance and commitment therapy. Drug & Alcohol Dependence, 143, 87–94.

Brown, D. W. (2010). Smoking prevalence among US veterans. *Journal of General Internal Medicine, 25*(2), 147–149.

Brown, R. A., Lejuez, C. W., Kahler, C. W., & Strong, D. R. (2002). Distress tolerance and duration of past smoking cessation attempts. *Journal of Abnormal Psychology, 111*(1), 180.

Brown, R. A., Palm, K. M., Strong, D. R., Lejuez, C. W., Kahler, C. W., Zvolensky, M. J., … Gifford, E. V. (2008). Distress tolerance treatment for early-lapse smokers rationale, program description, and preliminary findings. *Behavior Modification, 32*(3), 302–332.

Cahill, K., Stevens, S., Perera, R., & Lancaster, T. (2013). Pharmacological interventions for smoking cessation: An overview and network meta-analysis. *Cochrane Database of Systematic Reviews, 5*, 1–44.

Carey, M. P., Kalra, D. L., Carey, K. B., Halperin, S., & Richards, C. S. (1993). Stress and unaided smoking cessation: A prospective investigation. *Journal of Consulting and Clinical Psychology, 61*(5), 831.

Carter, B. D., Abnet, C. C., Feskanich, D., Freedman, N. D., Hartge, P., Lewis, C. E., … Jacobs, E. J. (2015). Smoking and mortality—Beyond established causes. *New England Journal of Medicine, 372*(7), 631–640.

Casetta, B., Videla, A. J., Bardach, A., Morello, P., Soto, N., Lee, K., … Ciapponi, A. (2016). Association between cigarette smoking prevalence and income level: A systematic review and meta-analysis. *Nicotine & Tobacco Research, 19*(12), 1401–1407.

Catchpole, R. E., McLeod, S. L., Brownlie, E. B., Allison, C. J., & Grewal, A. (2016). Cigarette smoking in youths with mental health and substance use problems: Prevalence, patterns, and potential for intervention. *Journal of Child & Adolescent Substance Abuse, 26*, 41–55.

Centers for Disease Control and Prevention (CDC). (2008). Annual smoking-attributable mortality, years of potential life lost, and economic costs--United States, 2000–2004. *MMWR. Morbidity and Mortality Weekly Report, 57*(45), 1226–1228.

Chaiton, M., Diemert, L., Cohen, J. E., Bondy, S. J., Selby, P., Philipneri, A., & Schwartz, R. (2016). Estimating the number of quit attempts it takes to quit smoking successfully in a longitudinal cohort of smokers. *BMJ Open, 6*(6), e011045.

Chen, D., & Wu, L. T. (2015). Smoking cessation interventions for adults aged 50 or older: A systematic review and meta-analysis. *Drug and Alcohol Dependence, 154*, 14–24.

Cnattingius, S. (2004). The epidemiology of smoking during pregnancy: Smoking prevalence, maternal characteristics, and pregnancy outcomes. *Nicotine & Tobacco Research, 6*(Suppl 2), S125–S140.

Cohen, S., & Lichtenstein, E. (1990). Perceived stress, quitting smoking, and smoking relapse. *Health Psychology, 9*(4), 466–478.

Croston, M. (2010). Motivational interviewing: An overview. *HIV Nursing, 10*(3), 15–18.

Dwyer-Lindgren, L., Mokdad, A. H., Srebotnjak, T., Flaxman, A. D., Hansen, G. M., & Murray, C. J. (2014). Cigarette smoking prevalence in US counties: 1996-2012. *Population Health Metrics, 12*(1), 1.

Ekpu, V. U., & Brown, A. K. (2015). The economic impact of smoking and of reducing smoking prevalence: Review of evidence. *Tobacco Use Insights, 8*, 1.

Eliasson, B. (2003). Cigarette smoking and diabetes. *Progress in Cardiovascular Diseases, 45*(5), 405–413.

Elwafi, H. M., Witkiewitz, K., Mallik, S., Thornhill, T. A., IV, & Brewer, J. A. (2013). Mindfulness training for smoking cessation: Moderation of the relationship between craving and cigarette use. *Drug and Alcohol Dependence, 130*(1), 222–229.

Fiore, M. C., Jaen, C. R., Baker, T., Bailey, W. C., Benowitz, N. L., Curry, S. E. E. A., … Henderson, P. N. (2008). *Treating tobacco use and dependence: 2008 update*. Rockville, MD: US Department of Health and Human Services.

Garey, L., Farris, S. G., Schmidt, N. B., & Zvolensky, M. J. (2016). The role of smoking-specific experiential avoidance in the relation between perceived stress and tobacco dependence, perceived barriers to cessation, and problems during quit attempts among treatment-seeking smokers. *Journal of Contextual Behavioral Science, 5*(1), 58–63.

Gifford, E. V., Kohlenberg, B. S., Hayes, S. C., Antonuccio, D. O., Piasecki, M. M., Rasmussen-Hall, M. L., & Palm, K. M. (2004). Acceptance-based treatment for smoking cessation. *Behavior Therapy, 35*(4), 689–705.

Gierisch, J. M., Bastian, L. A., Calhoun, P. S., McDuffie, J. R., & Williams, J. W. (2012). Smoking cessation interventions for patients with depression: A systematic review and meta-analysis. *Journal of General Internal Medicine, 27*(3), 351–360.

Goldstein, M. G., Whitlock, E. P., DePue, J., & Planning Committee of the Addressing Multiple Behavioral Risk Factors in Primary Care Project. (2004). Multiple behavioral risk factor interventions in primary care: Summary of research evidence. *American Journal of Preventive Medicine, 27*(2), 61–79.

Hall, S. M., Humfleet, G. L., Reus, V. I., Muñoz, R. F., & Cullen, J. (2004). Extended nortriptyline and psychological treatment for cigarette smoking. *American Journal of Psychiatry, 161*(11), 2100–2107.

Hall, S. M., Humfleet, G. L., Reus, V. I., Muñoz, R. F., Hartz, D. T., & Maude-Griffin, R. (2002). Psychological intervention and antidepressant treatment in smoking cessation. *Archives of General Psychiatry, 59*(10), 930–936.

Hall, S. M., Humfleet, G. L., Muñoz, R. F., Reus, V. I., Robbins, J. A., & Prochaska, J. J. (2009). Extended treatment of older cigarette smokers. *Addiction, 104*(6), 1043–1052.

Harrison, R., Preston, P., Bucur, C., & Fletcher, S. V. (2012). P205 smoking prevalence and smoking cessation amongst acute medical admissions. *Thorax, 67*(Suppl 2), A153–A154.

Hartmann-Boyce, J., Stead, L. F., Cahill, K., & Lancaster, T. (2014). Efficacy of interventions to combat tobacco addiction: Cochrane update of 2013 reviews. *Addiction, 109*(9), 1414–1425.

Haskins, B. L., Lesperance, D., Gibbons, P., & Boudreaux, E. D. (2017). A systematic review of smartphone applications for smoking cessation. *Translational Behavioral Medicine, 7*(2), 292–299.

Hayes, S. C., Strosahl, K. D., & Wilson, K. G. (1999). *Acceptance and commitment therapy: An experiential approach to behavior change*. New York: Guilford Press.

Heckman, C. J., Egleston, B. L., & Hofmann, M. T. (2010). Efficacy of motivational interviewing for smoking cessation: A systematic review and meta-analysis. *Tobacco Control, 19*(5), 410–416.

Heffner, J. L., Vilardaga, R., Mercer, L. D., Kientz, J. A., & Bricker, J. B. (2015). Feature-level analysis of a novel smartphone application for smoking cessation. *The American Journal of Drug and Alcohol Abuse, 41*(1), 68–73.

Hendricks, P. S., Delucchi, K. L., & Hall, S. M. (2010). Mechanisms of change in extended cognitive behavioral treatment for tobacco dependence. *Drug and Alcohol Dependence, 109*(1), 114–119.

Heppner, W. L., Spears, C. A., Correa-Fernández, V., Castro, Y., Li, Y., Guo, B., … Cinciripini, P. M. (2016). Dispositional mindfulness predicts enhanced smoking cessation and smoking lapse recovery. *Annals of Behavioral Medicine, 50*(3), 337–347.

Hettema, J. E., & Hendricks, P. S. (2010). Motivational interviewing for smoking cessation: A meta-analytic review. *Journal of Consulting and Clinical Psychology, 78*(6), 868–884.

Hoeppner, B. B., Hoeppner, S. S., Seaboyer, L., Schick, M. R., Wu, G. W., Bergman, B. G., & Kelly, J. F. (2015). How smart are smartphone apps for smoking cessation? A content analysis. *Nicotine & Tobacco Research, 118*(5), 1025–1031.

Hofmann, S. G., Asnaani, A., Vonk, I. J., Sawyer, A. T., & Fang, A. (2012). The efficacy of cognitive behavioral therapy: A review of meta-analyses. *Cognitive Therapy and Research, 36*(5), 427–440.

Jamal, A. (2016). Current cigarette smoking among adults—United States, 2005–2015. *MMWR. Morbidity and Mortality Weekly Report, 65*, 1205–1211.

Jha, P., Ramasundarahettige, C., Landsman, V., Rostron, B., Thun, M., Anderson, R. N., … Peto, R. (2013). 21st-century hazards of smoking and benefits of cessation in the United States. *New England Journal of Medicine, 368*(4), 341–350.

Kassel, J. D., Stroud, L. R., & Paronis, C. A. (2003). Smoking, stress, and negative affect: Correlation, causation, and context across stages of smoking. *Psychological Bulletin, 129*(2), 270.

King, B. A., Dube, S. R., Babb, S. D., & McAfee, T. A. (2013). Patient-reported recall of smoking cessation interventions from a health professional. *Preventive Medicine, 57*(5), 715–717.

Land, T. G., Rigotti, N. A., Levy, D. E., Schilling, T., Warner, D., & Li, W. (2012). The effect of systematic clinical interventions with cigarette smokers on quit status and the rates of smoking-related primary care office visits. *PLoS One, 7*(7), e41649.

Laude, J. R., Bailey, S. R., Crew, E., Varady, A., Lembke, A., McFall, D., … David, S. P. (2017). Extended treatment for cigarette smoking cessation: A randomized control trial. *Addiction, 112*, 1451–1459.

Lawson, P. J., Flocke, S. A., & Casucci, B. (2009). Development of an instrument to document the 5A's for smoking cessation. *American Journal of Preventive Medicine, 37*(3), 248–254.

Lee, E. B., An, W., Levin, M. E., & Twohig, M. P. (2015). An initial meta-analysis of Acceptance and Commitment Therapy for treating substance use disorders. *Drug and Alcohol Dependence, 155*, 1–7.

Leyro, T. M., Crew, E. E., Bryson, S. W., Lembke, A., Bailey, S. R., Prochaska, J. J., … Hall, S. M. (2016). Retrospective analysis of changing characteristics of treatment-seeking smokers: Implications for further reducing smoking prevalence. *BMJ Open, 6*(6), e010960.

Lichtenstein, E., Zhu, S. H., & Tedeschi, G. J. (2010). Smoking cessation quitlines: An underrecognized intervention success story. *American Psychologist, 65*(4), 252–261.

Lindson-Hawley, N., Thompson, T. P., & Begh, R. (2015). Motivational interviewing for smoking cessation. *Cochrane Database of Systematic Reviews, 3*, 1–61.

Miller, W. R. (2012). MI and psychotherapy. *MITRIP, 1*, 2–6.

Miller, W. R., & Rollnick, S. (2012). *Motivational interviewing: Preparing people for change* (3rd ed.). New York, NY: Guilford Press.

Nagelhout, G. E., de Korte-de Boer, D., Kunst, A. E., van der Meer, R. M., de Vries, H., van Gelder, B. M., & Willemsen, M. C. (2012). Trends in socioeconomic inequalities in smoking prevalence, consumption, initiation, and cessation between 2001 and 2008 in the Netherlands: Findings from a national population survey. *BMC Public Health, 12*(303), 1–9.

O'Donohue, W., & Maragakis, A. (Eds.). (2016). *Quality improvement in behavioral health*. New York: Springer.

Olaiya, O., Sharma, A. J., Tong, V. T., Dee, D., Quinn, C., Agaku, I. T., … Satten, G. A. (2015). Impact of the 5As brief counseling on smoking cessation among pregnant clients of Special Supplemental Nutrition Program for Women, Infants, and Children (WIC) clinics in Ohio. *Preventive Medicine, 81*, 438–443.

Papadakis, S., McDonald, P., Mullen, K. A., Reid, R., Skulsky, K., & Pipe, A. (2010). Strategies to increase the delivery of smoking cessation treatments in primary care settings: A systematic review and meta-analysis. *Preventive Medicine, 51*(3), 199–213.

Park, E. R., Gareen, I. F., Japuntich, S., Lennes, I., Hyland, K., DeMello, S., … Rigotti, N. A. (2015). Primary care provider-delivered smoking cessation interventions and smoking cessation among participants in the National Lung Screening Trial. *JAMA Internal Medicine, 175*(9), 1509–1516.

Payne, T. J., Gaughf, N. W., Sutton, M. J., Sheffer, C. E., Elci, O. U., Cropsey, K. L., … Crews, K. M. (2014). The impact of brief tobacco treatment training on practice behaviours, self-efficacy and attitudes among healthcare providers. *International Journal of Clinical Practice, 68*(7), 882–889.

Rollnick, S., Butler, C. C., Kinnersley, P., Gregory, J., & Mash, B. (2010). Competent novice: Motivational interviewing. *BMJ, 340*(7758), 1242–1245.

Rostron, B. L., Chang, C. M., & Pechacek, T. F. (2014). Estimation of cigarette smoking–Attributable morbidity in the United States. *JAMA Internal Medicine, 174*(12), 1922–1928.

Samet, J. M. (2013). Smoking cessation: Benefits versus risks of using pharmacotherapy to quit. *Circulation, 129*, 8–10.

Schuck, K., Otten, R., Kleinjan, M., Bricker, J. B., & Engels, R. C. (2014). Self-efficacy and acceptance of cravings to smoke underlie the effectiveness of quitline counseling for smoking cessation. *Drug and Alcohol Dependence, 142*, 269–276.

Shipton, D., Tappin, D. M., Vadiveloo, T., Crossley, J. A., Aitken, D. A., & Chalmers, J. (2009). Reliability of self reported smoking status by pregnant women for estimating smoking prevalence: A retrospective, cross sectional study. *BMJ, 339*, b4347.

Smith, A. (2015). U.S. smartphone use in 2015. Pew Research Center, Retrieved from http://www.pewinternet.org/2015/04/01/us-smartphone-use-in-2015/

Stead, L. F., Perera, R., & Lancaster, T. (2007). A systematic review of interventions for smokers who contact quitlines. *Tobacco Control, 16*(Suppl 1), i3–i8.

Steinberg, M. L., Williams, J. M., & Li, Y. (2015). Poor mental health and reduced decline in smoking prevalence. *American Journal of Preventive Medicine, 49*(3), 362–369.

Suls, J. M., Luger, T. M., Curry, S. J., Mermelstein, R. J., Sporer, A. K., & An, L. C. (2012). Efficacy of smoking-cessation interventions for young adults: A meta-analysis. *American Journal of Preventive Medicine, 42*(6), 655–662.

Thomas, K. H., Martin, R. M., Knipe, D. W., Higgins, J. P., & Gunnell, D. (2015). Risk of neuropsychiatric adverse events associated with varenicline: Systematic review and meta-analysis. *BMJ, 350*, h1109.

Thrul, J., Lipperman-Kreda, S., Grube, J. W., & Friend, K. B. (2014). Community-level adult daily smoking prevalence moderates the association between adolescents' cigarette smoking and perceived smoking by friends. *Journal of Youth and Adolescence, 43*(9), 1527–1535.

Thun, M. J., Carter, B. D., Feskanich, D., Freedman, N. D., Prentice, R., Lopez, A. D., ... & Gapstur, S. M. (2013). 50-year trends in smoking-related mortality in the United States. *New England Journal of Medicine, 368*(4), 351–364.

Tonstad, S. (2009). Cigarette smoking, smoking cessation, and diabetes. *Diabetes Research and Clinical Practice, 85*(1), 4–13.

Tran, B., Falster, M. O., Douglas, K., Blyth, F., & Jorm, L. R. (2015). Smoking and potentially preventable hospitalisation: The benefit of smoking cessation in older ages. *Drug and Alcohol Dependence, 150*, 85–91.

US Department of Health and Human Services. (2004). The health consequences of smoking: a report of the Surgeon General. Atlanta, GA: U.S. Department of Health and Human Services, Centers for Disease Control and Prevention, National Center for Chronic Disease Prevention and Health Promotion, Office on Smoking and Health.

U.S. Department of Health and Human Services (2014). The Health Consequences of Smoking—50 Years of Progress: A Report of the Surgeon General. Atlanta, GA: U.S. Department of Health and Human Services, Centers for Disease Control and Prevention, National Center for Chronic Disease Prevention and Health Promotion, Office on Smoking and Health.

Vidrine, J. I., Spears, C. A., Heppner, W. L., Reitzel, L. R., Marcus, M. T., Cinciripini, P. M., … Tindle, H. A. (2016). Efficacy of Mindfulness-Based Addiction Treatment (MBAT) for smoking cessation and lapse recovery: A randomized clinical trial. *Journal of Consulting and Clinical Psychology, 84*(9), 824–838.

Vozoris, N. T., & Stanbrook, M. B. (2011). Smoking prevalence, behaviours, and cessation among individuals with COPD or asthma. *Respiratory Medicine, 105*(3), 477–484.

Webb, M. S., de Ybarra, D. R., Baker, E. A., Reis, I. M., & Carey, M. P. (2010). Cognitive–behavioral therapy to promote smoking cessation among African American smokers: A randomized clinical trial. *Journal of Consulting and Clinical Psychology, 78*(1), 24.

Whitlock, E. P., Orleans, C. T., Pender, N., & Allan, J. (2002). Evaluating primary care behavioral counseling interventions: An evidence-based approach. *American Journal of Preventive Medicine, 22*(4), 267–284.

Whittaker, R., McRobbie, H., Bullen, C., Rodgers, A., & Gu, Y. (2016). Mobile phone-based interventions for smoking cessation (review). *Cochrane Database of Systematic Reviews, 4*, 1–46.

Xu, X., Bishop, E. E., Kennedy, S. M., Simpson, S. A., & Pechacek, T. F. (2015). Annual healthcare spending attributable to cigarette smoking: An update. *American Journal of Preventive Medicine, 48*(3), 326–333.

Zelman, D. C., Brandon, T. H., Jorenby, D. E., & Baker, T. B. (1992). Measures of affect and nicotine dependence predict differential response to smoking cessation treatments. *Journal of Consulting and Clinical Psychology, 60*, 943–952.

Ziedonis, D. M., Williams, J. M., & Smelson, D. A. (2003). Serious mental illness and tobacco addiction: A model program to address this common but neglected issue. *American Journal of the Medical Sciences, 326*, 223–230.

Chapter 13
Improving Sleep Quality Through Integrated Care

Jenna G. Renqvist and Adam D. Bramoweth

Introduction

There is substantial evidence that disordered sleep negatively impacts both physical and psychological health. The evidence for the negative effects of the two most prevalent sleep disorders, insomnia and obstructive sleep apnea (OSA), on overall health is particularly strong (Centers for Disease Control and Prevention, 2014; Edinger, Grubber, Ulmer, Zervakis, & Olsen, 2016). Insomnia is defined as dissatisfaction with sleep quantity or quality with severity of sleep onset latency (time awake before sleep onset), time awake after sleep onset, or early morning awakenings of at least 30 min, at a frequency of three or more nights per week, for a duration of three months or more that is not directly attributable to substance use or another psychiatric disorder (American Psychiatric Association, 2013). OSA is a condition during which five or more obstructive apneas or hypopneas, an occurrence during which the airway is either partially or fully closed, occur per hour of sleep, with the presence of nocturnal breathing disturbances (i.e., snoring, snorting/gasping, or breathing pauses) or daytime sleepiness, fatigue, or unrefreshing sleep (American Psychiatric Association, 2013).

Recent estimates suggest that up to 30% of adults suffer from insomnia (Budhiraja, Roth, Hudgel, Budhiraja, & Drake, 2011; Roth et al., 2011) and 17–22% of adults suffer from OSA (Franklin & Lindberg, 2015). Not only are these disorders prevalent but they also place individuals at risk for a wide variety of serious chronic health conditions, such as heart attack, stroke, and type 2 diabetes, as well as increased

J. G. Renqvist (✉)
Behavioral Health Department, VA Pittsburgh Healthcare System, Pittsburgh, PA, USA
e-mail: Jenna.Renqvist@va.gov

A. D. Bramoweth
Behavioral Health Department, VA Pittsburgh Healthcare System, Pittsburgh, PA, USA

Center for Health Equity Research and Promotion, Mental Illness Research, Education and Clinical Center, VA Pittsburgh Healthcare System, Pittsburgh, PA, USA
e-mail: Adam.Bramoweth@va.gov

M. P. Duckworth, W. T. O'Donohue (eds.), *Behavioral Medicine and Integrated Care*,
https://doi.org/10.1007/978-3-319-93003-9_13

risk of death compared to those without these disorders (Cappuccio, D'Elia, Strazzullo, & Miller, 2010b; Marshall, Wong, Cullen, Knuiman, & Grunstein, 2014; Taylor et al., 2007). Given the widespread impact untreated insomnia and OSA can have on overall health, it is not surprising that these disorders are associated with significant direct and indirect costs at both the individual and the societal level (AlGhanim, Comondore, Fleetham, Marra, & Ayas, 2008; Ayas et al., 2006; McCrae, Bramoweth, Williams, Roth, & Mosti, 2014; Ozminkowski, Wang, & Walsh, 2007).

The primary care setting likely provides the best opportunity to screen for common sleep disorders like insomnia and OSA, as this is often where sleep problems are first reported (Israel & Lieberman, 2004). In fact, OSA is most frequently diagnosed by primary care providers (PCPs) (Namen et al., 2002), and patients with insomnia typically first seek help in primary care (Aikens & Rouse, 2005). Estimates suggest that up to 50% of patients in primary care settings may be affected by insomnia (Arroll et al., 2012), and up to 10% of primary care patients are likely to meet the full criteria for an insomnia disorder (Arroll et al., 2012; Goodie & Hunter, 2014). Despite the frequency at which primary care patients experience disordered sleep, screening, assessment, and treatment/management of sleep disorders, like chronic insomnia and OSA, in the primary care setting, are often limited (Edinger et al., 2016; Lugtenberg, Zegers-van Schaick, Westert, & Burgers, 2009; Sake, Wong, Bartlett, & Saini, 2017). Infrequent assessment of sleep disorders in primary care results in as few as 1.2% of primary care patients being diagnosed with insomnia (Goodie & Hunter, 2014). These findings suggest that a substantial number of patients are not only at risk of their sleep disorders going undetected and untreated but are also at increased risk for developing chronic health problems related to their untreated sleep problems.

Behavioral medicine providers are well equipped to provide medical professionals and the general public with information about sleep disorders and associated health outcomes, assess for a variety of sleep complaints, facilitate inter-professional consultation and collaboration, and provide effective treatment for insomnia (Edinger et al., 2016; McDaniel et al., 2014). There is compelling evidence that providing behavioral medicine interventions within primary care instead of a specialty mental health clinic increases engagement in insomnia treatment (Bartels et al., 2004; Goodie & Hunter, 2014). Given insomnia and OSA are most often reported in primary care and given that patients are more likely to engage in behavioral medicine interventions offered in a primary care setting, offering a sleep-focused behavioral medicine evaluation for common sleep disorders in primary care clinics via an integrated behavioral medicine provider offers the best opportunity to engage patients in treatment.

The Negative Effects of Insomnia and Obstructive Sleep Apnea on Health

The definition of abnormal sleep duration varies widely; however, the National Sleep Foundation and the American Academy of Sleep Medicine/Sleep Research Society define normative sleep to be between 7 and 9 h per night (Hirshkowitz et al., 2015;

Watson et al., 2015). Definitions of short sleep in the research literature range from less than 7 h per night to less than 4 h per night, and long sleep definitions range from greater than 8 h per night to greater than 12 h per night (Cappuccio, Cooper, D'Elia, Strazzullo, & Miller, 2011; Cappuccio et al., 2010b). Abnormal sleep, which could be a consequence of insomnia, OSA, or other sleep, psychiatric, or medical disorders, has a variety of deleterious health effects. Both long and short sleep increase the risk for self-rated poor health, chronic disease, and mortality (Cappuccio et al., 2011, 2010b). While recent evidence suggests that long sleep (typically 9+ hours/night) may be more detrimental to health than short sleep (Cai et al., 2015), there is also a notable amount of data that suggests short sleep increases engagement in a variety of negative health behaviors (e.g., increased intake of unhealthy foods, physical inactivity, substance use) and increases risk for many negative health outcomes, such as obesity, high cholesterol, type 2 diabetes, hypertension, heart attacks, and death (Cappuccio et al., 2011; Gangwisch et al., 2010; Grandner, Patel, Gehrman, Perlis, & Pack, 2010; Liu et al., 2013; McKnight-Eily et al., 2011; Nebes, Buysse, Halligan, Houck, & Monk, 2009; Shankar, Charumathi, & Kalidindi, 2011; Vgontzas, Liao, Bixler, Chrousos, & Vela-Bueno, 2009). While an insomnia diagnosis does not require short sleep to be present, short sleep is often a consequence of an insomnia disorder (Fernandez-Mendoza, 2017; Vgontzas et al., 2009, 2010).

Chronic insomnia has strong associations with poor outcomes across a variety of medical symptoms and disorders. Specifically, individuals with insomnia symptoms have significantly lower cardiorespiratory fitness (Strand et al., 2012) and are more likely to experience breathing problems, urinary problems, gastrointestinal problems, chronic pain (Taylor et al., 2007), metabolic syndrome (Troxel et al., 2010), type 2 diabetes (Cappuccio, D'Elia, Strazzullo, & Miller, 2010a), cardiovascular symptoms, myocardial infarctions, and cardiovascular disease (Conley & Redeker, 2015; D. J. Taylor et al., 2007) than individuals without insomnia symptoms. Individuals with insomnia are significantly more likely to experience decreased cognitive and occupational functioning (Fernandez-Mendoza, 2017), depression (Baglioni et al., 2011; Fernandez-Mendoza, 2017), worse perceived health (Fernandez-Mendoza, 2017), and lower quality of life (Baglioni et al., 2011) than individuals without insomnia. There is strong evidence suggesting that patients with both short sleep and insomnia are at further increased risk for these negative health outcomes, particularly if they are men. Studies indicate that men with insomnia are up to four times more likely to experience the abovementioned health outcomes than men without insomnia symptoms, whereas the risk of negative health outcomes for women is less clear (Fernandez-Mendoza, 2017; Vgontzas et al., 2010).

Given the myriad of physiological, cognitive, and emotional symptoms associated with insomnia and OSA, it is not surprising that individuals with insomnia report a significantly lower quality of life, defined by the World Health Organization as a subjective evaluation of one's life within the context of larger culture in which they live and in relation to one's individual goals, values, expectations, and standards (The WHOQOL Group, 1995). Reviews of empirical studies evaluating quality of life using multidimensional self-report measures indicate that individuals with insomnia report significantly lower occupational, physical, emotional, and social functioning (Ishak et al., 2012; Leger et al., 2012). These studies indicate that all domains that compose an individual's quality of life are impacted by insomnia. In fact, the negative impact of insomnia on quality of life is so universal that similar findings are present in studies conducted throughout the world (Leger et al., 2012).

Untreated OSA is also associated with a number of negative health outcomes. Specifically, longitudinal studies suggest that untreated OSA is positively associated with body mass index (BMI), diabetes mellitus (Gottlieb et al., 2010), high systolic blood pressure, hypertension (Gottlieb et al., 2010; Redline et al., 2010), and low high-density lipoprotein cholesterol (HDL; i.e., "good" cholesterol; (Centers for Disease Control and Prevention, 2015; Gottlieb et al., 2010). Findings suggest that, for men, risk of heart failure and stroke increases as OSA severity increases (Gottlieb et al., 2010; Marshall et al., 2014; Redline et al., 2010). Individuals with moderate to severe OSA are also 2.5 times more likely to be diagnosed with cancer and 3.4 times more likely to die from cancer than individuals without OSA (Marshall et al., 2014). All-cause mortality risk is up to 4.2 times higher for men and women with moderate to severe OSA than those without OSA. As with risk for heart failure and stroke, mortality risk (e.g., risk of death) increases with severity of OSA. These findings suggest that identification and treatment of OSA can significantly reduce a patient's morbidity and mortality risk, especially for men (Gottlieb et al., 2010; Marshall et al., 2014; Redline et al., 2010). Studies evaluating the impact of untreated OSA on quality of life suggest that individuals with untreated OSA also report lower quality of life than both those without OSA (Yang et al., 2000) and those with OSA treated with continuous positive airway pressures (CPAP; (Batool-Anwar et al., 2016; Chai-Coetzer et al., 2013).

Untreated insomnia and OSA are both linked to a wide variety of negative health outcomes and decreased quality of life, suggesting that screening for sleep disorders and providing insomnia treatment in the primary care setting are important to maximize patient well-being and minimize risk for chronic disease. Behavioral medicine providers are particularly well equipped to perform both of these tasks. Greater integration of behavioral medicine providers and primary care significantly increases access to assessment of sleep disorders and non-pharmacological, evidence-based treatment of chronic insomnia that would otherwise only be accessible to patients receiving care in specialty mental health and sleep disorder clinics.

Insomnia Treatment: Recommendations and Practice

The American College of Physicians (Qaseem et al., 2016) suggests more efficient and effective delivery of adapted insomnia treatments provided by behavioral medicine providers (e.g., clinical psychologists, licensed clinical social workers) within the primary care setting is key to providing care to the largest number of patients suffering from insomnia with evidence-based treatment. Fortunately, behavioral medicine providers within primary care have a particularly effective tool with which to treat primary care patients with insomnia: cognitive behavioral therapy for insomnia (CBTI). CBTI is an evidence-based psychotherapy, typically delivered in individual sessions (20–50 min) as well as in group format (60–90 min). CBTI utilizes multiple components, including psychoeducation about sleep and insomnia, stimulus control, sleep restriction, cognitive therapy and cognitive restructuring, relaxation techniques, and sleep hygiene. Stimulus control in the context of CBTI involves strengthening the association of the bed and bedroom environment to sleep via going to bed and waking at specific times, getting out of bed when not sleeping and not returning until sleepy, and eliminating behaviors other than sleep and sexual activity in the bed. Sleep restriction involves temporarily restricting time in bed to approximate the duration of time the individual is currently sleeping and gradually expanding the total allowable time in bed until the individual reaches a satisfactory duration of quality of sleep. Cognitive therapy and cognitive restructuring involve enacting cognitive behavioral techniques to reduce worry about sleep and correcting inaccurate and maladaptive thoughts and beliefs about sleep, while relaxation techniques, such as progressive muscle relaxation and mindful breathing, are used to prepare the body for sleep. The sleep hygiene component of CBTI involves changing lifestyle factors that may be contributing to insomnia symptoms (e.g., use of caffeine or tobacco products close to bedtime, eating large meals close to bedtime, daytime napping). Individuals also typically maintain a daily sleep log that documents nightly bedtime, sleep onset latency, number of awakenings, and duration of time awake after sleep onset. This allows a clinician or, with education, the patient to calculate their time in bed, total sleep time, and sleep efficiency and to customize and titrate their prescribed sleep schedule.

CBTI has a strong evidence base (Jacobs, Pace-Schott, Stickgold, & Otto, 2004; Koffel, Koffel, & Gehrman, 2015; Mitchell, Gehrman, Perlis, & Umscheid, 2012; Morin, Culbert, & Schwartz, 1994; Morin et al., 2009; Smith et al., 2002; Taylor et al., 2014; Trauer, Qian, Doyle, Rajaratnam, & Cunnington, 2015; Wu, Appleman, Salazar, & Ong, 2015) and is effective in a variety of settings and formats (Manber et al., 2012; Trockel, Karlin, Taylor, & Manber, 2014). There is evidence that the benefits of CBTI extend beyond improving sleep quality to improvements in medical and psychological health (Baglioni et al., 2011; Blom et al., 2015; Conley & Redeker, 2015; Roane & Taylor, 2008; Troxel et al., 2010; Watanabe et al., 2011). Due to the strong evidence base, multiple health organizations and institutions recommend CBTI as the first-line treatment for insomnia, including the National Institutes of Health (National Institutes of Health, 2005), the Department of Veterans Affairs (2007), the British Association for Psychopharmacology (Wilson et al., 2010), and most recently the American College of Physicians (Qaseem et al., 2016). Treatment recommendations and guidelines disseminated by these institutions emphasize that CBTI be provided prior to pharmacologic interventions for most individuals with insomnia disorder.

A recent review of pharmacologic treatments for insomnia disorder conducted by the American College of Physicians outlines the existing evidence base for medications approved by the Federal Drug Administration (FDA) for use in the treatment of insomnia disorder (Wilt et al., 2016). The authors identified several classes of medications that are prescribed to treat insomnia disorders, including nonbenzodiazepine "Z" drugs (i.e., eszopiclone [Lunesta], zaleplon [Sonata], zolpidem [Ambien], zolpidem extended-release [Ambien CR], zolpidem sublingual [Edluar], and zolpidem sublingual [Intermezzo]), an orexin receptor antagonist (suvorexant [Belsomra]), melatonin, a melatonin receptor agonist (ramelteon [Rozerem], and a tricyclic antidepressant (doxepin [Silenor]), and benzodiazepines including estazolam (Prosom), flurazepam (Dalmane), quazepam (Doral), temazepam (Restoril), and triazolam (Halcion). Based on the reviewed evidence, the authors conclude that eszopiclone, zolpidem, and suvorexant may improve short-term global outcomes and sleep variables. However, they clarify that the absolute effect of these medications on insomnia symptoms were not sufficient to indicate remission of symptoms, and there was evidence for harms.

A subsequent comprehensive review and clinical practice guideline for the pharmacologic treatment of chronic insomnia in adults published by the American Academy of Sleep Medicine provides only weak recommendations for the use of suvorexant, eszopiclone, zaleplon, zolpidem, triazolam, temazepam, ramelteon, and doxepin for treatment of insomnia disorder (Sateia, Buysse, Krystal, Neubauer, & Heald, 2017). They clarify that while these medications may be more helpful than no treatment, CBTI has comparable efficacy and more durable treatment effects after treatment is discontinued than these medications. The authors recommend against the use of trazodone, tiagabine, diphenhydramine, melatonin, tryptophan, and valerian for treatment of insomnia disorder.

Despite the plethora of empirical evidence for CBTI as the recommended insomnia treatment over sleep medications (Manber et al., 2012; Sateia et al., 2017; Trockel et al., 2014; Wilson et al., 2010), CBTI is not consistently offered as the first-line treatment for insomnia. A recent review of VA electronic medical record data discovered that, of over 5000 veterans who received a recommendation for insomnia treatment, only 2% were referred to CBTI (Bramoweth et al., 2017). Improved integration of behavioral medicine and primary care has the potential to improve treatment of insomnia with CBTI and reduce referrals to specialty clinics. However, there are numerous barriers, at the provider, patient, and system level, which prevent adequate integration and implementation of both sleep disorder screening and CBTI within primary care.

Barriers to Integration

Provider-Level Barriers

A key provider barrier that can hinder implementation of evidence-based sleep treatments, especially insomnia, within the primary care setting is a lack of familiarity with current treatment recommendations (Edinger et al., 2016; Grol & Wensing, 2013; Lugtenberg et al., 2009; Sake et al., 2017). Research findings suggest that PCPs often do not evaluate for sleep-related problems during a typical exam (Edinger et al., 2016; Lugtenberg et al., 2009; Sake et al., 2017), in part due to lack of knowledge and training about sleep disorders and treatment (Edinger et al., 2016; Grol & Wensing, 2013; Lugtenberg et al., 2009; Sake et al., 2017) and in part due to insomnia symptoms not being a provider priority for patient care (Sake et al., 2017). Provider-reported barriers to implementing clinical guidelines for evaluation and treatment of sleep disorders include lack of awareness/familiarity with guidelines for treatment of sleep disorders, like those disseminated by the American Academy of Sleep Medicine (Schutte-Rodin, Broch, Buysse, Dorsey, & Sateia, 2008) and more recently the American College of Physicians (Qaseem et al., 2016), lack of agreement with guidelines/recommendations, and lack of outcome expectancy (Lugtenberg et al., 2009). A study which specifically assessed the management of insomnia within primary care suggested that, while 67% of primary care providers (PCPs) surveyed referred their patients with an insomnia complaint to a psychologist for "specific advice and treatment," 82% were hesitant to recommend non-pharmacological treatment, like CBTI, because they expected patients to decline more time-intensive treatments (Sake et al., 2017). Even when PCPs evaluate for sleep symptoms and determine that treatment for insomnia is needed, they often focus on identifying the underlying cause of insomnia (e.g., depression, PTSD, chronic low back pain, fibromyalgia) rather than considering insomnia as a diagnosis in need of its own treatment plan (Cheung, Bartlett, Armour, Glozier, & Saini, 2014; Davy, Middlemass, & Siriwardena, 2015). This is particularly problematic given that current diagnostic coding systems like the ICD-10 and the DSM-5 recognize insomnia as a disorder necessitating treatment independent of treatment for comorbid disorders (American Psychiatric Association, 2013; World Health Organization, 1992). These barriers often result in increased rates of prescription of sedative-hypnotic medications rather than referral to non-pharmacological treatments such as CBTI. Additionally, deprioritizing insomnia symptoms often leads to patients feeling frustrated, despite understanding that their insomnia may have multiple causes (Araujo, Jarrin, Leanza, Vallieres, & Morin, 2017; Davy et al., 2015).

Previous experiences and assumptions also influence PCPs willingness to discuss sleep problems with patients. In a recent survey, the vast majority of PCPs cited barriers to discussing sleep problems with patients, such as past experiences with prescription-seeking patients/beliefs that patients expect medications to be the only useful treatment for sleep problems (96%), patients wanting a "quick fix" (79%), patients being disinterested in changing their lifestyle, and patients being hesitant to engage in time-intensive non-pharmacological treatments (83%), as well as difficulty de-prescribing sedative-hypnotics (75%; (Sake et al., 2017). These findings are consistent with previous findings that 25–50% of PCPs perceive both patients' preferences for treatment and patients' ability (or inability) to engage in non-pharmacological treatment, like CBTI, are key barriers to implementing national standards of care for sleep disorders (Lugtenberg et al., 2009). Qualitative research indicates that providers often resort to prescribing sedative-hypnotic medications despite ambivalence about their use—perhaps to avoid confrontation with a patient or even to show sympathy (Cheung et al., 2014). Quantitative studies seem to support these perceptions as well. Secondary analyses of medical records data indicate that patients with sleep complaints are much more likely to be prescribed with sedative-hypnotic medications than to be referred to cognitive behavioral insomnia treatment (Bramoweth, 2017; Bramoweth et al., 2017). However, as providers become more aware of treatments like CBTI and these treatments become more easily accessible, the ratio of medications to CBTI will reduce.

Patient-Level Barriers

Research findings have identified the primary patient-level barrier to be poor communication and reporting of sleep-related complaints with providers. In fact, up to 52% patients with sleep disturbance are hesitant to discuss sleep problems with their PCP (Aikens & Rouse, 2005; Andrews, Coviello, Hurley, Rose, & Redeker, 2013), and as few as 5% of patients report symptoms or seek treatment for their sleep complaints from their healthcare providers (Erman, 2004). Counter to many PCPs' perceptions that patients are looking for "a quick fix" (Lugtenberg et al., 2009), patient hesitancy to discuss sleep problems was often related to fear that PCPs would prescribe "another pill," which is undesirable due to the adverse effects associated with sedative-hypnotic medications (Andrews et al., 2013). Also inconsistent with PCPs' perception that patients would be resistant to more time-intensive or non-pharmacological treatments (Lugtenberg et al., 2009; Sake et al., 2017), most patients with insomnia were interested in learning more about sleep and behavioral treatment strategies (Aikens & Rouse, 2005). This inconsistency between patient- and provider-reported barriers in discussing sleep problems and treatments is notable, as it indicates that a substantial number of patients may be interested in and benefit from non-pharmacological treatment, like CBTI, but are not provided with this opportunity simply due to inaccurate assumptions by both patient and provider and poor communication during health exams.

Systems-Level Barriers

A variety of systemic barriers can occur when implementing change, such as the integration of sleep disorder evaluations and delivery of CBTI or related treatments within primary care. These barriers can occur at numerous points in the integration process. Focus groups with PCPs indicate that systemic barriers to the implementation of clinical guidelines (e.g., American College of Physicians guidelines on management of chronic insomnia; Qaseem et al., 2016) and key recommendations for sleep disorders include lack of time, lack of resources, organizational constraints, and lack of reimbursement (Lugtenberg et al., 2009). Additional key limiting factors relate to physical infrastructure (e.g., lack of physical office space within primary care for a behavioral medicine clinician to conduct same-day evaluations for patients reporting insomnia/behavioral sleep problems during primary care appointments), poor clinic design (e.g., lack of clear local screening and/or treatment guidelines, CBTI provider offices located in a different building or within the general mental health clinic), and inadequate information technology (e.g., lack of or outdated electronic health records). Some provider-reported variables may also represent a lack of systemic support for the integration of behavioral medicine and primary care. Insufficient and inadequate opportunities for education and training on the value of assessing and treating sleep disorder may contribute to knowledge deficits, perceived ineffectiveness of treatments, and low self-efficacy to deliver sleep-related care. Similarly, provider-reported implementation barriers, such as failure to implement recommended sleep guidelines due to guidelines that are unclear, incomplete, outdated, or too complex, may represent systematic failures to provide clear, realistic, behavioral guidelines for sleep disorder screening and treatment. Limited support at the system level, whether related to financial constraints, limited physical resources, insufficient staffing, or inadequate clinic space all reduce the likelihood of successful integration of evidence-based sleep-related care with primary care.

Approaches to Integration

In recent years, a myriad of efforts to improve integration of evidence-based behavioral interventions in primary care have occurred. General approaches to improve integration include professional-oriented methods, organizational methods, and regulatory methods (Grol, Bosch, & Wensing, 2013). Provider-focused methods most frequently target improvements in education and information, as well as integration and implementation of evidence-based care. These methods have evidenced varying levels of success; no single strategy or program is effective or appropriate for all settings. Simply educating PCPs and the public about the symptoms, consequences, and treatment of sleep disorders and offering multidiscipline training opportunities can be helpful in increasing the effective and efficient integration of sleep medicine and primary care (Schmitz, 2016). Overcoming the education and information barriers about sleep can help to increase the frequency of sleep-related screening and assessment, improve accurate detection of symptoms, and facilitate treatment planning and initiation. Regular screening for sleep disorders is vital, given up to 95% of patients do not report or seek treatment for sleep complaints to their healthcare providers (Erman, 2004). Valid, reliable screening measures for sleep disorders include the Insomnia Severity Index (ISI; Bastien, Vallieres, & Morin, 2001; Morin, Belleville, Belanger, & Ivers, 2011), the Epworth Sleepiness Scale (ESS; Johns, 1991, 1992), and the STOP-BANG Questionnaire (Chung et al., 2012). The ISI is a 7-item questionnaire that assesses symptoms like difficulty falling asleep, staying asleep, and waking up too early as well as satisfaction with sleep and the impact of poor sleep on daytime function. A score $\geq$ 10 (range 0–28) is usually indicative of further assessment, and a score $\geq$ 15 indicates moderate–severe clinical symptoms. The ESS, an 8-item measure, is the most common assessment of daytime sleepiness, a key symptom of OSA and other sleep disorders. It assesses the likelihood of falling asleep in various situations, such as sitting and reading, watching TV, or while in the car stopped at a red light. A score > 10 (range 0–24) is indicative of excessive daytime sleepiness, and further evaluation is likely needed. The STOP-BANG is an 8-item questionnaire to assess risk for OSA and focuses on both self-reported or observed symptoms (i.e., snoring, daytime sleepiness, gasping or breathing pauses during sleep) and objective factors (i.e., high blood pressure, body mass index >35, age > 50, neck size >16 [female]/17 [male], gender [male]). Yes to three to four questions is considered intermediate risk of OSA, and five to eight is high risk.

Some common provider-level integration strategies include the distribution of educational materials, such as clinical practice guidelines, audiovisual materials, and printed handouts with information about current evidence and recommendations. Clinical practice guidelines, like those disseminated by the American Academy of Sleep Medicine (Schutte-Rodin et al., 2008) and the American College of Physicians (Qaseem et al., 2016), provide in-depth guidance about the treatment of insomnia utilizing cognitive behavioral interventions. However, helpful information is also available at sleep association websites like the Society of Behavioral Sleep Medicine (www.behavioralsleep.org), the American Academy of Sleep Medicine (www.aasmnet.org), and the National Sleep Foundation (sleepfoundation.org and sleep.org). Development of consensus strategies are challenging as each provider will have different learning style and learning preferences as well as access to different learning opportunities.

Conferences, lectures, and workshops that offer continuing education credits are also common approaches for making improvements and/or changes in clinical practice via provider education and training. The annual meeting of the Associated Professional Sleep Societies offers numerous opportunities to learn about advances in assessment and treatment of sleep disorders and to network with colleagues (sleepmeeting.org). Additionally, many academic societies like the Association for Behavioral and Cognitive Therapies (abct.org) and Society of Behavioral Medicine (www.sbm.org/about/special-interest-groups/sleep) now have special interest groups focused on sleep that provide opportunities to learn about evidence-based practices for insomnia and other sleep disorders. Evidence suggests that small-scale educational meetings (e.g., healthcare teams and clinics) and traditional methods, like grand rounds, are more helpful for implementing change in specific settings than large conferences or online learning (Wensing, Fluit, & Grol, 2013); localized application of educational strategies also allows for the development of implementation plans that are tailored to the individual needs of providers. For individualized and in-depth training, both basic and advanced, organizations like the Society of Behavioral Sleep Medicine (www.behavioralsleep.org) and the University of Pennsylvania (www.med.upenn.edu/bsm) offer training for community providers, and the Center for Deployment Psychology (deploymentpsych.org/training) and the Department of Veterans Affairs offer training for clinicians working with military service members and veterans.

The effectiveness of most educational methods is positive, but their effect is, at best, modest in magnitude (Wensing et al., 2013). Cochrane reviews suggest that educational interventions only result in an approximate 5% improvement in professional performance (Farmer et al., 2008; Forsetlund et al., 2009; O'Brien et al., 2007; Wensing et al., 2013). To be effective and influence change, information and education efforts about implementing innovative and evidence-based care typically need to be repeated at regular intervals and delivered in various modalities (Grol & Wensing, 2013). Ensuring the content provided is relevant to clinical practice, establishing specific learning goals (Burke & Hutchins, 2007), and increasing active participation in trainings (Beaudry, 1989) enhance motivation and learning (Burke & Hutchins, 2007). Education provided by key opinion leaders, individuals well respected by their peers and colleagues, as well as individuals with authority and prestige, can also enhance education and awareness efforts (Grol & Wensing, 2013). Overall, these findings indicate that, while improving provider knowledge and skills can be useful, education alone is rarely sufficient for successful integration.

Audit and feedback and clinical reminders are two additional methods that can improve the implementation of evidence-based care. Audit and feedback involves tracking clinical practice behaviors over a specific time period and providing clinicians with feedback about their performance (van der Weijden, Wensing, Eccles, & Grol, 2013). The existing research suggest that inclusion of data about the performance of a provider's colleagues as part of the feedback process, as well as provision of achievable benchmarks, improves the impact of feedback on behavior change (Balas et al., 1996; van der Weijden et al., 2013). Similar to some educational efforts, audit and feedback in the context of behavior change can also be enhanced if it is personalized, provided by a respected colleague, and related to patient-specific characteristics and outcomes rather than general health outcomes (Winkens et al., 1995, 1996; Winkens, Pop, Grol, Kester, & Knottnerus, 1992). Unfortunately, the optimal quantity of data for feedback has yet to be determined.

Clinical reminders are reminders to follow specific recommendations for clinical practices that are typically delivered verbally or electronically (van der Weijden et al., 2013). When using clinical reminders to improve integration, it is important to consider the costs and benefits of different reminder intervals, as the optimal timing of reminders differs based on the target behavior. For example, simultaneous reminders, provided at the moment of patient contact, can increase a desired behavior (e.g., screening for OSA and insomnia) or decrease an undesired behavior (e.g., writing a prescription for a sedative hypnotic prior to recommending CBTI). Reminders that occur between patient contacts can help to correct or improve patient care or assist with follow-up on important test results (e.g., discuss findings from an overnight sleep study). With advancements in electronic health records, clinical reminders are often easy to program and customize; however, it is important to consider the overall number and frequency of reminders, as they can become burdensome for providers. An overwhelming number or frequency of reminders may result in decreased completion rates, thereby decreasing their effectiveness as an integration tool. Considering the current knowledge and evidence, clinical reminders appear to be more feasible than audit and feedback for increasing adherence to clinical practice guidelines for insomnia (van der Weijden et al., 2013).

At the organizational and systemic level, improvement of evidence-based care can be facilitated by revision of professional roles—shifts and changes of job descriptions among health professionals and expansion of roles to include new tasks (e.g., CBTI delivered in primary care by nurses; (Grol et al., 2013). Additionally, primary care providers have indicated that brief, reliable screening instruments for sleep disorders (e.g., Insomnia Severity Index, Epworth Sleepiness Scale, STOP-BANG Questionnaire) and building a screening for sleep disorders into the check-in process would likely result in increased compliance with sleep-related guidelines (Sake et al., 2017). Formal integration of services, such as the integration of behavioral medicine and primary care, can also lead to better adoption of clinical practice guidelines (Falloon, Arroll, Elley, & Fernando 3rd, 2011). The optimal systemic approach or combination of approaches will likely vary by system.

Improving Integration Through Treatment Delivery Innovations

Numerous factors limit patient access to sleep disorder screening and CBTI, such as an insufficient availability of trained providers, distance to care and travel limitations, wait times for appointments, and method of treatment delivery (Manber, Simpson, & Bootzin, 2015). Stepped care models, in which patients are triaged and offered the least intensive treatment appropriate for their reported symptoms (O'Donohue & Draper, 2011), offer a variety of possible solutions to these barriers (Espie, 2009). Alternative treatment approaches to traditional CBTI, which is in-person, individual treatment delivered by a psychologist, can improve access to non-pharmacological insomnia treatments. Feasible alternatives include group-based treatment, briefer courses of treatment, and treatment via self-directed methods like workbooks, telephone, and the Internet. Offering a variety of treatments options can be especially valuable for improving access to insomnia treatment in an integrated care setting.

The qualifications and training necessary for a provider to deliver CBTI are frequently discussed topics in the field of behavioral sleep medicine, which is largely due to the widely recognized deficit of behavioral sleep medicine providers. Since at least the early 2000s, there have been several efforts to better understand the provider insufficiency problem and to develop solutions (Fields, Schutte-Rodin, Perlis, & Myers, 2013). Master's level providers (MLP), like nurse practitioners (NP) and physician assistants (PA), are promising CBTI providers due their ability to conduct medical assessments, make differential diagnoses and treatment plans, deliver care in both general and specialized settings, and conceptualize treatment in a biopsychosocial manner, all of which are important components of evaluating and treating insomnia. Also, insomnia treatment delivered by MLPs, specifically NPs and PAs, may appear to be more medical than mental health in nature to patients than treatment provided by psychologists or other MLPs like social workers or mental health counselors; this approach could reduce treatment-related stigma. While findings indicate that medical providers can effectively provide CBTI, provision of CBTI by non-doctoral level medical providers is not without its own challenges. For MLPs to be qualified to provide treatments, proper training in CBTI, as well as appropriate supervision, credentialing, and continuing education may be required (Manber et al., 2012); required qualifications for MLPs will likely differ across state and federal practice laws.

Group CBTI provided in a primary care setting can overcome several common barriers to the treatment of insomnia: provider availability, treatment accessibility, and mental health stigma. There is evidence that group CBTI lead by primary care nurses supervised by experienced psychologists can significantly reduce patients' insomnia symptoms (Espie et al., 2007). A recent meta-analysis of group-based CBTI suggests moderate to large effect sizes for reductions in sleep onset latency, times awake after sleep onset, and improvements in sleep efficiency, with improvements lasting 3–12 months (E. A. Koffel et al., 2015). Groups typically included less than ten individuals who attended four to eight 60–120-min sessions. Longer session and treatment duration was associated with larger treatment effects.

While group treatment can overcome many common barriers to care, key challenges associated with this modality, such as longer wait time and stigma, remain. There are often longer wait times for groups compared to individual treatment, as individuals may have to wait several weeks until the next series of sessions begins (Manber et al., 2015). This is particularly problematic because longer wait times could result in dropout before treatment even begins. Patient and provider perceptions about treatment may also interfere with the implementation of group treatment within the primary care setting. Despite evidence to the contrary, group treatment is often seen as less effective and credible than individual treatment by the patients and providers alike. Referring to group treatment as a workshop or class may reduce stigma and improve treatment acceptability and participation (Manber et al., 2015).

Brief treatments are a key part of a stepped care approach to treating insomnia (Espie, 2009). Several studies have focused on delivering CBTI in a briefer format. Evidence suggests that patients who engaged in a two-session CBTI group report feeling more rested and evidence lower insomnia severity and reduced time awake after sleep onset, as well as higher sleep efficiency and better sleep quality at 3-month follow-up compared to those attending two sleep hygiene groups (Edinger & Sampson, 2003). Brief behavioral treatment for insomnia (BBTI) was developed due to the known limitations of CBTI, namely, the lack of trained providers, and the duration, intensity, and cost of six to eight individual treatment sessions (Buysse et al., 2011; Troxel, Germain, & Buysse, 2012). The goal of BBTI was to develop a robust insomnia treatment that was relevant in a broad, general medical setting. BBTI is based on the behavioral components of CBTI—stimulus control and sleep restriction—and is intended to involve two in-person sessions and two phone follow-ups delivered by MLPs. The behavioral components of CBTI were reduced to four basic rules: (1) reduce time in bed; (2) get up at the same time every day, regardless of sleep duration,; (3) do not go to bed unless sleepy; and (4) do not stay in bed unless asleep (e.g., get out of bed if awake >30 min (Buysse et al., 2011)). These four rules are introduced in an initial in-person session lasting 45–60 min, followed by a brief ~30 min in-person follow-up 2 weeks later. Two brief, ~20 min, phone calls take place after each session and serve as opportunities to review treatment rules and adherence, as well as to adjust the prescribed sleep schedule. Evidence suggests that BBTI delivered by mental health MLPs and social workers effectively reduces insomnia symptoms (Buysse et al., 2011; Germain et al., 2014).

Alternative evidence-based methods for delivery of insomnia treatment, such as telephone-based care and self-directed care (e.g., paper and online/mobile-based care), can further help to increase access to care and fit well within a stepped care model. These interventions are often more readily accessible to patients and may be preferable for those who experience barriers related to distance to a provider or competing time demands due to work and/or child-care responsibilities. Others may simply want to try a lower intensity treatment with less contact with a provider that still offers a strong evidence base.

While treatment protocols, such as BBTI, involve phone care as a secondary or supportive aspect of care to in-person treatment delivery (Buysse et al., 2011), there is good preliminary support for CBTI delivered solely via telephone. One such study compared telephone-based CBTI, plus four information modules that were mailed to participants, to information that would typically be provided in a primary care setting (Arnedt et al., 2013). The four modules provided to patients included information on (1) behavioral strategies based on stimulus control and sleep restriction; (2) sleep hygiene focusing on education on how behaviors, substances, and environmental factors can impact sleep; (3) cognitive therapy focusing on dysfunctional beliefs about sleep that can contribute to insomnia; and (4) relapse prevention. Treatment involved 4–8 weekly 15–60-min phone calls with experienced clinical psychologists. The control group participants were mailed with informational material about CBTI, developed by the American Academy of Sleep Medicine (www.aasmnet.org/resources/pdf/products/understandinginsomnia_web.pdf) and received one 15–20-min phone call during which a clinician reviewed the provided information. Consistent with previous CBTI studies, patients in the treatment group achieved significant improvements, with large effect sizes, for sleep onset latency, time awake after sleep onset, and sleep efficiency, as well as for total sleep time and sleep quality, with continued treatment gains at 12-week follow-up. Although the information control condition resulted in significantly lower response and remission rates compared to the treatment condition, participants in the information control condition also evidenced a significant reduction in insomnia symptoms. This finding may indicate that an even less clinically intensive intervention, such as basic sleep hygiene guidelines or the four rules of BBTI, plus a brief phone call with a provider may be a useful entry-level treatment for many patients (Arnedt et al., 2013).

At the lowest level of the stepped-care pyramid exist interventions that provide the widest access to care and are easiest to disseminate—self-directed interventions. These approaches include written materials such as books and workbooks like *Quiet Your Mind and Get to Sleep* (Carney & Manber, 2009), *The Insomnia Answer* (Glovinsky & Spielman, 2006), *The Insomnia Workbook: A Comprehensive Guide to Getting the Sleep You Need* (Silberman, 2009), *No More Sleepless Nights* (Hauri

& Linde, 1996), *Say Good Night to Insomnia* (Jacobs, 2009), and *Improve Your Sleep: A Self-Guided Approach for Veterans with Insomnia* (Ulmer, Farrell-Carnahan, Hughes, Manber, & Tatum, 2016). Also, audiovisual interventions are available through interactive online and mobile platforms; two of the most well-studied are Sleep Healthy Using the Internet (SHUTi™; www.myshuti.com) and Sleepio ™ (www.sleepio.com). A meta-analysis of self-directed insomnia interventions found posttreatment improvements similar to other CBTI trials for key variables like sleep onset latency and sleep efficiency (Ho et al., 2015). Notably, some key methodological flaws in these studies, such as inconsistent use of intent-to-treat analyses and lower than usual dropout rates (e.g., some studies reported 0% drop out), may limit the generalizability of reported results (Manber et al., 2015). Evidence suggests that self-directed interventions that offered some clinician contact result in increased effectiveness. This may be due to the therapeutic elements of clinician contact, such as increased accountability, support and encouragement, added structure, ability to ask questions and voice concerns, and customization of treatment recommendations that are missing from purely self-directed approaches (Manber et al., 2015).

Perhaps the self-directed interventions with the most promise for wide dissemination are Internet- and mobile-based treatments. These interventions can serve as stand-alone treatments or as enhancements for in-person, and other, treatment modalities. Preliminary findings from the Department of Veterans Affairs shows that the use of the VA-developed mobile application, CBTI Coach, in conjunction with in-person treatment was acceptable to patients and did not compromise the effectiveness of in-person CBTI (Koffel et al., 2016). Two Internet-based interventions, SHUTi™ (Ritterband et al., 2009, 2017) and Sleepio™ (Espie et al., 2012), also offer robust treatment options, and both are supported by large randomized clinical trials, conducted in generalizable samples across several countries. Recently, a study using SHUTi showed continued treatment response at 1-year follow-up (Ritterband et al., 2017). With the ever-increasing availability of Internet access, these interventions may soon serve as the first-line treatment for many individuals. There is even preliminary evidence to suggest that Internet-based insomnia treatments can be effective when accessed through Internet connections provided in a community setting (e.g., library, community medical, or mental health center; Feuerstein et al., 2017). This could offer a cost-effective treatment option to individuals without regular Internet access.

Self-directed treatment approaches are not without their own challenges and limitations. One of the key limitations to self-directed approaches is the lack of follow-up procedures for those who experience a suboptimal treatment response. It is important that self-directed approaches to the treatment of insomnia offer information and advice about appropriate follow-up with a provider for those who do not experience a satisfactory response to treatment. If self-directed approaches are recommended by providers as a part of a stepped care approach, it is important that providers plan a timely follow-up to assess treatment response and evaluate the need for additional or alternative treatment.

Summary

As sleep disorders are most frequently reported and diagnosed in the primary care setting, the integration of behavioral medicine and primary care allows for the identification and treatment of sleep disorders to occur in a more efficient and effective manner. Untreated OSA and insomnia increase risk for chronic medical conditions and all-cause mortality and reduce quality of life; therefore, the negative impact of failing to provide treatment to individuals suffering from these disorders cannot be underestimated. Lack of provider knowledge about treatment guidelines and the efficacy of recommended treatments, de-prioritizing sleep concerns, and (potentially inaccurate) expectations about patient openness to non-pharmacological sleep treatments, particularly insomnia, serve as significant barriers to the provision of behavioral sleep treatments in the primary care setting. Patient hesitancy to discuss sleep-related concerns with their PCPs, barriers due to time, travel, finances, and competing demands, as well as limited willingness to engage in care due to stigma, serve as additional obstacles to care. Systematic barriers to integration of behavioral sleep medicine and evidence-based treatment guidelines for insomnia into the primary care setting often include infrastructure, resource, technology, and financial constraints.

Research findings suggest that a variety of different strategies may aid the integration of behavioral sleep medicine and primary care. Educating PCPs and the public about symptoms, consequences, and treatment of sleep disorder and offering appropriate and timely provider trainings related to the identification and treatment of sleep disorders are important but typically not sufficient successful integration. Some promising interventions involve educational efforts that provide recommendations that are applicable to a provider's clinical practice and can be delivered repeatedly over time. Providing feedback on specific performance metrics, the use of electronic clinical reminders, and the provision of financial incentives may also improve the implementation and integration of evidence-based care. Insomnia treatments have also been adapted to overcome numerous barriers and more easily integrate into the primary care environment, increase accessibility, and decrease provider burden; evidence supports CBTI delivered via group, telephone, and through Internet and mobile applications (either self-directed or therapist-assisted). CBTI can also be effectively delivered by MLPs in a briefer format, consisting of as few as two clinic visits.

Regardless of best efforts and improved practices at various levels, key components to successful integration of behavioral sleep medicine within primary care settings are the awareness of the innovation (i.e., assessment, diagnosis, and treatment of sleep disorder in primary care), consistent and continued systemic support for newly integrated clinical practices, interest in and involvement of providers (behavioral medicine and medical) and patients (Manber et al., 2015), and implementation of regular provider reminders and feedback. The methods described above will help to promote awareness of sleep disorders within primary care, emphasize the importance of screening for sleep disorders, and provide cognitive behavioral insomnia treatment to patients in primary care settings.

References

Aikens, J. E., & Rouse, M. E. (2005). Help-seeking for insomnia among adult patients in primary care. *The Journal of the American Board of Family Practice, 18*(4), 257–261 doi:18/4/257 [pii].

AlGhanim, N., Comondore, V. R., Fleetham, J., Marra, C. A., & Ayas, N. T. (2008). The economic impact of obstructive sleep apnea. *Lung, 186*(1), 7–12. https://doi.org/10.1007/s00408-007-9055-5

American Psychiatric Association. (2013). *Diagnostic and statistical manual of mental disorders* (5th ed.). Washington, DC: Author.

Andrews, L. K., Coviello, J., Hurley, E., Rose, L., & Redeker, N. S. (2013). "I'd eat a bucket of nails if you told me it would help me sleep:" Perceptions of insomnia and its treatment in patients with stable heart failure. *Heart & Lung: The Journal of Critical Care, 42*(5), 339–345. https://doi.org/10.1016/j.hrtlng.2013.05.003

Araujo, T., Jarrin, D. C., Leanza, Y., Vallieres, A., & Morin, C. M. (2017). Qualitative studies of insomnia: Current state of knowledge in the field. *Sleep Medicine Reviews, 31*, 58–69.

Arnedt, J. T., Cuddihy, L., Swanson, L. M., Pickett, S., Aikens, J., & Chervin, R. D. (2013). Randomized controlled trial of telephone-delivered cognitive behavioral therapy for chronic insomnia. *Sleep*. https://doi.org/10.5665/sleep.2448

Arroll, B., Fernando, A., 3rd, Falloon, K., Goodyear-Smith, F., Samaranayake, C., & Warman, G. (2012). Prevalence of causes of insomnia in primary care: A cross-sectional study. *The British Journal of General Practice: The Journal of the Royal College of General Practitioners, 62*(595), e99–e103. https://doi.org/10.3399/bjgp12X625157

Ayas, N. T., FitzGerald, J. M., Fleetham, J. A., White, D. P., Schulzer, M., Ryan, C. F., … Marra, C. A. (2006). Cost-effectiveness of continuous positive airway pressure therapy for moderate to severe obstructive sleep apnea/hypopnea. *Archives of Internal Medicine, 166*(9), 977–984 doi:166/9/977 [pii].

Baglioni, C., Battagliese, G., Feige, B., Spiegelhalder, K., Nissen, C., Voderholzer, U., … Riemann, D. (2011). Insomnia as a predictor of depression: A meta-analytic evaluation of longitudinal epidemiological studies. *Journal of Affective Disorders, 135*, 10–19. https://doi.org/10.1016/j.jad.2011.01.011

Balas, E. A., Boren, S. A., Brown, G. D., Ewigman, B. G., Mitchell, J. A., & Perkoff, G. T. (1996). Effect of physician profiling on utilization. Meta-analysis of randomized clinical trials. *Journal of General Internal Medicine, 11*(10), 584–590.

Bartels, S. J., Coakley, E. H., Zubritsky, C., Ware, J. H., Miles, K. M., Arean, P. A., … PRISM-E Investigators. (2004). Improving access to geriatric mental health services: A randomized trial comparing treatment engagement with integrated versus enhanced referral care for depression, anxiety, and at-risk alcohol use. *The American Journal of Psychiatry, 161*(8), 1455–1462. https://doi.org/10.1176/appi.ajp.161.8.1455

Bastien, C. H., Vallieres, A., & Morin, C. M. (2001). Validation of the insomnia severity index as an outcome measure for insomnia research. *Sleep Medicine, 2*, 297–307.

Batool-Anwar, S., Goodwin, J. L., Kushida, C. A., Walsh, J. A., Simon, R. D., Nichols, D. A., & Quan, S. F. (2016). Impact of continuous positive airway pressure (CPAP) on quality of life in patients with obstructive sleep apnea (OSA). *Journal of Sleep Research, 25*(6), 731–738. https://doi.org/10.1111/jsr.12430

Beaudry, J. S. (1989). The effectiveness of continuing medical education: A quantitative synthesis. *The Journal of Continuing Education in the Health Professions, 9*, 285–307.

Blom, K., Jernelöv, S., Kraepelien, M., Bergdahl, M. O., Jungmarker, K., Ankartjärn, L., … Kaldo, V. (2015). Internet treatment addressing either insomnia or depression, for patients with both diagnoses: A randomized trial. *Sleep, 38*(2), 267–277. https://doi.org/10.5665/sleep.4412

Bramoweth, A. D. (2017). A step in the right direction: Moving toward increased access to insomnia care. *Journal of Clinical Sleep Medicine: JCSM: Official Publication of the American Academy of Sleep Medicine, 13*(2), 161–162. https://doi.org/10.5664/jcsm.6432

Bramoweth, A. D., Luther, J. F., Hanusa, B. H., Walker, J. D., Atwood, C. W., & Germain, A. (2017). Clinical characterization of insomnia among veterans with PTSD: Identifying risk factors for diagnosis and treatment with sedative-hypnotics. *Defence and Peace Economics, Online* 12 July 2017. https://doi.org/10.1080/10242694.2017.1349633

Bramoweth, A. D., Renqvist, J. G., Hanusa, B. H., Walker, J. D., Germain, A., & Atwood, C. W., Jr. (2017). Identifying the demographic and mental health factors that influence insomnia treatment recommendations within a veteran population. *Behavioral Sleep Medicine*, 1–12. https://doi.org/10.1080/15402002.2017.1318752

Budhiraja, R., Roth, T., Hudgel, D. W., Budhiraja, P., & Drake, C. L. (2011). Prevalence and polysomnographic correlates of insomnia comorbid with medical disorders. *Sleep, 34*, 859–867. https://doi.org/10.5665/SLEEP.1114

Burke, L. A., & Hutchins, H. M. (2007). Training transfer: An integrative literature review. *Human Resources Development Review, 6*(3), 263–296. https://doi.org/10.1177/1534484307303035

Buysse, D. J., Germain, A., Moul, D. E., Franzen, P. L., Brar, L. K., Fletcher, M. E., … Monk, T. H. (2011). Efficacy of brief behavioral treatment for chronic insomnia in older adults. *Archives of Internal Medicine, 171*(10), 887–895.

Cai, H., Shu, X. O., Xiang, Y. B., Yang, G., Li, H., Ji, B. T., … Zheng, W. (2015). Sleep duration and mortality: A prospective study of 113 138 middle-aged and elderly Chinese men and women. *Sleep, 38*(4), 529–536. https://doi.org/10.5665/sleep.4564

Cappuccio, F. P., Cooper, D., D'Elia, L., Strazzullo, P., & Miller, M. A. (2011). Sleep duration predicts cardiovascular outcomes: A systematic review and meta-analysis of prospective studies. *European Heart Journal, 32*(12), 1484–1492. https://doi.org/10.1093/eurheartj/ehr007

Cappuccio, F. P., D'Elia, L., Strazzullo, P., & Miller, M. A. (2010a). Quantity and quality of sleep and incidence of type 2 diabetes: A systematic review and meta-analysis. *Diabetes Care, 33*(2), 414–420. https://doi.org/10.2337/dc09-1124

Cappuccio, F. P., D'Elia, L., Strazzullo, P., & Miller, M. A. (2010b). Sleep duration and all-cause mortality: A systematic review and meta-analysis of prospective studies. *Sleep, 33*(5), 585–592.

Carney, C. E., & Manber, R. (2009). *Quiet your mind and get to sleep: Solutions to insomnia for those with depression, anxiety or chronic pain*. Oakland, CA: New Harbinger Publications, Inc.

Centers for Disease Control and Prevention. (2014). Key sleep disorders. Retrieved from https://www.cdc.gov/sleep/about_sleep/key_disorders.html

Centers for Disease Control and Prevention. (2015). *LDL and HDL: "Bad" and "Good" cholesterol*. Retrieved from https://www.cdc.gov/cholesterol/ldl_hdl.htm

Chai-Coetzer, C. L., Antic, N. A., Rowland, L. S., Reed, R. L., Esterman, A., Catcheside, P. G., … McEvoy, R. D. (2013). Primary care vs specialist sleep center management of obstructive sleep apnea and daytime sleepiness and quality of life: A randomized trial. *JAMA, 309*(10), 997–1004. https://doi.org/10.1001/jama.2013.1823

Cheung, J. M., Bartlett, D. J., Armour, C. L., Glozier, N., & Saini, B. (2014). Insomnia patients' help-seeking experiences. *Behavioral Sleep Medicine, 12*(2), 106–122. https://doi.org/10.1080/15402002.2013.764529

Chung, F., Subramanyam, R., Liao, P., Sasaki, E., Shapiro, C., & Sun, Y. (2012). High STOP-bang score indicates a high probability of obstructive sleep apnoea. *British Journal of Anaesthesia, 108*(5), 768–775.

Conley, S., & Redeker, N. S. (2015). Cognitive behavioral therapy for insomnia in the context of cardiovascular conditions. *Current Sleep Medicine Reports, 1*(3), 157–165. https://doi.org/10.1007/s40675-015-0019-7

Davy, Z., Middlemass, J., & Siriwardena, A. N. (2015). Patients' and clinicians' experiences and perceptions of the primary care management of insomnia: Qualitative study. *Health Expectations: An International Journal of Public Participation in Health Care and Health Policy, 18*(5), 1371–1383. https://doi.org/10.1111/hex.12119

Department of Veterans Affairs. (2007). *Department of veterans affairs pharmacy benefits management service and medical advisory panel: Guidance for treatment of insomnia in veterans in the primary care setting*. Washington, DC: Department of Veterans Affairs.

Edinger, J. D., Grubber, J., Ulmer, C., Zervakis, J., & Olsen, M. (2016). A collaborative paradigm for improving management of sleep disorders in primary care: A randomized clinical trial. *Sleep, 39*(1), 237–247. https://doi.org/10.5665/sleep.5356

Edinger, J. D., & Sampson, W. S. (2003). A primary care friendly cognitive behavioral insomnia therapy. *Sleep, 26*(2), 177–182.

Erman, M. (2004). Clinical update – Diagnosis of insomnia in the primary care practice. Retrieved from http://www.medscape.org/viewarticle/478849

Espie, C. A. (2009). "stepped care": A health technology solution for delivering cognitive behavioral therapy as a first line insomnia treatment. *Sleep, 32*, 1549–1558.

Espie, C. A., Kyle, S. D., Williams, C., Ong, J. C., Douglas, N. J., Hames, P., & Brown, J. S. (2012). A randomized, placebo-controlled trial of online cognitive behavioral therapy for chronic insomnia disorder delivered via an automated media-rich web application. *Sleep, 35*, 769–781. https://doi.org/10.5665/sleep.1872

Espie, C. A., MacMahon, K. M., Kelly, H. L., Broomfield, N. M., Douglas, N. J., Engleman, H. M., … Wilson, P. (2007). Randomized clinical effectiveness trial of nurse-administered small-group cognitive behavior therapy for persistent insomnia in general practice. *Sleep, 30*(5), 574–584.

Falloon, K., Arroll, B., Elley, C. R., & Fernando, A., 3rd. (2011). The assessment and management of insomnia in primary care. *BMJ (Clinical Research Ed.), 342*, d2899.

Farmer, A. P., Legare, F., Turcot, L., Grimshaw, J., Harvey, E., McGowan, J. L., & Wolf, F. (2008). Printed educational materials: Effects on professional practice and health care outcomes. *The Cochrane Database of Systematic Reviews*, (3), CD004398. https://doi.org/10.1002/14651858.CD004398.pub2

Fernandez-Mendoza, J. (2017). The insomnia with short sleep duration phenotype: An update on its importance for health and prevention. *Current Opinion in Psychiatry, 30*(1), 56–63. https://doi.org/10.1097/YCO.0000000000000292

Feuerstein, S., Hodges, S. E., Keenaghan, B., Bessette, A., Forselius, E., & Morgan, P. T. (2017). Computerized cognitive behavioral therapy for insomnia in a community health setting. *Journal of Clinical Sleep Medicine, 13*(2), 267–274. https://doi.org/10.5664/jcsm.6460

Fields, B. G., Schutte-Rodin, S., Perlis, M. L., & Myers, M. (2013). Master's-level practitioners as cognitive behavioral therapy for insomnia providers: An underutilized resource. *Journal of Clinical Sleep Medicine: JCSM: Official Publication of the American Academy of Sleep Medicine, 9*(10), 1093–1096. https://doi.org/10.5664/jcsm.3096

Forsetlund, L., Bjorndal, A., Rashidian, A., Jamtvedt, G., O'Brien, M. A., Wolf, F., … Oxman, A. D. (2009). Continuing education meetings and workshops: Effects on professional practice and health care outcomes. *The Cochrane Database of Systematic Reviews*, (2), *CD003030*. https://doi.org/10.1002/14651858.CD003030.pub2

Franklin, K. A., & Lindberg, E. (2015). Obstructive sleep apnea is a common disorder in the population-a review on the epidemiology of sleep apnea. *Journal of Thoracic Disease, 7*(8), 1311–1322. https://doi.org/10.3978/j.issn.2072-1439.2015.06.11

Gangwisch, J. E., Malaspina, D., Babiss, L. A., Opler, M. G., Posner, K., Shen, S., … Ginsberg, H. N. (2010). Short sleep duration as a risk factor for hypercholesterolemia: Analyses of the national longitudinal study of adolescent health. *Sleep, 33*(7), 956–961.

Germain, A., Richardson, R., Stocker, R., Mammen, O., Hall, M., Bramoweth, A. D., … Buysse, D. J. (2014). Treatment for insomnia in combat-exposed OEF/OIF/OND military veterans: Preliminary randomized controlled trial. *Behaviour Research and Therapy, 61*, 78–88.

Glovinsky, P., & Spielman, A. (2006). *The insomnia answer: A personalized program for identifying and overcoming the three types of insomnia*. New York, NY: TarcherPerigee.

Goodie, J. L., & Hunter, C. L. (2014). Practical guidance for targeting insomnia in primary care settings. *Cognitive and Behavioral Practice, 21*(3), 261.

Gottlieb, D. J., Yenokyan, G., Newman, A. B., O'Connor, G. T., Punjabi, N. M., Quan, S. F., … Shahar, E. (2010). Prospective study of obstructive sleep apnea and incident coronary heart disease and heart failure: The sleep heart health study. *Circulation, 122*(4), 352–360. https://doi.org/10.1161/CIRCULATIONAHA.109.901801

Grandner, M. A., Patel, N. P., Gehrman, P. R., Perlis, M. L., & Pack, A. I. (2010). Problems associated with short sleep: Bridging the gap between laboratory and epidemiological studies. *Sleep Medicine Reviews, 14*(4), 239–247. https://doi.org/10.1016/j.smrv.2009.08.001

Grol, R., Bosch, M., & Wensing, M. (2013). Development and selection of strategies for improving patient care. In R. Grol, M. Wensing, M. Eccles, & D. Davis (Eds.), *Improving patient care* (2nd ed., pp. 165–184). Chichester, UK: Wiley. https://doi.org/10.1002/9781118525975.ch10

Grol, R., & Wensing, M. (2013). Dissemination of innovations. In R. Grol, M. Wensing, M. Eccles, & D. Davis (Eds.), *Improving patient care: The implementation of change in health care* (2nd ed., pp. 185–196). Chichester, UK: Wiley.

Hauri, P., & Linde, S. (1996). *No more sleepless nights* (Revised ed.). New York, NY: Wiley.

Hirshkowitz, M., Whiton, K., Albert, S. M., Alessi, C., Bruni, O., DonCarlos, L., … Adams Hillard, P. J. (2015). National sleep foundation's sleep time duration recommendations: Methodology and results summary. *Sleep Health: Journal of the National Sleep Foundation, 1*(1), 40–43 Retrieved from https://doi.org/10.1016/j.sleh.2014.12.010

Ho, F. Y., Chung, K. F., Yeung, W. F., Ng, T. H., Kwan, K. S., Yung, K. P., & Cheng, S. K. (2015). Self-help cognitive-behavioral therapy for insomnia: A meta-analysis of randomized controlled trials. *Sleep Medicine Reviews, 19*, 17–28. https://doi.org/10.1016/j.smrv.2014.06.010

Ishak, W. W., Bagot, K., Thomas, S., Magakian, N., Bedwani, D., Larson, D., … Zaky, C. (2012). Quality of life in patients suffering from insomnia. *Innovations in Clinical Neuroscience, 9*(10), 13–26.

Israel, A. G., & Lieberman, J. A., 3rd. (2004). Tackling insomnia: Diagnostic and treatment issues in primary care. *Postgraduate Medicine, 116*(6 Suppl Insomnia), 7–13. https://doi.org/10.3810/pgm.12.2004.suppl38.257

Jacobs, G. D. (2009). *Say good night to insomnia* (Revised ed.). New York, NY: Henry Holt and Company, LLC.

Jacobs, G. D., Pace-Schott, E. F., Stickgold, R., & Otto, M. W. (2004). Cognitive behavior therapy and pharmacotherapy for insomnia: A randomized controlled trial and direct comparison. *Archives of Internal Medicine, 164*(17), 1888–1896. https://doi.org/10.1001/archinte.164.17.1888

Johns, M. (1991). A new method for measuring daytime sleepiness: The Epworth sleepiness scale. *Sleep, 14*, 540–545.

Johns, M. (1992). Reliability and factor analysis of the Epworth sleepiness scale. *Sleep, 15*, 376–381.

Koffel, E., Kuhn, E., Petsoulis, N., Erbes, C. R., Anders, S., Hoffman, J. E., … Polusny, M. A. (2016). A randomized controlled pilot study of CBT-I coach: Feasibility, acceptability, and potential impact of a mobile phone application for patients in cognitive behavioral therapy for insomnia. *Health Informatics Journal*. epub ahead of print. https://doi.org/10.1177/1460458216656472

Koffel, E. A., Koffel, J. B., & Gehrman, P. R. (2015). A meta-analysis of group cognitive behavioral therapy for insomnia. *Sleep Medicine Reviews, 19*, 6–16. https://doi.org/10.1016/j.smrv.2014.05.001

Leger, D., Morin, C. M., Uchiyama, M., Hakimi, Z., Cure, S., & Walsh, J. K. (2012). Chronic insomnia, quality-of-life, and utility scores: Comparison with good sleepers in a cross-sectional international survey. *Sleep Medicine, 13*(1), 43–51. https://doi.org/10.1016/j.sleep.2011.03.020

Liu, Y., Croft, J. B., Wheaton, A. G., Perry, G. S., Chapman, D. P., Strine, T. W., … Presley-Cantrell, L. (2013). Association between perceived insufficient sleep, frequent mental distress, obesity and chronic diseases among US adults, 2009 behavioral risk factor surveillance system. *BMC Public Health, 13*, 84. https://doi.org/10.1186/1471-2458-13-84

Lugtenberg, M., Zegers-van Schaick, J. M., Westert, G. P., & Burgers, J. S. (2009). Why don't physicians adhere to guideline recommendations in practice? An analysis of barriers among Dutch general practitioners. *Implementation Science: IS, 4*, 54. https://doi.org/10.1186/1748-5908-4-54

Manber, R., Carney, C., Edinger, J., Epstein, D., Friedman, L., Haynes, P. L., … Trockel, M. (2012). Dissemination of CBTI to the non-sleep specialist: Protocol development and training issues. *Journal of Clinical Sleep Medicine: JCSM: Official Publication of the American Academy of Sleep Medicine, 8*, 209–218. https://doi.org/10.5664/jcsm.1786

Manber, R., Simpson, N. S., & Bootzin, R. R. (2015). A step towards stepped care: Delivery of CBT-I with reduced clinician time. *Sleep Medicine Reviews, 19*, 3–5. https://doi.org/10.1016/j.smrv.2014.09.003

Marshall, N. S., Wong, K. K., Cullen, S. R., Knuiman, M. W., & Grunstein, R. R. (2014). Sleep apnea and 20-year follow-up for all-cause mortality, stroke, and cancer incidence and mortality in the Busselton health study cohort. *Journal of Clinical Sleep Medicine: JCSM: Official Publication of the American Academy of Sleep Medicine, 10*(4), 355–362. https://doi.org/10.5664/jcsm.3600

McCrae, C. S., Bramoweth, A. D., Williams, J., Roth, A., & Mosti, C. (2014). Impact of cognitive behavioral treatment for insomnia on health care utilization and costs. *Journal of Clinical Sleep Medicine, 10*(2), 127–135.

McDaniel, S. H., Grus, C. L., Cubic, B. A., Hunter, C. L., Kearney, L. K., Schuman, C. C., … Johnson, S. B. (2014). Competencies for psychology practice in primary care. *The American Psychologist, 69*(4), 409–429. https://doi.org/10.1037/a0036072

McKnight-Eily, L. R., Eaton, D. K., Lowry, R., Croft, J. B., Presley-Cantrell, L., & Perry, G. S. (2011). Relationships between hours of sleep and health-risk behaviors in US adolescent students. *Preventive Medicine, 53*(4–5), 271–273. https://doi.org/10.1016/j.ypmed.2011.06.020

Mitchell, M. D., Gehrman, P., Perlis, M., & Umscheid, C. A. (2012). Comparative effectiveness of cognitive behavioral therapy for insomnia: A systematic review. *BMC Family Practice, 13*, 40. https://doi.org/10.1186/1471-2296-13-40

Morin, C. M., Belleville, G., Belanger, L., & Ivers, H. (2011). The insomnia severity index: Psychometric indicators to detect insomnia cases and evaluate treatment response. *Sleep, 34*, 601–608.

Morin, C. M., Culbert, J. P., & Schwartz, S. M. (1994). Nonpharmacological interventions for insomnia: A meta-analysis of treatment efficacy. *The American Journal of Psychiatry, 151*(8), 1172–1180. https://doi.org/10.1176/ajp.151.8.1172

Morin, C. M., Vallieres, A., Guay, B., Ivers, H., Savard, J., Merette, C., … Baillargeon, L. (2009). Cognitive behavioral therapy, singly and combined with medication, for persistent insomnia: A randomized controlled trial. *JAMA: The Journal of the American Medical Association, 301*, 2005–2015. https://doi.org/10.1001/jama.2009.682

Namen, A. M., Dunagan, D. P., Fleischer, A., Tillett, J., Barnett, M., McCall, W. V., & Haponik, E. F. (2002). Increased physician-reported sleep apnea: The national ambulatory medical care survey. *Chest, 121*(6), 1741–1747.

National Institutes of Health. (2005). *NIH state-of-the-science conference on manifestations and management of chronic insomnia*. Bethesda, MD: National Institutes of Health. Retrieved from http://consensus.nih.gov/2005/insomniastatement.pdf

Nebes, R. D., Buysse, D. J., Halligan, E. M., Houck, P. R., & Monk, T. H. (2009). Self-reported sleep quality predicts poor cognitive performance in healthy older adults. *The Journals of Gerontology.Series B, Psychological Sciences and Social Sciences, 64*(2), 180–187. https://doi.org/10.1093/geronb/gbn037

O'Brien, M. A., Rogers, S., Jamtvedt, G., Oxman, A. D., Odgaard-Jensen, J., Kristoffersen, D. T., … Harvey, E. L. (2007). Educational outreach visits: Effects on professional practice and health care outcomes. *The Cochrane Database of Systematic Reviews*, (4). https://doi.org/10.1002/14651858.CD000409.pub2

O'Donohue, W., & Draper, C. (2011). The case for evidence-based stepped care as a part of a reformed delivery system. In W. O'Donohue & C. Draper (Eds.), *Stepped care and e-health: Practical applications to behavioral disorders* (1st ed., pp. 1–16). New York: Springer.

Ozminkowski, R. J., Wang, S., & Walsh, J. K. (2007). The direct and indirect costs of untreated insomnia in adults in the United States. *Sleep, 30*(3), 263–273.

Qaseem, A., Kansagara, D., Forciea, M. A., Cooke, M., Denberg, T. D., & Clinical Guidelines Committee of the American College of Physicians. (2016). Management of chronic insomnia disorder in adults: A clinical practice guideline from the American college of physicians. *Annals of Internal Medicine, 165*(2), 125–133. https://doi.org/10.7326/M15-2175

Redline, S., Yenokyan, G., Gottlieb, D. J., Shahar, E., O'Connor, G. T., Resnick, H. E., … Punjabi, N. M. (2010). Obstructive sleep apnea-hypopnea and incident stroke: The sleep heart health study. *American Journal of Respiratory and Critical Care Medicine, 182*(2), 269–277. https://doi.org/10.1164/rccm.200911-1746OC

Ritterband, L. M., Thorndike, F. P., Gonder-Frederick, L. A., Magee, J. C., Bailey, E. T., Saylor, D. K., & Morin, C. M. (2009). Efficacy of an internet-based behavioral intervention for adults with insomnia. *Archives of General Psychiatry, 66*(7), 692–698.

Ritterband, L. M., Thorndike, F. P., Ingersoll, K. S., Lord, H. R., Gonder-Frederick, L., Frederick, C., … Morin, C. M. (2017). Effect of a web-based cognitive behavior therapy for insomnia intervention with 1-year follow-up: A randomized clinical trial. *JAMA Psychiatry, 74*(1), 68–75. https://doi.org/10.1001/jamapsychiatry.2016.3249

Roane, B. M., & Taylor, D. J. (2008). Adolescent insomnia as a risk factor for early adult depression and substance abuse. *Sleep, 31*, 1351–1356.

Roth, T., Coulouvrat, C., Hajak, G., Lakoma, M. D., Sampson, N. A., Shahly, V., … Kessler, R. C. (2011). Prevalence and perceived health associated with insomnia based on DSM-IV-TR; international statistical classification of diseases and related health problems, tenth revision; and research diagnostic criteria/international classification of sleep disorders, second edition criteria: Results from the america insomnia survey. *Biological Psychiatry, 69*, 592–600. https://doi.org/10.1016/j.biopsych.2010.10.023

Sake, F. T., Wong, K., Bartlett, D. J., & Saini, B. (2017). Insomnia management in the australian primary care setting. *Behavioral Sleep Medicine*, 1–15. https://doi.org/10.1080/15402002.2016.1266491

Sateia, M. J., Buysse, D. J., Krystal, A. D., Neubauer, D. N., & Heald, J. L. (2017). Clinical practice guideline for the pharmacologic treatment of chronic insomnia in adults: An American academy of sleep medicine clinical practice guideline. *Journal of Clinical Sleep Medicine: JCSM: Official Publication of the American Academy of Sleep Medicine, 13*(2), 307–349. https://doi.org/10.5664/jcsm.6470

Schmitz, M. F. (2016). The ACP guidelines for treatment of chronic insomnia: The challenge of implementation. *Behavioral Sleep Medicine, 14*(6), 699–700. https://doi.org/10.1080/15402002.2016.1220131

Schutte-Rodin, S., Broch, L., Buysse, D., Dorsey, C., & Sateia, M. (2008). Clinical guideline for the evaluation and management of chronic insomnia in adults. *Journal of Clinical Sleep Medicine: JCSM: Official Publication of the American Academy of Sleep Medicine, 4*, 487–504.

Shankar, A., Charumathi, S., & Kalidindi, S. (2011). Sleep duration and self-rated health: The national health interview survey 2008. *Sleep, 34*, 1173–1177. https://doi.org/10.5665/SLEEP.1232

Silberman, S. A. (2009). *The insomnia workbook: A comprehensive guide to getting the sleep you need*. Oakland, CA: New Harbinger Publications, Inc.

Smith, M. T., Perlis, M. L., Park, A., Smith, M. S., Pennington, J., Giles, D. E., & Buysse, D. J. (2002). Comparative meta-analysis of pharmacotherapy and behavior therapy for persistent insomnia. *The American Journal of Psychiatry, 159*, 5–11.

Strand, L. B., Laugsand, L. E., Wisløff, U., Nes, B. M., Vatten, L., & Janszky, I. (2012). Insomnia symptoms and cardiorespiratory fitness in healthy individuals: The Nord-tr\ondelag health study (HUNT). *Sleep*. https://doi.org/10.5665/sleep.2310

Taylor, D., Zimmerman, M., Gardner, C., Tatum, J., Bramoweth, A. D., Francetich, J., & Ruggero, C. (2014). A pilot randomized controlled trial of the effects of cognitive-behavioral therapy for insomnia on sleep and daytime functioning in college students. *Behavior Therapy, 45*(3), 376–389.

Taylor, D. J., Mallory, L. J., Lichstein, K. L., Durrence, H. H., Riedel, B. W., & Bush, A. J. (2007). Comorbidity of chronic insomnia with medical problems. *Sleep, 30*, 213–218.

The WHOQOL Group. (1995). The world health organization quality of life assessment (WHOQOL): Position paper from the world health organization. *Social Science & Medicine, 41*(10), 1403–1409.

Trauer, J. M., Qian, M. Y., Doyle, J. S., Rajaratnam, S. M., & Cunnington, D. (2015). Cognitive behavioral therapy for chronic insomnia: A systematic review and meta-analysis. *Annals of Internal Medicine, 163*(3), 191–204. https://doi.org/10.7326/M14-2841

Trockel, M., Karlin, B. E., Taylor, C. B., & Manber, R. (2014). Cognitive behavioral therapy for insomnia with veterans: Evaluation of effectiveness and correlates of treatment outcomes. *Behaviour Research and Therapy, 53*, 41–46. https://doi.org/10.1016/j.brat.2013.11.006

Troxel, W. M., Buysse, D. J., Matthews, K. A., Kip, K. E., Strollo, P. J., Hall, M., … Reis, S. E. (2010). Sleep symptoms predict the development of the metabolic syndrome. *Sleep, 33*(12), 1633–1640.

Troxel, W. M., Germain, A., & Buysse, D. J. (2012). Clinical management of insomnia with brief behavioral treatment (BBTI). *Behavioral Sleep Medicine, 10*, 266–279. https://doi.org/10.1080/15402002.2011.607200

Ulmer, C. S., Farrell-Carnahan, L., Hughes, J. M., Manber, R., Tatum, J., & the Mid-Atlantic (VISN 6) Mental Illness Research, Education and Clinical Center (MIRECC). (2016). *Improve your sleep: A self-guided approach for veterans with insomnia* (Version 1 ed.). Department of Veterans Affairs

van der Weijden, T., Wensing, M., Eccles, M., & Grol, R. (2013). Feedback and reminders. In R. Grol, M. Wensing, M. Eccles, & D. Davis (Eds.), *Improving patient care: The implementation of change in healthcare* (2nd ed., pp. 210–223). Chichester, UK: Wiley.

Vgontzas, A. N., Liao, D., Bixler, E. O., Chrousos, G. P., & Vela-Bueno, A. (2009). Insomnia with objective short sleep duration is associated with a high risk for hypertension. *Sleep, 32*(4), 491–497.

Vgontzas, A. N., Liao, D., Pejovic, S., Calhoun, S., Karataraki, M., Basta, M., … Bixler, E. O. (2010). Insomnia with short sleep duration and mortality: The penn state cohort. *Sleep, 33*(9), 1159–1164.

Watanabe, N., Furukawa, T. A., Shimodera, S., Morokuma, I., Katsuki, F., Fujita, H., … Perlis, M. L. (2011). Brief behavioral therapy for refractory insomnia in residual depression: An assessor-blind, randomized controlled trial. *The Journal of Clinical Psychiatry, 72*(12), 1651–1658.

Watson, N. F., Badr, M. S., Belenky, G., Bliwise, D. L., Buxton, O. M., Buysse, D., … Tasali, E. (2015). Recommended amount of sleep for a healthy adult: A joint consensus statement of the American academy of sleep medicine and sleep research society. *Sleep, 38*(6), 843–844. https://doi.org/10.5665/sleep.4716

Wensing, M., Fluit, C., & Grol, R. (2013). Educational strategies. In R. Grol, M. Wensing, M. Eccles, & D. Davis (Eds.), *Improving patient care: The implementation of change in health care* (2nd ed., pp. 197–209). Chichester, UK: Wiley.

Wilson, S. J., Nutt, D. J., Alford, C., Argyropoulos, S. V., Baldwin, D. S., Bateson, A. N., … Wade, A. G. (2010). British association for psychopharmacology consensus statement on evidence-based treatment of insomnia, parasomnias and circadian rhythm disorders. *Journal of Psychopharmacology, 24*(11), 1577–1601. https://doi.org/10.1177/0269881110379307

Wilt, T. J., MacDonald, R., Brasure, M., Olson, C. M., Carlyle, M., Fuchs, E., … Kane, R. L. (2016). Pharmacologic treatment of insomnia disorder: An evidence report for a clinical practice guideline by the American college of physicians. *Annals of Internal Medicine*, 1–10. https://doi.org/10.7326/M15-1781

Winkens, R. A., Pop, P., Bugter-Maessen, A. M., Grol, R. P., Kester, A. D., Beusmans, G. H., & Knottnerus, J. A. (1995). Randomised controlled trial of routine individual feedback to improve rationality and reduce numbers of test requests. *Lancet (London, England), 345*(8948), 498–502.

Winkens, R. A., Pop, P., Grol, R. P., Bugter-Maessen, A. M., Kester, A. D., Beusmans, G. H., & Knottnerus, J. A. (1996). Effects of routine individual feedback over nine years on general practitioners' requests for tests. *BMJ (Clinical Research Ed.), 312*(7029), 490.

Winkens, R. A., Pop, P., Grol, R. P., Kester, A. D., & Knottnerus, J. A. (1992). Effect of feedback on test ordering behaviour of general practitioners. *BMJ (Clinical Research Ed.), 304*(6834), 1093–1096.

World Health Organization. (1992). *The ICD-10 classification of mental and behavioural disorders: Clinical descriptions and diagnostic guidelines*. Geneva: World Health Organization.

Wu, J. Q., Appleman, E. R., Salazar, R. D., & Ong, J. C. (2015). Cognitive behavioral therapy for insomnia comorbid with psychiatric and medical conditions. *JAMA Internal Med.* https://doi.org/10.1001/jamainternmed.2015.3006

Yang, E. H., Hla, K. M., McHorney, C. A., Havighurst, T., Badr, M. S., & Weber, S. (2000). Sleep apnea and quality of life. *Sleep, 23*(4), 535–541.

Part V
Step-by-Step Guide to “Doing” Behavioral Health in the Context of Integrated Care

Chapter 14
Behavioral Health and Cancer

Claire C. Conley, Marlena M. Ryba, and Barbara L. Andersen

Introduction

Integrated care aims to connect the primary healthcare system with other human service systems in order to improve patient outcomes (Leutz, 1999). Behavioral medicine is an important addition as it integrates psychological, behavioral, and social factors into the prevention, treatment, and rehabilitation of illness and disease (Emmons, 2012; Keefe, 2011; Ruddy, Borresen, & Myerholtz, 2013; Valentijn, Schepman, Opheij, & Bruijnzeels, 2013). These efforts are important for cancer, as it is a disease having modifiable behavioral factors capable of reducing risk, morbidity, and premature cancer death.

We discuss contributions in the behavioral aspects of primary, secondary, and tertiary cancer prevention. For primary prevention, the focus is on modifiable behaviors for reducing exposure to cancer-causing substances, practices, and environments. For secondary prevention, behavioral aspects of usage and adherence to screening for breast, cervix, and colon cancers are discussed. As there is a large tertiary prevention literature, we focus on the detection and treatment of stress, anxiety, and depressive symptoms to reduce morbidity and mortality. We organize the three sections by the inclusion of (1) nature of the problem, (2) characteristics of individuals at risk, (3) barriers to prevention, and (4) guidelines for prevention or treatment. Also provided are discussion of (5) behavioral care, with an emphasis on efforts/interventions used in primary care settings; (6) behavioral interventions of low, moderate, and high intensity; and (7) the efficacy/effectiveness of interventions with individuals at risk. To begin, the cancer problem—incidence and mortality for adult males and female—is overviewed and, to end, commentary on the role of behavioral science in oncology is provided.

C. C. Conley · M. M. Ryba · B. L. Andersen (✉)
Department of Psychology, Ohio State University, Columbus, OH, USA
e-mail: Conley.405@osu.edu; MRyba@coastal.edu; Andersen.1@osu.edu

M. P. Duckworth, W. T. O'Donohue (eds.), *Behavioral Medicine and Integrated Care*,
https://doi.org/10.1007/978-3-319-93003-9_14

The Cancer Problem

The number of individuals affected by cancer continues to grow. In 2012 (the latest year for which information is available), it is estimated that 14.1 million new cancer cases occurred worldwide (Ferlay et al., 2015) with the burden expected to increase exponentially by 2030 due to increased population growth and longevity (Edwards et al., 2010).

In the U.S., roughly 1.7 million new cancer cases are diagnosed annually (American Cancer Society, 2016a). The most frequently diagnosed cancer sites are presented in Fig. 14.1. Survival rates are also increasing: the 5-year survival rate for all cancers diagnosed during 2005–2011 was 69%, up from 49% during 1975–1977 (American Cancer Society, 2016a). In 2016, more than 15.5 million children and adults with a history of cancer were alive (American Cancer Society, 2016c). By 2026, estimations suggest that the survivor population will increase to 20.3 million, with 10 million males and 10.3 million females. The majority of these individuals will be disease-free and return to primary care providers. Moreover, an oncologist shortage is predicted to occur by the year 2025 (Yang et al., 2014), further increasing the burden on primary care settings. Thus, improved survivorship will require an increased focus on integrated healthcare implemented for primary, secondary, and tertiary cancer prevention.

Estimated New Cases		Estimated Deaths	
Male	**Female**	**Male**	**Female**
Prostate 180,890 (21%)	Breast 246,660 (29%)	Lung & bronchus 85,920 (27%)	Lung & bronchus 72,160 (26%)
Lung & bronchus 117,920 (14%)	Lung & bronchus 106,470 (13%)	Prostate 26,120 (8%)	Breast 40,450 (14%)
Colon & rectum 70,820 (8%)	Colon & rectum 63,670 (8%)	Colon & rectum 26,020 (8%)	Colon & rectum 23,170 (8%)
Urinary bladder 58,950 (7%)	Uterine corpus 60,050 (7%)	Pancreas 21,450 (7%)	Pancreas 20,330 (7%)
Melanoma of the skin 46,870 (6%)	Thyroid 49,350 (6%)	Liver & intrahepatic bile duct 18,280 (6%)	Ovary 14,240 (5%)
Non-Hodgkin lymphoma 40,170 (5%)	Non-Hodgkin lymphoma 32,410 (4%)	Leukemia 14,130 (4%)	Uterine corpus 10,470 (4%)
Kidney & renal pelvis 39,650 (5%)	Melanoma of the skin 29,510 (3%)	Esophagus 12,720 (4%)	Leukemia 10,270 (4%)
Oral cavity & pharynx 34,780 (4%)	Leukemia 26,050 (3%)	Urinary bladder 11,820 (4%)	Liver & intrahepatic bile duct 8,890 (3%)
Leukemia 34,090 (4%)	Pancreas 25,400 (3%)	Non-Hodgkin lymphoma 11,520 (4%)	Non-Hodgkin lymphoma 8,630 (3%)
Liver & intrahepatic bile duct 28,410 (3%)	Kidney & renal pelvis 23,050 (3%)	Brain & other nervous system 9,440 (3%)	Brain & other nervous system 6,610 (2%)
All sites 841,390 (100%)	All sites 843,820 (100%)	All sites 314,290 (100%)	All sites 281,400 (100%)

Estimates are rounded to the nearest 10, and cases exclude basal cell and squamous cell skin cancers and in situ carcinoma except urinary bladder.

Fig. 14.1 Cancer incidence and mortality by site and gender. (American Cancer Society, *Cancer Facts and Figures*, 2016a)

Primary Prevention

Primary prevention is defined as altering behaviors or exposures that can lead to disease. While there are notable examples of genetic (e.g., BRCA1 in breast) and immune factors (e.g., non-Hodgkin's Lymphoma for those on immunosuppressive drugs, Kaposi's sarcoma for those with HIV immune suppression), the majority of cancers are not due to host factors. Environmental causes such as exposure to substances (asbestos, arsenic) or radiation are of low incidence as well. Instead, most cancers can be avoided through primary prevention (American Cancer Society, 2016b). Broadly, this consists of communications regarding cancer risk and promoting lifestyle interventions.

Cancer Risk Communication

Nature of the Problem Health communication is the first step in prevention and has the greatest potential to reduce cancer burden at individual, institutional, and societal levels (Fischhoff, Bostrom, & Quadrell, 1993; Kreps, 2003). For patients to make informed decisions about cancer, they have to be aware of their risk. Cancer prevention efforts typically involve the development and distribution of persuasive and informative educational material and programs as well as the development and use of behavioral intervention programs to initiate, promote, or change target health behaviors (Buller et al., 1999; Marcus et al., 2001; Pierce, Macaskill, & Hill, 1990). The ultimate aim is to prevent cancer initiation and/or speed its earliest detection (Kreps, 2003).

When health communication "goes wrong," it can impair both primary and secondary cancer prevention (Davis, Williams, Marin, Parker, & Glass, 2002) and may affect patient participation in cancer control programs (Michielutte, Alciati, & el Arculli, 1999). Participants in health communication focus groups frequently report awareness of cancer; however, their knowledge of cancer and cancer screening was often found to be limited, inaccurate, or confused (Davis, Arnold, Berkel, & Nandy, 1996; Davis et al., 2001; Davis, Holcombe, Berkel, Pramanik, & Divers, 1998; Lannin et al., 1998).

Characteristics of Individuals at Risk Patients' health literacy is increasingly recognized as a critical factor affecting patient-physician communication and health outcomes. Health literacy refers to individuals' capacity to obtain, process, and understand basic health information and services needed to make appropriate health decisions. Poor health literacy is common, especially among elderly patients. More than 33% of patients ages 65 and older have inadequate or marginal health literacy, as do up to 80% of patients in public hospital settings (Williams, Davis, Parker, & Weiss, 2002). Patients with poor health literacy report worse health status and have less understanding about their medical conditions and treatment; they may have increased hospitalization rates (Williams, Davis, Parker, & Weiss, 2002).

Barriers to Prevention A 2008 systematic review of health professionals' perceptions of patient-provider communication identified barriers (Légaré, Ratté, Gravel, & Graham, 2008). In 22 of 38 included studies, professionals identified time constraints as a barrier to discussion and shared decision-making. That is, despite knowledge of good communication and shared decision-making principles, providers believed that there was insufficient time to put said principles into practice (Rogers, 1995). Indeed, there is a general consensus that the growing demands and expectations of informed health consumers and societies pressure limited resources, including human resources (Kim, Salomon, Weinstein, & Goldie, 2006). Thus, time was cited as a barrier across many different cultural and organizational contexts (Légaré et al., 2008). However, results from more than a hundred randomized trials of patient-provider communication and shared decision-making provide no robust evidence that more time is required for prevention efforts in clinical practice than is usual care (Légaré et al., 2012, 2014; Stacey et al., 2014).

Providers also believed that such discussions were not applicable to their practice population (Cabana et al., 1999), either based on the characteristics of the patient (identified in 18 of 38 studies) or based on the clinical situation (identified in 16 of 38 studies) (Légaré et al., 2008). These results suggest that health professionals might be screening a priori which patients will prefer or benefit from shared decision-making. This is of some concern because physicians may misjudge patients' desire or ability to be actively involved in decision-making (Bruera, Sweeney, Calder, Palmer, & Benisch-tolley, 2001; Bruera, Willey, Palmer, & Rosales, 2002). Surveys consistently indicate that patients want more engagement than providers offer (Alston et al., 2012). Ironically, those patient populations that stand to benefit most from engaging in shared decision-making (e.g., older people, immigrants, people with lower levels of education, numeracy, and/or health literacy) report less interest in shared decision-making (Kiesler & Auerbach, 2006).

Although training programs for health professionals have been developed to address these barriers, they vary widely in what they deliver and how to implement them. In addition, evidence of their effectiveness is sparse (Légaré, Politi, Desroches, Stacey, & Bekker, 2012). Therefore, some have suggested that future interventions will need to target the public and patients directly (so-called patient-mediated interventions) in order to foster active patient participation in decisions (Légaré et al., 2008).

Behavioral Care: Options and Efficacy Authors (Davis et al., 2002; Mayeaux Jr. et al., 1996; Schapira, Nattinger, & McAuliffe, 2006; Schwartz, Woloshin, & Welch, 1999) have developed specific recommendations for effective risk communication. These recommendations incorporate not only clinicians but also institutions and other communicators (i.e., media or public health agencies).

- Clinicians should:
  - Slow down and use "living room language" that patients can understand.
  - Limit information given to patients at each interaction.
  - Review basic concepts of probability and their application to medical studies with patients.
  - Provide information based on a health belief model, rather than numerical probabilities.
  - Give priority to patient action, motivation, and self-empowerment.
  - Confirm patient understanding prior to ending an encounter.
- Institutions should:
  - Develop office-based tools to make up-to-date estimates of disease risk and treatment benefit easily available during office visits.
- All communicators (i.e., media or public health agencies) should:
  - Present data to the public in a clear and objective manner.
  - Use graphic displays to enhance quantitative risk communication.

Lifestyle Interventions

An estimated 75% of all cancers are due to modifiable, lifestyle risk factors: tobacco exposure, dietary intake (alcohol use, fat, low fruit and vegetable intake) and/or physical inactivity, sexual and reproductive lifestyle (unsafe sex, HPV exposure), and general environmental exposures (urban air pollution, household use of solid fuels) (Danaei, Vander Hoorn, Lopez, Murray, & Ezzati, 2005). Many of the targeted problems below are also ones related to the onset or worsening of other problems, such as cardiovascular disease, the leading cause of death and disability in the U.S. (Heron & Anderson, 2016).

Tobacco Use

Nature of the Problem Roughly 188,800 of the estimated 595,690 cancer deaths in 2016—32%—will be caused by tobacco use (American Cancer Society, 2016a). In addition to lung cancer (Alberg & Samet, 2003; U.S. Department of Health and Human Services, 2014), tobacco exposure increases risk for oral, laryngeal, pharyngeal, esophageal, gastric, pancreatic, renal, liver, bladder, uterine, cervical, colorectal, and ovarian cancers (Botteri et al., 2008; Castellsagué & Muñoz, 2003; Engeland, Andersen, Haldorsen, & Tretli, 1996; Hellberg & Stendahl, 2005; Iodice, Gandini, Maisonneuve, & Lowenfels, 2008; Liang, Chen, & Giovannucci, 2009; Sasco, Secretan, & Straif, 2004; Siegel et al., 2015). For many of these cancers, the risk conferred by tobacco exposure persists above and beyond other known risk factors (e.g., HPV exposure for cervical cancer). It should also be noted that tobacco users are less likely to engage in other health protective behaviors. For example, increased tobacco cravings are associated with low levels of physical activity (Haasova, Warren, Thompson, Ussher, & Taylor, 2016). Taken together, this may lead to an exponential increase in cancer risk. Thus, two of the most effective approaches to reduce cancer incidence are to reduce rates of tobacco use and exposure level through public health policy and behavioral interventions.

Comprehensive tobacco-control programs increase smoking cessation rates and also decrease initiation of smoking (*WHO report on the global tobacco epidemic,* 2013). In fact, public health policies, such as smoking bans and tax increases, have led to substantial decreases in the number of smokers over the last 50 years (U.S. Department of Health and Human Services, 2014). For example, youth (12–17 years) and adult (25 years and older) cigarette use declined dramatically with the start of anti-tobacco counter-marketing mass media campaigns (Farrelly, Davis, Haviland, Messeri, & Healton, 2005; Murphy-Hoefer, Hyland, & Rivard, 2010). Still, there is room for improvement with vigorous continuation of health policies: an estimated 30% reduction in the number of smokers could be achieved by doubling the inflation-adjusted price of cigarettes (Jha & Peto, 2015).

This potential for future gains occurs, however, when the technology of tobacco use itself is changing. Electronic cigarettes (or e-cigarettes) have been promoted as being more cost-effective, amenable to use in smoking-restricted environments, and socially acceptable than traditional cigarettes (Cobb, Byron, Abrams, & Shields, 2010; Henningfield & Zaatari, 2010; King, Alam, Promoff, Arrazola, & Sube, 2013). Between 2010 and 2013, the use of electronic cigarettes increased significantly across all demographic groups, although the use is highest among young adults ages 18–24 (McMillen, Gottlieb, Shaefer, Winickoff, & Klein, 2014). Among current smokers, e-cigarette use is associated with higher socioeconomic status, smoking more cigarettes, and having a quit attempt within the past year (Brown et al., 2014). However, 32.5% of current e-cigarette users are never or former smokers (McMillen, Gottlieb, Shaefer, Winickoff, & Klein, 2014). Thus, e-cigarettes contribute to primary nicotine addiction and to the renormalization of tobacco use (Fairchild, Bayer, & Colgrove, 2014). Akin to smoking bans, regulatory action is needed at the federal, state, and local levels to ensure that these products do not contribute to preventable chronic disease.

Characteristics of Individuals at Risk Large disparities in tobacco use remain across racial/ethnic groups and between groups defined by educational level, socioeconomic status, geographic region, sexual minorities (including GLBTQ individuals), and those with severe mental illness (U.S. Department of Health and Human Services, 2014). Specifically, daily use of tobacco is associated with female gender, White race, lower educational status, living at or above the poverty line, and living in the Midwest region of the U.S. (U.S. Department of Health and Human Services, 2014). Adults 18–25 and 26–44 years of age have the highest prevalence rates of tobacco use; tobacco use then declines with age. Furthermore, there is a continued rise in young adult smoking even as youth rates decline (Dietz, Sly, Lee, Arheart, & McClure, 2013). Finally, lifestyle (participation in organized activities, health status, use of other substances) and social variables (family members' and/or peers' tobacco use) also predict tobacco use (Pederson, Koval, Chan, & Zhang, 2007).

Barriers to Prevention Tobacco cessation interventions are underutilized in clinical practice despite being the most cost-effective health promotion strategy to reduce morbidity and mortality (Goldstein et al., 1998; Sarna et al., 2000; Vogt et al., 1998). This gap is illustrative of the "implementation cliff" or the lack of translation of effective interventions to clinical practice (Weisz, Ng, & Bearman, 2014). Self-identified barriers cited by oncology nurses and primary care physicians include limited knowledge and skills to do tobacco interventions, lack of time, lower patient priority compared to other clinical interventions, and the lack of consistent institutional expectations (Sarna, Wewers, Brown, Lillington, & Brecht, 2001; Sonmez et al., 2015). Additionally, a sizeable minority of nurses, general practitioners, and family physicians have negative beliefs and attitudes toward discussing smoking with their patients (Vogt, Hall, & Marteau, 2005). The most common negative beliefs are that such discussions are too time-consuming (weighted proportion, 42%) and are ineffective (38%). Other common negative beliefs include lacking confidence in one's ability to discuss smoking with patients (22%) or one's knowledge (16%) and feeling that such discussions are unpleasant (18%).

Guidelines for Prevention In 2008, the CDC's National Health Interview Survey reported that 20.6% of adults aged 18 years and older were current cigarette smokers. The U.S. Department of Health and Human Services has set the goal of decreasing this number to 12% by the year 2020 (U.S. Department of Health and Human Services Office of Disease Prevention and Health Promotion, 2016). In order to achieve this goal, the U.S. Preventive Services Task Force recommends that clinicians ask all adults about tobacco use and provide tobacco cessation interventions (including counseling and/or pharmacotherapy) for those who use tobacco products (U.S. Preventive Services Task Force, 2015).

Recently (2016) the National Comprehensive Cancer Network (NCCN) published smoking cessation treatment guidelines to be used by oncology professionals. For patients who are not ready to quit, providers should engage in motivational talk about smoking cessation, reviewing the health risks of smoking and the benefits of quitting and providing patient education. In addition, a patient's readiness to quit should be reassessed at each visit. For patients who are still smoking and say they want to quit, or for persons who have recently quit smoking, pharmacotherapy (such as short-acting nicotine replacement therapy [NRT]) and behavior therapy can be considered. Behavioral scientists have multiple skills (see concluding remarks below) that could aid facilities in meeting these guidelines.

Behavioral Care: Options and Efficacy Effectiveness of behavioral interventions for tobacco use has been reported for many types of interventions, including group behavioral therapy, individual therapy, physician counseling, telephone counseling, nursing interventions, and tailored self-help interventions (Lancaster & Stead, 2005; Lemmens, Oenema, Knut, & Brug, 2008; Lichtenstein, Glasgow, Lando, Ossip-Klein, & Boles, 1996; Strecher, 1999). These types of interventions are in line with treatment recommendations from the NCCN and USPSTF. Furthermore, the efficacy of behavioral treatments for smoking cessation is extremely reliable, in that 14 meta-analyses demonstrated 100% concordance on the presence/absence of efficacy of 17 different smoking cessation interventions (Hughes, 2009). However, the magnitude of effects of these interventions is not large (Hughes, 2009), and effects for maintenance are lower. Even the best tobacco use programs do not exceed a 50% abstinence rate (Piasecki, 2006). While intensive intervention, telephone counseling, and the use of pharmacotherapy have been found to improve outcomes to 24 months, they reach relatively few users (Ockene et al., 2000). Ockene et al. (2000) suggest that brief interventions during medical visits could be cost-effective and have high reach.

Tobacco use interventions delivered by healthcare providers have been of particular interest. Not only do smokers come into contact with the healthcare system on a frequent basis, smokers often cite the importance of physician advice in influencing their decision to quit smoking (Niaura & Abrams, 2002). Although there is little evidence that extensive physician training effects smoking cessation outcomes (Ferketich et al., 2014), there *is* a dose-dependent relationship between the intensity of physician contact and successful cessation outcome (Fiore, 2000). Evidence demonstrates that physician offers of assistance (e.g., behavioral support for cessation, offering nicotine replacement therapy) generate more quit attempts than physician merely giving advice to quit on medical grounds (Aveyard, Begh, Parsons, & West, 2012).

Alcohol Use

Nature of the Problem Like tobacco use, alcohol use is a modifiable risk factor. Praud et al. (2013) used global estimates of cancer causes and World Health Organization (WHO) estimates on the prevalence of drinkers to estimate the total number of alcohol-attributable cancer cases. Over the 10-year period considered, approximately 770,000 cancer cases could be attributed to alcohol consumption worldwide (5.5% of the total number of cancer cases). These authors concluded that a high burden of cancer morbidity is attributable to alcohol and that public health measures should be developed regarding alcohol consumption (Praud et al., 2013). However, it should be noted that the majority of these studies have examined heavy alcohol drinking; because of probable confounding, the role of light-to-moderate drinking remains unclear (Klatsky et al., 2015).

Characteristics of Individuals at Risk The so-called problem drinkers fall into two categories. Binge drinking is defined as consuming four or more alcoholic beverages per occasion for women or five or more drinks per occasion for men. According to national surveys, one in six U.S. adults binge drinks about four times a month, consuming about eight drinks per binge (Center for Disease Control, 2012). However, binge drinking is more common among men, among young adults aged 18–34 years, and among those with household incomes of $75,000 or more. Heavy drinking, on the other hand, is defined as consuming 8 or more alcoholic beverages per week for women or 15 or more alcoholic beverages per week for men. Although there are similarities between binge drinkers and heavy drinkers, a 2011 study by King and colleagues attempted to assess the unique characteristics of heavy drinkers via a prospective study. They demonstrated that, compared with light drinkers, heavy drinkers exhibited higher alcohol sensitivity, in terms of subjective stimulation and reward (liking and wanting), as well as lower sensitivity, in terms of subjective sedation and salivary cortisol reactivity (King, de Wit, McNamara, & Cao, 2011; King, Hasin, O'Connor, McNamara, & Cao, 2016). In behavioral economics terms, heavy drinkers simply find alcohol to be more rewarding than light drinkers (Tucker et al., 2016).

Barriers to Prevention Like tobacco use interventions, alcohol use interventions have been demonstrated to be efficacious in the context of primary care (Babor et al., 2007; Kaner et al., 2009; Madras et al., 2009; Vasilaki, Hosier, & Cox, 2006). However, physicians and nurses frequently identify barriers to implementation of alcohol use interventions (Coloma-Carmona, Carballo, & Tirado-González, 2016). Commonly reported barriers include the belief that patients will lie about their actual consumption and will not identify its negative consequences and the belief that patients will reject participating in an intervention for their alcohol consumption.

Guidelines for Prevention To reduce the risk of alcohol-related harms, the 2015–2020 U.S. Dietary Guidelines for Americans recommends that if alcohol is consumed, it should be consumed in moderation—up to one drink per day for women and two drinks per day for men. However, data from the 2008 National Survey on Drug Use and Health (NSDUH) demonstrate that 28.2% of adults aged 18 years and older reported that they drank excessively in the previous 30 days. Furthermore, only 8.2% of persons aged 12 years and older who needed alcohol treatment reported that they received specialty treatment for abuse or dependence in the past year in 2008.

The American Society of Addiction Medicine recommends a stepped care model for the treatment of alcohol use (American Society of Addiction Medicine, 1997). Specifically, they suggest that primary care providers routinely screen for the presence of alcohol use problems in patients, screen for risk factors for development of alcohol dependence, and provide appropriate interventions. For patients who drink alcohol at risk levels (the abovementioned "problem drinkers"), appropriate referrals should be provided.

Behavioral Care: Options and Efficacy Consistent with a stepped care model, treatments to reduce alcohol use come in two primary forms: brief intervention and extended intervention. Brief interventions typically consist of a single, 30-min session (Landy, Davey, Quintero, Pecora, & McShane, 2016); however, there is little evidence that such interventions are effective (Havard, Shakeshaft, Conigrave, & Doran, 2012; Landy, Davey, Quintero, Pecora, & McShane, 2016).

Extended interventions include three well-developed protocols with strong research backing: (1) 12-step programs, (2) cognitive behavioral therapy (CBT), and (3) motivational interviewing. First, there are a variety of 12-step approaches, including Alcoholics Anonymous (AA), but all are based on the assumption that substance dependence is a medical and/or spiritual disease (Nowinski, Baker, & Carroll, 1992). The 12-step approach consists of a brief, structured, manual-driven approach to facilitating recovery from alcohol abuse implemented over 12–15 sessions. These groups are widely available and are well known in many countries. Second, a variety of cognitive behavioral interventions for alcohol use have also been developed, differing in length, modality, content, and treatment setting (Morgenstern & Longabaugh, 2000). Despite differences, CBT for alcohol use has two core elements: a focus on Bandura's social-cognitive theory (e.g., deficits in coping skills serve to maintain excessive drinking) and coping skills training to address said deficits. Finally, motivational interviewing (MI) is a client-centered, directive method for enhancing intrinsic motivation to change by exploring and resolving ambivalence (Miller & Rollnick, 2002). Five key principles underlay MI. First, it emphasizes the individual's present interests and problems. Second, it involves selective responding to the client's speech in a way that resolves ambivalence and motivates the person to change. Third, it is a method of communication rather than a set of techniques. Fourth, it focuses on intrinsic motivation for change. Fifth, within this approach, change occurs because of its relevance to the person's own values (Mller & Rollnick, 2002).

These three treatments have been shown to be efficacious (Allen, Anton, Babor, & Carbonari, 1997), though the mechanisms for such are unclear despite study (Longabaugh et al., 2005; Morgenstern & Longabaugh, 2000). Therefore, the differentiation between programs may come from the ease of implementation and/or referral (Dennis, Perl, Huebner, & McLellan, 2000; Rieckmann, Kovas, Fussell, & Stettler, 2009; Roman & Johnson, 2002). In the context of primary care, screening for risky alcohol use in medical settings, providing brief interventions for those who drink above low risk drinking limits, and referring those at risk for an alcohol use disorder to specialized treatment (SBIRT) have proven effective for reducing alcohol use and alcohol-related consequences (Babor et al., 2007; Kaner et al., 2009; Madras et al., 2009; Vasilaki, Hosier, & Cox, 2006).

Physical Activity, Diet, and Nutrition

Nature of the Problem It has been estimated that 30–40% of all cancers can be prevented by physical activity, dietary changes, and maintenance of appropriate body weight (Renehan, Tyson, Egger, Heller, & Zwahlen, 2008; World Cancer Research Fund & American Institute for Cancer Research, 2007), and it is likely to be higher than this for some individual cancers. Increased body weight is associated with increased risk of many malignancies, although some of these associations differ based on gender. Among men, a 5 kg/m^2 increase in body mass index (BMI) has been related to increased risk of esophageal, thyroid, colorectal, and renal cancers (Renehan et al., 2008). In women, the same 5 kg/m^2 increase in BMI has been related to increased risk of endometrial, gallbladder, esophageal, and renal cancers (Renehan et al., 2008). Body fatness also increases the risk of breast cancer among postmenopausal women (Ligibel & Strickler, 2013; World Cancer Research Fund & American Institute for Cancer Research, 2007). Finally, there is preliminary evidence for a link between BMI and thyroid cancer (Peterson, De, & Nuttall, 2012).

The most common weight management interventions target physical activity and/or diet. Physical activity is a modifiable lifestyle risk factor that has the potential to reduce the risk of most major cancer sites (Friedenreich, Neilson, & Lynch, 2010). However, the positive effects of physical activity on cancer risk extend beyond overall reduction in body weight. Analyses controlling for body weight demonstrate that 4 or more hours per week of exercise results in a statistically significant reduction in cancer risk (Thune, Brenn, Lund, & Gaard, 1997). Hypothesized biological mechanisms include a likely effect of physical activity on insulin resistance, body composition, sex hormones, and metabolic hormones and a possible effect on vitamin D, adipokines, inflammation, and immune function (Friedenreich, Neilson, & Lynch, 2010; McTiernan, 2008).

The relationship between diet and cancer is also complex. While there is mixed evidence for the effects of specific micronutrients (e.g., vitamins, antioxidants, etc.) on cancer incidence (Bardia et al., 2008), several studies have demonstrated significant effects for types of foods eaten (e.g., fruits, vegetables, meat, fat, etc.). Specifically, high consumption of fiber (e.g., fruit, vegetables, and whole grains) is hypothesized to be protective, while high consumption of fat and meat is hypothesized to increase risk. Several studies have demonstrated a protective effect of fruit and vegetable consumption on cancer risk (Block, Patterson, & Subar, 1992; Chan, Gann, & Giovannucci, 2005; Gandini, Merzenich, Robertson, & Boyle, 2000; McGarr, Ridlon, & Hylemon, 2005; Slattery, Curtin, Edwards, & Schaffer, 2004). Furthermore, one case-control study demonstrated evidence supportive of the hypothesis that whole-grain intake protects against various cancers (Jacobs, Marquart, Slavin, & Kushi, 1998). On the other hand, high intake of animal fat and meat has been associated with an increased cancer risk (Kolonel, 2001; Sandhu, White, & McPherson, 2001). In summary, diet has been implicated in the etiology of cancer, but definitive etiologic evidence is lacking (Dagnelie, Schuurman, Goldbohm, & Van Den Brandt, 2004). Aside from following general dietary recommendations for healthy eating, there is no clear evidence that specific dietary components can effectively reduce cancer risk.

Characteristics of Individuals at Risk Overweight and obesity disproportionately affect certain demographic groups in the U.S. Overweight and obese adults are more likely to be male (70.9% of males vs. 61.9% of females), African-American (71.5% of African-Americans vs. 62.7% of Whites), and Hispanic or Latino (70.2% of Hispanic/Latino persons vs. 61.1% of non-Hispanic/non-Latino persons) (Ng et al., 2014; Nugent, Black, & Adams, 2016). Education and poverty status are also associated with higher rates of overweight and obesity, particularly when comparing the most extreme groups. For example, 71.2% of those with an educational level less than a high school diploma are overweight or obese, compared to 55.4% of those with a Master's degree, professional degree, or doctoral degree (Nugent et al., 2016). Similarly, 63% of those individuals living at or below the poverty line are overweight or obese, compared to 59.5% of those earning 400% of the poverty threshold or greater (Nugent et al., 2016).

Barriers to Prevention Several barriers to the successful implementation of weight loss programs exist. First, patient access to comprehensive programs is limited (Cole, Keppel, Andrilla, Cox, & Baldwin, 2016; Moyer, 2012; Ogden, Carroll, Kit, & Flegal, 2013), and in many cases, treatments are only partially covered by insurance (Koh & Sebelius, 2010; Madison, Schmidt, & Volpp, 2016; Weiner & Colameco, 2014). For example, Medicare only reimburses or pays for obesity counseling and treatment provided during in-person, face-to-face visits, creating potential financial barriers for patient participation in weight loss programs (Centers for Medicare and Medicaid Services, 2011). The coordinated infrastructure required to implement in-person comprehensive weight loss programs may serve as a barrier to health systems offering these successful programs. Thus, it is imperative to consider alternative approaches to providing these programs, such as remote programs delivered through mobile and web support (Appel et al., 2011; Hamar, Coberley, Pope, & Rula, 2014). Such interventions could minimize cost, location, and convenience as barriers to weight loss program participation (Jensen et al., 2014).

Second, barriers exist at the level of the physician. Primary care physicians report discomfort with discussing obesity and weight loss with patients, and only a minority of obese adults report having received weight loss counseling from a physician (Epling, Morley, & Ploutz-Snyder, 2011; Felix, West, & Bursac, 2008; Galuska, Will, Serdula, & Ford, 1999; Huang et al., 2004; Shiffman et al., 2009). When physicians do, it is often to prescribe weight loss medications not accompanied by appropriate counseling (Shiffman et al., 2009). Physician's insufficient guidance on weight management strategies may be due to inadequate counseling skills and/or lack of confidence (Huang et al., 2004).

Maintenance of effects poses a third and final barrier. Continued coach contact and self-monitoring are among a small number of strategies that can effectively prevent or reduce weight regain (Jeffery et al., 2000; Turk et al., 2009). However, their cost to implement (e.g., staffing requirements, participant burden) poses significant access and adherence barriers (Xiao, Yank, Wilson, Lavori, & Ma, 2013).

Guidelines for Prevention Between 2005 and 2008, only 30.8% of U.S. adults were considered to be at a healthy weight, and 33.9% were obese (U.S. Department of Health and Human Services Office of Disease Prevention and Health Promotion, 2016). By the year 2020, the national target is to increase the number of individuals at a healthy weight to 33.9%, while simultaneously decreasing the number of obese individuals to 30.5% (U.S. Department of Health and Human Services Office of Disease Prevention and Health Promotion, 2016).

Current physical activity guidelines suggest that adults should engage in both aerobic physical activity (a minimum of either 150 min at a moderate intensity or 75 min at a vigorous intensity) and muscle-strengthening activities (2 or more days per week) (U.S. Department of Health and Human Services, 2008). Furthermore, it is recommended that all adults should avoid inactivity. However, only 20% of adults meet the physical activity guidelines for aerobic and muscle-strengthening activity (U.S. Department of Health and Human Services and U.S. Department of Agriculture, 2015). Males are more likely to report doing regular physical activity compared to females (24% of males vs. 17% of females meet recommendations). Furthermore, about 30% of adults report engaging in no leisure time physical activity. Disparities also exist; individuals with lower income and those with lower educational attainment have lower rates of physical activity and are more likely to not engage in leisure time physical activity (U.S. Department of Health and Human Services and U.S. Department of Agriculture, 2015).

The U.S. Department of Agriculture published revised *Dietary Guidelines for Americans* in December 2015. These guidelines include five key recommendations that encourage healthy eating patterns: (1) follow a healthy eating pattern across the life span; (2) focus on variety, nutrient density, and amount; (3) limit calories from added sugars and saturated fats and reduce sodium intake; (4) shift to healthier food and beverage choices; and (5) support healthy eating patterns for all (U.S. Department of Health and Human Services and U.S. Department of Agriculture, 2015). Unfortunately, the typical eating patterns do not align with these dietary guidelines. Specifically, about three-fourths of the population has an eating pattern that is low in vegetables, fruits, dairy, and oils, while more than half of the population is meeting or exceeding total grain and total protein foods recommendations (U.S. Department of Health and Human Services and U.S. Department of Agriculture, 2015). In addition, most Americans exceed the recommendations for added sugars, saturated fats, and sodium, and the eating patterns of many are too high in calories. Taken together, the lack of adherence to physical activity and dietary recommendations may be responsible for the obesity epidemic in the U.S. (Wang & Beydoun, 2007).

Behavioral Care: Options and Efficacy The typical targets of behavioral weight management interventions are physical activity and dietary habits. Wadden, Brownell, and Foster (2002) proposed a three-stage process for selecting treatment for overweight and obesity (defined as a body mass index (BMI) greater than 25 kg/m^2). First, patients are divided into four levels based on BMI:

- Level 1: BMI < 27 kg/m^2
- Level 2: BMI 27–29 kg/m^2
- Level 3: BMI 30–39 kg/m^2
- Level 4: BMI ≥ 40 kg/m^2

All individuals are encouraged to control their weight, increasing their physical activity and making dietary changes. When this approach is not successful, more intensive intervention might be warranted, as in a "stepped care" model (Wadden, Brownell, & Foster, 2002). A matching decision is based on the individual's prior weight loss effort, treatment preferences, and need for weight reduction (as judged by the presence of comorbid conditions or other risk factors). Wadden and colleagues also recommend adjunct psychological counseling for these patients. Regardless of the treatment selected, the goal of treatment is attainment of a healthier weight.

Although behavioral weight management interventions achieve clinically significant weight losses of 8–10% (Butryn, Webb, & Wadden, 2011; Jeffery et al., 2000), only 40–60% of people achieve this goal (Unick, Jakicic, & Marcus, 2010). Furthermore, improving the maintenance of weight loss remains the critical challenge for all weight management approaches. Patients identify many barriers to maintenance of changes post-intervention (Morgan et al., 2016). In a classic series of studies, Perri and colleagues (Perri et al., 1988; Perri, Nezu, & Viegener, 1992) demonstrated that continuing behavioral care (provided via phone, mail, or in person) improved the maintenance of weight loss. However, patient participation in maintenance sessions tends to decline over time, requiring the development of innovative, integrated healthcare approaches in the long term.

Primary care weight management interventions illustrate a wide range of strategies but hold promise nonetheless (Ball, Leveritt, Cass, & Chaboyer, 2015; Bhattarai et al., 2013; Sanchez, Bully, Martinez, & Grandes, 2015; Simons-Morton, Calfas, Oldenburg, & Burton, 1998). In an illustrative example, Kallings, Leijon, Hellénius, and Ståhle (2008) investigated the efficacy of a physical activity intervention in the primary care context. Almost 500 patients were "prescribed" individualized physical activity programs by their primary care physician. Results demonstrated significant increases in self-reported physical activity and motivation for physical activity (Kallings, Leijon, Hellénius, & Ståhle, 2008). However, the consistency and clinical significance of primary care weight management interventions are unclear (Booth, Prevost, Wright, & Gulliford, 2014), and further research is needed to establish the optimal design and delivery (Ball, Leveritt, Cass, & Chaboyer, 2015; Gagliardi, Faulkner, Ciliska, & Hicks, 2015). For example, incorporating motivational interviewing techniques may increase long-term adherence (Hutchison, Breckon, & Johnston, 2009; McGrane, Galvin, Cusack, & Stokes, 2015). Additionally, long-term weight loss is increased when diet and physical activity are combined (Johns, Hartmann-Boyce, Jebb, & Aveyard, 2014). Thus, multicomponent interventions may yield the best results for maintenance of appropriate weight. Finally, Tulloch, Fortier, and Hogg (2006) suggest that stronger effects may come from interdisciplinary collaboration, in which providers refer patients to specialists.

Virus Exposure

Nature of the Problem Certain cancers are related to infectious agents, and exposures to these cancers could be avoided through education or vaccination (American Cancer Society, 2016b). Research suggests that almost all cervical cancer cases are caused by the human papillomavirus (HPV), for which two vaccines have been developed (Garland et al., 2007; Harper, 2008; The FUTURE II Study Group, 2007). Vaccination programs, along with education to reduce exposure risk (Anhang, Goodman, & Goldie, 2004; Fu, Bonhomme, Cooper, Joseph, & Zimet, 2014; Pierce Campbell, Menezes, Paskett, & Giuliano, 2012), would be an effective primary prevention strategy for cervical cancer. In fact, widespread HPV vaccination may reduce cervical cancer incidence by as much as 77% (Smith et al., 2007), and vaccination may be particularly important for populations at high risk for cervical cancer (Reiter, Katz, & Paskett, 2012).

Characteristics of Individuals at Risk Worldwide, the prevalence of HPV infections among women is about 10% (Clifford et al., 2005; De Sanjosé et al., 2007). However, there are significant age disparities in HPV prevalence, whereby women under the age of 35 years have the highest HPV prevalence (De Sanjosé et al., 2007). For instance, among college women in the U.S., HPV prevalence was 24.4% (Burk et al., 1996; Winer et al., 2003). In addition, individuals of Black or Hispanic ethnicity are at increased risk for HPV infection (Burk et al., 1996; Ley et al., 1991). Finally, the major behavioral risk factors for HPV infection are related to sexual activity (*IARC monographs on the evaluation of carcinogenic risks to human: Human papillomaviruses*, 2007), including acquisition of new male sexual partners, an increasing number of lifetime sexual partners in both females and their male partners (Burk et al., 1996; Karlsson et al., 1995; Kjaer et al., 1997, 2001; Ley et al., 1991; Vaccarella et al., 2006), having non-monogamous male partners, an increase in the age differences between women and their first sexual partner, long-term oral contraceptive use (Kjaer et al., 2001; Ley et al., 1991), and history of chlamydia infections (Kjaer et al., 1997).

Many of these risk factors can be accounted for by early age at first sexual intercourse (Kahn, Rosenthal, Succop, Ho, & Burk, 2002). In turn, sexual debut is predicted by a complex array of family, peer, and environmental factors (French & Dishion, 2003; James, Ellis, Schlomer, & Garber, 2016; Kaplan, Jones, Olson, & Yunzal-Butler, 2013). However, the proportion of adolescent females (ages 15–17) who report having ever had sexual intercourse differs by race, ethnicity, and socioeconomic status (U.S. Department of Health and Human Services Office of Disease

Prevention and Health Promotion, 2016). Specifically, a greater proportion of non-Hispanic White (34.7% vs. 26.2%) and higher socioeconomic status adolescents (33.1% vs. 26.9%) report having ever had sexual intercourse.

Furthermore, disparities in HPV vaccination uptake exist by location, race, and ethnicity. In 2014, Hispanic and Latinos had the highest vaccination rates, at 44.1% (U.S. Department of Health and Human Services Office of Disease Prevention and Health Promotion, 2016). This rate was 1.334 times the average rate for all other race/ethnicity groups, and 1.625 times the worst group rate (27.2% of the American Indian/Alaska Native population). This finding may be confounded with the disparities by geographic location: 34.7% of individuals living in a metropolitan location were vaccinated, compared to 32.2% of individuals living in a rural location (U.S. Department of Health and Human Services Office of Disease Prevention and Health Promotion, 2016).

Barriers to Prevention Behavioral factors have been related to HPV vaccination uptake. Patient-reported barriers include cost, feelings that vaccination was unnecessary, concerns that vaccination would promote adolescent sexual behavior, and concerns regarding vaccine safety and side effects (Brewer & Fazekas, 2007; Rambout, Tashkandi, Hopkins, & Tricco, 2014). Brewer and Fazekas (2007) found that vaccination acceptability was higher when people believed the vaccine was effective and that HPV infection was likely. Physician recommendation has also been identified as particularly important (Rosenthal et al., 2011). Thus, HPV vaccine programs in the U.S. should emphasize high vaccine effectiveness, the high likelihood of HPV infection, and physicians' recommendations, as well as addressing barriers to vaccination.

Guidelines for Prevention Current recommendations suggest that all females ages 11–12 receive the HPV vaccine (Petrosky et al., 2015). However, only 40% of 13- to 17-year-old females in the U.S. had received all 3 doses as of 2014 (Reagan-Steiner et al., 2015), and only 28.1% had done so by the recommended age of 15 (U.S. Department of Health and Human Services Office of Disease Prevention and Health Promotion, 2016). The U.S. Department of Health and Human Services has set the goal of increasing this number to 80% by the year 2020 (U.S. Department of Health and Human Services Office of Disease Prevention and Health Promotion, 2016).

Behavioral Care: Options and Efficacy Intervention strategies to address barriers to HPV vaccination, many of which can increase HPV vaccination coverage with modest cost (Smulian, Mitchell, & Stokley, 2016), include educational interventions and clinic-based interventions (Beavis & Levinson, 2016). Mixed results have been reported for purely educational interventions (Bennett et al., 2015; Foley et al., 2015; Gargano et al., 2013). Given the variability in results, it is unclear what impact educational interventions alone would ultimately have on HPV vaccine uptake (Fu, Bonhomme, Cooper, Joseph, & Zimet, 2014). Clinic-based interventions, on the other hand, have been encouraged by the Centers for Disease Control (CDC) as a way to bridge the gap between vaccine recommendations and uptake (U.S. Department of Health and Human Services Office of Disease Prevention and Health Promotion, 2016). For example, one cluster randomized controlled trial demonstrated that focused clinician education, electronic health record-based alerts, and quarterly performance feedback for physicians led to a modest increase in vaccine initiation (Fiks et al., 2013). Despite these promising results, authors caution that clinic-based interventions such as this should be considered an adjunct to a vaccine promotion program (Beavis & Levinson, 2016).

An Example: Primary Prevention of Cardiovascular Disease

An important barrier to the delivery of health behavior change interventions in primary care settings is the lack of an integrated screening and intervention approach that can cut across multiple risk factors and help clinicians and patients to address these risks in an efficient and productive manner (Goldstein, Whitlock, & DePue, 2004). Thus, in order to improve primary prevention of cancer, healthcare providers must systematically assess and address risk factors for the disease. While comprehensive, individualized programs in cancer control are rare, this approach is frequently utilized in prevention of cardiovascular disease (CVD). The approaches developed in the CVD literature may be easily translated to cancer control.

Clinicians and researchers in CVD often utilize the Framingham risk score algorithm to predict events related to coronary heart disease (CHD) (Wilson et al., 1998). This algorithm has been validated in various populations, and several modifiable risk factors emerge, including (1) hypertension, (2) high cholesterol, (3) obesity, (4) physical inactivity, and (5) smoking (Mendy & Vargas, 2015). Once a patient is assessed according to the Framingham risk score algorithm, he or she is referred for appropriate behavioral treatment. According to the American Heart Association, the best behavioral treatment for CHD patients involves comprehensive lifestyle changes, including increased physical activity and a high-fiber diet (Lichtenstein et al., 2006). Efficacious behavioral interventions have been designed to reduce CVD risk factors. A variety of behavioral interventions have been used, including physical activity, diet, and, smoking cessation, as well as a combination of these components (Belardinelli, Georgiou, Cianci, & Purcaro, 1999; Giannuzzi et al., 2008; Hu & Willett, 2002; Lisspers et al., 2005; O'Connor et al., 2009; Ornish et al., 1998; Pischke, Scherwitz, Weidner, & Ornish, 2008; Singh et al., 1992; Toobert, Glasgow, & Radcliffe, 2000; Wang et al., 2006).

The primary prevention behavioral interventions developed for high-risk CVD populations might be effectively applied in the context of cancer control. Akin to the American Society of Clinical Oncology's screening guidelines for depression and anxiety (Andersen et al., 2014), we present a decision tree for behavioral referrals in a primary prevention context (see Fig. 14.2). It is recommended that all patients in primary care be evaluated for risk factors for cancer at initiation of primary care and at periodic intervals in care provision. If multiple risk factors are identified, individuals should have further assessment to identify the nature and extent of problematic health behaviors. Following assessment, patients should be provided behavioral support according to their level of risk. In accordance with a stepped care model, patients are classified as low risk, moderate risk, and high risk. Furthermore, treatment tailoring is recommended: patients should receive intervention components that are relevant to their identified risk factors.

Patients designated as low risk will receive education-only support. Patients designated as moderate risk will be prescribed lifestyle changes tailored to their individual risk factors. Finally, patients designated as high risk will be prescribed a comprehensive, multiple behavior change intervention. Research supports the efficacy of multiple behavior change interventions in promoting lifestyle changes. Rather than hindering behavior change, additional behavioral components may in fact promote behavior change. Spring et al. (2009) reviewed evidence to determine the efficacy of a behavioral intervention to both promote smoking cessation and prevent weight gain among healthy adults. Meta-analytic results found that patients who received both smoking treatment and weight treatment showed increased abstinence and reduced weight compared with patients who received smoking treatment alone. These results have been extended to adults at risk for CHD (Steptoe, Kerry, Rink, & Hilton, 2001; Ward, White, & Druss, 2015), individuals at risk for type 2 diabetes (Greaves et al., 2011), and patients at risk for cancer (Spring, King, Pagoto, Van Horn, & Fisher, 2015). In short, multiple health behavior interventions may have additional value, above and beyond the additive effects of intervention components (Kirk, Penney, McHugh, & Sharma, 2012). This is reflected in the care map provided in Fig. 14.2.

Secondary Prevention

Secondary prevention aims to identify abnormal changes that precede the development of malignancy (Alberts & Hess, 2008), thus preventing the cancer from fully developing. This is done by detecting an existing disease prior to the appearance of symptoms (American Cancer Society, 2015). There is strong evidence that screening reduces mortality from breast, cervical, and colorectal cancers (American Cancer Society, 2015).[1]

[1] While screening is also shown to reduce mortality for lung cancer among long-term and/or heavy smokers (e.g., ≥30 pack-year smoking history), it is not recommended for the general population. For that reason, we have chosen not to review it here.

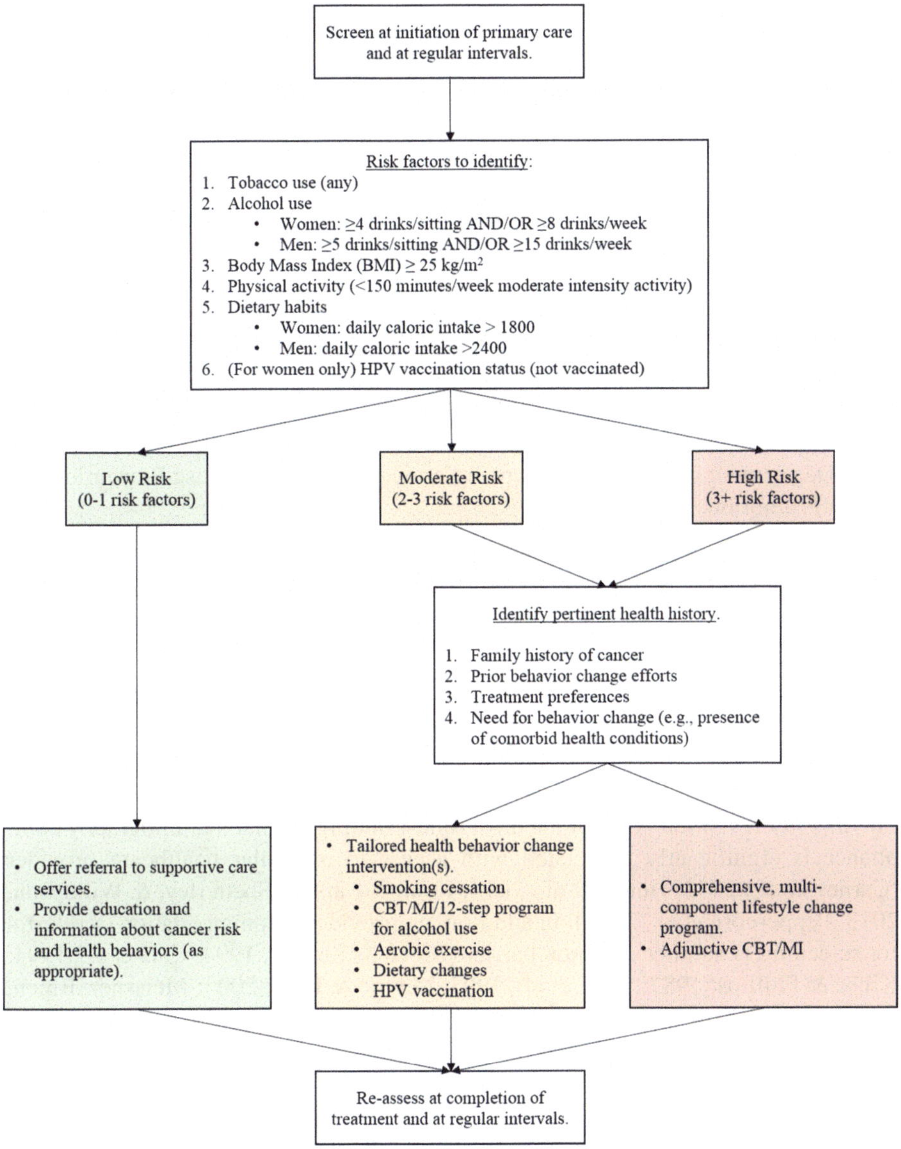

Fig. 14.2 Screening, assessment, and care recommendations for primary prevention of cancer

Breast Cancer

Nature of the Problem Mammography screening is the most effective early detection method (Henry, McDonald, Sherman, Kinney, & Stroup, 2014; Nelson et al., 2009).[2] Despite its efficacy, many remain unscreened (Onitilo et al., 2014). For women above 40 in the U.S., rates of mammography screening have remained between 50% and 80% since 2000 (Breen et al., 2007; Hirsch & Lyman, 2011; National Center for Health Statistics, 2012).

Characteristics of Individuals at Risk Compared to non-Hispanic White, U.S.-born women, minority and foreign-born women report lower rates of mammograms, even though they have increased risk breast cancer risk (Elewonibi, Thierry, & Miranda, 2016). In 2014, 73.3% of Whites had received a mammogram within the past 2 years, compared to 66.7% of the Hispanic or Latino population (U.S. Department of Health and Human Services Office of Disease Prevention and Health Promotion, 2016).

While mammography screening rates have improved nationally in the past 20 years (Doescher & Jackson, 2009), they are consistently lower among rural women (Engelman et al., 2002; Paskett et al., 2004), who are also less likely to be in line with recommended screening timeframes (Horner-Johnson, Dobbertin, & Iezzoni, 2015). *Healthy People 2020* highlights this discrepancy: 73.7% of urban women receive screening, compared to 61.7% of rural women (U.S. Department of Health and Human Services Office of Disease Prevention and Health Promotion, 2016).

Barriers to Prevention One of the most robust findings is that mammography compliance is significantly associated with access to a regular healthcare provider (Carney et al., 2012; Henry et al., 2014; Kempe, Larson, Shetterley, & Wilkinson, 2013; Peppercorn et al., 2015). In addition, no provider recommendation or referral for screening is another common barrier (Breen & Kessler, 1994; Carr et al., 1994; Kruse & Phillips, 1987; Love et al., 1993; Mayne & Earp, 2003; Meissner, Breen, Klabunde, & Vernon, 2006; Meissner, Klabunde, Breen, & Zapka, 2012; Rimer, Trock, Engstrom, Lerman, & King, 1991). Paskett et al. (2004) found that 67% of women reported that a physician had never encouraged them to receive a mammogram, even though 75% had reported receiving a regular checkup in the past year. This may be due to providers' attitudes: one study of rural primary care physicians identified the prevalent belief that patient factors (e.g., SES, low educational attainment, fatalism, lack of knowledge, etc.) will lead patients to non-compliance despite physicians' best efforts (Shell & Tudiver, 2004).

[2] Current U.S. Preventive Services Task Force (USPSTF) recommendations advise against clinicians teaching women how to perform breast self-examination (U.S. Preventive Services Task Force, 2016).

When mammography is recommended, other factors may impede it from occurring (Henry et al., 2014). Attitudes about the procedure (e.g., regarding the convenience, comfort) or its accuracy are important, as women having more favorable attitudes toward annual mammography also report stronger intentions to obtain one in the next year (Lantz, Weigers, & House, 1997; Steele & Porche, 2005). It is encouraging that positive change in attitudes is associated with mammography use (Rauscher, Hawley, & Earp, 2005). A second frequently identified barrier to screening is the time required to have a mammogram; in several surveys, time was endorsed as a barrier by as many as 24% of participants (Murimi & Harpel, 2010; Paskett et al., 2004; Peppercorn et al., 2015). Finally, limited health literacy is a barrier (Bennett & Chen, 2009; Cho, Lee, Arozullah, & Crittenden, 2008; Davis, Arnold, Berkel, & Nandy, 1996; White, Chen, & Atchison, 2008), as is lack of knowledge about breast cancer prevention (Elnicki, Morris, & Schockor, 1995).

Guidelines for Prevention The ACS and the United States Preventative Services Task Force (USPSTF) have published recommendations for the frequency of mammography (American Cancer Society, 2015; U.S. Preventive Services Task Force, 2016). While there is some discrepancy in recommendations, there is consensus that women should have biennial mammograms beginning in their 50s.

Behavioral Care: Options and Efficacy Sohl and Moyer (2007) conducted a meta-analysis of individual-level interventions (including telephone, print, and in-person interventions) for promoting mammography use. They found that women exposed to all three types of interventions were significantly more likely to get a mammogram ($p < 0.001$). Further, Davis et al. (2014) evaluated the effectiveness and cost-effectiveness of three additional, more intensive, individual-level interventions designed to promote mammography: enhanced care, health literacy-informed education of patients, and education plus nurse support. While mammography rates increased substantially over existing baseline rates in all three arms, the education plus nurse support arm was the most effective. However, in a meta-analysis of manuscripts published between 1984 and 1997, Legler et al. (2002) found that multilevel approaches to promote mammography had the greatest impact. Specifically, a combination of access-enhancing (e.g., transportation to appointments, facilitated scheduling, mobile vans, vouchers, and reduced cost mammograms) and individual-directed strategies (e.g., one-on-one counseling, letters and reminders, and telephone counseling) demonstrated the strongest effects (an estimated 27% increase in mammography use across nine studies [95% confidence interval: 9.9%–43.9%]). Therefore, both individual and multilevel behavioral interventions for increasing mammography rates have promise.

Cervical Cancer

Nature of the Problem The Papanicolaou, or Pap smear, screening test is used to detect precancerous changes within the cervix (Everett, Bryant, Griffin, Martin-hirsch, & Carol, 2014). The incidence of cervical cancer is reduced by 93.5%, 92.5%, 90.8%, 83.6%, and 64.1% if women have screening every year, every 2 years, every 3 years, every 5 years, and every 10 years, respectively; these screening intervals would mean women having 50, 25, 16, 10, and 5 smear tests, respectively, in their lifetime (IARC Working Group on Cervical Cancer Screening Programs, 1986). Despite its effectiveness, only 84.5% of females aged 21–65 years were compliant with cervical cancer screening guidelines in 2008 (U.S. Department of Health and Human Services Office of Disease Prevention and Health Promotion, 2016).

In this context, it is clear that the most efficacious and most cost-effective strategy is HPV vaccine prior to the onset of sexual activity (i.e., 11–12 years). As this occurs, the need for (and dollars expended on) Pap smears will decline.

Characteristics of Individuals at Risk Several risk factors for cervical cancer have been identified (Chelimo, Wouldes, Cameron, & Elwood, 2013). Though the most important of these is HPV exposure (see discussion above), other risk factors include smoking (see discussion above), dietary factors (see discussion above), body weight (see discussion above), age at first sexual intercourse (Louie et al., 2009; Plummer, Peto, & Franceschi, 2012), immunosuppression (Dugue, Rebolj, Garred, & Lynge, 2016), chlamydia infection (Silva, Cerqueiera, & Medeiros, 2014), prenatal exposure to diethylstilbestrol (DES) (Troisi et al., 2016), long-term use of oral contraceptives (Gierisch et al., 2013; La Vecchia & Boccia, 2014), having multiple (≥3) full-term pregnancies (Muñoz et al., 2002), being younger than 17 at first full-term pregnancy (Louie et al., 2009), and socioeconomic status (Froment, Gomez, Roux, Derouen, & Kidd, 2014; Singh, Azuine, & Siahpush, 2012; Ward et al., 2004).

Furthermore, significant disparities in cervical cancer screening exist by race, ethnicity, geographic location, education, and disability status. Specifically, women are less likely to have received a Pap test within the past 3 years if they are non-White (78%, compared to 82.7% of Whites), have a less than high school educational level (68.5%, compared to 87.5% of individuals with an advanced degree), live in a rural area (77.4%, compared to 81.2% of individuals in a metropolitan area), or have a disability (77.8%, compared to 81.7% of persons without disabilities) (U.S. Department of Health and Human Services Office of Disease Prevention and Health Promotion, 2016).

Barriers to Prevention Several studies have examined behavioral predictors of cervical cancer screening for rarely or never-screened women (Hatcher, Studts, Dignan, Turner, & Schoenberg, 2011; Studts, Tarasenko, & Schoenberg, 2013). Factors increasing likelihood of being rarely or never screened included belief that cervical cancer has symptoms, not having a regular source of medical care, belief that screening tests cause worry, employment status, knowing where to access screening, believing that screening is too expensive, and willingness to get a Pap test if one's physician recommended it (Hatcher, Studts, Dignan, Turner, & Schoenberg, 2011). Education, perceived income inadequacy, health status, and type of health insurance coverage were each associated with at least one perceived barrier (Studts, Tarasenko, & Schoenberg, 2013). To further complicate matters, other research has shown that women have poor recall of their history of cervical cancer screening, both in terms of timing and results (Newell, Girgis, Sanson-Fisher, & Ireland, 2000). Of women who reported being adequately screened, 28% were actually inadequately screened. Further, 11% of patients who reported a normal Pap test actually had abnormal or inadequate results. Thus, knowledge of one's history is an additional barrier to appropriate cervical cancer screening.

Guidelines for Prevention The American Cancer Society recommends that cervical cancer screening should begin at age 21 (American Cancer Society, 2015). Screening should occur every 3 years for women 21–29 and every 5 years thereafter. Women should not be screened after age 65. The American Society of Clinical Oncology recommends a slightly different screening pattern: women should be screened every 5 years from age 25 to age 65 (Jeronimo et al., 2016). However, in 2008 only 84.5% of females aged 21–65 years had received cervical cancer screening within the past 3–5 years (U.S. Department of Health and Human Services Office of Disease Prevention and Health Promotion, 2016).

As discussed previously, a large percentage of the U.S. population has not been vaccinated in accordance with current recommendations. Although several national agencies (including the American Cancer Society [ACS], the U.S. Preventative Services Task Force [USPSTF], the American College of Obstetricians and Gynecologists [ACOG], and the Society of Gynecologic Oncology [SCG]) state that vaccination status should not affect cervical cancer screening schedule (Centers for Disease Control and Prevention, 2016), statistical simulation suggests that unvaccinated women may optimally require screening two to three times more frequently than vaccinated women (Accetta et al., 2010; Naber, Matthijsse, Rozemeijer, Penning, & Inge, 2016).

Behavioral Care: Options and Efficacy Behavioral interventions may increase uptake of cervical cancer screening. A Cochrane review of such interventions identified 38 trials (Everett et al., 2014). While heterogeneity between trials limited statistical pooling of data, there seems to be substantial support for invitation letters in increasing uptake. There is limited evidence to support the use of educational materials alone (Everett et al., 2014). Furthermore, physician-based strategies, especially manual and computer-generated reminders, appear to be a very effective approach in the implementation of cervical cancer screening (Kupets & Covens, 2001). Kupets and Covens identified the number of reminders needed to intervene for cervical cancer screening; approximately three physicians need to be exposed to a reminder notice before one physician actually orders the appropriate screening test(s). Thus, authors have suggested that any of these strategies alone may not increase cervical cancer screening to desired rates; rather, multilevel interventions may be necessary (Bastani et al., 2002).

Colorectal Cancer

Nature of the Problem There are two primary methods for screening for colorectal cancer (CRC): fecal occult blood test (FOBT) and colonoscopy. Randomized controlled trials have shown that FOBT can reduce CRC incidence and mortality, and observational studies suggest colonoscopy is effective as well (Walsh & Terdiman, 2003). However, the use of both FOBT and colonoscopy is well below optimal (Meissner, Breen, Klabunde, & Vernon, 2006). Only 52.1% of adults aged 50–75 years received a colorectal cancer screening based on the most recent guidelines in 2008 (U.S. Department of Health and Human Services Office of Disease Prevention and Health Promotion, 2016).

Characteristics of Individuals at Risk Individuals are less likely to have been screened for colorectal cancer if they live in a rural area (55.1%, compared to 58.7% of individuals in a metropolitan area) or have a disability (57.3%, compared to 61.8% of persons without disabilities). When recommended, women are more likely than men (59.1% vs. 57.2%) to be compliant with screening (U.S. Department of Health and Human Services Office of Disease Prevention and Health Promotion, 2016).

Barriers to Prevention Multiple behavioral barriers to screening exist, of which some are remediable (Weitzman, Zapka, Estabrook, & Goins, 2001). Knowledge about colorectal cancer is low, and misperceptions are common (Weitzman, Zapka, Estabrook, & Goins, 2001). For example, two consistent barriers to screening are the beliefs that (a) the test is not needed and (b) the test is embarrassing. (Janz, Wren, Schottenfeld, & Guire, 2003). Furthermore, the psychosocial factor that has been identified as one of the strongest predictors of adherence across studies is knowledge of family history of colorectal cancer (Gili, Roca, Ferrer, Obrador, & Cabeza, 2006; Vernon, 1997). One study compared "users," "attempters," and non-users of colorectal cancer screening (Janz et al., 2007). The importance of psychological decisional factors (e.g., discomfort, concern about complications, anxiety, embarrassment, fear of results) differed significantly by screening status, such that more non-users and attempters reported psychological decisional factors as important compared to users. Among factors interfering with test completion, 38.5% attempting FOBT reported they "forgot" whereas 29.8% attempting colonoscopy were "afraid of pain" (Janz et al., 2007). Finally, preparation for (24-h intake restriction, consumption of bowel pre-liquid) and the time commitment (24 h for preparation, test, and recovery) of screening poses scheduling difficulties and financial drawbacks (e.g., lost wages) for many (Kiviniemi, Bennett, Zaiter, & Marshall, 2011).

Guidelines for Prevention The American Cancer Society currently recommends either fecal occult blood testing (FOBT) every year or colonoscopy every 10 years for all average risk individuals aged 50 years or older (American Cancer Society, 2015). At present, the available evidence does not currently support choosing one test over another. In 2008, only 52.1% of adults aged 50–75 years had received either type of recommended colorectal cancer screening (U.S. Department of Health and Human Services Office of Disease Prevention and Health Promotion, 2016). The U.S. Department of Health and Human Services has set the goal of increasing this number to 70.5% by the year 2020.

Behavioral Care: Options and Efficacy Several effective interventions to promote CRC screening have been identified (Rawl, Menon, Burness, & Breslau, 2012). Morrow, Dallo, and Julka (2010) found that interventions to increase CRC screening had the most robust effects compared to controls when they included patient mailings and/or telephone outreach components. Such interventions were hypothesized to increase awareness among individuals eligible for CRC screening. Holden, Jonas, Porterfield, Reuland, and Harris (2010) and Sabatino et al. (2012) found similar effects for interventions that included patient reminders. Furthermore, there is strong effectiveness evidence for interventions including individual communications to patients by clinic staff, elimination of structural barriers (e.g., simplifying access to FOBT cards, providing FOBT tests and instructions for home use), or system-level changes (e.g., systematic rather than opportunistic screening) (Holden, Jonas, Porterfield, Reuland, & Harris, 2010). As discussed in regards to breast and cervical cancer screening, multifactor interventions that target more than one level of the CRC screening process are likely to have larger effects (Power et al., 2009).

More recently, it has been suggested that the evidence base for improving CRC screening supports a new model of primary care delivery (Klabunde et al., 2007). With it, primary care practices implementing effective systems and procedures for screening are key for improving screening rates. Active engagement and support of practices (i.e., using a team approach, establishment of information systems, increasing patient involvement, changing reimbursement policies, etc.) are essential for the potential of colorectal cancer screening to be realized (Klabunde et al., 2007).

Tertiary Prevention

Tertiary prevention aims to reduce morbidity and minimize the impact of a disease among already-affected individuals. The goal is to reduce or delay disease-related complications, reduce stress, and achieve mental, physical, and social recovery. To do so, research shows biobehavioral interventions can improve tertiary care and reduce disease burden.

Stress

There is enormous stress and quality of life disruption with a cancer diagnosis and treatment. It promotes a cascade of negative sequelae—some biologic, others behavioral—which have their own negative consequences (Andersen, Kiecolt-Glaser, & Glaser, 1994; Golden-Kreutz et al., 2005) and impact the "whole cancer patient" (Adler, Page, & National Institute of Medicine (U.S.). Committee on Psychosocial Services to Cancer Patients/Families in a Community Setting, 2008). If left untreated, stress occurring at the time of cancer diagnosis contributes to lower quality of life, increased depressive and anxiety symptoms, increased adverse effects, and more physical symptoms. In fact, stress and stress-related biologic alterations can elicit symptoms but also "generate" depressive or anxiety disorders (Wu & Andersen, 2010).

CBT has been used for problems such as insomnia and fatigue, and interestingly, depression and anxiety symptoms often improve. For example, CBT for insomnia (CBT-I) (Dirksen & Epstein, 2008; Espie et al., 2008; Fiorentino et al., 2010; Garland et al., 2014; Savard, Simard, Ivers, & Morin, 2005) uses cognitive strategies, education and provision of sleep hygiene information, relaxation training, stimulus control, and sleep restriction. Improvements in subjective (Espie et al., 2008; Fiorentino et al., 2010) and objective (Espie et al., 2008; Fiorentino et al., 2010; Garland et al., 2014) sleep indices, lower frequency of medicated nights (Fiorentino et al., 2010; Savard et al., 2005), and better sleep quality (Fiorentino et al., 2010; Garland et al., 2014) have been reported along with significant reductions in anxiety (Dirksen & Epstein, 2008; Savard et al., 2005) and depressive symptoms (Dirksen & Epstein, 2008; Savard et al., 2005), as well as improvements in mood (Garland et al., 2014) have been found post-treatment. Similarly, CBT for fatigue (Kangas, Bovbjerg, & Montgomery, 2008) uses cognitive restructuring for negative beliefs about fatigue and behavioral strategies such as activity scheduling or increasing exercise. Patients report improvements in fatigue (Gielissen, Verhagen, & Bleijenberg, 2007; Kangas, Bovbjerg, & Montgomery, 2008; Lee, Lim, Yoo, & Kim, 2011; Montgomery et al., 2014), quality of life (Lee, Lim, Yoo, & Kim, 2011), and psychological distress (Gielissen, Verhagen, & Bleijenberg, 2007).

Psychopathology

Nature of the Problem Psychiatric disorders are more prevalent among cancer patients than among those with any other chronic illness (Evans et al., 2005). Though studies vary, the point prevalence estimates are 38.2% for any mood disorder, 20.7% for all types of depression, 10.3% for anxiety disorders, and 19.4% for any adjustment disorder (Mitchell et al., 2011). By comparison, the World Health Organization World Mental Health reports *12-month* prevalence estimates for the U.S. as 9.7% for mood disorders and 19.0% for anxiety disorders (Kessler et al., 2009). Among cancer patients, major depressive disorder (MDD) is the most common psychiatric disorder, with prevalence rates ranging from 10% to 50% (Croyle & Rowland, 2003; Fann et al., 2008; Massie, Gagnon, & Holland, 1994). Anxiety is also common, with prevalence rates ranging from 25% to 48% (Brintzenhofe-Szoc et al., 2009; Burgess et al., 2005; Stark et al., 2002). As is the case for those without concurrent physical illness, depression and anxiety often co-occur among cancer patients. Stark et al. (2002) found that 38% of cancer patients with an anxiety disorder also have MDD.

Tertiary prevention for cancer patients with comorbid psychiatric disorders is imperative, particularly in the case of depression. Functional impairment accompanying major depressive disorder (MDD) is significant and includes poorer physical health, more pain, increased anxiety, substance use, and low quality of life in the areas of relationships, self-care, physical activities, sexual functioning, and sleep, among others (Burgess et al., 2005; Chida, Hamer, Wardle, & Steptoe, 2008; Ciaramella & Poli, 2001; Evans et al., 2005; Fortner, Stepanski, Wang, Kasprowicz, & Durrence, 2002; Lev et al., 2001; Lundberg & Passik, 1997; Williamson, 2000). Economic issues also are consequential in that cancer patients with depression spend more time with physicians, have more frequent hospital and primary care visits, and have higher healthcare costs (Carlson & Bultz, 2004; Chirikos, Mph, & Jacobsen, 2008; Hewitt & Rowland, 2002). In general, depression is a risk factor for premature mortality (RR = 1.22–1.39) (Kang et al., 2009; Mozaffari et al., 2009), but this is particularly true for cancer patients (Chida, Hamer, Wardle, & Steptoe, 2008). For breast cancer patients, for example, both cancer death (RR = 1.18) (Kang et al., 2009) and all-cause death rates (RR = 1.31) (Standish et al., 2008) are elevated; conversely, a decrease in depressive symptoms is associated with longer survival (Wiltschke et al., 1995).

Characteristics of Individuals at Risk Risk factors for psychiatric disorders include familial history (positive), gender (female), partner/marital status (alone), low socioeconomic status (SES), and others, such as a pre-cancer history of mood and anxiety disorders (Breitbart, 1995; Morasso et al., 2001) (see Table 14.1). Additionally, data show that high levels of stress and/or depressive symptoms at diagnosis/treatment are long-term limiting factors and place individuals at risk for future symptoms (Andersen, Goyal, Westbrook, Bishop, & Carson, 2017). Even when early symptoms decline, patients may experience no further improvement in stress and/or return to earlier, higher depressive symptom levels. These patterns underscore the importance of tertiary prevention and the recommendation to screen patients at the time of diagnosis for symptoms of depression and anxiety (Andersen et al., 2014). The data also show that the absolute levels of symptoms at diagnosis/treatment best predict risk. Thus, patients with higher stress levels are in need of early, evidence-based, psychological treatment not only to lower current stress but to prevent its maintenance and the poorer quality of life which follows (Andersen et al., 2004, 2008, 2010).

Barriers While it is known that both depression and anxiety are prevalent among cancer patients, discussions about psychosocial difficulties and referral to psychosocial services often do not occur. It is estimated that 7.6 million cancer survivors in the U.S. have not discussed their psychosocial functioning with healthcare providers (Forsythe et al., 2013) in spite of Institute of Medicine (IOM) recommendations for providers to have such discussions. Studies suggest that patients are aware of their need to deal with emotional problems, want their medical team to ask and offer emotional help (Miller, Pittman, & Strong, 2003), and have generally positive views of psychosocial services (Owen, Goldstein, Lee, Breen, & Rowland, 2007). However, except for the most obvious symptoms such as suicidal ideation (Oquendo et al., 2004), diagnostic criteria for depression and other disorders may not be known by a medical team (Fallowfield, Ratcliffe, Jenkins, & Saul, 2001), symptoms may be trivialized as a "normal" reaction or interpreted as due only to impaired physical status (Evans et al., 2005). Studies show that even when significant symptoms are detected, their severity is underestimated or undertreated (Keller et al., 2000, 2004; McDonald et al., 1999; Newell, Sanson-Fisher, Girgis, & Bonaventura, 1998; Singer et al., 2011). In addition to lack of symptom relief, the absence of treatment brings further sequelae (Fann et al., 2008)—more symptom distress (Mystakidou et al., 2005; Sadler et al., 2002; Smith, Gomm, & Dickens, 2003), less meaning in life (Carver & Antoni, 2004; Simonelli, Fowler, Maxwell, & Andersen, 2008), less social support (Parker, Baile, de Moor, & Cohen, 2003; Schroevers, Ranchor, & Sanderman, 2003), maladaptive coping (Carver et al., 1993), and employment absenteeism (Shelby, Golden-Kreutz, & Andersen, 2008), among others. Treatments can successfully address these problems (Faller et al., 2013; Stanton, 2006) and has the potential to reduce the risk of recurrence (Andersen et al., 2008) or cancer death (Andersen et al., 2010; Giese-Davis et al., 2011; Hjerl et al., 2003; Pinquart & Duberstein, 2010). Unfortunately, evidence-based treatments (EBTs) are underutilized in clinical practice as dissemination of EBTs has been extremely slow and training opportunities for providers scarce. This is in spite of the hundreds of RCTs (Andersen, 1992, 2002; Osborn, Demoncada, & Feuerstein, 2006) that have tested psychosocial treatments and found them efficacious for cancer patients.

Guidelines Two national forces provide impetus for recognition of psychopathology and provision of treatment. In 2012 the Commission on Cancer of the American College of Surgeons (CoC) defined stringent new patient-centered quality standards for accreditation of 1500+ cancer clinics and hospitals. According to Standard 3.2, all cancer clinics must provide psychosocial services to cancer patients and document the efficacy of doing so. The second is the American Society of Clinical Oncology (ASCO) guidelines (Andersen et al., 2014), specifying that all patients be evaluated for symptoms of depression (Kroenke, Spitzer, & Williams, 2001) and anxiety (Spitzer, Kroenke, Williams, & Löwe, 2006) at periodic times across the trajectory of care. In Table 14.1 the guidelines are summarized. Assessment should be performed using validated, published measures and procedures. Depending on levels of symptoms and supplementary information, differing treatment pathways are recommended: "Psychological and psychosocial interventions should derive from relevant treatment manuals for empirically supported treatments specifying the content and guiding the structure, delivery mode, and duration of the intervention." Taken together, CoC specifies the necessity and ASCO specifies the means for cancer centers—large and small and urban and rural—to assess and provide treatment when indicated.

Behavioral Care: Options and Efficacy Efficacious treatments exist for moderate to severe symptoms (Cuijpers et al., 2014; Delgado & Zarkowski, 2004; Rapaport et al., 2006). Among psychotherapies, cognitive behavioral therapy (CBT) (Butler, Chapman, Forman, & Beck, 2006; Dimidjian et al., 2006) is the treatment of choice and is an effective treatment for both mood and anxiety disorders (Hofmann, Asnaani, Vonk, Sawyer, & Fang, 2012). CBT is more effective than control conditions (Beltman, Oude Voshaar, & Speckens, 2010; Hofmann, Asnaani, Vonk, Sawyer, & Fang, 2012; van Straten, Geraedts, Verdonck-de Leeuw, Andersson, & Cuijpers, 2010) and in RCTs, as effective as antidepressant medication (ADM) (Strunk & DeRubeis, 2001). Even among the severely depressed, Hollon et al. (2005) found that both CBT and ADM produced comparable results (about 58% treatment responders) during the acute phase, but when discontinued, patients treated with CBT were at lower risk for relapse for upward of 2 years than those treated with ADM.

CBT for depression has three components (Beck, Rush, Shaw, & Emery, 1979). *Behavioral activation* involves efforts to increase patients' engagement in activities and contexts that may allow them to experience pleasure or a sense of accomplishment; behavioral activation is also done to promote cognitive change (Jacobson, Martell, & Dimidjian, 2001). Secondly, *correcting negative automatic thoughts* is a collaborative process when therapist and client work together to identify and evaluate depressive thinking accompanying patients' negative mood states. Once patients have mastered these and other basic skills (e.g., problem solving, assertive communication), therapists assist clients to *identify and change core beliefs and schemas*, which, more generally, underlie a depressed patient's pervasive, negative beliefs. Research suggests that all three components are important, although some studies show that behavioral therapy, such as behavioral activation, is sufficient (Dimidjian et al., 2006).

Table 14.1 American Society of Clinical Oncology recommendations for screening, assessment, and treatment in the management of symptoms of depression and anxiety in adults with cancer

Screening, assessment, and treatment: Depression in adults with cancer		
Level of symptomatology determined by the PHQ-9[a]	Further assessment	Treatment
None/mild Score 1–7		Offer referral to supportive care services
Moderate Score 8–14 or Moderate to severe Score 15–19 or Severe Score 20–27	Identify pertinent history/ specific risk factors for depression: Family history Prior depressive disorder Psychiatric history Disease severity Gender Partner status Presence of other chronic illness Employment/SES	Moderate: low-intensity intervention options include Individually guided self-help based on CBT Group-based CBT for depression Group-based psychosocial interventions Structured physical activity program Pharmacologic intervention, as appropriate
		Moderate to severe: high-intensity intervention options include Individual psychotherapy (CBT, interpersonal therapy) Pharmacologic intervention Combination of psychotherapy and pharmacologic intervention
Screening, assessment, and treatment: Anxiety in adults with cancer		
Level of symptomatology determined by the GAD-7[b]	Further assessment	Treatment
None/mild Score 0–4, 5–9		Offer referral to supportive care services
Moderate Score 10–14 or Moderate to severe Score 15–21	Identify pertinent history/ specific risk factors for (generalized) anxiety: Family history Psychiatric history History/presence of alcohol or substance abuse Presence of other chronic illness	Moderate: low-intensity intervention options include Education and active monitoring Non-facilitated or guided self-help based on CBT Group psychosocial intervention Pharmacologic intervention, as appropriate
		Moderate to severe: high-intensity intervention options include Individual psychotherapy (CBT, applied relaxation) Pharmacologic intervention Combination of psychotherapy and pharmacologic intervention

[a]*PHQ-9* Patient Health Questionnaire Nine-Symptom Depression Scale (Kroenke et al., 2001)
[b]*GAD-7* Generalized Anxiety Disorder 7-item (Spitzer et al., 2006)

An Example: CBT for Cancer Patients with Mood and Anxiety Disorders

A number of meta-analyses have examined the efficacy of psychotherapy for depressed breast cancer patients and generally report moderate effectiveness in reducing symptoms of depression, anxiety, and pain (Fann et al., 2008; Lepore & Coyne, 2006; Newell, Sanson-Fisher, & Savolainen, 2002; Sheard & Maguire, 1999; Williams & Dale, 2006). However, the majority of outcome studies for both depression and anxiety have been criticized as using subsyndromal and unsystematically diagnosed samples (Hopko, Colman, & Carvalho, 2008; Newell, Sanson-Fisher, & Savolainen, 2002; Osborn, Demoncada, & Feuerstein, 2006; Sheard & Maguire, 1999). We provide two exceptions below. These two examples are unique in adapting cognitive behavioral therapy for patients with comorbid MDD.

Cognitive Behavioral Therapy for Cancer Patients (Brothers, Yang, Strunk, & Andersen, 2011). Brothers, Yang, Strunk, and Andersen (2011) combined elements of the biobehavioral intervention (BBI; Andersen, 2002; Andersen et al., 2004) for cancer patients with the core strategies of CBT for depression with cancer survivors ($N = 36$) diagnosed with MDD in a single-arm study. CBT components were, namely, behavioral activation (daily activity/symptom log, activity scheduling, review of successes/obstacles), cognitive reappraisal (thought records, generating alternative thoughts, maintenance), and efficacious components of biobehavioral treatment (progressive muscle relaxation, social support, and assertive communication). A 12–16 session treatment was developed and tested with a mixed gender and mixed disease site and stage (I–IV; recurrence) sample, all meeting criteria for MDD. As is common for those with depression, 53% of the sample had a comorbid anxiety disorder (e.g., generalized anxiety disorder) and 50% had a prior depressive episode. Results showed significant improvement in depressive symptoms as measured by both the Beck Depression Inventory-II (BDI-II; Beck, Steer, & Brown, 1996) and the clinician-rated Hamilton Rating Scale for Depression (HRSD; Williams, 1988), fatigue, and quality of life. Clinically significant reductions occurred for 61% of the patients using the BDI-II criterion and 69% using the HRSD criterion. Importantly, 90% of the treatment completers met criteria for depression remission.

Brief Behavioral Activation Treatment for Depression (*BATD;* Lejuez, Hopko, LePage, Hopko, & McNeil, 2001). Hopko et al. (2008) conducted a RCT comparing behavioral activation component of CBT with problem solving with breast cancer patients ($N = 80$) with diagnosed with MDD using the Anxiety Disorders Interview Schedule-IV (ADIS-IV; Brown, DiNardo, & Barlow, 1994). In BATD, behavioral activation uses structured attempts at engendering increases in overt behaviors that are likely to bring patients into contact with reinforcing environmental contingencies and produce corresponding improvements in thoughts, mood, and overall quality of life (Hopko, Lejuez, Ruggiero, & Eifert, 2003). Initial sessions involved assessing the function of depressed behavior, establishing patient rapport, motivational exercises focused on behavioral change, depression psychoeducation, understanding the relationship between depression and breast cancer, and discussion of the treatment rationale. Subsequent sessions focused on systematically increasing activities with reinforcing environmental contingencies—a necessary precursor toward the reduction of overt and covert depressed behavior. BATD was compared to problem-solving therapy (PST). Problem-solving therapy largely is based on research suggesting that a range of life events or problems have a strong association with psychological well-being (Nezu, 1987). It is designed to attenuate depressive symptoms by assisting patients in generating and developing skills that alleviate life events or problems that interfere with psychosocial functioning (Hegel, Barrett, & Oxman, 2000). Overall, both treatments resulted in improvement across all outcome measures, including self-reported depression (BDI-II), clinician-rated depression (HRSD), somatic anxiety, bodily pain, quality of life, and social functioning. Treatment gains were maintained at the 12-month follow-up, with those in the BATD arm having more post-treatment improvements than those in the PST arm. Follow-up analyses (Hopko et al., 2013) found that both treatments significantly decreased suicidal ideation and increased hopefulness at post-treatment, and this too was maintained at the 12-month follow-up. Based on response (50% reduction in baseline symptoms) and remission criteria (BDI-II < 10), 75% of patients exhibited clinically significant reductions in depression.

These studies provide two different successful demonstrations of CBT for cancer patients with MDD. They suggest that CBT, with or without all of the standard components, is effective for MDD and can be tailored to the unique needs of individuals with a comorbid cancer diagnosis.

Concluding Remarks: Integration of Behavioral Scientists into Primary and Secondary Prevention and Tertiary Cancer Care

The role of the behavioral scientist (psychologist) differs considerably across the levels of cancer prevention reviewed here. For primary prevention, the majority of the efforts occur in public health or community health venues, with fewer in primary care and the fewest within oncology settings. In secondary prevention, cancer screening uptake and follow-up occurs largely in primary care settings. The work of tertiary prevention described above has occurred thus far primarily in large regional centers (i.e., Veterans Affairs hospitals (VAH), comprehensive cancer centers) with little work having come from community facilities or practices. Unlike other chronic illnesses, such as diabetes or cardiovascular disease, current management for oncology patients is remaining in specialty oncology centers or practices with the shift to primary care, even for long-time survivors, occurring very slowly. Thus, behavioral scientists in oncology will contribute in different ways, driven by the level of prevention within which they are focused. Specifically, those in primary prevention will be within public health and system change venues. As such, training, level of integration, barriers to integration, financial considerations, and policy for behavioral scientists are largely level dependent. For this discussion, focus is on behavioral scientists in secondary and tertiary prevention as their roles may have the greatest overlap.

In the literature reviewed, the contributions of behavioral scientists have been within three contexts (Fisher & Dickinson, 2014). First, there is the traditional role of provider to individual patients. This might also include selective consultations with MDs, for example, or meeting with family members. These psychologists often regard themselves as mental health providers rather than health providers. This type of service delivery is the most vulnerable to future continuance, due to its (expensive) requirement of professional time, difficulty with reimbursement (see below), and limited patient access (Kazdin, 2008). A second role for behavioral scientists—and the one in which the greatest contribution have been made—is to develop, apply, and make operational behavioral/psychological assessments and develop, validate, and deliver evidence-based, secondary and tertiary prevention programs or treatments. The third key role has been for behavioral scientists to develop behavioral care for high-risk patient groups. Related to this could be assisting in care coordination, particularly for patients with behavioral issues who may also be high users of health services. However, behavioral scientists in oncology have not taken the lead in this latter area despite their expertise to do so. There are other roles for behavioral scientists (e.g., clinical consultation to the staff, working to improve the organization's functioning in the areas of patient flow, staffing, etc.; Fisher & Dickinson, 2014), but examples of such in oncology are not obvious.

Training

Currently there is no training paradigm that integrates behavioral science and cancer. Perhaps more serious is that psychology's current training programs are not producing sufficient numbers of psychologists trained in patient-centered integrated care in general or that in oncology specifically (Weil et al., 2015). As has been suggested, psychologists need to be competent in integrating psychological services into healthcare settings and practice (Johnson, 2013; Johnson & Marrero, 2016). Training in oncology is limited at both the pre- and postdoctoral levels, with predoctoral training limited to the few graduate programs, primarily in clinical psychology, that have oncology researchers within specialty training in behavioral medicine (e.g., University of Miami) or health psychology (e.g., Ohio State University, University of California—Los Angeles). The extent to which this training provides a readiness for entry into integrated care within internal medicine or oncology environments is variable. Minimum training requirements might include the following: (a) a rigorous "Cancer 101" understanding, e.g., epidemiology, behavioral responses and trajectories, cancer treatments, etc.; (b) familiarity with the behavioral oncology knowledge base, particularly that for empirically supported interventions, and an awareness of oncology-relevant behavioral guidelines; (c) awareness that primary care and oncology settings are ones of high volume where time-focused, circumscribed interventions are normative; and (d) clinical opportunities in which psychology trainees are a part of multidisciplinary primary healthcare teams.

At the postdoctoral level, there have been NIH F32 (National Research Service Award (NRSA) for individual postdoctoral fellows), F99/100 (pathway to independence), or K07 (career independent) awards; however, these are primarily focused on research (rather than clinical) development, training, and mentorship. However, VAH postdoctoral positions often have substantial (e.g., $\geq 50\%$) time dedicated to clinical training and service provision.

Expertise and Role of the Psychologist

Many health system administrators and medical professionals are unaware of what psychologists have to offer (Johnson & Marrero, 2016). Thus, it seems reasonable to ask, "What does the psychologist bring to oncology integrated medical care?" There are three key, unique domains of accomplishment and expertise. They are considered in the context of Raghavan, Bright, and Shadoin's (2008) model showing "patient encounter" in a center circle surrounded by larger, concentric ones of organization, agency, and social policy contributions.

The first key skill is the ability of the behavioral scientist to conceptualize the person, i.e., human behavior and psychological processes, and the environment. This skill is most obvious in providers of behavioral services to the individual, but the skills are generalizable to group and systems. This enables the behavioral scientist to contribute substantively to "macro" assessment, evaluation, and decision-making in departments, larger units, systems of care, and policy. The second key skill is expertise in conceptualizing the assessment of health behaviors and psychological processes. A foundation of clinical psychology is expertise in assessment, be it individuals, groups, or environments. Again, the obvious exemplar is assessment of behavior, cognitions, and psychological responses of the individual patient, but the foundational training of the scientist in assessment, psychometrics, research design, and statistics can be the guideposts for determining patient-reported outcomes, system outcomes, or data for policy decision-making. The third key skill is that to develop, evaluate, and, for some, provide empirically supported behavioral and psychological care. These key areas are made even more contributory by the expertise of behavioral scientists to conceptualize, research, analyze, and interpret data to develop and enhance behavioral healthcare.

Financial Issues in Service Delivery

At present, behavioral healthcare and general physical care are usually supported by different health insurance funding mechanisms, with the former being an insurance "carve out" within general health insurance coverage for the latter. Each has different restrictions on frequency and type of service offered with the fee model being charges for individual visits or "procedures." This is a service model rewarding providers for the volume of services, per se, with no linkage to quality of care. This has been seen as one of the most important external challenges to achieving high-quality patient-centered integrated care. As U.S. healthcare is not a single-payer system but one of thousands, changing the payment model is a major challenge. There are newer models (Kathol, Butler, McAlpine, & Kane, 2010; O'Donnell, Williams, & Kilbourne, 2013) such as the Medicare Payment Advisory Commission (MedPAC) endorsement of "bundled" payments, i.e., managing a patient with cancer is achieved by a set fee, a "bundled payment," for all the services of the healthcare team of which a behavioral scientist might be a part. Another approach might include pay-for-performance or gain-sharing arrangements that are designed to reward providers for efficiently delivering appropriate care (Korda & Eldridge, 2011). Suffice it to say, these issues are evolving; a more complete discussion of these complex issues can be found in Kessler (this volume).

Concluding Remarks

Behavioral scientists must advocate for the integration of behavioral health into cancer prevention and control. Prior accomplishments, particularly those relevant to the delivery of empirically supported treatments, may have little value added, however, unless there is a translation from the research environments of their development and testing to the diversity of clinical settings in oncology where they are needed. Addressing this longstanding gap ("implementation cliff") is complex (Backer, David, & Soucy, 1995; Barlow & McHugh, 2012). There are recent efforts in oncology to conceptualize this problem (Andersen & Dorfman, 2016) and train (Brothers et al., 2015) and support community providers to achieve EBT usage (Ryba, Brothers, & Andersen, 2017). Ultimately, the challenges in the dissemination and implementation of cancer prevention and control behavioral measures are two (Herschell, Kolko, Baumann, & Davis, 2010): (1) Can psychologists in the community be trained and become knowledgeable and skillful in new prevention and control treatment implementations? And (2) how do behavioral scientists' usage of new knowledge/skills improve outcomes for oncology patients? Behavioral scientists have the skills to meet these two challenges.

References

Accetta, G., Biggeri, A., Carreras, G., Lippi, G., Carozzi, F. M., Confortini, M., … Paci, E. (2010). Is human papillomavirus screening preferable to current policies in vaccinated and unvaccinated women? A cost-effectiveness analysis. *Journal of Medical Screening, 17*(4), 181–189.

Adler, N. E., Page, A., & National Institute of Medicine (U.S.). Committee on Psychosocial Services to Cancer Patients/Families in a Community Setting. (2008). *Cancer care for the whole patient: Meeting psychosocial health needs*. Washington, DC: National Academies Press.

Alberg, A. J., & Samet, J. M. (2003). Epidemiology of lung cancer. *Chest, 123*, 21–49.

Alberts, D. S., & Hess, L. M. (Eds.). (2008). *Fundamentals of cancer prevention* (2nd ed.). Berlin, Germany: Springer.

Allen, J., Anton, R. F., Babor, T. F., & Carbonari, J. (1997). Project MATCH secondary a priori hypotheses. *Addiction, 92*(12), 1671–1698.

Alston, C., Paget, L., Halvorson, G., Novelli, B., Guest, J., Mccabe, P., … Rohrbach, V. (2012). *Communicating with patients on health care evidence*. Washington, DC: Institute of Medicine of the National Academies Retrieved from https://nam.edu/wp-content/uploads/2015/06/VSRT-Evidence.pdf

American Cancer Society. (2015). *Guidelines for the early detection of cancer. www.Cancer.Org*. Atlanta, GA: American Cancer Society.

American Cancer Society. (2016a). *Cancer facts & figures*. Atlanta, GA. American Cancer Society

American Cancer Society. (2016b). *Cancer prevention & early detection facts & figures*. Atlanta, GA: American Cancer Society, Inc.

American Cancer Society. (2016c). *Cancer treatment & survivorship facts & figures*. Atlanta, GA: American Cancer Society, Inc.

American Society of Addiction Medicine. (1997). *Public policy statement: On screening for addiction in primary care settings*. Chevy Chase, MD. ASAM News

Andersen, B. L. (1992). Psychological interventions for cancer patients to enhance the quality of life. *Ambulatory Pediatrics, 60*(4), 552–568.

Andersen, B. L. (2002). Biobehavioral outcomes following psychological interventions for cancer patients. *Journal of Consulting and Clinical Psychology, 70*(3), 590–610.

Andersen, B. L., DeRubeis, R. J., Berman, B. S., Gruman, J., Champion, V. L., Massie, M. J., … Rowland, J. H. (2014). Screening, assessment, and care of anxiety and depressive symptoms in adults with cancer: An American Society of Clinical Oncology guideline adaptation. *Journal of Clinical Oncology, 32*(15), 1605–1619.

Andersen, B. L., & Dorfman, C. S. (2016). Evidence-based psychosocial treatment in the community: Considerations for dissemination and implementation. *Psycho-Oncology, 25*(5), 482–490.

Andersen, B. L., Farrar, W. B., Golden-Kreutz, D. M., Glaser, R., Emery, C. F., Crespin, T. R., … Carson, W. E. (2004). Psychological, behavioral, and immune changes after a psychological intervention: A clinical trial. *Journal of Clinical Oncology, 22*(17), 3570–3580.

Andersen, B. L., Kiecolt-Glaser, J. K., & Glaser, R. (1994). A biobehavioral model of cancer stress and disease course. *American Psychologist, 49*(5), 389–404.

Andersen, B. L., Thornton, L. M., Shapiro, C. L., Farrar, W. B., Mundy, B. L., Yang, H. C., & Carson, W. E. (2010). Biobehavioral, immune, and health benefits following recurrence for psychological intervention participants. *Clinical Cancer Research, 16*(12), 3270–3278.

Andersen, B. L., Yang, H.-C., Farrar, W. B., Golden-Kreutz, D. M., Emery, C. F., Thornton, L. M., … Carson, W. E. (2008). Psychologic intervention improves survival for breast cancer patients. *Cancer, 113*(12), 3450–3458.

Andersen, B. L., Godiwala Goyal, N., Westbrook, T. D., Bishop, B., & Carson, W. E., III. (2017). Trajectories of stress, depressive symptoms, and immunity in cancer survivors: Diagnosis to 5 years. *Clinical Cancer Research, 23*(1), 52–61.

Anhang, R., Goodman, A., & Goldie, S. J. (2004). HPV communication: Review of existing research and recommendations for patient education. *CA: a Cancer Journal for Clinicians, 54*(5), 248–259.

Appel, L., Clark, J., Yeh, H.-C., Wang, N.-Y., Coughlin, J., Daumit, G., … Brancati, F. (2011). Comparative effectiveness of weight-loss interventions in clinical practice. *New England Journal of Medicine, 365*(21), 1959–1968.

Aveyard, P., Begh, R., Parsons, A., & West, R. (2012). Brief opportunistic smoking cessation interventions: A systematic review and meta-analysis to compare advice to quit and offer of assistance. *Addiction, 107*(6), 1066–1073.

Babor, T., McRee, B. G., Kassebaum, P. A., Grimaldi, P. L., Ahmed, K., & Bray, J. (2007). Screening, Brief Intervention, and Referral to Treatment (SBIRT): Toward a public health approach to the management of substance abuse. *Substance Abuse, 28*(3), 7–30.

Backer, T. E., David, S. L., & Soucy, G. P. (1995). *Reviewing the behavioral science knowledge base on technology transfer*. United States Government Printing. Rockville, MD.

Ball, L., Leveritt, M., Cass, S., & Chaboyer, W. (2015). Effect of nutrition care provided by primary health professionals on adults' dietary behaviours: A systematic review. *Family Practice, 32*(6), 605–617.

Bardia, A., Tleyjeh, I. M., Cerhan, J. R., Sood, A. K., Limburg, P. J., Erwin, P. J., & Montori, V. M. (2008). Efficacy of antioxidant supplementation in reducing primary cancer incidence and mortality: Systematic review and meta-analysis. *Mayo Clinic Proceedings, 83*(1), 23–34.

Barlow, D. H., & McHugh, R. K. (2012). *Dissemination and implementation of evidence-based psychological interventions*. Oxford, UK: Oxford University Press.

Bastani, R., Berman, B. a., Belin, T. R., Crane, L. A., Marcus, A. C., Nasseri, K., … Henneman, C. E. (2002). Increasing cervical cancer screening among underserved women in a large urban county health system: Can it be done? What does it take? *Medical Care, 40*(10), 891–907.

Beavis, A. L., & Levinson, K. L. (2016). Preventing cervical cancer in the United States: Barriers and resolutions for HPV vaccination. *Frontiers in Oncology, 6*(February), 1–9.

Beck, A. T., Rush, A. J., Shaw, B. F., & Emery, G. (1979). *Cognitive therapy of depression*. New York, NY: Guilford Press.

Beck, A. T., Steer, R. A., & Brown, G. K. (1996). *Manual for beck depression inventory-II*. San Antonio, TX: The Psychological Corporation.

Belardinelli, R., Georgiou, D., Cianci, G., & Purcaro, A. (1999). Randomized, controlled trial of long-term moderate exercise training in chronic heart failure: Effects on functional capacity, quality of life, and clinical outcome. *Circulation, 99*(9), 1173–1182.

Beltman, M. W., Oude Voshaar, R. C., & Speckens, A. E. (2010). Cognitive-behavioural therapy for depression in people with a somatic disease: Meta-analysis of randomised controlled trials. *British Journal of Psychiatry, 197*(1), 11–19.

Bennett, A. T., Patel, D. A., Carlos, R. C., Zochowski, M. K., Pennewell, S. M., Chi, A. M., & Dalton, V. K. (2015). Human papillomavirus vaccine uptake after a tailored, online educational intervention for female university students: A randomized controlled trial. *Journal of Women's Health, 24*(11), 950–957.

Bennett, I., & Chen, J. (2009). The contribution of health literacy to disparities in self-rated health status and preventive health behaviors in older adults. *The Annals of Family Medicine, 7*(3), 204–211.

Bhattarai, N., Prevost, A. T., Wright, A. J., Charlton, J., Rudisill, C., & Gulliford, M. C. (2013). Effectiveness of interventions to promote healthy diet in primary care: Systematic review and meta-analysis of randomised controlled trials. *BMC Public Health, 13*, 1203.

Block, G., Patterson, B., & Subar, A. (1992). Fruit, vegetables, and cancer prevention: A review of the epidemiological evidence. *Nutrition and Cancer, 18*(1), 1–29.

Booth, H. P., Prevost, T. A., Wright, A. J., & Gulliford, M. C. (2014). Effectiveness of behavioural weight loss interventions delivered in a primary care setting: A systematic review and meta-analysis. *Family Practice, 31*(6), 643–653.

Botteri, E., Iodice, S., Bagnardi, S., Raimondi, A. B., Lowenfels, M., & Maisonneuve, P. (2008). Smoking and colorectal Cancer. *JAMA, 300*(23), 2765–2778.

Breen, N., Cronin, K. A., Meissner, H. I., Taplin, S. H., Tangka, F. K., Tiro, J. A., & McNeel, T. S. (2007). Reported drop in mammography: Is this cause for concern? *Cancer, 109*(12), 2405–2409.

Breen, N., & Kessler, L. (1994). Changes in the use of screening mammography: Evidence from the 1987 and 1990 National Health Interview Surveys. *American Journal of Public Health, 84*(1), 62–67.

Breitbart, W. (1995). Identifying patients at risk for, and treatment of major psychiatric complications of cancer. *Supportive Care in Cancer: Official Journal of the Multinational Association of Supportive Care in Cancer, 3*(1), 45–60.

Brewer, N. T., & Fazekas, K. I. (2007). Predictors of HPV vaccine acceptability: A theory-informed, systematic review. *Preventive Medicine, 45*(2–3), 107–114.

Brintzenhofe-Szoc, K. M., Levin, T. T., Yuelin Li, B., Kissane, D. W., Zabora, J. R., & Levin, T. (2009). Mixed anxiety/depression symptoms in a large cancer cohort: Prevalence by cancer type. *Psychosomatics, 50*(4), 383–391.

Brothers, B. M., Carpenter, K. M., Shelby, R. A., Thornton, L. M., Frierson, G. M., Patterson, K. L., & Andersen, B. L. (2015). Dissemination of an evidence-based treatment for cancer patients: Training is the necessary first step. *Translational Behavioral Medicine, 5*(1), 103–112.

Brothers, B. M., Yang, H.-C., Strunk, D. R., & Andersen, B. L. (2011). Cancer patients with major depressive disorder: Testing a biobehavioral/cognitive behavior intervention. *Journal of Consulting and Clinical Psychology, 79*(2), 253–260.

Brown, J., West, R., Beard, E., Michie, S., Shahab, L., & McNeill, A. (2014). Prevalence and characteristics of e-cigarette users in Great Britain: Findings from a general population survey of smokers. *Addictive Behaviors, 39*(6), 1120–1125.

Brown, T. A., DiNardo, P. A., & Barlow, D. H. (1994). *Anxiety disorders interview schedule for DSM-IV (ADIS-IV)*. San Antonio, TX: Psychological Corporation.

Bruera, E., Sweeney, C., Calder, K., Palmer, L., & Benisch-tolley, S. (2001). Patient preferences versus physician perceptions of treatment decisions in cancer care. *Journal of Clinical Oncology, 19*(11), 2883–2885.

Bruera, E., Willey, J. S., Palmer, J. L., & Rosales, M. (2002). Treatment decisions for breast carcinoma: Patient preferences and physician perceptions. *Cancer, 94*, 2076–2080.

Buller, D. B., Morrill, C., Taren, D., Aickin, M., Sennott-Miller, L., Buller, M. K., … Wentzel, T. M. (1999). Randomized trial testing the effect of peer education at increasing fruit and vegetable intake. *Journal of the National Cancer Institute, 91*(17), 1491–1500.

Burgess, C., Cornelius, V., Love, S., Graham, J., Richards, M., & Ramirez, A. (2005). Depression and anxiety in women with early breast cancer: Five year observational cohort study. *British Medical Journal, 330*(7493), 702.

Burk, R. D., Ho, G. Y., Beardsley, L., Lempa, M., Peters, M., & Bierman, R. (1996). Sexual behavior and partner characteristics are the predominant risk factors for genital human papillomavirus infection in young women. *The Journal of Infectious Diseases, 174*(4), 679–689.

Butler, A. C., Chapman, J. E., Forman, E. M., & Beck, A. T. (2006). The empirical status of cognitive-behavioral therapy: A review of meta-analyses. *Clinical Psychology Review, 26*(1), 17–31.

Butryn, M. L., Webb, V., & Wadden, T. A. (2011). Behavioral treatment of obesity. *Psychiatric Clinics of North America, 34*(4), 841–859.

Cabana, M., Rand, C., Powe, N., Wu, A. W., Wilson, M., Abboud, P.-A. C., & Rubin, H. (1999). Why don't physicians follow clinical practice guidelines. *JAMA: The Journal of the American Medical Association, 282*, 1458–1465.

Carlson, L. E., & Bultz, B. D. (2004). Efficacy and medical cost offset of psychosocial interventions in cancer care: Making the case for economic analyses. *Psycho-Oncology, 13*(12), 837–849.

Carney, P. A., O'Malley, J., Buckley, D. I., Mori, M., Lieberman, D. A., Fagnan, L. J., … Morris, C. (2012). Influence of health insurance coverage on breast, cervical, and colorectal cancer screening in rural primary care settings. *Cancer, 118*(24), 6217–6225.
Carr, W. P., Maldonado, G., Leonard, P. R., Halberg, J. U., Church, T. R., Mandel, J. H., … Mandel, J. S. (1994). Mammogram utilization among farm women. *The Journal of Rural Health, 12*(4), 278–290.
Carver, C. S., & Antoni, M. H. (2004). Finding benefit in breast cancer during the year after diagnosis predicts better adjustment 5 to 8 years after diagnosis. *Health Psychology: Official Journal of the Division of Health Psychology, American Psychological Association, 23*(6), 595–598.
Carver, C. S., Pozo, C., Harris, S. D., Noriega, V., Scheier, M. F., Robinson, D. S., … Clark, K. C. (1993). How coping mediates the effect of optimism on distress: A study of women with early stage breast cancer. *Journal of Personality and Social Psychology, 65*(2), 375–390.
Castellsagué, X., & Muñoz, N. (2003). Chapter 3: Cofactors in human papillomavirus carcinogenesis--role of parity, oral contraceptives, and tobacco smoking. *Journal of the National Cancer Institute. Monographs, 31*, 20–28.
Center for Disease Control. (2012). Vital signs: Binge drinking prevalence, frequency, and intensity among adults — United States, 2010. *Morbidity and Mortality Weekly Report, 61*(1), 14–19.
Centers for Disease Control and Prevention. (2016). *Cervical cancer screening guidelines for average-risk women [Internet]*. Bethesda, MD: Centers for Disease Control [cited August 15, 2016]. Available from: https://www.cdc.gov/cancer/cervical/pdf/guidelines.pdf
Centers for Medicare and Medicaid Services. (2011). *Decision memo for intensive behavioral therapy for obesity [Internet]*. Baltimore, MD: Centers for Medicare and Medicaid Services [cited August 15, 2016]. Available from: https://www.cms.gov/medicare-coveragedatabase/details/nca-decision-memo.aspx?&NcaName=Intensive%20Behavioral%20Therapy%20for%20Obesity&bc=ACAAAAAAIAAA&NCAId=253
Chan, J. M., Gann, P. H., & Giovannucci, E. L. (2005). Role of diet in prostate cancer development and progression. *Journal of Clinical Oncology, 23*(32), 8152–8160.
Chelimo, C., Wouldes, T. A., Cameron, L. D., & Elwood, J. M. (2013). Risk factors for and prevention of human papillomaviruses (HPV), genital warts and cervical cancer. *Journal of Infection, 66*(3), 207–217.
Chida, Y., Hamer, M., Wardle, J., & Steptoe, A. (2008). Do stress-related psychosocial factors contribute to cancer incidence and survival? *Nature Clinical Practice Oncology, 5*(8), 466–475.
Chirikos, T. N., Mph, A. R., & Jacobsen, P. B. (2008). Functional impairment and the economic consequences of female breast Cancer. *Women & Health, 242*(May 2015), 37–41.
Cho, Y. I., Lee, S.-Y. D., Arozullah, A. M., & Crittenden, K. S. (2008). Effects of health literacy on health status and health service utilization amongst the elderly. *Social Science & Medicine, 66*(8), 1809–1816.
Ciaramella, A., & Poli, P. (2001). Assessment of depression among cancer patients: The role of pain, cancer type and treatment. *Psycho-Oncology, 10*(2), 156–165.
Clifford, G., Gallus, S., Herrero, R., Munoz, N., Snijders, P. J. F., Vaccarella, S., … Franceschi, S. (2005). Worldwide distribution of human papillomavirus types in cytologically normal women in the International Agency for Research on Cancer HPV prevalence surveys: A pooled analysis. *Lancet, 366*, 991–998.
Cobb, N. K., Byron, M. J., Abrams, D. B., & Shields, P. G. (2010). Novel nicotine delivery systems and public health: The rise of the E-cigarette. *American Journal Public Health, 100*(12), 2340–2342.
Cole, A. M., Keppel, G. A., Andrilla, H. A., Cox, C. M., & Baldwin, L.-M. (2016). Primary care patients' willingness to participate in comprehensive weight loss programs: From the WWAMI region practice and research network. *The Journal of the American Board of Family Medicine, 29*(5), 572–580.
Coloma-Carmona, A., Carballo, J. L., & Tirado-González, S. (2016). Barriers for identification and treatment of problem drinkers in primary care. *Gaceta Sanitaria, xx*, 5–9.

Croyle, R. T., & Rowland, J. H. (2003). Mood disorders and cancer: A National Cancer Institute perspective. *Biological Psychiatry, 54*(3), 191–194.
Cuijpers, P., Sijbrandij, M., Koole, S., Huibers, M., Berking, M., & Andersson, G. (2014). Psychological treatment of generalized anxiety disorder: A meta-analysis. *Clinical Psychology Review, 34*(2), 130–140.
Dagnelie, P. C., Schuurman, A. G., Goldbohm, R. A., & Van Den Brandt, P. A. (2004). Diet, anthropometric measures and prostate cancer risk: A review of prospective cohort and intervention studies. *BJU International, 93*(8), 1139–1150.
Danaei, G., Vander Hoorn, S., Lopez, A. D., Murray, C. J. L., & Ezzati, M. (2005). Causes of cancer in the world: Comparative risk assessment of nine behavioural and environmental risk factors. *Lancet, 366*(9499), 1784–1793.
Davis, T. C., Arnold, C., Berkel, H., & Nandy, I. (1996). Knowledge and attitude on screening mammography among low-literate, low-income women. *Cancer, 78*, 1912–1920.
Davis, T. C., Dolan, N. C., Ferreira, M. R., Tomori, C., Green, K. W., Sipler, A. M., & Bennett, C. L. (2001). The role of inadequate health literacy skills in colorectal cancer screening. *Cancer Investigation, 19*(2), 193–200.
Davis, T. C., Holcombe, R. F., Berkel, H. J., Pramanik, S., & Divers, S. G. (1998). Informed consent for clinical trials: A comparative study of standard versus simplified forms. *Journal of the National Cancer Institute, 90*(9), 668–674.
Davis, T. C., Rademaker, A., Bennett, C. L., Wolf, M. S., Carias, E., Reynolds, C., … Arnold, C. L. (2014). Improving mammography screening among the medically underserved. *Journal of General Internal Medicine, 29*(4), 628–635.
Davis, T. C., Williams, M. V., Marin, E., Parker, R. M., & Glass, J. (2002). Health literacy and cancer communication. *CA: a Cancer Journal for Clinicians, 52*(3), 134–149.
De Sanjosé, S., Diaz, M., Castellsagué, X., Cliff, G., Bruni, L., Muñoz, N., & Bosch, F. X. (2007). Worldwide prevalence and genotype distribution of cervical human papillomavirus DNA in women with normal cytology : A meta-analysis. *The Lancet Infectious Diseases, 7*, 453–459.
Delgado, P. L., & Zarkowski, P. (2004). Treatment of mood disorders. In D. J. Panksepp (Ed.), *Textbook of biological psychiatry* (pp. 231–266). Hoboken, NJ: Wiley-Liss.
Dennis, M. L., Perl, H. I., Huebner, R. B., & McLellan, A. T. (2000). Twenty-five strategies for improving the design, implementation and analysis of health services research related to alcohol and other drug abuse treatment. *Addiction (Abingdon, England), 95 Suppl, 3*(February), S281–S308.
Dietz, N. A., Sly, D. F., Lee, D. J., Arheart, K. L., & McClure, L. A. (2013). Correlates of smoking among young adults: The role of lifestyle, attitudes/beliefs, demographics, and exposure to anti-tobacco media messaging. *Drug and Alcohol Dependence, 130*(1–3), 115–121.
Dimidjian, S., Hollon, S. D., Dobson, K. S., Schmaling, K. B., Kohlenberg, R. J., Addis, M. E., … Jacobson, N. S. (2006). Randomized trial of behavioral activation, cognitive therapy, and antidepressant medication in the acute treatment of adults with major depression. *Journal of Consulting and Clinical Psychology, 74*(4), 658–670.
Dirksen, S. R., & Epstein, D. R. (2008). Efficacy of an insomnia intervention on fatigue, mood and quality of life in breast cancer survivors. *Journal of Advanced Nursing, 61*(6), 664–675.
Doescher, M. P., & Jackson, J. E. (2009). Trends in cervical and breast cancer screening practices among women in rural and urban areas of the United States. *Journal of Public Health Management and Practice, 15*(3), 200–209.
Dugue, P.-A., Rebolj, M., Garred, P., & Lynge, E. (2016). Immunosuppression and risk of cervical cancer. *Expert Review of Anticancer Therapy, 13*(1), 29–42.
Edwards, B. K., Ward, E., Kohler, B. A., Eheman, C., Zauber, A. G., Anderson, R. N., … Ries, L. A. G. (2010). Annual report to the nation on the status of cancer, 1975-2006, featuring colorectal cancer trends and impact of interventions (risk factors, screening, and treatment) to reduce future rates. *Cancer, 116*(3), 544–573.

Elewonibi, B. R., Thierry, A. D., & Miranda, P. Y. (2016). Examining mammography use by breast cancer risk, race, nativity, and socioeconomic tatus. *Journal of Immigrant and Minority Health. 20*(1), 59–65

Elnicki, D. M., Morris, D. K., & Schockor, W. T. (1995). Patient-perceived barriers to preventive health care among indigent, rural appalachian patients. *Archives of Internal Medicine, 155*, 421–424.

Emmons, K. M. (2012). Behavioral medicine and the health of our nation: Accelerating our impact. *Annals of Behavioral Medicine, 43*(2), 153–161.

Engeland, A., Andersen, A., Haldorsen, T., & Tretli, S. (1996). Smoking habits and risk of cancers other than lung cancer: 28 years' follow-up of 26,000 Norwegian men and women. *Cancer Causes & Control: CCC, 7*(3), 497–506.

Engelman, K. K., Hawley, D. B., Gazaway, R., Mosier, M. C., Ahluwalia, J. S., & Ellerbeck, E. F. (2002). Impact of geographic barriers on the utilization of mammograms by older rural women. *Journal of the American Geriatrics Society, 50*(1), 62–68.

Epling, J. W., Morley, C. P., & Ploutz-Snyder, R. (2011). Family physician attitudes in managing obesity: A cross-sectional survey study. *BMC Research Notes, 4*, 473.

Espie, C. A., Fleming, L., Cassidy, J., Samuel, L., Taylor, L. M., White, C. A., … Paul, J. (2008). Randomized controlled clinical effectiveness trial of cognitive behavior therapy compared with treatment as usual for persistent insomnia in patients with cancer. *Journal of Clinical Oncology, 26*(28), 4651–4658.

Evans, D. L., Charney, D. S., Lewis, L., Golden, R. N., Gorman, J. M., Krishnan, K. R. R., … Valvo, W. J. (2005). Mood disorders in the medically ill: Scientific review and recommendations. *Biological Psychiatry, 58*(3), 175–189.

Everett, T., Bryant, A., Griffin, M. F., Martin-hirsch, P. P. L., & Carol, A. (2014). Interventions targeted at women to encourage the uptake of cervical screening. *Cochrane Database of Systematic Reviews*, (5), CD002834

Fairchild, A. L., Bayer, R., & Colgrove, J. (2014). The renormalization of smoking? E-cigarettes and the tobacco "endgame". *New England Journal of Medicine, 370*(4), 293–295.

Faller, H., Schuler, M., Richard, M., Heckl, U., Weis, J., & Kuffner, R. (2013). Effects of psycho-oncologic interventions on emotional distress and quality of life in adult patients with cancer: Systematic review and meta-analysis. *Journal of Clinical Oncology, 31*(6), 782–793.

Fallowfield, L., Ratcliffe, D., Jenkins, V., & Saul, J. (2001). Psychiatric morbidity and its recognition by doctors in patients with cancer. *British Journal of Cancer, 84*(8), 1011–1015.

Fann, J. R., Thomas-Rich, A. M., Katon, W. J., Cowley, D., Pepping, M., McGregor, B. A., & Gralow, J. (2008). Major depression after breast cancer: A review of epidemiology and treatment. *General Hospital Psychiatry, 30*(2), 112–126.

Farrelly, M. C., Davis, K. C., Haviland, M. L., Messeri, P., & Healton, C. G. (2005). Evidence of a dose-response relationship between "truth" antismoking ads and youth smoking prevalence. *American Journal of Public Health, 95*(3), 425–431.

Felix, H., West, D. S., & Bursac, Z. (2008). Impact of USPSTF practice guidelines on clinician weight loss counseling as reported by obese patients. *Preventive Medicine, 47*(4), 394–397.

Ferketich, A. K., Pennell, M., Seiber, E. E., Wang, L., Farietta, T., Jin, Y., & Wewers, M. E. (2014). Provider-delivered tobacco dependence treatment to medicaid smokers. *Nicotine and Tobacco Research, 16*(6), 786–793.

Ferlay, J., Soerjomataram, I., Dikshit, R., Eser, S., Mathers, C., Rebelo, M., … Bray, F. (2015). Cancer incidence and mortality worldwide: Sources, methods and major patterns in GLOBOCAN 2012. *International Journal of Cancer, 136*(5), E359–E386.

Fiks, A. G., Grundmeier, R. W., Mayne, S., Song, L., Feemster, K., Karavite, D., … Localio, A. R. (2013). Effectiveness of decision support for families, clinicians, or both on HPV vaccine receipt. *Pediatrics, 131*, 1114–1124.

Final Update Summary: Tobacco Use in Adults and Pregnant Women: Counseling and Interventions. U.S.Preventive Services Task Force. July 2015. https://www.uspreventiveservicestaskforce.org/Page/Document/UpdateSummaryFinal/tobacco-use-in-adults-andpregnant-women-counseling-and-interventions.

Fiore, M. C. (2000). A clinical practice guideline for treating tobacco use and dependence: A US public health service report. *Journal of the American Medical Association, 283*(24), 3244–3254.

Fiorentino, L., Mcquaid, J. R., Liu, L., Natarajan, L., He, F., Lawton, S., … Ancoli-israel, S. (2010). Cancer survivors: A randomized controlled crossover pilot study. *Nature and Science of Sleep, 2*, 1–8.

Fischhoff, B., Bostrom, A., & Quadrell, M. J. (1993). Risk perception and communication. *Annual Review of Public Health, 14*, 183–203.

Fisher, L., & Dickinson, W. P. (2014). Psychology and primary care: New collaborations for providing effective care for adults with chronic health conditions. *The American Psychologist, 69*(4), 355–363.

Foley, O. W., Birrer, N., Rauh-Hain, J. A., Clark, R. M., DiTavi, E., & del Carmen, M. G. (2015). Effect of educational intervention on cervical cancer prevention and screening in hispanic women. *Journal of Community Health, 40*(6), 1178–1184.

Forsythe, L. P., Kent, E. E., Weaver, K. E., Buchanan, N., Hawkins, N. A., Rodriguez, J. L., … Rowland, J. H. (2013). Receipt of psychosocial care among cancer survivors in the United States. *Journal of Clinical Oncology : Official Journal of the American Society of Clinical Oncology, 31*(16), 1961–1969.

Fortner, B. V., Stepanski, E. J., Wang, S. C., Kasprowicz, S., & Durrence, H. H. (2002). Sleep and quality of life in breast cancer patients. *Journal of Pain and Symptom Management, 24*(5), 471–480.

French, D. C., & Dishion, T. J. (2003). Predictors of early initiation of sexual intercourse among high-risk adolescents. *Journal of Early Adolescence, 23*(3), 295–315.

Friedenreich, C. M., Neilson, H. K., & Lynch, B. M. (2010). State of the epidemiological evidence on physical activity and cancer prevention. *European Journal of Cancer, 46*(14), 2593–2604.

Froment, M., Gomez, S. L., Roux, A., Derouen, M. C., & Kidd, E. A. (2014). Impact of socioeconomic status and ethnic enclave on cervical cancer incidence among Hispanics and Asians in California. *Gynecologic Oncology, 133*(3), 409–415.

Fu, L. Y., Bonhomme, L. A., Cooper, S. C., Joseph, J. G., & Zimet, G. D. (2014). Educational interventions to increase HPV vaccination acceptance: A systematic review. *Vaccine, 32*(17), 1901–1920.

Gagliardi, A. R., Faulkner, G., Ciliska, D., & Hicks, A. (2015). Corrigendum to "Factors contributing to the effectiveness of physical activity counselling in primary care: A realist systematic review" [Patient Educ. Couns. 98 (4) (2015) 412–419]. *Patient Education and Counseling, 98*(7), 923. https://doi.org/10.1016/j.pec.2014.11.020

Galuska, D. A., Will, J. C., Serdula, M. K., & Ford, E. S. (1999). Are health care professionals advising obese patients to lose weight? *Journal of the American Medical Association, 282*(16), 1576.

Gandini, S., Merzenich, H., Robertson, C., & Boyle, P. (2000). Meta-analysis of studies on breast cancer risk and diet. *European Journal of Cancer, 36*(5), 636–646.

Gargano, L. M., Herbert, N. L., Painter, J. E., Sales, J. M., Morfaw, C., Rask, K., … Hughes, J. M. (2013). Impact of a physician recommendation and parental immunization attitudes on receipt or intention to receive adolescent vaccines. *Human Vaccines and Immunotherapeutics, 9*(12), 2627–2633.

Garland, S. M., Hernandez-Avila, M., Wheeler, C. M., Perez, G., Harper, D. M., Leodolter, S., … Koutsky, L. a. (2007). Quadrivalent vaccine against human papillomavirus to prevent anogenital diseases. *The New England Journal of Medicine, 356*(19), 1928–1943.

Garland, S. N., Carlson, L. E., Stephens, A. J., Antle, M. C., Samuels, C., & Campbell, T. S. (2014). Mindfulness-based stress reduction compared with cognitive behavioral therapy for the treatment of insomnia comorbid with cancer: A randomized, partially blinded, noninferiority trial. *Journal of Clinical Oncology, 32*(5), 449–457.

Giannuzzi, P., Temporelli, P. L., Marchioli, R., Maggioni, A. P., Balestroni, G., Ceci, V., … Vanuzzu, D. (2008). Global secondary prevention strategies to limit event recurrence after myocardial infarction: Results of the GOSPEL study, a multicenter, randomized controlled trial. *Archives of Internal Medicine, 168*(20), 2194–2204.

Gielissen, M. F. M., Verhagen, C. A. H. H. V. M., & Bleijenberg, G. (2007). Cognitive behaviour therapy for fatigued cancer survivors: Long-term follow-up. *British Journal of Cancer, 97*(5), 612–618.

Gierisch, J. M., Coeytaux, R. R., Urrutia, R. P., Havrilesky, L. J., Moorman, P. G., Lowery, W. J., ... Myers, E. R. (2013). Oral contraceptive use and risk of breast, cervical, colorectal, and endometrial cancers: A systematic review. *Cancer Epidemiology Biomarkers & Prevention, 22*(11), 1931–1944.

Giese-Davis, J., Collie, K., Rancourt, K. M. S., Neri, E., Kraemer, H. C., & Spiegel, D. (2011). Decrease in depression symptoms is associated with longer survival in patients with metastatic breast cancer: A secondary analysis. *Journal of Clinical Oncology, 29*(4), 413–420.

Gili, M., Roca, M., Ferrer, V., Obrador, A., & Cabeza, E. (2006). Psychosocial factors associated with the adherence to a colorectal cancer screening program. *Cancer Detection and Prevention, 30*(4), 354–360.

Golden-Kreutz, D. M., Thornton, L. M., Gregorio, S. W., Frierson, G. M., Jim, H. S., Carpenter, K. M., ... Andersen, B. L. (2005). Traumatic stress, perceived global stress, and life events: Prospectively predicting quality of life in breast cancer patients. *Health Psychology, 24*(3), 288–296.

Goldstein, M. G., Depue, J. D., Monroe, A. D., Lessne, C. W., Rakowski, W., Prokhorov, A., ... Dube, C. E. (1998). A population-based survey of physician smoking cessation. *Preventive Medicine, 27*, 720–729.

Goldstein, M. G., Whitlock, E. P., & DePue, J. (2004). Multiple behavioral risk factor interventions in primary care: Summary of research evidence. *American Journal of Preventive Medicine, 27*(SUPPL), 61–79.

Greaves, C. J., Sheppard, K. E., Abraham, C., Hardeman, W., Roden, M., Evans, P. H., & Schwarz, P. (2011). Systematic review of reviews of intervention components associated with increased effectiveness in dietary and physical activity interventions. *BMC Public Health, 11*(1), 119.

Haasova, M., Warren, F. C., Thompson, T., Ussher, M., & Taylor, A. H. (2016). The association between habitual physical activity and cigarette cravings, and influence of smokers' characteristics in disadvantaged smokers not ready to quit. *Psychopharmacology, 233*(14), 2765–2774.

Hamar, B., Coberley, C., Pope, J., & Rula, E. (2014). Initial evaluation of a scalable lifestyle program for sustained weight loss. *Journal of Obesity & Weight Loss Therapy,* S4, 005

Harper, D. M. (2008). Impact of vaccination with Cervarix(TM) on subsequent HPV-16/18 infection and cervical disease in women 15-25 years of age. *Gynecologic Oncology, 110*, S11–S17.

Hatcher, J., Studts, C. R., Dignan, M. B., Turner, L. M., & Schoenberg, N. E. (2011). Predictors of cervical cancer screening for rarely or never screened rural Appalachian women. *Journal of Health Care for the Poor and Underserved, 22*(1), 176–193.

Havard, A., Shakeshaft, A. P., Conigrave, K. M., & Doran, C. M. (2012). Randomized controlled trial of mailed personalized feedback for problem drinkers in the emergency department: The shortterm impact. *Alcoholism: Clinical & Experimental Research, 36*(3), 523–531.

Hellberg, D., & Stendahl, U. (2005). The biological role of smoking, oral contraceptive use and endogenous sexual steroid hormones in invasive squamous epithelial cervical cancer. *Anticancer Research, 25*(4), 3041–3046.

Hegel, M. T., Barrett, J. E., & Oxman, T. E. (2000). Training therapists in problem-solving treatment of depressive disorders in primary care: Lessons learned from the "Treatment Effectiveness Project". *Families, Systems, & Health, 18*(4), 423–435.

Henningfield, J. E., & Zaatari, G. S. (2010). Electronic nicotine delivery systems: Emerging science foundation for policy. *Tobacco Control: An International Journal, 19*(2), 89–90.

Henry, K. A., McDonald, K., Sherman, R., Kinney, A. Y., & Stroup, A. M. (2014). Association between individual and geographic factors and nonadherence to mammography screening guidelines. *Journal of Women's Health, 23*(8), 664–674.

Heron, M., & Anderson, R. N. (2016). *Changes in the leading cause of death: Recent patterns in heart disease and cancer mortality, NCHS Data Brief (Vol. 254)*. Hyattsville, MD. U.S.: Department of Health and Human Services.

Herschell, A. D., Kolko, D. J., Baumann, B. L., & Davis, A. C. (2010). The role of therapist training in the implementation of psychosocial treatments: A review and critique with recommendations. *Clinical Psychology Review, 30*(4), 448–466.

Hewitt, M., & Rowland, J. H. (2002). Mental health service use among adult cancer survivors: Analyses of the National Health Interview Survey. *Journal of Clinical Oncology, 20*(23), 4581–4590.

Hirsch, B. R., & Lyman, G. H. (2011). Breast cancer screening with mammography. *Current Oncology Reports, 13*(1), 63–70.

Hjerl, K., Andersen, E. W., Keiding, N., Mouridsen, H. T., Mortensen, P. B., & Jørgensen, T. (2003). Depression as a prognostic factor for breast cancer mortality. *Psychosomatics, 44*(1), 24–30.

Hofmann, S. G., Asnaani, A., Vonk, I. J. J., Sawyer, A. T., & Fang, A. (2012). The efficacy of cognitive behavioral therapy: A review of meta-analyses. *Cognitive Therapy Research, 36*(5), 427–440.

Holden, D. J., Jonas, D. E., Porterfield, D. S., Reuland, D., & Harris, R. (2010). Systematic review: Enhancing the use and quality of colorectal cancer screening. *Annals of Internal Medicine, 152*, 668–676.

Hollon, S. D., DeRubeis, R. J., Shelton, R. C., Amsterdam, J. D., Salomon, R. M., O'Reardon, J. P., … Gallop, R. (2005). Prevention of relapse following cognitive therapy vs medications in moderate to severe depression. *Archives of General Psychiatry, 62*(4), 417–422.

Hopko, D. R., Bell, J. L., Armento, M. E. A., Robertson, S. M., Mullane, C., Wolf, N., & Lejuez, C. W. (2008). Cognitive-behavior therapy for depressed cancer patients in a medical care setting. *Behavior Therapy, 39*(2), 126–136.

Hopko, D. R., Colman, L., & Carvalho, J. P. (2008). Depression in cancer patients: Prevalence, impact, assessment, and intervention. *Depression: Mind and Body, 4*, 51–62.

Hopko, D. R., Funderburk, J. S., Shorey, R. C., McIndoo, C. C., Ryba, M. M., File, A. A., … Vitulano, M. (2013). Behavioral activation and problem-solving therapy for depressed breast cancer patients: Preliminary support for decreased suicidal ideation. *Behavior Modification, 37*(6), 747–767.

Hopko, D. R., Lejuez, C. W., Ruggiero, K. J., & Eifert, G. H. (2003). Contemporary behavioral activation treatments for depression: Procedures, principles, and progress. *Clinical Psychology Review, 23*(5), 699–717.

Horner-Johnson, W., Dobbertin, K., & Iezzoni, L. I. (2015). Disparities in receipt of breast and cervical cancer screening for rural women age 18 to 64 with disabilities. *Women's Health Issues : Official Publication of the Jacobs Institute of Women's Health, 25*(3), 246–253.

Hu, F. B., & Willett, W. C. (2002). Optimal diets for prevention of coronary heart disease. *JAMA, 288*(20), 2569–2578.

Huang, J., Yu, H., Marin, E., Brock, S., Carden, D., & Davis, T. (2004). Physicians' weight loss counseling in two public hospital primary care clinics. *Academic Medicine : Journal of the Association of American Medical Colleges, 79*(2), 156–161.

Hughes, J. R. (2009). How confident should we be that smoking cessation treatments work? *Addiction, 104*(10), 1637–1640.

Hutchison, A. J., Breckon, J. D., & Johnston, L. H. (2009). Physical activity behavior change interventions based on the transtheoretical model: A systematic review. *Health Education & Behavior, 36*(5), 829–845.

International Agency for Research on Cancer. (2007). *IARC monographs on the evaluation of carcinogenic risks to humans: Human papillomaviruses (Volume 90)*. Lyon, France: World Health Organization.

IARC Working Group on Cervical Cancer Screening Programs. (1986). Screening for squamous cervical cancer: Duration of low risk after negative results of cervical cytology and its implication for screening policies. *British Medical Journal, 293*(6548), 659–664.

Iodice, S., Gandini, S., Maisonneuve, P., & Lowenfels, A. B. (2008). Tobacco and the risk of pancreatic cancer: A review and meta-analysis. *Langenbeck's Archives of Surgery, 393*(4), 535–545.

Jacobs, D. R., Marquart, L., Slavin, J., & Kushi, L. H. (1998). Whole-grain intake and cancer: An expanded review and meta-analysis. *Nutrition and Cancer, 30*(2), 85–96.

Jacobson, N. S., Martell, C. R., & Dimidjian, S. (2001). Behavioral activation treatment for depression: Returning to contextual roots. *Clinical Psychology: Science and Practice, 8*(3), 255–270.

James, J., Ellis, B. J., Schlomer, G. L., & Garber, J. (2016). Sex-specific pathways to early puberty, sexual debut, and sexual risk taking: Tests of an integrated evolutionary-developmental model. *Developmental Psychology, 48*(3), 687–702.

Janz, N. K., Lakhani, I., Vijan, S., Hawley, S. T., Chung, L. K., & Katz, S. J. (2007). Determinants of colorectal cancer screening use, attempts, and non-use. *Preventive Medicine, 44*(5), 452–458.

Janz, N. K., Wren, P. A., Schottenfeld, D., & Guire, K. E. (2003). Colorectal cancer screening attitudes and behavior: A population-based study. *Preventive Medicine, 37*(6), 627–634.

Jeffery, R. W., Drewnowski, A., Epstein, L. H., Stunkard, A. J., Wilson, G. T., Wing, R. R., & Hill, D. R. (2000). Long-term maintenance of weight loss: Current status. *Health Psychology : Official Journal of the Division of Health Psychology, American Psychological Association, 19*(1), 5–16.

Jensen, M. D., Ryan, D. H., Apovian, C. M., Ard, J. D., Comuzzie, A. G., Donato, K. A., ... Yanovski, S. Z. (2014). 2013 AHA/ACC/TOS guideline for the management of overweight and obesity in adults: A report of the American college of cardiology/American heart association task force on practice guidelines and the obesity society. *Journal of the American College of Cardiology, 63*(25 PART B), 2985–3023.

Jeronimo, J., Castle, P. E., Temin, S., Denny, L., Gupta, V., Kim, J. J., ... Shastri, S. S. (2016). Secondary prevention of cervical cancer: ASCO resource-stratified clinical practice guideline. *Journal of Global Oncology., 3*(5), 635–657.

Jha, P., & Peto, R. (2015). Global effects of smoking, of quitting, and of taxing tobacco — NEJM. *New England Journal of Medicine, 370*, 60–68.

Johns, D. J., Hartmann-Boyce, J., Jebb, S. A., & Aveyard, P. (2014). Diet or exercise interventions vs combined behavioral weight management programs: A systematic review and meta-analysis of directcom parisons. *Journal of the Academy of Nutrition and Dietetics, 114*(10), 1557–1568.

Johnson, S. B. (2013). Increasing psychology's role in health research and health care. *The American Psychologist, 68*(5), 311–321.

Johnson, S. B., & Marrero, D. (2016). Innovations in healthcare delivery and policy: Implications for the role of the psychologist in preventing and treating diabetes. *American Psychologist, 71*(7), 628–637.

Kahn, J. A., Rosenthal, S., Succop, P. A., Ho, G. Y. F., & Burk, R. D. (2002). The interval between menarche and age of first sexual intercourse as a risk factor for subsequent HPV infection in adolescent and young adult women. *Journal of Pediatric Medicine, 141*, 718–723.

Kallings, L. V., Leijon, M., Hellénius, M.-L., & Ståhle, A. (2008). Physical activity on prescription in primary health care: A follow-up of physical activity level and quality of life. *Scandinavian Journal of Medicine & Science in Sports, 18*(2), 154–161.

Kaner, E. F. S., Dickinson, H. O., Beyer, F., Pienaar, E., Schlesinger, C., Campbell, F., ... Heather, N. (2009). The effectiveness of brief alcohol interventions in primary care settings: A systematic review. *Drug and Alcohol Review, 28*(3), 301–323.

Kang, D., Weaver, M., Park, N., Smith, B., McArdle, T., & Carpenter, J. (2009). Significant impairment in immune recovery after cancer treatment. *Nursing Research, 58*(2), 105–114.

Kangas, M., Bovbjerg, D. H., & Montgomery, G. H. (2008). Cancer-related fatigue: A systematic and meta-analytic review of non-pharmacological therapies for cancer patients. *Psychological Bulletin, 134*(5), 700–741.

Kaplan, D. L., Jones, E. J., Olson, C., & Yunzal-Butler, C. B. (2013). Early age of first sex and health risk in an urban adolescent population. *Journal of School Health, 83*, 350–356.
Karlsson, R., Jonsson, M., Edlund, K., Evander, M., Gusavasson, A., Boden, E., … Waddel, G. (1995). Lifetime number of partners as the only independent risk factor or human papillomavirus infection: A population-based study. *Sexually Transmitted Diseases, 22*(2), 119–127.
Kathol, R. G., Butler, M., McAlpine, D. D., & Kane, R. L. (2010). Barriers to physical and mental condition integrated service delivery. *Psychosomatic Medicine, 72*(6), 511–518.
Kazdin, A. E. (2008). Evidence-based treatment and practice – New opportunities to bridge clinical research and practice, enhance the knowledge base, and improve patient care. *American Psychologist, 63*(3), 146–159.
Keefe, F. J. (2011). Behavioral medicine: A voyage to the future. *Annals of Behavioral Medicine, 41*(2), 141–151.
Keller, M., Sommerfeldt, S., Fischer, C., Knight, L., Riesbeck, M., Löwe, B., … Lehnert, T. (2004). Recognition of distress and psychiatric morbidity in cancer patients: A multi-method approach. *Annals of Oncology, 15*(8), 1243–1249.
Keller, M. B., McCullough, J. P., Klein, D. N., Arnow, B., Dunner, D. L., Gelenberg, A. J., … Zajecka, J. (2000). A comparison of nefazodone, the cognitive behavioral-analysis system of psychotherapy, and their combination for the treatment of chronic depression. *New England Journal of Medicine, 342*(20), 1462–1470.
Kempe, K. L., Larson, R. S., Shetterley, S., & Wilkinson, A. (2013). Breast cancer screening in an insured population: Whom are we missing? *The Permanente Journal, 17*(1), 38–44.
Kessler, R. C., Aguilar-Gaxiola, S., Alonso, J., Chatterji, S., Lee, S., Ormel, J., … Wang, P. (2009). The global burden of mental disorders: An update from the WHO World Mental Health (WMH) surveys. *Epidemiologia e Psichiatria Sociale, 18*(1), 23–33.
Kiesler, D. J., & Auerbach, S. M. (2006). Optimal matches of patient preferences for information, decision-making and interpersonal behavior: Evidence, models, and interventions. *Patient Education and Counseling, 61*, 319–341.
Kim, J. J., Salomon, J. A., Weinstein, M. C., & Goldie, S. J. (2006). Packaging health services when resources are limited: The example of a cervical cancer screening visit. *PLoS Medicine, 3*(11), e434.
King, A. C., de Wit, H., McNamara, P. J., & Cao, D. (2011). Rewarding, stimulant, and sedative alcohol responses and relationship to future binge drinking. *Archives of General Psychiatry, 68*(4), 389–399.
King, A. C., Hasin, D., O'Connor, S. J., McNamara, P. J., & Cao, D. (2016). A prospective 5-year re-examination of alcohol response in heavy drinkers progressing in alcohol use disorder. *Biological Psychiatry, 79*(6), 489–498.
King, B. A., Alam, S., Promoff, G., Arrazola, R., & Sube, S. R. (2013). Awareness and ever use of electronic cigarettes among U.S. adults, 2010-2011. *Nicotine & Tobacco Research, 15*(9), 1623–1627.
Kirk, S. F. L., Penney, T. L., McHugh, T.-L. F., & Sharma, A. M. (2012). Effective weight management practice: A review of the lifestyle intervention evidence. *International Journal of Obesity, 36*(2), 178–185.
Kiviniemi, M. T., Bennett, A., Zaiter, M., & Marshall, J. R. (2011). Individual-level factors in colorectal cancer screening: A review of the literature on the relation of individual-level health behavior constructs and screening behavior. *Psycho-Oncology, 20*(10), 1023–1033.
Kjaer, S. K., Chackerian, B., van den Brule, A. J. C., Svare, E. I., Paull, G., Walbomers, J. M. M., … Meijer, C. L. M. (2001). High-risk human papillomavirus is sexually transmitted: Evidence from a follow-up study of virgins starting sexual activity (intercourse). *Cancer Epidemiology Biomarkers & Prevention, 10*, 101–106.
Kjaer, S. K., Van Den Brule, A. J. C., Bock, J. E., Poll, P. A., Engholm, G., Sherman, M. E., … Meijer, C. J. L. M. (1997). Determinants for genital human papillomavirus (HPV) infection in 1000 randomly chosen young Danish women with normal pap smear: Are there different risk

profiles for oncogenic and nononcogenic HPV types? *Cancer Epidemiology Biomarkers & Prevention, 6*, 799–805.
Klabunde, C. N., Lanier, D., Breslau, E. S., Zapka, J. G., Fletcher, R. H., Ransohoff, D. F., & Winawer, S. J. (2007). Improving colorectal cancer screening in primary care practice: Innovative strategies and future directions. *Journal of General Internal Medicine., 22*(8), 1195–1205.
Klatsky, A. L., Li, Y., Nicole Tran, H., Baer, D., Udaltsova, N., Armstrong, M. A., & Friedman, G. D. (2015). Alcohol intake, beverage choice, and cancer: A cohort study in a large kaiser permanente population. *The Permanente Journal, 19*(2), 28–34.
Koh, H. K., & Sebelius, K. G. (2010). Promoting prevention through the Affordable Care Act. *New England Journal of Medicine, 363*(14), 1296–1299.
Kolonel, L. N. (2001). Fat, meat, and prostate cancer. *Epidemiologic Reviews, 23*(1), 72–81.
Korda, H., & Eldridge, G. N. (2011). Payment incentives and integrated care delivery: Levers for health system reform and cost containment. *Inquiry, 48*(4), 277–287.
Kreps, G. L. (2003). The impact of communication on cancer risk, incidence, morbidity, mortality, and quality of life. *Health Communication, 15*(2), 161–169.
Kroenke, K., Spitzer, R. L., & Williams, J. B. W. (2001). The PHQ-9. *Journal of General Internal Medicine, 16*(9), 606–613.
Kruse, J., & Phillips, D. M. (1987). Factors influencing women's decision to undergo mammography. *Obstetrics & Gynecology, 70*(5), 744–748.
Kupets, R., & Covens, a. (2001). Strategies for the implementation of cervical and breast cancer screening of women by primary care physicians. *Gynecologic Oncology, 83*(2), 186–197.
La Vecchia, C., & Boccia, S. (2014). Oral contraceptives, human papillomavirus and cervical cancer. *European Journal of Cancer Prevention, 23*, 110–112.
Lancaster, T., & Stead, L. F. (2005). Individual behavioural counselling for smoking cessation. *Cochrane Database of Systematic Reviews*, (2), CD001292.
Landy, M. S. H., Davey, C. J., Quintero, D., Pecora, A., & McShane, K. E. (2016). A systematic review on the effectiveness of brief interventions for alcohol misuse among adults in emergency departments. *Journal of Substance Abuse Treatment, 61*, 1–12.
Lannin, D. R., Mathews, H. F., Mitchell, J., Swanson, M. S., Swanson, F. H., & Edwards, M. S. (1998). Influence of socioeconomic and cultural factors on racial differences in late-stage presentation of breast cancer. *JAMA : The Journal of the American Medical Association, 279*(22), 1801–1807.
Lantz, P. M., Weigers, M. E., & House, J. S. (1997). Education and income differentials in breast and cervical cancer screening. Policy implications for rural women. *Medical Care, 35*(3), 219–236.
Lee, H., Lim, Y., Yoo, M.-S., & Kim, Y. (2011). Effects of a nurse-led cognitive-behavior therapy on fatigue and quality of life of patients with breast cancer undergoing radiotherapy: An exploratory study. *Cancer Nursing, 34*(6), E22–E30.
Légaré, F., Politi, M. C., Desroches, S., Stacey, D., & Bekker, H. (2012). Training health professionals in shared decision-making: An international environmental scan. *Patient Education and Counseling, 88*, 159–169.
Légaré, F., Ratté, S., Gravel, K., & Graham, I. D. (2008). Barriers and facilitators to implementing shared decision-making in clinical practice: Update of a systematic review of health professionals' perceptions. *Patient Education and Counseling, 73*(3), 526–535.
Légaré, F., Stacey, D., Turcotte, S., Cossi, M. J., Kryworuchko, J., Graham, I. D., … Elwyn, G. (2014). Interventions for improving the adoption of shared decision making by healthcare professionals (Review). *Cochrane Database of Systematic Reviews*, (9), CD006732.
Légaré, F., Turcotte, S., Dawn, S., Ratté, S., Kryworuchko, J., & Graham, I. D. (2012). Patients' perceptions of sharing in decisions: A systematic review of interventions to enhance shared decision making in routine clinical practice. *The Patient - Patient-Centered Outcomes Research, 5*(1), 1–19.

Legler, J., Meissner, H. I., Coyne, C., Breen, N., Chollette, V., & Rimer, B. K. (2002). The effectiveness of interventions to promote mammography among women with historically lower rates of screening. *Cancer Epidemiology Biomarkers and Prevention, 11*(1), 59–71.
Lejuez, C. W., Hopko, D. R., LePage, J. P., Hopko, S. D., & McNeil, D. W. (2001). A brief behavioral activation treatment for depression. *Cognitive and Behavioral Practice, 8*, 164–175.
Lemmens, V., Oenema, A., Knut, I. K., & Brug, J. (2008). Effectiveness of smoking cessation interventions among adults: A systematic review of reviews. *European Journal of Cancer Prevention: The Official Journal of the European Cancer Prevention Organisation (ECP), 17*(6), 535–544.
Lepore, S. J., & Coyne, J. C. (2006). Psychological interventions for distress in cancer patients: A review of reviews. *Annals of Behavioral Medicine: A Publication of the Society of Behavioral Medicine, 32*(2), 85–92.
Leutz, W. N. (1999). Five laws for integrating medical and social services: Lessons from the United States and the United Kingdom. *The Milbank Quarterly, 77*(1), 77–110, iv–v.
Lev, E. L., Daley, K. M., Conner, N. E., Reith, M., Fernandez, C., & Owen, S. V. (2001). An intervention to increase quality of life and self-care self-efficacy and decrease symptoms in breast cancer patients. *Scholarly Inquiry for Nursing Practice, 15*(3), 277–294.
Ley, C., Bauer, H. M., Reingold, A., Schiffman, M. H., Chambers, J. C., Tashiro, C. J., & Manos, M. M. (1991). Determinants of genital human papillomavirus infection in young women. *Journal of the National Cancer Institute, 83*, 997–1003.
Liang, P. S., Chen, T., & Giovannucci, E. (2009). Cigarette smoking and colorectal cancer incidence and mortality: Systematic review and meta-analysis. *International Journal of Cancer. Journal International Du Cancer, 124*(10), 2406–2415.
Lichtenstein, A. H., Appel, L. J., Brands, M., Carnethon, M., Daniels, S., Franch, H. A., … Wylie-Rosett, J. (2006). Diet and lifestyle recommendations revision 2006: A scientific statement from the American heart association nutrition committee. *Circulation, 114*(1), 82–96.
Lichtenstein, E., Glasgow, R. E., Lando, H. A., Ossip-Klein, D. J., & Boles, S. M. (1996). Telephone counseling for smoking cessation: Rationales and meta-analytic review of evidence. *Health Education Research, 11*(2), 243–257.
Ligibel, J. A., & Strickler, H. D. (2013). Obesity and its impact on breast cancer: Tumor incidence, recurrence, survival, and possible interventions. In *American Society of Clinical Oncology Educational Book/ASCO. American Society of Clinical Oncology. Meeting, 2013* (pp. 52–59).
Lisspers, J., Sundin, O., Ohman, A., Hofman-Bang, C., Rydén, L., & Nygren, A. (2005). Long-term effects of lifestyle behavior change in coronary artery disease: Effects on recurrent coronary events after percutaneous coronary intervention. *Health Psychology: Official Journal of the Division of Health Psychology, American Psychological Association, 24*(1), 41–48.
Longabaugh, R., Donovan, D. M., Karno, M. P., McCrady, B. S., Morgenstern, J., & Tonigan, J. S. (2005). Active ingredients: How and why evidence-based alcohol behavioral treatment interventions work. *Alcoholism, Clinical and Experimental Research, 29*(2), 235–247.
Louie, K., de Sanjose, S., Diaz, M., Castellsague, X., Herrero, R., Meijer, C. J., … Rica, C. (2009). Early age at first sexual intercourse and early pregnancy are risk factors for cervical cancer in developing countries. *British Journal of Cancer, 100*, 1191–1197.
Love, R. R., Brown, R. L., Davis, J. E., Baumann, L. J., Fontana, S. A., & Sanner, L. A. (1993). Frequency and determinants of screening for breast cancer in primary care group practice. *Archives of Internal Medicine, 153*(18), 2113–2117.
Lundberg, J. C., & Passik, S. D. (1997). Alcohol and cancer: A review for psycho-oncologists. *Psycho-Oncology, 6*(4), 253–266.
Madison, K., Schmidt, H., & Volpp, K. R. (2016). Smoking, obesity, health insurance, and health incentives in the Affordable Care Act. *JAMA: The Journal of the American Medical Association, 310*(2), 143–144.
Madras, B. K., Compton, W. M., Avula, D., Stegbauer, T., Stein, J. B., & Clark, H. W. (2009). Screening, brief interventions, referral to treatment (SBIRT) for illicit drug and alcohol use

at multiple healthcare sites: Comparison at intake and 6 months later. *Drug and Alcohol Dependence, 99*(1–3), 280–295.

Marcus, A. C., Heimendinger, J., Wolfe, P., Fairclough, D., Rimer, B. K., Morra, M., … Wooldridge, J. (2001). A randomized trial of a brief intervention to increase fruit and vegetable intake: A replication study among callers to the CIS. *Preventive Medicine, 33*(3), 204–216.

Massie, M. J., Gagnon, P., & Holland, J. C. (1994). Depression and suicide in patients with cancer. *Journal of Pain and Symptom Management, 9*(5), 325–340.

Mayeaux, E. J., Jr., Murphy, P. W., Arnold, C., Davis, T. C., Jackson, R. H., & Sentell, T. (1996). Improving patient education for patients with low literacy skills. *American Family Physician, 53*(1), 205–211.

Mayne, L., & Earp, J. (2003). Initial and repeat mammography screening: Different behaviors/ different predictors. *The Journal of Rural Health, 19*(1), 63–71.

McDonald, M. V., Passik, S. D., Dugan, W., Rosenfeld, B., Theobald, D. E., & Edgerton, S. (1999). Nurses' recognition of depression in their patients with cancer. *Oncology Nursing Forum, 26*(3), 593–599.

McGarr, S. E., Ridlon, J. M., & Hylemon, P. B. (2005). Diet, anaerobic bacterial metabolism, and colon cancer: A review of the literature. *Journal of Clinical Gastroenterology, 39*(2), 98–109.

McGrane, N., Galvin, R., Cusack, T., & Stokes, E. (2015). Addition of motivational interventions to exercise and traditional physiotherapy: A review and meta-analysis. *Physiotherapy (United Kingdom), 101*(1), 1–12.

McMillen, R. C., Gottlieb, M. A., Shaefer, R. M. W., Winickoff, J. P., & Klein, J. D. (2014). Trends in electronic cigarette use among U.S. adults: Use is increasing in both smokers and nonsmokers. *Nicotine & Tobacco Research, 17*(10). https://doi.org/10.1093/ntr/ntu213

McTiernan, A. (2008). Mechanisms linking physical activity with cancer. *Nature Reviews Cancer, 8*(3), 205–211.

Meissner, H. I., Breen, N., Klabunde, C. N., & Vernon, S. W. (2006). Patterns of colorectal cancer screening uptake among men and women in the United States. *Cancer Epidemiology Biomarkers and Prevention, 15*(2), 389–394.

Meissner, H. I., Klabunde, C. N., Breen, N., & Zapka, J. M. (2012). Breast and colorectal cancer screening: U.S. primary care physicians' reports of barriers. *American Journal of Preventive Medicine, 43*(6), 584–589.

Mendy, V. L., & Vargas, R. (2015). Trends in major risk factors for cardiovascular disease among adults in the Mississippi Delta region, Mississippi behavioral risk factor surveillance system, 2001-2010. *Preventing Chronic Disease, 12*, E21.

Michielutte, R., Alciati, M. H., & el Arculli, R. (1999). Cancer control research and literacy. *Journal of Health Care for the Poor and Underserved, 10*(3), 281–297.

Miller, B. E., Pittman, B., & Strong, C. (2003). Gynecologic cancer patients' psychosocial needs and their views on the physician's role in meeting those needs. *International Journal of Gynecological Cancer, 13*(2), 111–119.

Miller, W. R., & Rollnick, S. (2002). *Motivational interviewing: Preparing people for change* (2nd ed.). New York, NY: Guilford Press.

Mitchell, A. J., Chan, M., Bhatti, H., Halton, M., Grassi, L., Johansen, C., & Meader, N. (2011). Prevalence of depression, anxiety, and adjustment disorder in oncological, haematological, and palliative-care settings: A meta-analysis of 94 interview-based studies. *The Lancet Oncology, 12*(2), 160–174.

Mller, W. R., & Rollnick, S. (2002). *Motivational interviewing: Preparing people for change. Journal of chemical information and modeling* (2nd ed.). New York, NY: Guilford Press.

Montgomery, G. H., David, D., Kangas, M., Green, S., Sucala, M., Bovbjerg, D. H., … Schnur, J. B. (2014). Randomized controlled trial of a cognitive-behavioral therapy plus hypnosis intervention to control fatigue in patients undergoing radiotherapy for breast cancer. *Journal of Clinical Oncology, 32*(6), 557–563.

Morasso, G., Costantini, M., Viterbori, P., Bonci, F., Del Mastro, L., Musso, M., ... Venturini, M. (2001). Predicting mood disorders in breast cancer patients. *European Journal of Cancer (Oxford, England : 1990), 37*(2), 216–223.

Morgan, F., Battersby, A., Weightman, A. L., Searchfield, L., Turley, R., Morgan, H., ... Ellis, S. (2016). Adherence to exercise referral schemes by participants – What do providers and commissioners need to know? A systematic review of barriers and facilitators. *BMC Public Health, 16*, 1–11.

Morgenstern, J., & Longabaugh, R. (2000). Cognitive-behavioral treatment for alcohol dependence: A review of evidence for its hypothesized mechanisms of action. *Addiction, 95*(10), 1475–1490.

Morrow, J. B., Dallo, F. J., & Julka, M. (2010). Community-based colorectal cancer screening trials with multi-ethnic groups: A systematic review. *Journal of Community Health, 35*(6), 592–601.

Moyer, V. (2012). Screening for and management of obesity in adults: U.S. preventive services task force recommendation statement. *Annals of Internal Medicine, 157*, 373–378.

Mozaffari, F., Lindemalm, C., Choudhury, A., Granstam-Björneklett, H., Lekander, M., Nilsson, B., ... Mellstedt, H. (2009). Systemic immune effects of adjuvant chemotherapy with 5-fluorouracil, epirubicin and cyclophosphamide and/or radiotherapy in breast cancer: A longitudinal study. *Cancer Immunology and Immunotherapy, 58*(1), 111–120.

Muñoz, N., Franceschi, S., Bosetti, C., Moreno, V., Herrero, R., Smith, J. S., & Shah, K. V. (2002). Role of parity and human papillomavirus in cervical cancer: The IARC multicentric case-control study. *Lancet, 359*, 1093–1101.

Murimi, M. W., & Harpel, T. (2010). Practicing preventive health: The underlying culture among low-income rural populations. *Journal of Rural Health, 26*(3), 273–282.

Murphy-Hoefer, R., Hyland, A., & Rivard, C. (2010). The influence of tobacco countermarketing ads on college students' knowledge, attitudes, and beliefs. *Journal of American College Health : J of ACH, 58*(4), 373–381.

Mystakidou, K., Tsilika, E., Parpa, E., Katsouda, E., Galanos, A., & Vlahos, L. (2005). Assessment of anxiety and depression in advanced cancer patients and their relationship with quality of life. *Quality of Life Research, 14*(8), 1825–1833.

Naber, S. K., Matthijsse, S. M., Rozemeijer, K., Penning, C., & Inge, M. C. (2016). Cervical cancer screening in partly HPV vaccinated cohorts – A cost-effectiveness analysis. *PLoS One, 11*(1), 1–15.

National Center for Health Statistics. (2012). *Health, United States, 2011: With special feature on socioeconomic status and health*. Hyattsville, MD. U.S. Department of Health and Human Services

National Comprehensive Cancer Network (NCCN). (2016). *Smoking Cessation*. https://doi.org/10.1002/14651858.CD000146.pub2

Nelson, H. D., Tyne, K., Naik, A., Bougatsos, C., Chan, B. K., & Humphrey, L. (2009). Screening for breast cancer: An update for the U.S. preventive services task force. *Annals of Internal Medicine, 151*(10), 727–737.

Newell, S., Girgis, A., Sanson-Fisher, R., & Ireland, M. (2000). Accuracy of patients' recall of pap and cholesterol screening. *American Journal of Public Health, 90*(9), 1431–1435.

Newell, S., Sanson-Fisher, R. W., Girgis, A., & Bonaventura, A. (1998). How well do medical oncologists' perceptions reflect their patients' reported physical and psychosocial problems?: Data from a survey of five oncologists. *Cancer, 83*(8), 1640–1651.

Newell, S. A., Sanson-Fisher, R. W., & Savolainen, N. J. (2002). Systematic review of psychological therapies for cancer patients: Overview and recommendations for future research. *Journal of the National Cancer Institute, 94*(8), 558–584.

Nezu, A. M. (1987). A problem-solving formulation of depression: A literature review and proposal of a pluralistic model. *Clinical Psychology Review, 7*(2), 121–144.

Ng, M., Fleming, T., Robinson, M., Thomson, B., Graetz, N., Margono, C., ... Gakidou, E. (2014). Global, regional, and national prevalence of overweight and obesity in children and adults during 1980-2013: A systematic analysis for the global burden of disease study 2013. *The Lancet, 384*(9945), 766–781.

Niaura, R., & Abrams, D. B. (2002). Smoking cessation: Progress, priorities, and prospectus. *Journal of Consulting and Clinical Psychology, 70*(3), 494–509.

Nowinski, J., Baker, S., & Carroll, K. (1992). *Twelve step facilitation therapy manual: A clinical research guide for therapists treating individuals with alcohol abuse and dependence, Project MATCH Monograph Series (Vol. 1)*. Rockville, MD: NIAA Project MATCH Monograph Series.

Nugent, C., Black, L., & Adams, P. (2016). *Tables of adult health behaviors, body weight: National Health Interview Survey, 2011–2014 [Internet]*. Bethesda, MD: U.S. Department of Health and Human Services, National Center for Health Statistics [cited August 15, 2016]. Available from: http://www.cdc.gov/nchs/nhis/SHS/tables.htm.

O'Connor, C. M., Whellan, D. J., Lee, K. L., Keteyian, S. J., Cooper, L. S., Ellis, S. J., … Pina, I. L. (2009). Efficacy and safety of exercise training in patients with chronic heart failure: HF-ACTION randomized controlled trial. *JAMA, 301*(14), 1439–1450.

O'Donnell, A. N., Williams, M., & Kilbourne, A. M. (2013). Overcoming roadblocks: Current and emerging reimbursement strategies for integrated mental health services in primary care. *Journal of General Internal Medicine, 28*(12), 1667–1672.

Ockene, J. K., Emmons, K. M., Mermelstein, R. J., Perkins, K. a., Bonollo, D. S., Voorhees, C. C., & Hollis, J. F. (2000). Relapse and maintenance issues for smoking cessation. *Health Psychology: Official Journal of the Division of Health Psychology, American Psychological Association, 19*(1 Suppl), 17–31.

Ogden, C. L., Carroll, M. D., Kit, B. K., & Flegal, K. M. (2013). Prevalence of obesity among adults: United States, 2011-2012. *NCHS Data Brief, 131*(131), 1–8.

Onitilo, A. A., Liang, H., Stankowski, R. V., Engel, J. M., Broton, M., Doi, S. A., & Miskowiak, D. A. (2014). Geographical and seasonal barriers to mammography services and breast cancer stage at diagnosis. *Rural and Remote Health, 14*(3), 1–13.

Oquendo, M. A., Galfalvy, H. C., Russo, S., Ellis, S. P., Grunebaum, M. F., Burke, A. K., & Mann, J. J. (2004). Prospective study of clinical predictors of suicidal acts after a major depressive episode in patients with major depressive disorder or bipolar disorder. *American Journal of Psychiatry, 161*(8), 1433–1441.

Ornish, D., Scherwitz, L. W., Billings, J. H., Gould, K. L., Merritt, T. A., Sparler, S., Armstrong, W. T., Ports, T. A., Kirkeeide, R. L., Hogeboom, C., & Brand, R. J. (1998). Intensive lifestyle changes for reversal of coronary heart disease. *JAMA, 280*(23), 2001.

Osborn, R. L., Demoncada, A. C., & Feuerstein, M. (2006). Psychosocial interventions for depression, anxiety, and quality of life in cancer survivors: Meta-analyses. *International Journal of Psychiatry in Medicine, 36*(1), 13–34.

Owen, J. E., Goldstein, M. S., Lee, J. H., Breen, N., & Rowland, J. H. (2007). Use of health-related and cancer-specific support groups among adult cancer survivors. *Cancer, 109*(12), 2580–2589.

Parker, P. A., Baile, W. F., de Moor, C., & Cohen, L. (2003). Pyschosocial and demographic predictors of quality of life in a large sample of cancer patients. *Psycho-Oncology, 12*(2), 183–193.

Paskett, E. D., Tatum, C., Rushing, J., Michielutte, R., Bell, R., Foley, K. L., … Dickinson, S. (2004). Racial differences in knowledge, attitudes, and cancer screening practices among a triracial rural population. *Cancer, 101*(11), 2650–2659.

Pederson, L. L., Koval, J. J., Chan, S. S. H., & Zhang, X. (2007). Variables related to tobacco use among young adults: Are there differences between males and females? *Addictive Behaviors, 32*(2), 398–403.

Peppercorn, J., Houck, K., Beri, N., Villagra, V., Wogu, A. F., Lyman, G. H., & Wheeler, S. B. (2015). Breast cancer screening utilization and understanding of current guidelines among rural U.S. women with private insurance. *Breast Cancer Research and Treatment, 153*(3), 659–667.

Perri, M. G., McAllister, D. a., Gange, J. J., Jordan, R. C., McAdoo, G., & Nezu, A. M. (1988). Effects of four maintenance programs on the long-term management of obesity. *Journal of Consulting and Clinical Psychology, 56*(4), 529–534.

Perri, M. G., Nezu, A. M., & Viegener, B. J. (1992). *Improving the long-term management of obesity: Theory, research, and clinical guidelines*. New York, NY: John Wiley & Sons.

Peterson, E., De, P., & Nuttall, R. (2012). BMI, diet and female reproductive factors as risks for thyroid cancer: A systematic review. *PLoS One, 7*(1), e29177.

Petrosky, E., Bocchini, J. A., Hariri, S., Chesson, H., Curtis, C. R., Saraiya, M., … Markowitz, L. E. (2015). Use of 9-valent human papillomavirus (HPV) vaccine: Updated HPV vaccination recommendations of the advisory committee on immunization practices. *MMWR. Morbidity and Mortality Weekly Report, 64*(11), 300–304.

Piasecki, T. M. (2006). Relapse to smoking. *Clinical Psychology Review, 26*(2), 196–215.

Pierce Campbell, C. M., Menezes, L. J., Paskett, E. D., & Giuliano, A. R. (2012). Prevention of invasive cervical cancer in the United States: Past, present, and future. *Cancer Epidemiology Biomarkers and Prevention., 21*(9), 1402–1408.

Pierce, J. P., Macaskill, P., & Hill, D. (1990). Long-term effectiveness of mass media led antismoking campaigns in Australia. *American Journal of Public Health, 80*(5), 565–569.

Pinquart, M., & Duberstein, P. R. (2010). Depression and cancer mortality: A meta-analysis. *Psychological Medicine, 40*(11), 1797–1810.

Pischke, C. R., Scherwitz, L., Weidner, G., & Ornish, D. (2008). Long-term effects of lifestyle changes on well-being and cardiac variables among coronary heart disease patients. *Health Psychology, 27*(5), 584–592.

Plummer, M., Peto, J., & Franceschi, S. (2012). Time since first sexual intercourse and the risk of cervical cancer. *International Journal of Cancer, 130*, 2638–2644.

Power, E., Miles, A., Von Wagner, C., Robb, K., Wardle, J., & Oncology, F. (2009). Uptake of colorectal cancer screening: System, provider and individual factors and strategies to improve participation. *Colorectal Cancer, 5*, 1371–1388.

Praud, D., Rota, M., Rehm, J., Shield, K., Zatonski, W., Hashibe, M., … Boffetta, P. (2013). Cancer incidence and mortality attributable to alcohol consumption. *International Journal of Cancer, 138*, 1380–1387.

Raghavan, R., Bright, C. L., & Shadoin, A. L. (2008). Toward a policy ecology of implementation of evidence-based practices in public mental health settings. *Implementation Science : IS, 3*, 26.

Rambout, L., Tashkandi, M., Hopkins, L., & Tricco, A. C. (2014). Self-reported barriers and facilitators to preventive human papillomavirus vaccination among adolescent girls and young women: A systematic review. *Preventive Medicine, 58*(1), 22–32.

Rapaport, M. H., Gharabawi, G. M., Canuso, C. M., Mahmoud, R. A., Keller, M. B., Bossie, C. A., … Nemeroff, C. B. (2006). Effects of risperidone augmentation in patients with treatment-resistant depression: Results of open-label treatment followed by double-blind continuation. *Neuropsychopharmacology: Official Publication of the American College of Neuropsychopharmacology, 31*(11), 2505–2513.

Rauscher, G. H., Hawley, S. T., & Earp, J. A. L. (2005). Baseline predictors of initiation vs. maintenance of regular mammography use among rural women. *Preventive Medicine, 40*(6), 822–830.

Rawl, S. M., Menon, U., Burness, A., & Breslau, E. S. (2012). Interventions to promote colorectal cancer screening: An integrative review. *Nursing Outlook, 60*(4), 172–181 e13.

Reagan-Steiner, S., Yankey, D., Jeyarajah, J., Elam-Evans, L. D., Singleton, J. A., Curtis, C. R., … Stokley, S. (2015). National, regional, state, and selected local area vaccination coverage among adolescents aged 13–17 years — United States, 2014. *Morbidity and Mortality Weekly Report, 64*(29), 784–792.

Reiter, P. L., Katz, M. L., & Paskett, E. D. (2012). HPV vaccination among adolescent females from Appalachia: Implications for cervical cancer disparities. *Cancer Epidemiology Biomarkers and Prevention, 21*(12), 2220–2230.

Renehan, A. G., Tyson, M., Egger, M., Heller, R. F., & Zwahlen, M. (2008). Body-mass index and incidence of cancer: A systematic review and meta-analysis of prospective observational studies. *Lancet, 371*(November), 569–578.

Rieckmann, T. R., Kovas, A. E., Fussell, H. E., & Stettler, N. M. (2009). Implementation of evidence-based practices for treatment of alcohol and drug disorders: The role of the state authority. *The Journal of Behavioral Health Services & Research : Official Publication of the National Council for Community Behavioral Healthcare, 36*(4), 407–419.

Rimer, B. K., Trock, B., Engstrom, P. F., Lerman, C., & King, E. (1991). Why do some women get regular mammograms? *American Journal of Preventive Medicine, 7*(2), 69–74.

Rogers, E. (1995). *Diffusion of innovations* (4th ed.). New York, NY: The Free Press.

Roman, P. M., & Johnson, J. A. (2002). Adoption and implementation of new technologies in substance abuse treatment. *Journal of Substance Abuse Treatment, 22*(4), 211–218.

Rosenthal, S. L., Weiss, T. W., Zimet, G. D., Ma, L., Good, M. B., & Vichnin, M. D. (2011). Predictors of HPV vaccine uptake among women aged 19-26: Importance of a physician's recommendation. *Vaccine, 29*(5), 890–895.

Ruddy, N. B., Borresen, D., & Myerholtz, L. (2013). Win/win: Creating collaborative training opportunities for behavioral health providers within family medicine residency programs. *International Journal of Psychiatry in Medicine, 45*(4), 367–376.

Ryba, M. M., Brothers, B. M., & Andersen, B. L. (2017). Implementation of an evidence-based biobehavioral treatment for cancer patients. *Translational Behavioral Medicine, 7*(4), 648–656.

Sabatino, S. A., Lawrence, B., Elder, R., Mercer, S. L., Wilson, K. M., DeVinney, B., … Glanz, K. (2012). Effectiveness of interventions to increase screening for breast, cervical, and colorectal cancers: Nine updated systematic reviews for the guide to community preventive services. *American Journal of Preventive Medicine, 43*(1), 97–118.

Sadler, I., Jacobsen, P. B., Booth-Jones, M., Belanger, H., Weitzner, M., & Fields, K. K. (2002). Preliminary evaluation of a clinical syndrome approach to assessing cancer-related fatigue. *Journal of Pain and Symptom Management, 23*(5), 406–416.

Sanchez, A., Bully, P., Martinez, C., & Grandes, G. (2015). Effectiveness of physical activity promotion interventions in primary care: A review of reviews. *Preventive Medicine, 76*(S), S56–S67.

Sandhu, M. S., White, I. R., & McPherson, K. (2001). Systematic review of the prospective cohort studies on meat consumption and colorectal cancer risk: A meta-analytical approach. *Cancer Epidemiology, Biomarkers & Prevention : A Publication of the American Association for Cancer Research, 10*, 439–446.

Sarna, L., Brown, J. K., Lillington, L., Rose, M., Wewers, M. E., & Brecht, M. L. (2000). Tobacco interventions by oncology nurses in clinical practice: Report from a national survey. *Cancer, 89*(4), 881–889.

Sarna, L., Wewers, M. E., Brown, J. K., Lillington, L., & Brecht, M. L. (2001). Barriers to tobacco cessation in clinical practice: Report from a national survey of oncology nurses. *Nursing Outlook, 49*(4), 166–172.

Sasco, A. J., Secretan, M. B., & Straif, K. (2004). Tobacco smoking and cancer : A brief review of recent epidemiological evidence. *Lung Cancer, 45*(S2), S3–S9.

Savard, J., Simard, S., Ivers, H., & Morin, C. M. (2005). Randomized study on the efficacy of cognitive-behavioral therapy for insomnia secondary to breast cancer, part I: Sleep and psychological effects. *Journal of Clinical Oncology, 23*(25), 6083–6096.

Schapira, M. M., Nattinger, A. B., & McAuliffe, T. L. (2006). The influence of graphic format on breast cancer risk communication. *Journal of Health Communication, 11*(6), 569–582.

Schroevers, M. J., Ranchor, A. V., & Sanderman, R. (2003). The role of social support and self-esteem in the presence and course of depressive symptoms: A comparison of cancer patients and individuals from the general population. *Social Science and Medicine, 57*(2), 375–385.

Schwartz, L. M., Woloshin, S., & Welch, H. G. (1999). Risk communication in clinical practice: Putting cancer in context. *Journal of the National Cancer Institute Monographs, 25*, 124–133.

Sheard, T., & Maguire, P. (1999). The effect of psychological interventions on anxiety and depression in cancer patients: Results of two meta-analyses. *British Journal of Cancer, 80*(11), 1770–1780.

Shelby, R. A., Golden-Kreutz, D. M., & Andersen, B. L. (2008). PTSD diagnoses, subsyndromal symptoms, and comorbidities contribute to impairments for breast cancer survivors. *Journal of Traumatic Stress, 21*(2), 165–172.
Shell, R., & Tudiver, F. (2004). Barriers to cancer screening by rural Appalachian primary care providers. *Journal of Rural Health, 20*(4), 368–373.
Shiffman, S., Sweeney, C. T., Pillitteri, J. L., Sembower, M. A., Harkins, A. M., & Wadden, T. A. (2009). Weight management advice: What do doctors recommend to their patients? *Preventive Medicine, 49*(6), 482–486.
Siegel, R. L., Jacobs, E. J., Newton, C. C., Feskanich, D., Freedman, N. D., Prentice, R. L., & Jemal, A. (2015). Deaths due to cigarette smoking for 12 smoking-related cancers in the United States. *JAMA Internal Medicine, 4*, E1–E3.
Silva, J., Cerqueiera, F., & Medeiros, R. (2014). Chlamydia trachomatis infection: Implications for HPV status and cervical cancer. *Archives of Gynecology and Obstetrics, 289*, 715–723.
Simonelli, L. E., Fowler, J., Maxwell, G. L., & Andersen, B. L. (2008). Physical sequelae and depressive symptoms in gyneacologic cancer survivors: Meaning in life as a mediator. *Annals of Behavioral Medicine., 35*(3), 275–284.
Simons-Morton, D. G., Calfas, K. J., Oldenburg, B., & Burton, N. W. (1998). Effects of interventions in health care settings on physical activity or cardiorespiratory fitness. *American Journal of Preventive Medicine, 15*(4), 413–430.
Singer, S., Brown, A., Einenkel, J., Hauss, J., Hinz, A., Klein, A., … Brähler, E. (2011). Identifying tumor patients' depression. *Supportive Care in Cancer, 19*(11), 1697–1703.
Singh, G. K., Azuine, R. E., & Siahpush, M. (2012). Global inequalities in cervical cancer incidence and mortality are linked to deprivation, low socioeconomic status, and human development. *Interntional Journal of MCH and AIDS, 1*(1), 17–30.
Singh, R. B., Rastogi, S. S., Verma, R., Laxmi, B., Singh, R. B., Ghosh, S., & Niaz, M. A. (1992). Randomised controlled trial of cardioprotective diet in patients with recent acute myocardial infarction: Results of one year follow up. *BMJ (Clinical Research Ed.), 304*(6833), 1015–1019.
Slattery, M. L., Curtin, K. P., Edwards, S. L., & Schaffer, D. M. (2004). Plant foods, fiber, and rectal cancer. *The American Journal of Clinical Nutrition, 79*(2), 274–281.
Smith, E. M., Gomm, S. a., & Dickens, C. M. (2003). Assessing the independent contribution to quality of life from anxiety and depression in patients with advanced cancer. *Palliative Medicine, 17*(6), 509–513.
Smith, J. S., Lindsay, L., Hoots, B., Keys, J., Franceschi, S., Winer, R., & Clifford, G. M. (2007). Human papillomavirus type distribution in invasive cervical cancer and high-grade cervical lesions: A meta-analysis update. *International Journal of Cancer, 121*(3), 621–632.
Smulian, E., Mitchell, K., & Stokley, S. (2016). Interventions to increase HPV vaccination coverage: A systematic review. *Human Vaccines & Immunotherapeutics, 5515 12*(ePub ahead of print) *12*(6), 1566–1588.
Sohl, S. J., & Moyer, A. (2007). Tailored interventions to promote mammography screening: A meta-analytic review. *Preventive Medicine, 45*(4), 252–261.
Sonmez, C. I., Aydin, L. Y., Turker, Y., Baltaci, D., Dikici, S., Sariguzel, Y. C., … Demir, M. (2015). Comparison of smoking habits, knowledge, attitudes and tobacco control interventions between primary care physicians and nurses. *Tobacco Induced Diseases, 13*(1), 37.
Spitzer, R. L., Kroenke, K., Williams, J. B. W., & Löwe, B. (2006). A brief measure for assessing generalized anxiety disorder: The GAD-7. *Archives of Internal Medicine, 166*(10), 1092–1097.
Spring, B., Howe, D., Berendsen, M., McFadden, H. G., Hitchcock, K., Rademaker, A. W., & Hitsman, B. (2009). Behavioral intervention to promote smoking cessation and prevent weight gain: A systematic review and meta-analysis. *Addiction, 104*(9), 1472–1486.
Spring, B., King, A., Pagoto, S., Van Horn, L., & Fisher, J. (2015). Fostering multiple healthy lifestyle behaviors for primary prevention of cancer. *The American Psychologist, 70*(2), 75–90.
Stacey, D., Légaré, F., Col, N. F., Bennett, C. L., Barry, M. J., Eden, K. B., … Holmes-rovner, M. (2014). Decision aids for people facing health treatment or screening decisions. *Cochrane Database of Systematic Reviews*, (1), Art. No.: CD001431.

Standish, L., Torkelson, C., Hamill, F., Yim, D., Hill-Force, A., Fitzpatrick, A., ... Martzen, M. (2008). Immune defects in breast cancer patients after radiotherapy. *Journal of the Society for Integrative Oncology, 6*(3), 110–121.

Stanton, A. L. (2006). Psychosocial concerns and interventions for cancer survivors. *Journal of Clinical Oncology, 24*(32), 5132–5137.

Stark, D., Kiely, M., Smith, A., Velikova, G., House, A., & Selby, P. (2002). Anxiety disorders in cancer patients: Their nature, associations, and relation to quality of life. *Journal of Clinical Oncology, 20*(14), 3137–3148.

Steele, S. K., & Porche, D. J. (2005). Testing the theory of planned behavior to predict mammography intention. *Nursing Research, 54*(5), 332–338.

Steptoe, A., Kerry, S., Rink, E., & Hilton, S. (2001). The impact of behavioral counseling on stage of change in fat intake, physical activity, and cigarette smoking in adults at increased risk of coronary heart disease. *American Journal of Public Health, 91*(2), 265–269.

Strecher, V. J. (1999). Computer-tailored smoking cessation materials: A review and discussion. *Patient Education and Counseling, 36*(2), 107–117.

Strunk, D. R., & DeRubeis, R. J. (2001). Cognitive therapy for depression: A review of its efficacy. *Journal of Cognitive Psychotherapy, 15*(4), 289–297.

Studts, C. R., Tarasenko, Y. N., & Schoenberg, N. E. (2013). Barriers to cervical cancer screening among middle-aged and older rural appalachian women. *Journal of Community Health, 38*(3), 500–512.

The FUTURE II Study Group. (2007). Quadrivalent vaccine against human pappilomavirus to prevent high-grade cervical lesions. *The New England Journal of Medicine, 356*(19), 1915–1927.

Thune, I., Brenn, T., Lund, E., & Gaard, M. (1997). Physical activity and the risk of breast cancer. *The New England Journal of Medicine, 336*(18), 1269–1275.

Toobert, D. J., Glasgow, R. E., & Radcliffe, J. L. (2000). Physiologic and related behavioral outcomes from the Women's lifestyle heart trial. *Annals of Behavioral Medicine : A Publication of the Society of Behavioral Medicine, 22*(1), 1–9.

Troisi, R., Hatch, E. E., Palmer, J. R., Titus, L., Robboy, S. J., Strohsnitter, W. C., ... Hoover, R. N. (2016). Prenatal diethystilbestrol exposure and high-grade squamous cell neoplasia of the lower genital tract. *The American Journal of Obstetrics & Gynecology, 215*(3), 322.e1–322.e8.

Tucker, J. A., Cheong, J. W., Chandler, S. D., Lambert, B. H., Kwok, H., & Pietrzak, B. (2016). Behavioral economic indicators of drinking problem severity and initial outcomes among problem drinkers attempting natural recovery: A cross-sectional naturalistic study. *Addiction, 111*, 1956–1965.

Tulloch, H., Fortier, M., & Hogg, W. (2006). Physical activity counseling in primary care: Who has and who should be counseling? *Patient Education and Counseling, 64*(1–3), 6–20.

Turk, M. W., Yang, K., Hravnak, M., Sereika, S. M., Ewing, L. J., & Burke, L. E. (2009). Randomized clinical trials of weight-loss maintenance: A review. *Journal of Cardiovascular Nursing, 24*(1), 58–80.

U.S. Department of Health and Human Services. (2008). *Physical activity guidelines for Americans*. Retrieved from https://health.gov/paguidelines/pdf/paguide.pdf

U.S. Department of Health and Human Services. (2014). *The health consequences of smoking—50 years of progress: A report of the surgeon general* (pp. 1–36). U S Department of Health and Human Services,Centers for Disease Control and Prevention National Center for Chronic Disease Prevention and Health Promotion Health, Office on Smoking and Health.

U.S. Department of Health and Human Services and U.S. Department of Agriculture. (2015). *2015–2020 dietary guidelines for Americans* (8th ed.). https://doi.org/10.1097/NT.0b013e31826c50af

U.S. Department of Health and Human Services Office of Disease Prevention and Health Promotion. (2016). *Healthy people 2020 [Internet]*. Washington, DC: U.S. Department of Health and Human Services, Office of Disease Prevention and Health Promotion [cited August 15, 2016]. Available from: https://www.healthypeople.gov/2020/topics-objectives/topic/cancer

U.S. Preventive Services Task Force. (2016, January). *Final update summary: Breast cancer: Screening*. U.S. Preventive Services Task Force. https://www.uspreventiveservicestaskforce.org/Page/Document/UpdateSummaryFinal/breast-cancer-screening

Unick, J. L., Jakicic, J. M., & Marcus, B. H. (2010). Contribution of behavior intervention components to 24-month weight loss. *Medicine & Science in Sports & Exercise, 42*(4), 745–753.

Vaccarella, S., Franceschi, S., Herrero, R., Mun, N., Snijders, P. J. F., Clifford, G. M., ... Group, S. (2006). Sexual behavior, condom use, and human papillomavirus: Pooled analysis of the IARC human papillomavirus prevalence surveys. *Cancer Epidemiology Biomarkers & Prevention, 15*, 326–333.

Valentijn, P. P., Schepman, S. M., Opheij, W., & Bruijnzeels, M. A. (2013). Understanding integrated care: A comprehensive conceptual framework based on the integrative functions of primary care. *International Journal of Integrated Care, 13*(4), e010.

van Straten, A., Geraedts, A., Verdonck-de Leeuw, I., Andersson, G., & Cuijpers, P. (2010). Psychological treatment of depressive symptoms in patients with medical disorders: A meta-analysis. *Journal of Psychosomatic Research, 69*(1), 23–32.

Vasilaki, E. I., Hosier, S. G., & Cox, W. M. (2006). The efficacy of motivational interviewing as a brief intervention for excessive drinking: A meta-analytic review. *Alcohol and Alcoholism, 41*(3), 328–335.

Vernon, S. W. (1997). Participation in colorectal cancer screening: A review. *Journal of the National Cancer Institute, 89*(19), 1406–1422.

Vogt, F., Hall, S., & Marteau, T. M. (2005). General practitioners' and family physicians' negative beliefs and attitudes towards discussing smoking cessation with patients: A systematic review. *Addiction, 100*(10), 1423–1431.

Vogt, T., Hollis, J., Lichtenstein, E., Stevens, V., Glasgow, R., & Whitlock, E. (1998). The medical care system and prevention: The need for a new paradigm. *HMO Practice, 12*(1), 5–13.

Wadden, T. a., Brownell, K. D., & Foster, G. D. (2002). Obesity: Responding to the global epidemic. *Journal of Consulting and Clinical Psychology, 70*(3), 510–525.

Walsh, J. M. E., & Terdiman, J. P. (2003). Colorectal cancer screening: Scientific review. *JAMA: The Journal of the American Medical Association, 289*(10), 1288–1296.

Wang, C., Harris, W. S., Chung, M., Lichtenstein, A. H., Balk, E. M., Kupelnick, B., ... Lau, J. (2006). nΣ3 fatty acids from fish or fish-oil supplements, but not linolenic acid, benefit cardiovascular disease outcomes in primary- and secondary-prevention studies: A systematic review. *The American Journal of Clinical Nutrition, 84*(Cvd), 5–17.

Wang, Y., & Beydoun, M. A. (2007). The obesity epidemic in the United States – Gender, age, socioeconomic, racial/ethnic, and geographic characteristics: A systematic review and meta-regression analysis. *Epidemiologic Reviews, 29*(1), 6–28.

Ward, E., Jemal, A., Cokkinides, V., Singh, G. K., Cardinez, C., Ghafoor, A., & Thun, M. (2004). Cancer disparities by race/ethnicity and socioeconomic status. *CA: a Cancer Journal for Clinicians, 54*, 78–93.

Ward, M. C., White, D. T., & Druss, B. G. (2015). A meta-review of lifestyle interventions for cardiovascular risk factors in the general medical population. *The Journal of Clinical Psychiatry, 76*(4), e477–e486.

Weil, A. M., Wolfe, C. R., Reyna, V. F., Widmer, C. L., Cedillos-Whynott, E. M., & Brust-Renck, P. G. (2015). Proficiency of FPPI and objective numeracy in assessing breast cancer risk estimation. *Learning and Individual Differences, 43*, 149–155.

Weiner, J., & Colameco, C. (2014). Essential health benefits: 50-state variations on a theme. Princeton, NJ: RobertWood Johnson Foundation.

Weisz, J., Ng, M., & Bearman, S. (2014). Odd couple? Reenvisioning the relation between science and practice in the dissemination-implementation era. *Clinical Psychological Science, 2*(1), 58–74.

Weitzman, E. R., Zapka, J., Estabrook, B., & Goins, K. V. (2001). Risk and reluctance: Understanding impediments to colorectal cancer screening. *Preventive Medicine, 32*, 502–513.

White, S., Chen, J., & Atchison, R. (2008). Relationship of preventive health practices and health literacy: A national study. *American Journal of Health Behavior, 32*(3), 227–242.
WHO report on the global tobacco epidemic. (2013). *Enforcing bans on tobacco advertising, promotion and sponsorship*. Geneva, Switzerland. World Health Organization.
Williams, J. W. (1988). A structured interview guide for the Hamilton depression rating scale. *Archives of General Psychiatry, 45*(8), 742–747.
Williams, M. V., Davis, T., Parker, R. M., & Weiss, B. D. (2002). The role of health literacy in patient-physician communication. *Family Medicine, 34*(5), 383–389.
Williams, S., & Dale, J. (2006). The effectiveness of treatment for depression/depressive symptoms in adults with cancer: A systematic review. *British Journal of Cancer, 94*(3), 372–390.
Williamson, G. M. (2000). Extending the activity restriction model of depressed affect: Evidence from a sample of breast cancer patients. *Health Psychology: Official Journal of the Division of Health Psychology, American Psychological Association, 19*(4), 339–347.
Wilson, P. W., D'Agostino, R. B., Levy, D., Belanger, A. M., Silbershatz, H., & Kannel, W. B. (1998). Prediction of coronary heart disease using risk factor categories. *Circulation, 97*(18), 1837–1847.
Wiltschke, C., Krainer, M., Budinsky, A., Berger, A., Müller, C., Zeillinger, R., … Zielinski, C. (1995). Reduced mitogenic stimulation of peripheral blood mononuclear cells as a prognostic parameter for the course of breast cancer: A prospective longitudinal study. *British Journal of Cancer, 71*(6), 1292–1296.
Winer, R. L., Lee, S., Hughes, J. P., Adam, D. E., Kiviat, N. B., & Koutsky, L. A. (2003). Genital human papillomavirus infection: Incidence and risk factors in a cohort of female university students. *American Journal of Epidemiology, 157*(3), 218–226.
World Cancer Research Fund, & American Institute for Cancer Research. (2007). Food, nutrition, physical activity, and the prevention of cancer: A global perspective. In *Cancer research*. American Institute for Cancer Research, Washington, DC.
Wu, S. M., & Andersen, B. L. (2010). Stress generation over the course of breast cancer survivorship. *Journal of Behavioral Medicine, 33*(3), 250–257.
Xiao, L., Yank, V., Wilson, S. R., Lavori, P. W., & Ma, J. (2013). Two-year weight-loss maintenance in primary care-based diabetes prevention program lifestyle interventions. *Nutrition & Diabetes, 3*(2), e76.
Yang, W., Williams, J. H., Hogan, P. F., Bruinooge, S. S., Rodriguez, G. I., Kosty, M. P., … Goldstein, M. (2014). Projected supply of and demand for oncologists and radiation oncologists through 2025: An aging, better-insured population will result in shortage. *Journal of Oncology Practice/American Society of Clinical Oncology, 10*(1), 39–45.

Chapter 15
Behavioral Health and Chronic Pain

Tony Iezzi, Melanie P. Duckworth, Gwendolyn Carlson, and Dennis C. Turk

Behavioral Health and Chronic Pain

Pain is prevalent in the general population and is among the most common symptom presentations in primary care, emergency room, and hospital settings (National Center for Health Statistics, 2016). Chronic pain is costly to persons experiencing it and to society and is associated with significant morbidity, mortality, healthcare utilization, and lost work days. Because chronic pain occurs in a biopsychosocial context, the assessment and management of chronic pain is best accomplished with using an integrated behavioral health management approach (Flor & Turk, 2011; Gatchel, Peng, Peters, Fuchs, & Turk, 2007). This chapter presents an overview of the literature addressing the scope and significance of chronic pain and provides brief reviews and clinical recommendations related to (1) the assessment and management of chronic pain in primary care settings, (2) the role of primary care providers and psychologists in addressing the key care needs of chronic pain patients, (3) the role of opioids and medical cannabis in pain management, and (4) the management of chronic pain through brief psychosocial interventions, formal stepped care interventions, and interdisciplinary pain management programs.

T. Iezzi (✉)
Behavioral Medicine Service, London Health Sciences Center, London, ON, Canada
e-mail: tony.iezzi@lhsc.on.ca

M. P. Duckworth
Department of Psychology, University of Nevada, Reno, Reno, NV, USA
e-mail: melanied@unr.edu

G. Carlson
Department of Psychology, University of Nevada, Reno, Reno, NV, USA

D. C. Turk
Department of Anesthesiology & Pain Medicine, University of Washington, Seattle, WA, USA
e-mail: turkdc@uw.edu

M. P. Duckworth, W. T. O'Donohue (eds.), *Behavioral Medicine and Integrated Care*,
https://doi.org/10.1007/978-3-319-93003-9_15

Scope and Significance of Chronic Pain

Pain is a universal and complex phenomenon. As defined by the International Association for the Study of Pain, pain is "an unpleasant sensory and emotional experience associated with actual or potential tissue damage, or described in terms of such damage" (p. 210) and is always a subjective experience (Merskey & Bogduk, 1994). The Institute of Medicine (2011) has proposed a view of pain as a multidimensional experience that is influenced by a number of biological, psychological, social, and cultural factors.

Pain that is experienced on a more protracted basis is identified as chronic pain. Chronic pain is typically defined as pain that persists for greater than 3 months or beyond the expect period of healing; for research purposes, a cutoff of greater than 6 months is often used (Merskey & Bogduk, 1994). Individuals experiencing chronic pain also begin to report changes in all life domains (i.e., vocational, housekeeping and house maintenance, recreational, social, familial, and interpersonal activities). These changes lead to significant emotional distress, which contributes to disability and suffering.

Prevalence and Cost

The scope and significance of chronic pain was recently captured by the Global Burden of Disease Study 2013 (Vos et al., 2015). This study encompassed a comprehensive investigation of diseases across the world conducted over a 23-year period. Rice, Smith, and Blyth (2016) provide a synopsis of the key findings related to chronic pain. They noted that chronic pain and disability due to pain are featured prominently on the list of the most impactful diseases. In a list of 59 chronic conditions, recurrent tension headache, migraine headache, low back pain, neck pain, and other musculoskeletal conditions were ranked 2nd, 7th, 12th, 17th, and 32th, respectively. Even more significant is the impact of chronic pain in terms of years lived with disability (YLD). The authors state that YLD, which takes into account the prevalence and severity of a condition, gives a more accurate impression of the impact of any condition. The single greatest source of YLD across the world is chronic low back pain (accounting for greater than 146 million YLD), with major depressive disorder serving as the second greatest source of YLD (greater than 51 million YLD). Other rankings include chronic neck pain ranked 4th (greater than 34 million years), migraine headache ranked 6th (greater than 28 million years), other musculoskeletal disorders ranked 10th (greater than 22 million years), osteoarthritis ranked 13th (greater than 12 million years), and medication overuse leading to headache ranked 18th (greater than 9 million years). Rice et al. (2016) concluded that chronic pain has become the most significant cause of current and future morbidity and disability across the world. Chronic pain also represents one of the most prevalent and disabling medical conditions in the United States. More than 100 million adult

Americans experience chronic pain (Gaskin & Richard, 2012). It has been estimated that 56% of the adult population has experienced pain and 40% of the adult population experienced severe pain during the previous 3 months (Nahin, 2015). The cause of pain varies, with an estimated 22% of US adults experiencing arthritic conditions, 20% experiencing low back pain, nearly 18% experiencing non-arthritic joint pain, 14% experiencing neck pain, and 10% experiencing sciatica (Clarke, Nahin, Barnes, & Stussman, 2016). Chronic pain is prevalent in children and adolescents as well, with international estimates ranging from 11% to 38% of the general pediatric population (King et al., 2011), with severe and disabling pain reported by 5% to 8% of children and adolescents (Huguet & Miro, 2008).

Chronic pain is also the leading cause of long-term disability in the United States (National Institutes of Health, 2013). It is estimated that pain-related costs totaled between 560 and 635 billion in 2010, a sum greater than the total annual cost for heart disease, cancer, and diabetes (Gaskin & Richard, 2012). Gaskin and Richard found that the annual lost productivity costs associated with pain range from $297 billion to $336 billion and the annual healthcare costs associated with pain range from $261 billion to $300 billion. To determine the cost of pain at the individual patient level, Gannon, Finn, O'Gorman, Ruane, and McGuire (2013) examined chronic pain patient's medical expenses at a tertiary pain management clinic. Results revealed that the annual total cost per patient was $24,043. Gannon and colleagues found that the annual indirect costs per patient totaled $13,252, with lost days of work accounting for 39% of the total indirect costs. The annual direct healthcare costs per patient totaled $10,791, with inpatient and outpatient hospital care accounting for 44% and 19% of direct healthcare costs, respectively. The total direct cost of moderate to severe pediatric chronic pain in the United States is estimated to be $19.5 billion per year (Groenewald, Essner, Wright, Fesinmeyer, & Palermo, 2014; Groenewald, Wright, & Palermo, 2015). Collectively, these findings demonstrate the degree to which chronic pain burdens affected individuals, their significant others, and the larger society.

Risk Factors

While chronic pain occurs at high rates, chronic pain is not evenly distributed across the general population. A number of subpopulations have been identified as being at higher risk for developing chronic pain conditions. Individuals over age 65 are at increased risk for chronic pain (Ortman, Velkoff, & Hogan, 2014). Since it is estimated that the US population of persons 65 years or older will nearly double from 43.1 million in 2012 to 83.7 million in 2050 (Institute of Medicine, 2011), the absolute number of individuals with chronic pain will escalate accordingly. Other sociodemographic factors are also associated with the presence of chronic pain. In addition to age, sex and ethnicity have also been identified as risk factors for developing chronic pain, with women and non-Hispanics being more likely to report pain and Asians being less likely to report pain (Nahin, 2015). Additionally, low socioeconomic status is associated with a greater likelihood of experiencing pain and disability as a result of pain (Brekke, Hjortdahl, & Kvien, 2002; Dorner et al., 2011). Moreover, treatments received have been found to vary in relation to these cultural factors, these differences likely contributing to the significant disparities that exist in healthcare delivery and outcomes (Grol-Prolopczyk, 2017).

Medical conditions and injuries have also been identified as predictors of chronic pain. Numerous medical conditions are associated with chronic pain (e.g., osteoarthritis, fibromyalgia, diabetic peripheral neuropathy, cancer) (Johannes, Le, Zhou, Johnston, & Dworkin, 2010). Pain appears to be more common among individuals with a history of injury or trauma (e.g., a history of physical and sexual abuse, involvement in motor vehicle collisions) (Ellsberg, Jansen, Heise, Watts, & Garcia-Moreno, 2008; Giummarra et al., 2016; Sachs-Ericsson, Kendall-Tackett, & Hernandez, 2007). Although there are a variety of circumstances that can lead to injury, the development of post-injury chronic pain is best predicted by the severity of the injury, pain experienced in the immediate aftermath of injury, the number of pain sites reported, the level of pain interference, and the injured person's beliefs and expectations about the limits and requirements of recovery (Duckworth & Iezzi, 2010; Hu et al., 2016; Iezzi, Duckworth, Mercer, & Vuong, 2007; Platts-Mills et al., 2016; Turk, Fillingim, Ohrbach, & Patel, 2016). Post-traumatic stress disorder has also been reported to be associated with persistence and intensity of pain as well as prolonged disability (Brennstuhl, Tarquinio, & Montel, 2015; Demyttenaere et al., 2007; Duckworth & Iezzi, 2010; Pedler, Kamper, & Sterling, 2016).

Although some risk factors are immutable and cannot be modified by healthcare providers (e.g., sociodemographic variables), other risk factors for chronic pain are more malleable. These risk factors include beliefs (e.g., catastrophizing, self-efficacy) and coping behaviors (e.g., pain avoidance) that are among the best predictors of short- and long-term recovery. Greater catastrophizing, anxiety, and depression have consistently predicted the presence of acute and chronic postsurgical pain (Jackson, Tian, Wang, Iezzi, & Xie, 2016; Theunissen, Peters, Bruce, Gramke, & Marcus, 2012). It is hypothesized that, in the presence of acute pain, some patients will avoid engaging in behaviors they believe will increase pain and engage in behavior they believe will reduce pain. These beliefs are often not accurate, can disrupt recovery, and contribute to the development of chronic pain (Crombez, Eccleston, Van Damme, Vlaeyen, & Karoly, 2012). As a result, cognitive and behavioral risk factors are highly predictive of pain trajectories and chronic pain development.

Pain-Related Disability

Identifying risk factors for chronic pain is important for prevention and early intervention. Chronic pain patients are at an increased risk of experiencing a variety of physical, psychological, occupational, and financial consequences (Duckworth &

Iezzi, 2010). Pain has been shown to contribute to physical disability, with pain associated with reductions in strength, stamina, mobility, and range of motion (Ratzon, Froom, Friedman, & Amit, 2013). In comparison to patients without chronic pain, patients with chronic pain spend significantly more time lying down and significantly less time sitting and standing, and evidence significantly lower average and peak movement intensity (Raijmakers, Nieuwenhuizen, Beckerman, & de Groot, 2015). Due to pain-related limitations, chronic pain has been shown to predict greater interference with daily activities as well as reduced physical functioning and health-related quality of life (Kawai, Kawai, Wollan, & Yawn, 2017; Vartiainen, Heiskanen, Sintonen, Roine, & Kalso, 2016).

While there are clear physical effects of chronic pain, these effects are often accompanied by negative psychological consequences. Psychological disorders, including anxiety, depression, and post-traumatic stress disorder (PTSD), are predictive of poorer recovery among chronic pain patients (Brennstuhl et al., 2015; Demyttenaere et al., 2007; Duckworth & Iezzi, 2010). Prevalence estimates for chronic pain and psychiatric comorbidity vary greatly. Rates of anxiety among chronic pain patients range from 18% to 55% (Ho, Li, Ng, Tsui, & Ng, 2011; Sagheer, Khan, & Sharif, 2013), rates of depression range from 12% to 72% (Ho et al., 2011; Poole, White, Blake, Murphy, & Bramwell, 2009; Proctor, Estroff, Empting, Shearer-Williams, & Hoffmann, 2013; Sagheer et al., 2013), and rates of PTSD range from nearly 5% to 29% (Ho et al., 2011; Proctor et al., 2013). Emotional distress has consistently been shown to predict greater pain interference and greater impairment among chronic pain patients (Chisari & Chilcot, 2017; Valentine, Gerber, Nobles, Shtasel, & Marques, 2016). These factors often account for greater proportions of the variance in disability than physical pathology (e.g., Carragee, Alamin, Miller, & Carragee, 2005). It appears that while psychological distress can occur as a result of pain onset, the relationship between pain and psychological distress is bidirectional (Edwards, Dworkin, Sullivan, Turk, & Wasan, 2016; Turk et al., 2016). Psychological distress can exacerbate the pain experience and lead to further impairment among chronic pain patients.

Given the negative functional and psychological consequences associated with chronic pain, many individuals with chronic pain have a difficult time engaging in activities of daily living, including occupational and social activities. In their review of the costs and consequences associated with chronic pain, Andrew, Derry, Taylor, Straube, and Phillips (2014) found chronic pain to be predictive of greater work disability and decreased work efficiency. In addition to the financial hardship associated with work disability, chronic pain patients who do not return to work are likely to report greater physical impairment and psychological distress (Jackson, Iezzi, & Lafreniere, 1996, 1997; Jackson, Iezzi, Lafreniere, & Narduzzi, 1998; Outcalt et al., 2015; Sullivan et al., 2017). These findings are consistent with the larger unemployment literature, which indicates that unemployment contributes to deterioration in physical and mental health and greater mortality (Laditka & Laditka, 2016; Strandh, Winefield, Nilsson, & Hammarström, 2014).

Assessment and Management of Chronic Pain in the Primary Care Setting

As patients transition from acute pain to chronic pain, the level of assessment and management of pain will escalate in terms of effort, time, skill set, and complexity of service. The integrated care team has become the standard for chronic pain management. Chronic pain management in the primary care setting or hospitals and pain clinics is guided by the biopsychosocial model (Duckworth, Iezzi, & Sewell, 2009; Flor & Turk, 2011; Gatchel et al., 2007). This model views chronic pain as an experience that is influenced by the interplay of biological, psychological, and social factors. Successful management of chronic pain requires that all aspects of the chronic pain experience be addressed.

The Role of the Primary Care Physician

Assessment and management of chronic pain patients usually begins in the primary care setting. Primary care providers (PCPs) take patient histories, identify symptoms, conduct a physical examination, and develop an initial treatment plan. PCPs initially focus on establishing the location, duration, intensity, and quality of the patient's pain experience and relating the reported pain to physical injuries, disease conditions, and/or other medical history. In such settings, the PCP's goals for pain assessments include determining whether further diagnostic testing is indicated, establishing a medical diagnosis, determining if medical findings can account for the patient's report of pain, and forwarding treatment options (Dansie & Turk, 2013).

As part of an integrated approach to pain management in the primary care setting, PCPs may enlist the assistance of other service providers who can aid in the assessment and management of chronic pain patients. These service providers may include nurses, physiotherapists, occupational therapists, and psychologists. The PCP's role is to oversee the management of the chronic pain patient, including the prescription and use of pain medications and the use and benefit derived from various rehabilitation efforts. In the absence of a complete response to these pain management efforts, and in the presence of persistent pain, the most function-preserving message from the PCP to the patient is to maintain as normal a life as possible in spite of pain, to be active, and to moderate expectations for pain reduction (Duckworth et al., 2009). In addition, the PCP needs to provide reassurance about the patient's prognosis, be especially conservative in recommending pharmacotherapy or other invasive pain treatments, and avoid overmedicalizing or overpathologizing the pain patient, thereby preventing the development of a host of other problems (e.g., medication abuse; Duckworth et al., 2009).

The Role of the Psychologist

The primary role of the psychologist is to not only assist in the psychological assessment and management of chronic pain patients but to guide and support PCPs and other service providers involved in the management of chronic pain patients (Duckworth et al., 2009). For example, psychologists are central in evaluating psychological distress in chronic pain patients and in recommending treatment strategies that may complement more traditional pharmacological and physically oriented treatments. Psychologists can also identify and problem-solve around maladaptive attitudes, beliefs, and expectations (e.g., fear of pain or injury, catastrophizing) as well as inappropriate coping strategies (e.g., activity avoidance), all of which are among the best predictors of poor prognosis. Psychologists are most qualified to perform a detailed analysis of pain-related functional limitations and support needs and shape a pain treatment plan that will result in more optimal outcomes for such patients.

Psychologists are skilled in the conduct of detailed chronic pain assessments via the use of semi-structured interviews and psychological testing (for a comprehensive review, see Turk & Melzack, 2011). Psychological assessments in primary care settings tend to be shorter in length. Brief screening instruments that evaluate the presence and impact of certain pain-relevant behaviors are frequently employed. Measures of pain intensity include numeric, verbal, and visual rating scales that provide anchors (e.g., 0 = no pain and 5 = severe pain) to be used by patients in communicating the intensity of pain experienced, while measures of pain-relevant behavior are likely to include functional abilities, pain beliefs and expectations, psychological distress, and pain coping styles and strategies. Relatively brief and standardized measures of these pain- and mood-relevant constructs include the West Haven-Yale Multidimensional Pain Inventory (MPI; Kerns, Turk, & Rudy, 1985), Medical Outcomes Study Short-Form (SF-36; Ware, Snow, Kosinski, & Gandek, 1993), Pain Disability Index (PDI; Tait, Pollard, Margolis, Duckro, & Krause, 1987), Coping Strategies Questionnaire (CSQ; Keefe, Crisson, Urban, & Williams, 1990), Beck Depression Inventory-II (BDI-II; Beck, Steer, & Brown, 1996), and Beck Anxiety Inventory (BAI; Beck & Steer, 1993). For reviews, see Taylor et al. (2016), Turk et al. (2016), and Turk and Melzack (2011).

Psychological assessments that are undertaken in hospitals and pain clinics can rely on more extensive personality testing aimed at capturing the complexity of pain presentations. Commonly administered personality tests include the following: Minnesota Multiphasic Personality Inventory-2 (MMPI-2; Butcher, Dalhstrom, Graham, Tellegen, & Kaemmer, 1989), Millon Clinical Multiaxial Inventory-II (MCMI; Millon, Millon, Davis, & Grossman, 1994), Personality Assessment Inventory (PAI; Morey, 1991), Pain Behavior Checklist (PBC; Richards, Nepomuceno, Riles, & Suer, 1982), Sickness Impact Profile (SIP; Bergner, Bobbitt, Carter, & Gilson, 1981), and Chronic Pain Acceptance Questionnaire (CPAQ; McCracken, Vowles, & Eccleston, 2004). For reviews of both brief and more extensive measures of pain and pain-relevant behaviors, see Taylor et al. (2016), Turk et al. (2016), and Turk and Melzack (2011).

The Role of Opioids and Medical Cannabis in Pain Management

Perhaps the mainstays of treatment for patients with chronic pain are pharmacological. Opioids have been used for thousands of years, while the use of medical cannabis is a more recent phenomenon. The prescription of these drugs has generated an enormous amount of concern and controversy among chronic pain patients, PCPs, and the United States population at large.

Between the years 2000 and 2010, the number of opioid analgesic prescriptions in the United States increased from 43.8 million to 89.2 million (Sites, Beach, & Davis, 2014). From 1999 to 2008, sales of opioid pain relievers in the United States nearly quadrupled (Centers for Disease Control and Prevention, 2011). The number of opioid-related overdose deaths in the United States has increased by 200% from 2000 to 2014 (Rudd, Aleshire, Zibbell, & Gladden, 2016). As a result of the increase in both the prescription of opioids and opioid-related deaths, substance use among chronic pain patients has received greater research attention in recent years. It is important to recognize that the statistics regarding opioid use and opioid-related deaths are based on the general population and not on patients medically prescribed opioids. Problems arise related to access of opioids in society and not solely to patients for whom these drugs are prescribed, per se.

Problematic opioid use can be sorted into the following three categories: misuse, abuse, and addiction. Opioid misuse is characterized by use that contradicts its prescribed pattern of use, and adverse effects may or may not be present. Opioid abuse is characterized by intentional use for a purpose that is not medical in nature. Opioid addiction is characterized by a pattern of use that is associated with the experience of harms or the potential to experience harms; for a full review of opioid misuse, abuse, and addiction definitions, see Jones, Baldwin, Manocchio, White and Mack (2016), O'Connor et al. (2013), & Smith et al. (2013).

In a systematic review, Vowles et al. (2015) examined problematic opioid use among chronic pain patients. Findings revealed that rates of opioid misuse, abuse, and addiction varied greatly among chronic pain patients, with misuse ranging from less than 2% to 56.3% in high-quality studies and from less than 1% to 81% in low-quality studies. These large differences in the estimated rates of opioid abuse and misuse may be attributable to differences among the definitions of abuse and misuse used, the methods and criteria used to assess and label these problems, as well as the populations sampled. However, given the large variability in prevalence rates, determining which chronic pain patients are at an increased risk of engaging in problematic opioid use is a significant challenge for both physicians and psychologists.

An important caveat is that not all or even the majority of patients prescribed opioids for medical problems will misuse these drugs. Findings from the empirical literature suggest there are multiple factors that serve to increase the likelihood that chronic pain patients will engage in problematic opioid use. These factors include co-occurring symptoms of anxiety or depression (Manchikanti et al., 2007, 2012), preexisting psychological disorders, and prior history of illicit drug and alcohol abuse (Hser et al., 2017; Ives et al., 2006; Turk, Swanson, & Gatchel, 2008). A patient's understanding of opioids may also be an important variable in the development of problematic opioid use. Stumbo, Yarborough, McCarty, Weisner, and Green (2017) examined pathways to opioid use disorders (OUDs) among patients with opioid dependence diagnoses. In addition to a substance abuse history, qualitative analyses revealed that patients identified and described the following pathways to OUDs: inadequately managed chronic pain (i.e., high pain severity), the use of opioids during acute pain episodes, recreational opioid use, and the use of opioids to manage emotional distress. These findings suggest that misperceptions about the purpose of opioids may contribute to opioid misuse among some chronic pain patients.

Regardless of patient risk factors, ongoing assessment at regularly scheduled visits will allow physicians and psychologists to observe any changes that may increase a chronic pain patient's risk of problematic opioid use. It is also critical that physicians, psychologists, and other members of an integrated care team meet regularly to collect information regarding the consistency and accuracy of patient reporting. All members of the integrated care team should also provide consistent education about opioids and their role in optimizing patient functioning, not eliminating pain. The perception that pain is not being adequately controlled may be a pathway to problematic opioid use (Stumbo et al., 2017). Chou et al. (2009) recommended that patients complete an informed consent document to demonstrate that they have been oriented to the risks associated with opioids and the expectations for treatment. If patients have the expectation that their pain should be eliminated, they may be inclined to take a greater dosage than what was medically prescribed in an effort to minimize their pain. Proper orientation to opioids and their role in reducing pain interference to increase engagement in meaningful activities can reduce the likelihood of unintentional opioid misuse.

Medical cannabis has been not only proposed as a less harmful alternative to opioids in the management of chronic pain but also has promise as a group of therapeutic agents (Savage et al., 2016). Lachenmeier and Rehm (2015) found the typical recreational dose of cannabis to be significantly less lethal than the typical recreational dose for opioids including heroine and methadone. Boehnke, Litinas, and Clauw (2016) examined the impact of medical cannabis use on health outcomes and opioid use among a sample of chronic pain patients. Results revealed that medical cannabis use was associated with a 45% increase in self-reported quality life and a 64% decrease in opioid use. Chronic pain patients also reported using fewer medications after initiating cannabis use across the following medication classes: nonsteroidal anti-inflammatory drugs, disease-modifying antirheumatic drugs, antidepressants, serotonin-norepinephrine reuptake inhibitors, and selective serotonin reuptake inhibitors. These findings are consistent with previous studies that have found medical cannabis use to be associated with decreases in subjective pain experiences among patients with chronic pain conditions (Abrams et al., 2007; Corey-Bloom et al., 2012; Ware et al., 2010). These collective findings, as well as the significantly lower overdose risk associated with cannabis use, have contributed to its appeal as an alternative to opioids in the management of chronic pain.

Because of the documented risks associated with recreational cannabis use (Solowij et al., 2002; Tashkin, 2013), researchers have begun to question the utility of cannabis in the management of chronic pain conditions. The current research literature regarding the long-term, physiological effects of medical cannabis use is limited; however, findings from those studies that have been performed suggest that medical cannabis may be associated with more non-serious adverse effects but does not convey any increased risk of serious adverse effects.

The immediate consequences of cannabis use are not as severe as the risks associated with opioid use, but the long-term effects of medical cannabis use are unclear. Patients should be oriented to the risks associated with each treatment option, and these potential risks should be weighed against the potential functional gains the patients may experience as a result of opioid or cannabis prescription. Strategies to better ensure a successful recovery include a thorough and systematic assessment of substance misuse risk factors, education about the role of medication in pain management, and the establishment of clear and function-based treatment goals (Chou et al., 2009, 2015; Dowell, Haegerich, & Chou, 2016).

The use of pharmacotherapy to manage chronic pain requires a cost-benefit analysis. The decision to medicate chronic pain patients is not simple nor are the decisions regarding the type of medication to be administered (e.g., opioids or cannabis), the appropriate dosage, or the length of administration. There is no medication regimen that can be universally applied (Nuckols et al., 2014). These decisions will depend on each patient's level of functioning and each patient's treatment goals as they pertain to future functioning. There are consequences associated with under medication, such as patients being unable to engage in activities in daily living due to pain interference. There are also consequences associated with overmedication. In the case of opioids, overmedication may increase a patient's risk of addiction and overdose (Vowles et al., 2015). In summary, integrated care team members and patients should discuss the costs and benefits of medication as part of a comprehensive, integrated approach to pain management, and medication should be utilized to the degree that it optimizes a patient's functioning.

Management of Chronic Pain in Integrated Care Settings: From Brief, Self-Guided Psychological Interventions to Interdisciplinary Pain Management Programs

The management of chronic pain often depends on home care and care provided in clinical setting. The majority of chronic pain patients self-manage their symptoms at home with over-the-counter interventions (e.g., nonsteroidal anti-inflammatory agents, acetaminophen, heat, rest) and are treated in primary care settings (Breuer, Cruciani, & Portenoy, 2010). Primary care settings allow for a more flexible and adaptable model of care that attends to the more specific needs of chronic pain patients, while hospital and pain clinic settings often offer a more cohesive, comprehensive, and collaborative intervention; intervention of this level is usually required for more difficult and intractable pain presentations. Even when in receipt of care in such specialty care settings, the majority of patients will return to the primary care setting for maintenance and monitoring.

Interventions used to manage chronic pain may be placed on a continuum from least intensive, invasive, and restrictive to most intensive, invasive, and restrictive. Offering a self-management intervention for home use and in the primary care setting might be considered the least intensive and restrictive interventions, whereas an interdisciplinary pain program in a hospital/pain clinic setting would be considered a more intensive and restrictive intervention. It is not likely that any single treatment will be optimally effective for all of those affected. Given the range of treatment needs of chronic pain patients and the variety of interventions available for chronic pain patients, opportunities for customized treatments abound (Turk, 2005). In terms of providing empirically supported behavioral interventions in primary care settings and within a stepped care framework, there are a number of interventions that can be considered, including bibliotherapy, group interventions, and technological options (e.g., Internet, smartphones). The following sections will describe these triage alternatives for chronic pain patients.

Bibliotherapy and eHealth Interventions for Chronic Pain Patients

Bibliotherapy is an easy accessible resource for chronic pain patients and service providers. Bibliotherapy allows access to treatment within the patient's home and completion of treatment at a pace that respects the patient's physical and psychological needs. Self-help interventions based on cognitive-behavioral principles including cognitive-behavioral therapy (CBT) and variants such as acceptance and commitment therapy (ACT) and mindfulness-based stress reduction (MBSR) have been shown to significantly improve physical and emotional functioning, satisfaction, acceptance, and quality of life and decrease pain (e.g., Johnston, Foster, Shennan, Starkey, & Johnson, 2010; Lorig, Lubeck, Kraines, Seleznick, & Holman, 1985; Thorsell et al., 2011). See Sturgeon (2014) for a review of the distinctions among ACT, CBT, and MBSR that adhere to cognitive-behavioral principles. CBT protocols have been adapted to book and workbook formats as easily disseminable treatment options for chronic pain patients. Guided self-help education programs have been receiving empirical support. A meta-analysis of 16 studies that evaluated guided self-help education programs revealed such programs to have a small but robust effect on pain severity and disability in chronic pain patients (Liegl, Boeckle, Leitner, & Pieh, 2016).

Pain workbooks have also been developed and their effectiveness evaluated. Dear et al. (2017) used a randomized controlled trial to compare the effectiveness achieved by a chronic pain management program delivered remotely via an online or workbook format. A sample of 178 chronic pain patients were assigned to the two treatment groups (online group versus workbook group), with treatment lasting 8 weeks, and with all participants having access to a psychologist on a weekly basis via email and telephone throughout the treatment. Significant posttreatment improvements in disability status, depression, and anxiety were noted; however, no differences in treatment effectiveness between the two treatment groups were found.

In addition to bibliotherapy, eHealth resources are readily avaiable and can serve to educate patients. eHealth resources often take the form of web-based or app-based interventions (e.g., Macea, Gajos, Calil, & Fregni, 2010; Rini et al., 2015; Ruehlman, Karoly, & Enders, 2012). Patients can be encouraged to visit research-based websites such as the Centers for Disease Control and Prevention, National Institutes of Health, and Mayo Clinic. It is important that service providers orient patients to scientifically-valid, web-based resources to reduce the likelihood of accessing inaccurate or harmful information from nonscientific web-based resources (Sundararaman, Edwards, Ross, & Jamison, 2017).

Web-based and app-based interventions have recently been used to effectively treat chronic pain (Macea et al., 2010; Rini et al., 2015; Ruehlman et al., 2012). Several recent reviews have examined the evidence for the utility of these applications (e.g., Lalloo, Jibb, Rivera, Agarwal, & Stinson, 2015; Sundararaman et al., 2017). Lalloo et al. conducted a review of self-management apps for pain, identifying hundreds of apps that address pain management in some form. These authors noted that in attempting to select among many untested pain management apps, patients should aim to identify those apps that contain intervention components that have proven beneficial in the larger pain intervention context. Sundararaman et al. caution about the research limitations of the studies in this field and emphasize the need for rigorous studies to establish the relation of mobile Health technology (mHealth) use to improved quality of life, functional autonomy, and decreased hospital use. Lalloo et al. identified five specific components in pain self-management apps: self-care skills training, education, self-monitoring, social support, and goal setting. Healthcare providers should consider these components when recommending eHealth and mHealth options to chronic pain patients.

Brief Psychotherapies

Brief psychological interventions have been created and proved effective for the management of chronic pain. These therapies require more involvement by a psychologist. Included among the brief psychotherapies that are particularly amenable to pain management in the integrated care context are motivational interviewing and mindfulness-based interventions.

Motivational interviewing is a person-centered approach that resolves ambivalence about behavior change by strengthening motivation and commitment to change. It is an ideal intervention for the psychologist because of its brevity, and it can be administered over the phone or in person. This intervention is especially suited for addressing adherence issues in the management of chronic pain (e.g., opioid medication schedule). There is preliminary evidence supporting the potential utility of this approach with chronic pain patients (Alperstein & Sharpe, 2016; Romano & Peters, 2015). Mindfulness-based interventions have been reported to have significant nonspecific effects on both pain reduction and improvement of emotional distress (Chiesa & Serretti, 2011). Although the standard program formally requires that patients attend weekly, 2-h sessions over a period of 8 weeks, mindfulness-based interventions can be customized to meet the care needs of patients treated in integrated care settings. In such settings, the psychologist assumes the role of a mindfulness coach, with the bulk of mindfulness-based practice being self-guided and occurring outside of the treatment setting. Findings from a recent randomized control trial and a recent meta-analysis found that a MBSR and ACT had similar effect as CBT on catastrophizing, self-efficacy, and acceptance for low back pain (Turner et al., 2016; Veehof, Trompetter, Bohlmeijer, & Schreurs, 2016). Thus, although different techniques may be used with these variants, they all tend to have a basis in cognitive-behavioral principles of self-management, with attention paid to maladaptive beliefs and behaviors that contribute to the maintenance and exacerbation of pain and related disability.

Group Interventions

In addition to the individual interventions that have been described, group interventions for chronic pain are available and can prove a cost-saving treatment option for the large number of patients who present for management of pain (e.g., Keefe, Baupre, Rumble, Kelleher, & Van Denburg, 2018; Lamb et al., 2010). The initial aim of a group intervention should be orienting members to the structure and processes of the group intervention and expectations related to members' active participation in the group intervention. This would involve a discussion of the number of scheduled sessions, the duration of each session, participation during group sessions, completion of homework assignments between sessions, and commitment to maintaining the confidentiality of other group members. Another early aim of the group intervention should be patient education related to physical, occupational, social, and psychological consequences of chronic pain conditions and the identification of treatment goals that address each of those domains of function (Keefe et al., 2018).

Following the establishment of individual goals, group sessions should address those physical (e.g., pain and physiological arousal), cognitive (e.g., unhelpful thinking strategies), and affective (e.g., depression and anxiety) variables that are associated with and often serve to maintain and/or exacerbate chronic pain (Kamper et al., 2012; Keefe et al., 2018; Valentine et al., 2016). It should be recognized that pain patients typically do not engage in excessive rest or excessively strenuous activities each day (Andrews, Strong, & Meredith, 2012). Group leaders should orient group members to increasing assertiveness and communication skills to help them cope with the social consequences that often accompany chronic pain and the ongoing need for patients to act as their own healthcare advocates (Cegala, McClure, Marinelli, & Post, 2000). Lastly, relaxation training should be used to manage the physiological arousal associated with pain as well as pain-related psychological, occupational, and social stressors.

Formal Stepped Care Pain Interventions

Formal models of stepped care can be characterized as promoting methodical assessment of the match between a patient's reported symptoms and the treatment deemed to be both the most appropriate and least invasive strategy for managing the reported symptoms. (Dobscha et al., 2009; Otis, MacDonald, & Dobscha, 2006; Plagge, Lu, Lovejoy, Karl, & Dobscha, 2013). The most effective stepped care approaches to pain management emphasize a sequenced intervention that (Duckworth, Iezzi, & Carlson, 2018):

1. Addresses patients' pain-related worries and concerns about pain, provides psychoeducation aimed at imparting accurate information about the patient's diagnosis, corrects misconceptions about the nature of pain, promotes a return to normal functioning, and discourages activity avoidance
2. Provides structured support for self-management efforts such as physical exercise and activity engagement
3. Provides more intensive psychological intervention aimed at addressing clinically significant emotional distress and lifestyle impairment

Otis et al. (2006) have forwarded a three-step approach to pain management. In Step 1, intervention strategies are aimed at recognizing and addressing patient concerns about pain and enhancing patient readiness for self-care. Step 1 interventions tend to work best for chronic pain patients who tend to experience less intense pain and less emotional distress, rely less on medication, and are more active across a variety of lifestyle domains. In Step 2, an escalation in the involvement of psychologists is indicated. Psychologists at this step try to determine which additional intervention strategies might serve best in maximizing treatment outcome, for example, including patient participation in a psychoeducational group and/or brief individual therapy. Step 3 involves the use of more intensive psychological interventions aimed at managing psychological distress and addressing lifestyle impairments across occupational, interpersonal, and social domains of function. Step 3 is most helpful to patients who have not responded optimally to early interventions and who continue to report significant levels of pain, pain-related disability, and clinically significant emotional distress.

Although empirical examinations of the utility of stepped and integrated approaches to the management of chronic pain are few in number, several studies provide clear support for these approaches and are presented in more extensive detail. Dobscha et al. (2009) conducted an empirical study of the effectiveness of integrated care for chronic pain patients. Participants were recruited via Veterans Administration primary care facilities that served as recruitment sites for the study. The researchers randomly assigned 42 PCPs and 401 chronic pain patients served by these clinicians to either an assistance with pain treatment group or a treatment as usual group. The assistance with pain treatment group was structured to (1) provide clinicians with a two-session education program in which feedback and recommendations were provided and specialty care referrals were facilitated by the integrated care team and (2) provide patients with assessment as well as a variety of pain management strategies, all as part of a four-session workshop. A full-time psychologist, a case manager, and an internist formed the integrated care team and were available one day per week. The treatment as usual group consisted of clinicians and patients who had treatment as usual in terms of access to the pain clinic and associated services. At 1-year follow-up, greater improvements in pain-related disability, pain intensity, and depression and greater impressions of positive change were noted in the assistance with pain treatment group.

In a more recent but uncontrolled study, Plagge et al. (2013) evaluated the effectiveness of integrated care in managing comorbid pain and post-traumatic stress disorder experienced by veterans of the Iraq and Afghanistan wars. Integrated care management was defined as the provision of eight sessions of behavioral activation by a care team comprised of a PCP, psychologist, and physiatrist. Findings indicated that patients improved across a host of outcomes, including pain severity, pain interference, quality of life, post-traumatic stress symptoms, depression, and general emotional well-being. The stepped care model has also been used successfully to increase PCPs' knowledge related to pain conditions, use of opioid treatment agreements and urine drug screens, implementation of pain treatments, and engagement in ongoing evaluation of pain and its consequences (Anderson et al., 2016). Overall, preliminary results support the utility of formal stepped care interventions and integrative approaches in identifying and tailoring empirically supported healthcare services to chronic pain patients.

Interdisciplinary Pain Management Programs

The interdisciplinary pain management program is still the gold standard for the comprehensive treatment of chronic pain patients. The therapeutic and cost-saving benefits of interdisciplinary pain management programs have been well supported from an empirical perspective (Gatchel, McGeary, McGeary, & Lippe, 2014; Gatchel & Okifuji, 2006; Turk & Okifuji, 2002). Interdisciplinary pain management programs are characterized by greater coordination of services that involve a number of providers that work under the same roof. It is also the case that the team comes together to provide a treatment plan with common rehabilitation goals. Interdisciplinary programs are the most intensive type of intervention in terms of patients and service providers. Treatment tends to focus on improving quality of life, fostering return to work, reducing healthcare utilization and medication reliance, and reducing impairment and disability. The emphasis on returning to work and reducing disability is highly important as the biggest cost associated with chronic pain is in not being able to return to work and remaining on disability payments.

Gatchel et al. (2014) note that *interdisciplinary* pain management programs are not the same as multidisciplinary pain management programs. Multidisciplinary pain programs usually involve several healthcare providers (e.g., physician, psychologist, physiotherapist, and occupational therapist), and their communication and integration of services tends to be limited by virtue of not being in the same location. Multidisciplinary service providers tend to administer treatment somewhat independently of each other. More importantly, compared to interdisciplinary programs, multidisciplinary programs have not been found to be as effective in the treatment of chronic pain (Scascighini, Toma, Dober-Spielman, & Sprott, 2008). In general, although pain programs have been found effective, there is still some debate as to which treatment components contribute most positive patient outcomes. There is a need for more studies examining the complex array of patient factors (e.g., gender, race, and education), treatment orientations (e.g., operant, cognitive-behavioral), settings (e.g., inpatient versus outpatient, hospital versus community), modalities (e.g., individual versus group, office versus the web), and funding sources (e.g., Worker's Compensation and Veterans Administration) that predict patients' long-term adjustment to pain and pain-related impairments.

Despite the strong empirical evidence demonstrating that interdisciplinary pain programs are not more costly than other interventions (Gatchel & Okifuji, 2006), the actual number of interdisciplinary programs has dwindled over the last 20 years. Over time, an increasing number of barriers have served to impede access to interdisciplinary pain programs (Gatchel et al., 2014; Gatchel & Okifuji, 2006; Janke, Cheatle, Keefe, & Dhingra, 2017). Third-party payers perceive interdisciplinary pain programs to be expensive and tend to refuse or limit access to such programs. Third-party payers tend to prefer single modality medical procedures (e.g., injections, surgeries, and pharmacotherapy). The use of fee for service payment is also incompatible with a holistic approach to pain management. These pain programs are also more difficult to access for people of ethnic and racial diversity and people from rural areas. Professionals involved in these pain programs are not always appropriately trained in pain management.

Conclusion

Chronic pain is clearly a debilitating and demoralizing condition with many consequences. Chronic pain patients present with a range of needs that can be best addressed by an interdisciplinary team of healthcare service providers who are capable of administering a range of interventions in a comprehensive, coordinated and cost-effective manner. More research identifying exactly what interventions and for whom is indicated. It is clear that chronic pain management is changing and is being influenced by technological advancements (e.g., web- and app-based interventions). Chronic pain management is also being influenced by convenience; for example, a prescription for pain medication is an easier intervention to follow than a 12-week physical exercise or meditation-exercise program. But the recent increase in opioid use has led to serious iatrogenic effects, and the fallout will occur for years to come. Although the use of medical cannabis has some advantages, its use needs to be monitored carefully to avoid unanticipated complications. It is time to view chronic pain as a problem that presents a challenge to the entire existence of the individual with persistent pain. More clinical research aimed at reducing the suffering experienced by chronic pain patients is needed. Particularly needed is research aimed at reducing the burden experienced by persons with chronic pain who represent culturally diverse and disenfranchised groups.

References

Abrams, D. I., Jay, C. A., Shade, S. B., Vizoso, H., Reda, H., Press, S., … Petersen, K. L. (2007). Cannabis in painful HIV-associated sensory neuropathy: A randomized placebo-controlled trial. *Neurology, 68*, 515–521.

Alperstein, D., & Sharpe, L. (2016). The efficacy of motivational interviewing in adults with chronic pain: A meta-analysis and systematic review. *Journal of Pain, 17*, 393–403.

Anderson, D. R., Zlateva, I., Coman, E. N., Khatri, K., Tian, T., & Kerns, R. D. (2016). Improving pain care through implementation of stepped care model at a multisite community health center. *Journal of Pain Research, 9*, 1021–1029.

Andrew, R., Derry, S., Taylor, R. S., Straube, S., & Phillips, C. J. (2014). The costs and consequences of adequately managed chronic non-cancer pain and chronic neuropathic pain. *Pain Practice, 14*(1), 79–94.

Andrews, N. E., Strong, J., & Meredith, P. J. (2012). Activity pacing, avoidance, endurance, and associations with patient functioning in chronic pain: A systematic review and meta-analysis. *Archives of Physical Medicine and Rehabilitation, 93*, 2109–2121.

Beck, A. T., & Steer, R. A. (1993). *Beck anxiety inventory manual*. San Antonio, TX: The Psychological Corporation.

Beck, A. T., Steer, R. A., & Brown, G. K. (1996). *The Beck depression inventory-II*. San Antonio, TX: Psychological Corporation.

Bergner, M., Bobbitt, R. A., Carter, W. B., & Gilson, B. S. (1981). The sickness impact profile: Development and final revision of a health measure. *Medical Care, 8*, 787–805.

Boehnke, K. F., Litinas, E., & Clauw, D. J. (2016). Medical cannabis use is associated with decreased opiate medication use in a retrospective cross-sectional survey of patients with chronic pain. *Journal of Pain, 17*, 739–744.

Brekke, M., Hjortdahl, P., & Kvien, T. K. (2002). Severity of musculoskeletal pain: Relations to socioeconomic inequality. *Social Science & Medicine, 54*(2), 221–228.

Brennstuhl, M. J., Tarquinio, C., & Montel, S. (2015). Chronic pain and PTSD: Evolving views on their comorbidity. *Perspectives in Psychiatric Care, 51*(4), 295–304.

Breuer, B., Cruciani, R., & Portenoy, R. K. (2010). Pain management by primary care physicians, pain physicians, chiropractors, and acupuncturists: A national survey. *Southern Medical Journal, 103*(8), 738–747.

Butcher, J. N., Dalhstrom, W. G., Graham, J. R., Tellegen, A., & Kaemmer, B. (1989). *Manual for the administration and scoring the Minnesota multiphasic personality inventory-2*. Minneapolis, MN: University of Minnesota Press.

Carragee, E. J., Alamin, T. F., Miller, J. L., & Carragee, J. M. (2005). Discograhic, MRI and psychosocial determinants of low back pain disability and remission: A prospective study in subjects with benign persistent back pain. *The Spine Journal, 5*, 24–35.

Cegala, D. J., McClure, L., Marinelli, T. M., & Post, D. M. (2000). The effects of communication skills training on patients' participation during medical interviews. *Patient Education and Counseling, 41*(2), 209–222.

Centers for Disease Control and Prevention. (2011). Vital signs: Overdoses of prescription opioid pain relievers---United States, 1999–2008. *MMWR. Morbidity and Mortality Weekly Report, 60*, 1487–1492.

Chiesa, A., & Serretti, A. (2011). Mindfulness-based interventions for chronic pain: A systematic review of the evidence. *Journal of Alternative and Complementary Medicine, 17*, 83–93.

Chisari, C., & Chilcot, J. (2017). The experience of pain severity and pain interference in vulvodynia patients: The role of cognitive-behavioural factors, psychological distress and fatigue. *Journal of Psychosomatic Research, 93*, 83–89.

Chou, R., Fanciullo, G. J., Fine, P. G., Adler, J. A., Ballantyne, J. C., Davies, P., … Gilson, A. M. (2009). Clinical guidelines for the use of chronic opioid therapy in chronic noncancer pain. *Journal of Pain, 10*, 113–130.

Chou, R., Turner, J. A., Devine, E. B., Hansen, R. N., Sullivan, S. D., Blazina, I., … Deyo, R. A. (2015). The effectiveness and risks of long-term opioid therapy for chronic pain: A systematic review for a National Institutes of Health pathways to prevention workshop. *Annals of Internal Medicine, 162*, 276–286.

Clarke, T. C., Nahin, R. L., Barnes, P. M., & Stussman, B. J. (2016). *Use of complementary health approaches for musculoskeletal pain disorders among adults: United States, 2012.* . National Health Statistics Reports; no 98. Hyattsville, MD: National Center for Health Statistics.

Corey-Bloom, J., Wolfson, T., Gamst, A., Jin, S., Marcotte, T. D., Bentley, H., & Gouaux, B. (2012). Smoked cannabis for spasticity in multiple sclerosis: A randomized, placebo-controlled trial. *Canadian Medical Association Journal, 184*, 1143–1150.

Crombez, G., Eccleston, C., Van Damme, S., Vlaeyen, J. W., & Karoly, P. (2012). Fear-avoidance model of chronic pain: The next generation. *Clinical Journal of Pain, 28*(6), 475–483.

Dansie, E. J., & Turk, D. C. (2013). Assessment of patients with chronic pain. *British Journal of Anaesthesia, 111*, 19–25.

Dear, B. F., Gandy, M., Ricciardi, T., Fogliati, V. J., McDonald, S., Staples, L. G., … Titov, N. (2017). The pain course: A randomized controlled trial comparing a remote-delivered chronic pain management program when provided in online and workbook formats. *Pain, 158*, 1289–1301.

Demyttenaere, K., Bruffaerts, R., Lee, S., Posada-Villa, J., Kovess, V., Angermeyer, M. C., … Lara, C. (2007). Mental disorders among persons with chronic back or neck pain: Results from the world mental health surveys. *Pain, 129*(3), 332–342.

Dobscha, S. K., Corson, K., Perrin, N. A., Hanson, G. C., Leibowitz, R. Q., Doak, M. N., et al. (2009). Collaborative care for chronic pain in primary care. *Journal of the American Medical Association, 301*, 1242–1252.

Dorner, T. E., Muckenhuber, J., Stronegger, W. J., Ràsky, É., Gustorff, B., & Freidl, W. (2011). The impact of socio-economic status on pain and the perception of disability due to pain. *European Journal of Pain, 15*(1), 103–109.

Dowell, D., Haegerich, T. M., & Chou, R. (2016). CDC guideline for prescribing opioids for chronic pain—United States, 2016. *JAMA, 315*, 1624–1645.

Duckworth, M. P., & Iezzi, T. (2010). Physical injuries, pain, and psychological trauma: Pathways to disability. *Psychological Injury and Law, 3*, 241–253.

Duckworth, M. P., Iezzi, T., & Carlson, G. (2018). Meeting the care needs of patients with multiple chronic conditions. In M. P. Duckworth & W. T. O'Donohue (Eds.), *Behavioral medicine and integrated care: Efficient delivery of the most effective treatments*. New York, NY: Springer Publishing.

Duckworth, M. P., Iezzi, T., & Sewell, T. (2009). Assessing and managing chronic pain in the primary care setting. In L. James & W. T. O'Donohue (Eds.), *The primary care consultant toolkit: Tools for behavioral medicine* (pp. 183–197). New York, NY: Springer Press.

Edwards, R. R., Dworkin, R. H., Sullivan, M. D., Turk, D. C., & Wasan, A. D. (2016). The role of psychosocial processes in the development and maintenance of chronic pain disorders. *Journal of Pain, 17*(9, Suppl. 2), T70–T92.

Ellsberg, M., Jansen, H. A., Heise, L., Watts, C. H., & Garcia-Moreno, C. (2008). Intimate partner violence and women's physical and mental health in the WHO multi-country study on women's health and domestic violence: An observational study. *Lancet, 371*(9619), 1165–1172.

Flor, H., & Turk, D. C. (2011). *Chronic pain: An integrated biobehavioral approach*. Seattle, WA: IASP Press.

Gannon, B., Finn, D. P., O'gorman, D., Ruane, N., & McGuire, B. E. (2013). The cost of chronic pain: An analysis of a regional pain management service in Ireland. *Pain Medicine, 14*(10), 1518–1528.

Gaskin, D. J., & Richard, P. (2012). The economic cost of pain in the United States. *Journal of Pain, 13*, 715–724.

Gatchel, R. J., McGeary, D. D., McGeary, C. A., & Lippe, B. (2014). Interdisciplinary chronic pain management: Past, present, and future. *American Psychologist, 69*, 119–130.

Gatchel, R. J., & Okifuji, A. (2006). Evidence-based scientific data documenting the treatment and the cost-effectiveness of comprehensive pain programs for chronic nonmalignant pain. *Journal of Pain, 7*, 779–793.

Gatchel, R. J., Peng, Y. B., Peters, M. L., Fuchs, P. N., & Turk, D. C. (2007). The biopsychosocial approach to chronic pain: Scientific advances and future directions. *Psychological Bulletin, 133*, 581–624.

Giummarra, M. J., Ioannou, L., Ponsford, J., Cameron, P. A., Jennings, P. A., Gibson, S. J., & Georgiou-Karistianis, N. (2016). Chronic pain following motor vehicle collision. *Clinical Journal of Pain, 32*(9), 817–827.

Groenewald, C. B., Essner, B. S., Wright, D., Fesinmeyer, M. D., & Palermo, T. M. (2014). The economic costs of chronic pain among a cohort of treatment-seeking adolescents in the United States. *Journal of Pain, 15*(9), 925–933.

Groenewald, C. B., Wright, D. R., & Palermo, T. M. (2015). Health care expenditures associated with pediatric pain-related conditions in the United States. *Pain, 156*, 951–957.

Grol-Prolopczyk, H. (2017). Sociodemographic disparities in chronic pain, based on 12-year longitudinal data. *Pain, 159*, 313–322.

Ho, P. T., Li, C. F., Ng, Y. K., Tsui, S. L., & Ng, K. F. J. (2011). Prevalence of and factors associated with psychiatric morbidity in chronic pain patients. *Journal of Psychosomatic Research, 70*(6), 541–547.

Hser, Y. I., Mooney, L. J., Saxon, A. J., Miotto, K., Bell, D. S., & Huang, D. (2017). Chronic pain among patients with opioid use disorder: Results from electronic health records data. *Journal of Substance Abuse Treatment, 77*, 26–30.

Hu, J., Bortsov, A. V., Ballina, L., Orrey, D. C., Swor, R. A., Peak, D., … Hendry, P. (2016). Chronic widespread pain after motor vehicle collision typically occurs through immediate development and nonrecovery: Results of an emergency department-based cohort study. *Pain, 157*(2), 438–444.

Huguet, A., & Miro, J. (2008). The severity of chronic pediatric pain: An epidemiological study. *Journal of Pain, 9*(3), 226–236.

Iezzi, T., Duckworth, M. P., Mercer, V., & Vuong, L. (2007). Chronic pain and head injury following motor vehicle collisions: A double whammy or different sides of a coin. *Psychology, Health & Medicine, 12*(2), 197–212.

Institute of Medicine (US) Committee on Advancing Pain Research, Care, and Education. (2011). *Relieving pain in America: A blueprint for transforming prevention, care, education, and research*. Washington, D.C: National Academies Press (US).

Ives, T. J., Chelminski, P. R., Hammett-Stabler, C. A., Malone, R. M., Perhac, J. S., Potisek, N. M., … Pignone, M. P. (2006). Predictors of opioid misuse in patients with chronic pain: A prospective cohort study. *BMC Health Services Research, 6*, 46–56.

Jackson, T., Iezzi, A., & Lafreniere, K. (1996). The differential effects of employment status in chronic pain and healthy comparison groups. *International Journal of Behavioral Medicine, 3*, 354–369.

Jackson, T., Iezzi, A., & Lafreniere, K. (1997). The impact of psychosocial features of employment status on emotional distress in chronic pain and healthy control samples. *Journal of Behavioral Medicine, 20*, 241–256.

Jackson, T., Iezzi, A., Lafreniere, K., & Narduzzi, K. (1998). Relations of employment status to emotional distress among chronic pain patients: A path analysis. *Clinical Journal of Pain, 14*, 55–60.

Jackson, T., Tian, P., Wang, Y., Iezzi, T., & Xie, W. (2016). Toward identifying moderators of associations between presurgery emotional distress and postoperative pain outcomes: A meta-analysis of longitudinal studies. *Journal of Pain, 17*, 874–888.

Janke, E. A., Cheatle, M. D., Keefe, F. J., & Dhingra, L. K. (2017). *Improving access to psychosocial care for individuals with persistent pain: The National Pain Strategy call for interdisciplinary pain care*. New York, NY: Society of Behavioral Medicine.

Johannes, C. B., Le, T. K., Zhou, X., Johnston, J. A., & Dworkin, R. H. (2010). The prevalence of chronic pain in United States adults: Results of an internet-based survey. *Journal of Pain, 11*(11), 1230–1239.

Johnston, M., Foster, M., Shennan, J., Starkey, N. J., & Johnson, A. (2010). The effectiveness of an acceptance and commitment therapy self-help intervention for chronic pain. *Clinical Journal of Pain, 26*(5), 393–402.

Jones, C. M., Baldwin, G. T., Manocchio, T., White, J. O., & Mack, K. A. (2016). Trends in methadone distribution for pain treatment, methadone diversion, and overdose deaths-United States, 2002-2014. *MMWR: Morbidity and Mortality Weekly Report, 65*, 667–671.

Kamper, S. J., Maher, C. G., Costa, L. D. C. M., McAuley, J. H., Hush, J. M., & Sterling, M. (2012). Does fear of movement mediate the relationship between pain intensity and disability in patients following whiplash injury? A prospective longitudinal study. *Pain, 153*, 113–119.

Kawai, K., Kawai, A. T., Wollan, P., & Yawn, B. P. (2017). Adverse impacts of chronic pain on health-related quality of life, work productivity, depression and anxiety in a community-based study. *Family Practice, 34*(6), 656–661 cmx034.

Keefe, F. J., Baupre, P. M., Rumble, M. E., Kelleher, S. A., & Van Denburg, A. (2018). Group therapy for patients with chronic pain. In D. C. Turk & R. J. Gatchel (Eds.), *Psychological treatments for pain: A practitioner's handbook* (3rd ed.). New York: Guilford.

Keefe, F. J., Crisson, J., Urban, B. J., & Williams, D. (1990). Analyzing chronic low back pain: The relative contribution of pain coping strategies. *Pain, 40*, 293–301.

Kerns, R. D., Turk, D. C., & Rudy, T. E. (1985). The west haven-Yale multidimensional pain inventory. *Pain, 23*, 345–356.

King, S., Chambers, C. T., Huguet, A., MacNevin, R. C., McGrath, P. J., Parker, L., & MacDonald, A. J. (2011). The epidemiology of chronic pain in children and adolescents revisited: A systematic review. *Pain, 152*, 2729–2738.

Lachenmeier, D. W., & Rehm, J. (2015). Comparative risk assessment of alcohol, tobacco, cannabis and other illicit drugs using the margin of exposure approach. *Scientific Reports, 5*, 8126. https://doi.org/10.1038/srep0812

Laditka, J. N., & Laditka, S. B. (2016). Unemployment, disability and life expectancy in the United States: A life course study. *Disability and Health Journal, 9*(1), 46–53.

Lalloo, C., Jibb, L. A., Rivera, J., Agarwal, A., & Stinson, J. N. (2015). "There's a pain app for that": Review of patient-targeted smartphone applications for pain management. *Clinical Journal of Pain, 31*, 557–563.

Lamb, S. E., Hansen, Z., Lall, R., Castelnuovo, E., Withers, E. J., Nichols, V., … Back Skills Training Trial, i. (2010). Group cognitive behavioural treatment for low-back pain in primary care: A randomised controlled trial and cost-effectiveness analysis. *Lancet, 375*(9718), 916–923.

Liegl, G., Boeckle, M., Leitner, A., & Pieh, C. (2016). A meta-analytic review of brief guided self-help education for chronic pain. *European Journal of Pain, 20*, 1551–1562.
Lorig, K., Lubeck, D., Kraines, R. G., Seleznick, M., & Holman, H. R. (1985). Outcomes of self-help education for patients with arthritis. *Arthritis and Rheumatism, 28*(6), 680–685.
Macea, D. D., Gajos, K., Calil, Y. A. D., & Fregni, F. (2010). The efficacy of web-based cognitive behavioral interventions for chronic pain: A systematic review and meta-analysis. *Journal of Pain, 11*, 917–929.
Manchikanti, L., Abdi, S., Atluri, S., Balog, C. C., Benyamin, R. M., Boswell, M. V., … Burton, A. W. (2012). American Society of Interventional Pain Physicians (ASIPP) guidelines for responsible opioid prescribing in chronic non-cancer pain: Part I--evidence assessment. *Pain Physician, 15*(3 Suppl), S1–S65.
Manchikanti, L., Giordano, J., Boswell, M. V., Fellows, B., Manchukonda, R., & Pampati, V. (2007). Psychological factors as predictors of opioid abuse and illicit drug use in chronic pain patients. *Journal of Opioid Management, 3*, 89–100.
McCracken, L. M., Vowles, K. E., & Eccleston, C. (2004). Acceptance of chronic pain: Component analysis and a revised assessment method. *Pain, 107*, 159–166.
Merskey, H., & Bogduk, N. (1994). *Classification of chronic pain: Descriptions of chronic pain syndromes and definitions of pain terms*. Seattle, WA: IASP Press.
Millon, T., Millon, C., Davis, R., & Grossman, S. (1994). *Millon clinical inventory-III manual*. Minneapolis, MN: National Computer Systems.
Morey, L. C. (1991). *The personality assessment inventory: Professional manual*. Odessa, FL: Psychological Assessment Resources.
Nahin, R. L. (2015). Estimates of pain prevalence and severity in adults: United States, 2012. *Journal of Pain, 16*, 769–780.
National Center for Health Statistics. (2016). *National center for health statistics* (September 25, 2016.) Table 11. Twenty leading principal reasons for office visits, by patient's sex: United States, 2012. Retrieved from: http://www.cdc.gov/nchs/data/ahcd/namcs_summary/2012_namcs_web_tables.pdf
National Institutes of Health. (2013). *Fact sheet: Pain management*. Retrieved from: https://report.nih.gov/nihfactsheets/Pdfs/PainManagement(NINR).pdf
Nuckols, T. K., Anderson, L., Popescu, I., Diamant, A. L., Doyle, B., Di Capua, P., & Chou, R. (2014). Opioid prescribing: A systematic review and critical appraisal of guidelines for chronic pain. *Annals of Internal Medicine, 160*, 38–47.
O'Connor, A. B., Turk, D. C., Dworkin, R. H., Katz, N. P., Colucci, R., Haythornthwaite, J. A., … Reisfield, G. (2013). Abuse liability measures for use in analgesic clinical trials in patients with pain: IMMPACT recommendations. *Pain, 154*, 2324–2334 *Journal of Pain, 16*, 769-–780.
Ortman, J. M., Velkoff, V. A., & Hogan, H. (2014). *An aging nation: The older population in the United States, Current population reports* (pp. 25–1140). Washington, DC: U.S. Census Bureau.
Otis, J. D., MacDonald, A., & Dobscha, S. K. (2006). Integration and coordination of pain management in primary care. *Journal of Clinical Psychology, 62*, 1333–1343.
Outcalt, S. D., Kroenke, K., Krebs, E. E., Chumbler, N. R., Wu, J., Yu, Z., & Bair, M. J. (2015). Chronic pain and comorbid mental health conditions: Independent associations of post-traumatic stress disorder and depression with pain, disability, and quality of life. *Journal of Behavioral Medicine, 38*(3), 535–543.
Pedler, A., Kamper, S. J., & Sterling, M. (2016). Addition of posttraumatic stress and sensory hypersensitivity more accurately estimates disability and pain than fear avoidance measures alone after whiplash injury. *Pain, 157*(8), 1645–1654.
Plagge, J. M., Lu, M. W., Lovejoy, T. I., Karl, A. I., & Dobscha, S. K. (2013). Treatment of comorbid pain and PTSD in returning veterans: A collaborative approach utilizing behavioral activation. *Pain Medicine, 14*, 1164–1172.
Platts-Mills, T. F., Flannigan, S. A., Bortsov, A. V., Smith, S., Domeier, R. M., Swor, R. A., … Lee, D. C. (2016). Persistent pain among older adults discharged home from the emergency department after motor vehicle crash: A prospective cohort study. *Annals of Emergency Medicine, 67*(2), 166–176.

Poole, H., White, S., Blake, C., Murphy, P., & Bramwell, R. (2009). Depression in chronic pain patients: Prevalence and measurement. *Pain Practice, 9*(3), 173–180.

Proctor, S. L., Estroff, T. W., Empting, L. D., Shearer-Williams, S., & Hoffmann, N. G. (2013). Prevalence of substance use and psychiatric disorders in a highly select chronic pain population. *Journal of Addiction Medicine, 7*(1), 17–24.

Raijmakers, B. G., Nieuwenhuizen, M. G., Beckerman, H., & de Groot, S. (2015). Differences in the course of daily activity level between persons with and without chronic pain. *American Journal of Physical Medicine & Rehabilitation, 94*(2), 101–113.

Ratzon, N. Z., Froom, P., Friedman, S., & Amit, Y. (2013). Functional capacity evaluation of work performance among individuals with pelvic injuries following motor vehicle accidents. *Work, 45*(2), 191–200.

Rice, A. S. C., Smith, B. H., & Blyth, F. M. (2016). Pain and the global burden of disease. *Pain, 157*, 791–796.

Richards, J. S., Nepomuceno, C., Riles, M., & Suer, Z. (1982). Assessing pain behavior: The UAB pain behavior scale. *Pain, 14*, 393–398.

Rini, C., Porter, L. S., Somers, T. J., McKee, D. C., DeVellis, R. F., Smith, M., … Keefe, F. J. (2015). Automated internet-based pain coping skills training to manage osteoarthritis pain: A randomized controlled trial. *Pain, 156*(5), 837–848.

Romano, M., & Peters, L. (2015). Evaluating the mechanisms of change in motivational interviewing in the treatment of mental health problems: A review and meta-analysis. *Clinical Psychology Review, 38*, 1–12.

Rudd, R. A., Aleshire, N., Zibbell, J. E., & Gladden, R. M. (2016). Increases in drug and opioid overdose deaths—United States, 2000–2014. *American Journal of Transplantation, 16*, 1323–1327.

Ruehlman, L. S., Karoly, P., & Enders, C. (2012). A randomized controlled evaluation of an online chronic pain self-management program. *Pain, 153*(2), 319–330.

Sachs-Ericsson, N., Kendall-Tackett, K., & Hernandez, A. (2007). Childhood abuse, chronic pain, and depression in the National Comorbidity Survey. *Child Abuse & Neglect, 31*(5), 531–547.

Sagheer, M. A., Khan, M. F., & Sharif, S. (2013). Association between chronic low back pain, anxiety and depression in patients at a tertiary care Centre. *Journal of the Pakistan Medical Association, 63*(6), 688–690.

Savage, S. R., Romero-Sandoval, A., Schatman, M., Wallace, M., Fanciullo, G., McCarberg, B., & Ware, M. (2016). Cannabis in pain treatment: Clinical and research considerations. *Journal of Pain, 17*, 654–668.

Scascighini, L., Toma, V., Dober-Spielman, S., & Sprott, H. (2008). Multidisciplinary treatment for chronic pain: A systematic review of interventions and outcomes. *Rheumatology, 47*, 670–678.

Sites, B. D., Beach, M. L., & Davis, M. (2014). Increases in the use of prescription opioid analgesics and the lack of improvement in disability metrics among users. *Regional Anesthesia and Pain Medicine, 39*, 6–12.

Smith, S. M., Dart, R. C., Katz, N. P., Paillard, F., Adams, E. H., Comer, S. D., … Jones, C. M. (2013). Classification and definition of misuse, abuse, and related events in clinical trials: ACTTION systematic review and recommendations. *Pain, 154*, 2287–2296.

Solowij, N., Stephens, R. S., Roffman, R. A., Babor, D. T., Kadden, R., Miller, M., … Vendetti, J. (2002). Cognitive functioning of long-term heavy cannabis users seeking treatment. *JAMA, 287*, 1123–1131.

Strandh, M., Winefield, A., Nilsson, K., & Hammarström, A. (2014). Unemployment and mental health scarring during the life course. *European Journal of Public Health, 24*(3), 440–445.

Stumbo, S. P., Yarborough, B. J. H., McCarty, D., Weisner, C., & Green, C. A. (2017). Patient-reported pathways to opioid use disorders and pain-related barriers to treatment engagement. *Journal of Substance Abuse Treatment, 73*, 47–54.

Sturgeon, J. A. (2014). Psychological therapies for the management of chronic pain. *Psychology Research and Behavior Management, 7*, 115–124.

Sullivan, M., Adams, H., Thibault, P., Moore, E., Carriere, J. S., & Larivière, C. (2017). Return to work helps maintain treatment gains in the rehabilitation of whiplash injury. *Pain, 158*(5), 980–987.

Sundararaman, L. V., Edwards, R. R., Ross, E. L., & Jamison, R. N. (2017). Integration of mobile health technology in the treatment of chronic pain: A critical review. *Regional Anesthesia and Pain Medicine, 42*, 488–498.

Tait, R. C., Pollard, C. A., Margolis, R. B., Duckro, P. N., & Krause, S. J. (1987). The pain disability index: Psychometric and validity data. *Archives of Physical Medicine and Rehabilitation, 68*, 438–441.

Tashkin, D. P. (2013). Effects of marijuana smoking on the lung. *Annals of the American Thoracic Society, 10*, 239–247.

Taylor, A. M., Phillips, K., Patel, K. V., Turk, D. C., Dworkin, R. H., Beaton, D., … Witter, J. (2016). Assessment of physical function and participation in chronic pain clinical trials: IMMPACT/OMERACT recommendations. *Pain, 157*, 1836–1850.

Theunissen, M., Peters, M. L., Bruce, J., Gramke, H. F., & Marcus, M. A. (2012). Preoperative anxiety and catastrophizing: A systematic review and meta-analysis of the association with chronic postsurgical pain. *Clinical Journal of Pain, 28*(9), 819–841.

Thorsell, J., Finnes, A., Dahl, J., Lundgren, T., Gybrant, M., Gordh, T., & Buhrman, M. (2011). A comparative study of 2 manual-based self-help interventions, acceptance and commitment therapy and applied relaxation, for persons with chronic pain. *Clinical Journal of Pain, 27*, 716–723.

Turk, D. C. (2005). The potential of treatment matching for subgroups of patients with chronic pain: Lumping versus splitting. *Clinical Journal of Pain, 21*, 44–55.

Turk, D. C., Fillingim, R. B., Ohrbach, R., & Patel, K. V. (2016). Assessment of psychosocial and functional impact of chronic pain. *Journal of Pain, 17*(9, Suppl. 2), T21–T49.

Turk, D. C., & Melzack, R. (2011). *Handbook of pain assessment* (3rd ed.). New York, NY: Guilford Press.

Turk, D. C., & Okifuji, A. (2002). Psychological factors in chronic pain: Evolution and revolution. *Journal of Consulting and Clinical Psychology, 70*, 678–690.

Turk, D. C., Swanson, K. S., & Gatchel, R. J. (2008). Predicting opioid misuse by chronic pain patients: A systematic review and literature synthesis. *Clinical Journal of Pain, 24*, 497–508.

Turner, J. A., Anderson, M. L., Balderson, B. H., Cook, A. J., Sherman, K. J., & Cherkin, D. C. (2016). Mindfulness-based stress reduction and cognitive behavioral therapy for chronic low back pain: Similar effects on mindfulness, catastrophizing, self-efficacy, and acceptance in a randomized controlled trial. *Pain, 157*, 2434–2444.

Valentine, S. E., Gerber, M. W., Nobles, C. J., Shtasel, D. L., & Marques, L. (2016). Longitudinal study of mental health and pain-related functioning following a motor vehicle collision. *Health Psychology, 35*, 742–750.

Vartiainen, P., Heiskanen, T., Sintonen, H., Roine, R. P., & Kalso, E. (2016). Health-related quality of life and burden of disease in chronic pain measured with the 15D instrument. *Pain, 157*(10), 2269–2276.

Veehof, M. M., Trompetter, H. R., Bohlmeijer, E. T., & Schreurs, K. M. (2016). Acceptance- and mindfulness-based interventions for the treatment of chronic pain: A meta-analytic review. *Cognitive and Behavior Therapy, 45*(1), 5–31.

Vos, T., Barber, R. M., Bell, B., Bertozzi-Villa, A., Birukov, S., Bollinger, I., … Murray, C. G. J. (2015). Global, regional, and national incidence, prevalence, and years lived with disability for 301 acute and chronic diseases and injuries in 188 countries 1990-2013: A systematic analysis for the global burden of disease study 2013. *Lancet, 386*, 743–800.

Vowles, K. E., McEntee, M. L., Julnes, P. S., Frohe, T., Ney, J. P., & van der Goes, D. N. (2015). Rates of opioid misuse, abuse, and addiction in chronic pain: A systematic review and data synthesis. *Pain, 156*, 569–576.

Ware, J. E., Snow, K. K., Kosinski, M., & Gandek, B. (1993). *SF-36 health survey: Manual and interpretation guide*. Boston, MA: The Health Institute, New England Medical Center.

Ware, M. A., Wang, T., Shapiro, S., Robinson, A., Ducruet, T., Huynh, T., … Collet, J. P. (2010). Smoked cannabis for chronic neuropathic pain: A randomized controlled trial. *Canadian Medical Association Journal, 182*, E694–E701.

Chapter 16
Promoting the Behavioral Health of Persons with Neurocognitive Disorders

Jonathan Singer, Adrienne Chong, Ryan Hisaka, and Jane E. Fisher

It is estimated that the worldwide number of individuals with dementia will reach 135 million by 2050 (Rahman, 2017; Rizzi, Rosset, & Roriz-Cruz, 2014) without any indication of a cure on the horizon. The label "dementia" is a summary term for a group of symptoms that include decline from previous levels of functioning, difficulties in expressive and receptive language, impaired judgment, impaired ability to acquire and remember new information, and impaired visuospatial abilities (McKhann et al., 2011). The most prevalent neurocognitive disorders leading to dementia are Alzheimer's disease (AD) (77%; Barker et al., 2002; Hebert, Weuve, Scherr, & Evans, 2013), vascular dementia (VaD) (15–20%; Barker et al., 2002; Centers for Disease Control and Prevention, 2006), and dementia with Lewy bodies (10–26%; Barker et al., 2002; Jellinger & Attems, 2011), with over 30% of dementia cases involving mixed neuropathology (e.g., AD with cerebrovascular disease or AD with Lewy body), (Jellinger & Attems, 2011; LoGiudice & Watson, 2014). Importantly, diagnostic labels generally are not informative for describing an individual patient's current level of functioning or predicting the rate of disease progression. Increasing evidence indicates that lifestyle, general health status, and environmental factors such as caregivers' skill and emotional well-being significantly impact the functioning and quality of life of persons with neurocognitive disorders (Lwi, Ford, Casey, Miller, & Levenson, 2017; Vance & Struzick, 2007). This chapter will describe a model of person-centered care for promoting the quality of life and behavioral health of persons with neurocognitive disorders and their families.

J. Singer (✉) · A. Chong · R. Hisaka · J. E. Fisher
Department of Psychology, University of Nevada, Reno, Reno, NV, USA
e-mail: rshsaka@nevada.unr.edu; akchong@nevada.unr.edu; jonathan.singer@nevada.unr.edu; fisher@unr.edu

M. P. Duckworth, W. T. O'Donohue (eds.), *Behavioral Medicine and Integrated Care*,
https://doi.org/10.1007/978-3-319-93003-9_16

The decline in memory and verbal functioning, which are predominant in the majority of neurocognitive disorders, present significant assessment and treatment challenges as patients eventually become unable to describe their internal physiological and psychological states (e.g., whether they are experiencing pain, discomfort, or changes therein following treatment of comorbid condition). The integration of specialty care focused both on the accuracy of diagnosis and support for optimizing the quality of life for the patient and his/her family is now considered to be best practice (Galvin & Sadowsky, 2012; van Hout, Vernooij-Dassen, & Stalman, 2007). Primary care providers have a particularly important role in promoting the safety and quality of life of patients with dementia as they are on the front lines for responding to (a) patient and family members' concerns regarding changes in cognition, affect, and behavior prior to the diagnosis of a neurocognitive disorder, (b) guiding patients and their families through the diagnostic process, c) responding to patients' and/or family members' reports of changes in functioning and the detection and treatment of comorbid conditions following diagnosis, and (d) collaborating with patients and their families over the course of what can be years of disease progression (Boustani, Peterson, Hanson, Harris, & Lohr, 2003).

Epidemiology and Diagnosis of Neurocognitive Disorders

Diagnostic Challenges and Age-Associated Complications Neurocognitive disorders are age-associated diseases, with the majority of patients developing symptomatology after the age of 65 and the highest incidence rate in individuals between the ages of 80 and 84 (Prince et al., 2013). Recent improvements in detection sensitivity have resulted in a higher rate of early onset neurocognitive disease diagnosis, i.e., disease onset prior to age 65 (Lambert et al., 2014). Early onset of a neurocognitive disease can present diagnostic challenges as memory lapses are less likely to be salient to younger adults, and thus they are less inclined to seek assessment by a healthcare provider. The base rates of early onset neurocognitive disease are very low; the "typical" patient with a neurocognitive disorder is older (Hebert et al., 2013), is retired (Lambert et al., 2014), and has a higher number of comorbid conditions (Abizanda et al., 2014).

Differential diagnosis of specific neurocognitive disorders is crucial for treatment planning, understanding expected changes vs. unexpected changes in disease trajectory, and optimizing quality of life for patients. In 2012 the National Institute on Aging published updated diagnostic criteria in an effort to improve the diagnostic accuracy of all neurocognitive disorders (see McKhann, Albert, & Sperling, 2012). The revised criteria are based on a continuous model of differential diagnosis and now include guidelines for assessing the transition from no cognitive decline to mild cognitive impairment to meeting the criteria for dementia. Second, the revised criteria allow for the possibility that impairment in memory may not be the primary symptom in individuals presenting with neurocognitive decline and that patients' predominant symptomatology may involve language, spatial ability, or executive function. Third, additional causes of cognitive impairment have been incorporated within the criteria (e.g., Lewy bodies, frontotemporal lobar degeneration).

Unfortunately, reliance on non-evidence-based diagnostic procedures (e.g., brief cognitive screening alone, diagnosis absent neurological examination, and neuroimaging) continues to be a problem in the field (Paterson, Takada, & Geschwind, 2012). A recent study by Beach, Monsell, Phillips, and Kukull (2012) evaluated clinical and neuropathology autopsy data for more than 1100 subject. The researchers found that, between 2005 and 2010, specificity of the exact disease ranged from 44.3% to 70.8%, depending on the diagnostic criteria used. The wide variability in diagnostic specificity speaks to the challenge of accurately identifying the etiology of neurocognitive symptoms. In contrast to standard practice, the integrated care model incorporates the expertise of specialists (neurologists, neuropsychologists), resulting in a more thorough and accurate diagnostic evaluation (Villars et al., 2010).

An integrated model of healthcare is characterized by a high degree of collaboration and communication between health professionals with the shared goal of optimizing patient health through a variety of prevention and intervention strategies. Treatment planning is comprehensive in addressing the biological, psychological, and social needs of the patient. Integrated healthcare teams include a diverse group of members (e.g., physicians, nurses, psychologists, social workers, and other health professionals; American Psychological Association, 2017). While involvement of an interdisciplinary team may increase healthcare costs in the short term, a pilot study investigated integrated care and found it to be economically effective in reducing costs in the long term (Bandurska et al., 2017). Reduced costs in the long term are realized through effective detection and management of comorbid conditions and associated prevention of excess disability, (Looman, Huijsman, Bouwmans-Frijters, Stolk, & Fabbricotti, 2016) and the prevention or delay of institutionalization (Dramé et al., 2011).

Unique Issues in the Treatment of Persons with Dementia

Dementia-Specific Challenges in Polypharmacy Polypharmacy, defined as the use of two or more medications (see Brown, 2016; Gnjidic et al., 2012; Hovstadius & Petersson, 2012), is highly prevalent within geriatric healthcare, with more than one third of prescriptions in the United States being filled by individuals over the age of 65 (Marcum, Driessen, Thorpe, Gellad, & Donohue, 2014). Polypharmacy increases the risk of drug reactions and severe side effects (Brown, 2016; Norgaard, Jensen-Dahm, Gasse, Hansen, & Waldemar, 2017). Pharmacological intervention with patients with dementia typically includes both cognitive enhancing and psychotropic medications in addition to medications prescribed for comorbid age-associated conditions. A recent study of over 250,000 older adults found that individuals with a neurocognitive disorder had a significantly higher rate of polypharmacy, even when controlling for age, gender, and comorbidities, and that individuals experiencing polypharmacy were at higher risk for migraines, dizziness, and hypertension (Clague, Mercer, McLean, Reynish, & Guthrie, 2016).

Pharmacological Approaches to Cognitive Enhancement Currently, there are four medications that have been approved by the FDA for individuals with neurocognitive disorder: donepezil, galantamine, rivastigmine, and memantine (Di Santo, Prinelli, Adorni, Caltagirone, & Musicco, 2013; Tan et al., 2014). A Cochrane meta-analysis was performed to evaluate treatment effects, including effects of these four medications on cognition and activities of daily living (ADLs). Thirty-four (34) RCTs fit the criteria that included being written in English, published before 2012, and evaluated treatment effects of the four medications on individuals with neurocognitive disorders. Memantine had the greatest treatment effect throughout all studies, with the other three medications producing equivocal results when compared to the placebo (Di Santo et al., 2013). Many of the studies included within the meta-analysis did not examine patient functioning beyond 3 months, and therefore, long-term effects were not analyzed. The RCTs that did report long-term outcomes showed the medications had little to no effect on cognitive decline. Moreover, Geldmacher (2003) and Lopez et al. (2009) reported moderate improvement in cognition for individuals with Alzheimer's disease using "cognitive enhancing" medications but found only minimal effects in 40% of the entire sample.

Several side effects (e.g., urinary incontinence, fatigue, dizziness, nausea) have been reported for each of the currently approved cognitive enhancing medications (Bond et al., 2012; Kim, Brown, Ding, Kiel, & Berry, 2011). Additionally, the cognitive enhancing medications have been reported to exacerbate confusion and increase the risk of falls and sleep problems, which already occur at high rates for patients with neurocognitive disorder (Kim et al., 2011; McKhann et al., 2011). The verbal deficits that develop during the course of degenerative neurocognitive disorders present challenges when family healthcare advocates and healthcare providers analyze the risks and benefits of medication and drug effects/side effects.

Pharmacological Management of Behavioral and Affective Changes In recent years, the treatment of individuals with a neurocognitive disorder has become increasingly controversial due to the prevalent use of psychotropic medication for the management of what are commonly referred to as "non-cognitive psychiatric symptoms." Over 25% of older adults diagnosed with a neurocognitive disorder are medicated with two or more psychotropic drugs (Norgaard et al., 2017). Antipsychotic medications have been the primary intervention for behavioral or "non-cognitive psychiatric symptoms" related to neurocognitive disorders (Chiu, Bero, Hessol, Lexchin, & Harrington, 2015; Kales, Gitlin, & Lyketsos, 2015; Molinari et al., 2010; Vasudev et al., 2015) despite FDA black box warnings against their use in the care of elderly persons with dementia due to the risk of serious adverse effects (Centers for Medicare & Medicaid Services, 2013; U.S. Food and Drug Administration, 2008). A recent study (Norgaard et al., 2017) reported that 25% of individuals with dementia were prescribed antipsychotic medication despite studies reporting that antipsychotics increase mortality and yield little, if any, positive effects (see Ballard et al., 2009; Maust et al., 2015). Alarmingly, a study of 559 individuals who were diagnosed with a neurocognitive disorder and prescribed psychotropic medication found that only 10% of the prescription and/or management of psychotropic drug use was appropriate. The three major categories of inappropriate use of psychotropic medications involved indication, inadequate evaluation, and therapy duration (van der Spek et al., 2016).

Maust et al. (2015) investigated mortality rates of 90,786 individuals over the age of 65 who were diagnosed with dementia and administered at least one antipsychotic, such as haloperidol, olanzapine, risperidone, and quetiapine. Outcome measures included the absolute change in mortality risk and the Veteran's Affairs registries, based on mortality data obtained from the US National Death Index. The mortality risk of haloperidol and risperidone users was found to be almost double than that of nonusers. Moreover, findings at the 180-day outcome demonstrated the use of haloperidol for individuals with dementia was associated with 1 additional death for every 26 patients. In general, both antipsychotics and antidepressants statistically increased the risk of mortality for individuals with dementia, in comparison to nonusers (e.g., Ballard et al., 2009; Wang et al., 2014).

Numerous studies have evaluated both the short- and long-term effects of antipsychotics on behavioral and psychological symptoms for persons with dementia (e.g., Tampi, Tampi, Balachandran, & Srinivasan, 2016). Tampi and colleagues (2016) conducted a systematic review of meta-analyses that examined the use of antipsychotics in individuals with forms of dementia, including Alzheimer's disease, Lewy bodies, and VaD. Inclusion criteria included being published in a peer-reviewed journal and examining psychotropic medication's effect on individuals with dementia. Based on the eight studies included in the meta-analysis, Tampi and colleagues (2016) concluded that the use of antipsychotic drugs resulted in moderate improvements in psychosis (delusions and hallucinations) and improvements in agitation (i.e., physical aggression, verbal aggression, excitability, oppositional behavioral, and excessive motor activity) within the first 4 weeks; however, there were no long-term improvements, and severe adverse events were reported (e.g., cerebrovascular adverse events, Parkinsonism, sedation, gait disturbance, cognitive decline, pneumonia). These results further indicate that antipsychotics are contraindicated for the treatment of behavioral problems in persons with dementia, as there are limited short-term benefits and serious adverse effects, including premature death.

As mentioned earlier, monitoring of treatment effects (either positive or negative) is a significant challenge in the care of verbally impaired individuals. Monitoring the effects of antipsychotic medications presents a unique challenge as several of the side effects of antipsychotic medications mirror the symptoms of degenerative neurocognitive disorders (e.g., confusion, loss of language, etc.). Schneider, Dagerman, and Insel (2005) reported sedation (15–24% of the participants with dementia), confusion (11–18%), and cognitive disturbances (5–7%) as common adverse events related to atypical antipsychotic treatment, concluding that "adverse events offset the advantages in the efficacy of atypical antipsychotic drugs" (p. 1525). The most recent American Geriatric Society (AGS) Beers consensus criteria for safe medication use in the elderly recommend avoiding antipsychotics in the treatment of elderly with dementia, due to the increased mortality and cerebrovascular accident risk (Campanelli, 2012).

Healthcare Implications of Judgments of Quality of Life in Patients with Dementia

Quality of life (QoL) is a broad and multidimensional construct that encompasses physical, mental, social, and role functioning and health perceptions (Bowling et al., 2015). The World Health Organization defines QoL as an "…individual's perceptions of their position in life in the context of the culture and value systems in which they live, and in relation to their goals, expectations, standards and concerns" (Bowling, 2001; World Health Organization, 1997). The importance of clear criteria and procedures for evaluating the QoL of persons with neurocognitive disorders is critical, as medical proxies often make decisions to treat or discontinue treatment of comorbid conditions based on their perceptions of the patient's QoL. If a patient is experiencing excess disability (e.g., the patient appears to be in the advanced stage of a neurocognitive disorder but is actually evidencing the effects of sedation due to overmedication), the medical proxy may decide to discontinue treatment of a comorbid based on an incorrect condition(s). Additionally, care facilities are increasingly requiring that their staff measure QoL to create goals specifically focused on improving QoL for individuals with neurocognitive disorders (Beerens et al., 2014; Beerens, Zwakhalen, Verbeek, Ruwaard, & Hamers, 2013).

The American Academy of Neurology (Doody et al., 2001) and the World Alzheimer's report (Prince, Comas-Herrera, Knapp, Guerchet, & Karagiannidou, 2016) propose that interventions to improve QoL should encompass comprehensive integrated care. As stated above, accurate diagnosis is crucial for developing an appropriate treatment plan. Yet research has consistently found that the diagnosis and treatment of individuals with dementia is often suboptimal for reasons including lack of differential diagnosis, inadequate treatment of comorbid conditions, and misattribution of excess disability due to treatable adverse medical or environmental events (see Doody et al., 2001; Odenheimer et al., 2013).

A "Contextual" Model of Dementia Care

The significant variability in functioning and rate of disease progression within neurocognitive disease diagnostic groups strongly suggests that lifestyle, environmental, and genetic variables impact the health and quality of life of persons with dementia (Brown, Lockwood, & Sonawane, 2005; Van Duijn et al., 1994). The contextual model of behavior posits that behavior is context bound and based on an interaction of the person's learning and genetic histories with the current environment that sets the occasion for the production of the behavior (Catania, 1996). When applied to the functioning of persons with dementia, the goal of intervention is to support the maintenance of behavior in an individual who will inevitably experience devastating losses due to neurodegeneration. Strategies for promoting behavioral health are identified through an assessment of the individual's learning history, current physiological status and behavioral repertoire, and the features of the current environment that support or inhibit the patient's repertoire (Fisher, Drossel, Yury, & Cherup, 2007). A substantial body of literature indicates that the functioning of persons with neurocognitive disorders is influenced by environmental factors, including the affective responding of persons around them as well as sensory stimuli (see Buchanan, Christenson, Houlihan, & Ostrom, 2011; Fleming, Goodenough, Low, Chenoweth, & Brodaty, 2016). Following diagnosis, the behavior of patients with dementia is often misattributed to the underlying neuropathology, even when contextually appropriate. For example, if a verbally impaired patient responds in a distressed or "agitated" manner to negative affect and corrective feedback by a family member, the patient's reaction (which would be considered a normal reaction to rude behavior in a cognitively healthy individual) is highly likely to be pathologized as a symptom of the disease. The administration of medications to reduce what is judged to be a behavioral "symptom" may accelerate reduction of the patient's already diminishing repertoire (Garrison-Diehn, Rummel, & Fisher, 2013).

Numerous non-pharmacological interventions focused on supporting adaptive behavior and/or preventing problem behaviors by identifying and treating the underlying cause (e.g., pain, discomfort, over or understimulation, punitive caregiver behavior) have been shown to be efficacious (see Buchanan et al., 2011; Gitlin, Kales, & Lyketsos, 2012; Gitlin, Winter, Dennis, Hodgson, & Hauck, 2010).

Maintaining Adaptive Behavior While Preventing Excess Disability

Excess disability involves a decline in functioning that exceeds what would be expected based on an individual's underlying medical condition (Dawson, Wells, & Kline, 1993). Over the course of degenerative neurocognitive disorders, excess disability is manifested in the premature loss of behavior (e.g., when a medication causes impairment in language or increased confusion; Yury & Fisher, 2007). Promoting behavioral health in persons with neurocognitive disorders often requires the detection, reduction, or prevention of premature declines in functioning and maintaining or restoring function (Fisher et al., 2007).

Behaviors that are viewed as challenging are commonly treated with approaches that aim to reduce or eliminate the behavior (Enns, Rhemtulla, Ewa, Fruetel, & Holroyd-Leduc, 2014) through environmental, physical, and/or chemical restraints.

However, studies have demonstrated that these "restraint based" interventions can have serious adverse effects on individual with dementia including increased risk of falls and serious injury and premature death (see Baert, Gorus, Mets, Geerts, & Bautmans, 2011; Ballard et al., 2009; Neufeld et al., 1999).

Chemical restraints are defined as "any drug used for discipline or convenience and not required to treat medical symptoms" (U.S. Department of Health and Human Services, 2005). As explicated above, antipsychotics are commonly used to reduce behaviors that are judged to be a problem or "neuropsychiatric symptom" among individuals diagnosed with a neurocognitive disorder, despite evidence of an increased risk of mortality associated with use of antipsychotics in this population (Ballard et al., 2009). The use of medication to decrease any behavior in individuals with a neurocognitive disorder is particularly concerning, even when targeting behavior that is viewed as problematic. The inappropriate use of medications for chemical restraint can lead to excess disability in the form of a premature reduction in an individual's behavioral and verbal repertoire (Fisher et al., 2007).

Unlike restraint-based approaches, treatment goals within the contextual model of dementia care focus on maintaining an individual's behavioral repertoire. Within the behavioral model, effective approaches to treatment assess the functional relevance of all behaviors, including ones labeled as challenging. Treatments focused on supporting adaptive behavior and preventing rather than eliminating challenging behavior ultimately reduce excess disability or prevent it altogether.

Family caregivers play a critically important role in promoting the health of persons with dementia as they are in a position of observing and reporting information about changes in cognitive and behavioral health (e.g., as reflected in changes in the patient's verbal responding and ability to complete self-care and more complex tasks such as managing finances and medications) and safety (e.g., based on observations of impaired driving and/or confusion in the use of potentially dangerous machinery and household appliances). To illustrate, abrupt changes in long-standing high-frequency behaviors may help family caregivers and healthcare providers detect adverse medical and/or environmental events (an abrupt decline in a patient's appetite, verbal expressiveness, or activity level may indicate an acute condition such as an infection or medication side effect). In addition, family caregivers and their relationship (both the relationship history and current relationship) with the patient are critical features of the context of the patient's experience.

Barriers to Maintaining Adaptive Behavior

The multifaceted nature of dementia symptoms and comorbidities in individuals with a neurocognitive disorder contribute to the difficulty in detecting adverse effects. Adverse events may be physiological and psychological (Andreassi, 2013; Fauth & Gibbons, 2014). Psychological events include, but are not limited to, depression, anxiety, hallucinations (mostly seen in dementia with Lewy Bodies), and apathy (Fauth & Gibbons, 2014). Physiological adverse events include, but are not limited to, pain, insomnia, and confusion (Andreassi, 2013). Both psychological and physiological adverse events have been reported as significant barriers to maintaining adaptive behavior in individuals with neurocognitive disorder.

Depression Depression occurs at significantly higher rates in elderly persons with dementia when compared to cognitively healthy elderly. A recent study of rates of depression (depression assessed using the Cornell Scale of Depression) within a sample of 1000 individuals with dementia found that 50.2% of participants had a score that was considered in the clinically significant range for depression (Knapskog, Barca, & Engedal, 2014). A 34-site prospective study found that individuals with dementia were more than twice as likely than those with normal cognition to be diagnosed with depression (Snowden et al., 2015). Despite these high rates, a recent study found that only 18% of individuals who have depression and a neurocognitive disorder receive any form of treatment (Goodarzi, Mele, Roberts, & Holroyd-Leduc, 2017). The undertreatment of depression in this population may be due to the difficulties with detecting depression in a verbally impaired population and the misattribution of depression symptoms (e.g., social withdrawal, decline in activity, sleep disturbance, etc.) to neurodegeneration. This is troubling, as depression can have serious negative effects on an individual with neurocognitive impairment, including interfering with adaptive behavior. Beyond the personal suffering an individual with a neurocognitive disorder experiences, depression can exacerbate the symptoms of neurocognitive disorder (Alexopoulos, 2005). Moreover, the comorbid depression in individuals with neurocognitive disorder can interfere with the individuals' ability to complete activities and maintain healthy relationships with people around them, both of which have been shown to improve QoL.

Pain It is estimated that over 50% of individuals over the age of 65 experience regular pain (Achterberg et al., 2013). Pain is one of the most common precursors of excess disability and behavioral disturbance in individuals with a neurocognitive disorder. Progressive impairment in the ability to verbally label and report private experiences such as pain or discomfort presents a significant barrier to the health and quality of life of persons with dementia (see Achterberg et al., 2013; Husebo et al., 2008). As discussed earlier, these medications have been found to have substantial side effects including mortality, cerebrovascular events, and increased risk of falls (Ballard, Smith, Corbett, Husebo, & Aarsland, 2011). Moreover, the pain interferes with adaptive behavior, such as utilization of coping strategies, and acts as a catalyst to increase behavioral changes. In order to reduce and detect pain behaviors in a more strategic way, Achterberg and colleagues (2013) recommended the utilization of "pain teams" as opportunities for staff to consult with experts in neurocognitive care settings to develop collaborative treatment recommendations. Utilizing an integrated healthcare model would be potentially valuable in ensuring future improvements in the effective management of pain in individuals with neurocognitive disorder.

Promotion of Health to Improve Wellness for Individuals with Dementia

Behavioral activation is an evidence-based treatment for depression that has been found to be effective for every age group (Yon & Scogin, 2008). The key component of behavior activation is behavioral repertoire to increase contact with positive consequences. This may include engaging in more activities rather than being inactive, withdrawn, and avoidant (Snarski et al., 2011). Behavioral activation has been found to be efficacious for geriatric populations (Moss, Scogin, Di Napoli, & Presnell, 2012; Snarski et al., 2011; Yon & Scogin, 2008), which is important due to the high rates of isolation and decreases in engagement in activities for this population. The advantage of using a treatment such as behavioral activation to increase health and wellness is that it is a short-term therapy and easy to understand, due to its basic adherence of behavioral principles (Snarski et al., 2011). However, there are only a limited number of studies that have investigated behavioral activation with individuals with dementia. In a study of mental disorders in an older cohort, Snarski and colleagues (2011) found that behavioral activation decreased rates of depression for all mental disorders; however, there were only nine participants who were diagnosed with dementia, and there was no between group analysis. To our knowledge, there is no RCT that has investigated behavioral activation in individuals with any neurocognitive disorder. Notwithstanding, in promoting health and wellness in individuals with dementia, exercise (a possible activity for behavioral activation) has been found to be efficacious with this population.

Activity level tends to be inversely correlated with age but highly correlated with quality of life, mood, and cognitive health in the elderly including those with a neurocognitive disorder (Rolland et al., 2007). Due to the heuristic that individuals with neurocognitive disorder are "fragile" and "too cognitively impaired" to participate in any type of exercise, these individuals are not given the opportunity to partake in exercises (Bauman, Merom, Bull, Buchner, & Fiatarone Singh, 2016). Teri and colleagues (2003) found that just 60 min of exercise per week for individuals with Alzheimer's disease resulted in improved physical health and mood. Moreover, Rolland and colleagues (2007) conducted an RCT and found similar results as Teri et al. (2003). It was demonstrated that 1 h a day of exercise for individuals with Alzheimer's disease resulted in a decrease in rates of decline in ADLs.

There has been a growing amount of research addressing mindfulness to improve and promote health and wellness in the medical setting. Mindfulness-based stress reduction (MBSR) is a protocol-based intervention that has been shown in numerous RCTs to be effective in reducing chronic pain (Hilton et al., 2017), cancer (Rush & Sharma, 2016), fibromyalgia (Lauche, Cramer, Dobos, Langhorst, & Schmidt, 2013), vascular disease (Abbott et al., 2014), HIV/AIDS (Riley & Kalichman, 2015), and depression (Gu, Strauss, Bond, & Cavanagh, 2015). An examination of the literature found that studies have used MBSR with older adults. Paller and colleagues (2015) conducted a unique study that evaluated the MBSR protocol in both individuals with dementia and their caregivers. This was a small prospective study

($n = 17$ patients; $n = 20$ caregivers) that found significant improvements in caregivers and individuals with dementia's QoL and depression from pre- to posttest ($p < 0.05$). Moreover, the caregivers' distress improved significantly from pre- to posttest ($p < 0.05$). To our knowledge, this pilot study was the first study that has demonstrated that MBSR can have a positive effect on both the caregiver and the individual with a neurocognitive disorder. This is important as studies have found that caregiver's distress and mood can have an effect on the individual with the neurocognitive disorder (Thomas et al., 2006; Wetzels, Zuidema, De Jonghe, Verhey, & Koopmans, 2010).

Promoting the health and wellness of individuals with neurocognitive disorder should be a priority. As pharmaceutical interventions have been shown to have little effect and may cause a decrease health and wellness in individuals with neurocognitive impairment, a non-pharmaceutical approach is warranted. The studies above illustrate the positive effects of non-pharmaceutical interventions, including behavioral activation, exercise, and MBSR.

Promote Family Members/Caregiver QoL and Neurocognitive Education

Family members and/or caregivers for individuals with neurocognitive disorders play an intricate role in the care of these individuals as this disorder can cause severe disability (Gallagher-Thompson et al., 2012). It is estimated that 14.9 million people in the United States currently care for someone who has some form of dementia (Alliance, 2012). There are negative effects that have been associated with being a caregiver of an individual with a neurocognitive disorder, including increases in depression, anxiety, family conflict, social isolation, and role captivity (Judge, Yarry, Looman, & Bass, 2013; Molinari, 2006). These negative effects can create a strain on the caregiver-care receipt relationship and negatively affect the health of the care recipient. Numerous studies have evaluated different interventions designed to promote the behavioral health and quality of life of caregivers of individuals with neurocognitive disorder (see Judge et al., 2013; Schultz et al., 2003). The Resources for Enhancing Alzheimer's Caregiver Health (REACH; Schultz et al., 2003) clinical trial and the Acquiring New Skills While Enhancing Remaining Strengths (ANSWERS; Judge et al., 2013) both investigated interventions for caregivers of individuals with Alzheimer's disease. The trials of the interventions were rooted from a cognitive behavioral approach to psychoeducation and support of individuals with Alzheimer's disease.

The REACH trial, a multicentered (six sites) trial, aimed to evaluate the effectiveness of social and behavioral interventions for caregivers of individuals with Alzheimer's disease and other memory disorders (Schultz et al., 2003). The interventions that were utilized included individual information and support strategies, group support and family systems therapy, psychoeducational and skill-based training approaches, home-based environmental interventions, and enhanced technology support symptoms. These interventions were hypothesized to decrease grief and depression symptoms. All of the interventions yielded a statistically significant effect on normal grief symptoms. When examining the intervention components, cognitive and behavioral strategies were found to be most effective at reducing levels of complicated grief. Information and emotional support were most effective for addressing normal grief, and environmental modifications were most effective for ameliorating depressive symptoms (Holland, Currier, & Gallagher-Thompson, 2009). The results illustrate that a multitude of interventions may be warranted, based on the caregiver's clinical repertoire and the care recipient's risk factors.

The ANSWERS trial investigated interventions including education about dementia and memory loss, effective communication, managing memory, staying active, and recognizing emotions and behaviors for family caregivers of individuals with dementia. Interventions aimed at alleviating and reducing caregivers' negative outcomes included educational and skill-based interventions, heightening caregiving efficacy, and reducing strain for family caregivers (Judge et al., 2013). The researchers found that the interventions were efficacious in improving key strain and psychosocial outcomes for caregivers. It should be noted that a strength-based approach was utilized when developing and implementing care goals, as well as educating the caregivers about neurocognitive disorders.

These two trials have set the groundwork for interventions in promoting family member's/caregiver's health and QoL. These trials investigated different interventions and demonstrated that non-pharmaceutical interventions (e.g., neurocognitive education, group support, family systems therapy, psychoeducational interventions) are efficacious in positively affecting the caregiver-care recipient relationship and improving QoL. More importantly, these positive effects were found with little to no side effects.

References

Abbott, R. A., Whear, R., Rodgers, L. R., Bethel, A., Coon, J. T., Kuyken, W., … Dickens, C. (2014). Effectiveness of mindfulness-based stress reduction and mindfulness based cognitive therapy in vascular disease: A systematic review and meta-analysis of randomised controlled trials. *Journal of Psychosomatic Research, 76*(5), 341–351.

Abizanda, P., Romero, L., Sanchez-Jurado, P. M., Martinez-Reig, M., Alfonso-Silguero, S. A., & Rodriguez-Manas, L. (2014). Age, frailty, disability, institutionalization, multimorbidity or comorbidity. Which are the main targets in older adults? *The Journal of Nutrition, Health & Aging, 18*(6), 622.

Achterberg, W. P., Pieper, M. J., van Dalen-Kok, A. H., De Waal, M. W., Husebø, B., Lautenbacher, S., … Corbett, A. (2013). Pain management in patients with dementia. *Clinical Interventions in Aging, 8*, 1471–1482.

Alexopoulos, G. S. (2005). Depression in the elderly. *The Lancet, 365*(9475), 1961–1970.

Alliance, F. C. (2012). *Fact sheet: Selected caregiver statistics*. San Francisco, CA: Family Caregiver Alliance.

American Psychological Association. (2017). *Integrated Health Care*. Retrieved from http://www.apa.org/health/integrated-health-care.aspx

Andreassi, J. L. (2013). *Psychophysiology: Human behavior & physiological response*. Mahwah, NJ: Lawrence Erlbaum Associates, Inc.

Baert, V., Gorus, E., Mets, T., Geerts, C., & Bautmans, I. (2011). Motivators and barriers for physical activity in the oldest old: A systematic review. *Ageing Research Reviews, 10*(4), 464–474.

Ballard, C., Hanney, M. L., Theodoulou, M., Douglas, S., McShane, R., Kossakowski, K., ... Jacoby, R. (2009). The dementia antipsychotic withdrawal trial (DART-AD): Long-term follow-up of a randomised placebo-controlled trial. *The Lancet Neurology, 8*(2), 151–157.

Ballard, C., Smith, J., Corbett, A., Husebo, B., & Aarsland, D. (2011). The role of pain treatment in managing the behavioural and psychological symptoms of dementia (BPSD). *International Journal of Palliative Nursing, 17*(9), 420–424.

Bandurska, E., Damps-Konstanska, I., Popowski, P., Jedrzejczyk, T., Janowiak, P., Swietnicka, K., ... Jassem, E. (2017). Impact of Integrated Care Model (ICM) on Direct Medical Costs in Management of Advanced Chronic Obstructive Pulmonary Disease (COPD). *Medical Science Monitor, 23*, 2850–2862.

Barker, W. W., Luis, C. A., Kashuba, A., Luis, M., Harwood, D. G., Loewenstein, D., ... Graff-Radford, N. (2002). Relative frequencies of Alzheimer disease, Lewy body, vascular and frontotemporal dementia, and hippocampal sclerosis in the state of Florida brain Bank. *Alzheimer Disease & Associated Disorders, 16*(4), 203–212.

Bauman, A., Merom, D., Bull, F. C., Buchner, D. M., & Fiatarone Singh, M. A. (2016). Updating the evidence for physical activity: Summative reviews of the epidemiological evidence, prevalence, and interventions to promote "active aging". *The Gerontologist, 56*(Suppl_2), S268–S280.

Beach, T. G., Monsell, S. E., Phillips, L. E., & Kukull, W. (2012). Accuracy of the clinical diagnosis of Alzheimer disease at National Institute on Aging Alzheimer disease centers, 2005–2010. *Journal of Neuropathology & Experimental Neurology, 71*(4), 266–273.

Beerens, H. C., Sutcliffe, C., Renom-Guiteras, A., Soto, M. E., Suhonen, R., Zabalegui, A., ... RightTimePlaceCare Consortium. (2014). Quality of life and quality of care for people with dementia receiving long term institutional care or professional home care: The European RightTimePlaceCare study. *Journal of the American Medical Directors Association, 15*(1), 54–61.

Beerens, H. C., Zwakhalen, S. M., Verbeek, H., Ruwaard, D., & Hamers, J. P. (2013). Factors associated with quality of life of people with dementia in long-term care facilities: A systematic review. *International Journal of Nursing Studies, 50*(9), 1259–1270.

Bond, M., Rogers, G., Peters, J., Anderson, R., Hoyle, M., Miners, A., ... Jeffreys, M. (2012). The effectiveness and cost-effectiveness of donepezil, galantamine, rivastigmine and memantine for the treatment of Alzheimer's disease (review of technology appraisal no. 111): A systematic review and economic model. *Health Technology Assessment (Winchester, England), 16*(21), 1–470.

Boustani, M., Peterson, B., Hanson, L., Harris, R., & Lohr, K. N. (2003). Screening for dementia in primary care: A summary of the evidence for the US preventive services task force. *Annals of Internal Medicine, 138*(11), 927–937.

Bowling, A. (2001). Measuring disease. In *A review of disease-specific quality of life measurement scales*. Buckingham, UK: Open University Press.

Bowling, A., Rowe, G., Adams, S., Sands, P., Samsi, K., Crane, M., ... Manthorpe, J. (2015). Quality of life in dementia: A systematically conducted narrative review of dementia-specific measurement scales. *Aging & Mental Health, 19*(1), 13–31.

Brown, L. G. (2016). Untangling polypharmacy in older adults. *Medsurg Nursing, 25*(6), 408–412.

Brown, R. C., Lockwood, A. H., & Sonawane, B. R. (2005). Neurodegenerative diseases: An overview of environmental risk factors. *Environmental Health Perspectives, 113*(9), 1250–1256.

Buchanan, J. A., Christenson, A., Houlihan, D., & Ostrom, C. (2011). The role of behavior analysis in the rehabilitation of persons with dementia. *Behavior Therapy, 42*(1), 9–21.

Campanelli, C. M. (2012). American Geriatrics Society updated beers criteria for potentially inappropriate medication use in older adults: The American Geriatrics Society 2012 beers criteria update expert panel. *Journal of the American Geriatrics Society, 60*(4), 616.

Catania, A. C. (1996). On the origins of behavior structure. *Advances in Psychology, 117*, 3–12.

Centers for Medicare & Medicaid Services. (2013). *Atypical Antipsychotic Medications: Use in Adults*. Retrieved from https://www.cms.gov/medicaremedicaid-coordination/fraud-prevention/medicaid-integrity-education/pharmacy-education-materials/downloads/atyp-antipsych-adult-factsheet.pdf

Chapman, D. P., Williams, S. M., Strine, T. W., Anda, R. F., & Moore, M. J. (2006). Dementia and its implications for public health. *Preventing Chronic Disease, 3*(2), A34.

Chiu, Y., Bero, L., Hessol, N. A., Lexchin, J., & Harrington, C. (2015). A literature review of clinical outcomes associated with antipsychotic medication use in north American nursing home residents. *Health Policy, 119*(6), 802–813.

Clague, F., Mercer, S. W., McLean, G., Reynish, E., & Guthrie, B. (2016). Comorbidity and polypharmacy in people with dementia: Insights from a large, population-based cross-sectional analysis of primary care data. *Age and Ageing, 46*(1), 33–39.

Dawson, P., Wells, D. L., & Kline, K. (1993). *Enhancing the abilities of persons with Alzheimer's and related dementias: A nursing perspective*. New York, NY: Springer Publishing Company.

Di Santo, S. G., Prinelli, F., Adorni, F., Caltagirone, C., & Musicco, M. (2013). A meta-analysis of the efficacy of donepezil, rivastigmine, galantamine, and memantine in relation to severity of Alzheimer's disease. *Journal of Alzheimer's Disease, 35*(2), 349–361.

Doody, R. S., Stevens, J. C., Beck, C., Dubinsky, R. M., Kaye, J. A., Gwyther, L. M. S. W., … Cummings, J. L. (2001). Practice parameter: Management of dementia (an evidence-based review) report of the quality standards Subcommittee of the American Academy of neurology. *Neurology, 56*(9), 1154–1166.

Dramé, M., Fierobe, F., Lang, P. O., Jolly, D., Boyer, F., Mahmoudi, R., … Voisin, T. (2011). Predictors of institution admission in the year following acute hospitalisation of elderly people. *The Journal of Nutrition. Health & Aging, 15*(5), 399–403.

Enns, E., Rhemtulla, R., Ewa, V., Fruetel, K., & Holroyd-Leduc, J. M. (2014). A controlled quality improvement trial to reduce the use of physical restraints in older hospitalized adults. *Journal of the American Geriatrics Society, 62*(3), 541–545.

Fauth, E. B., & Gibbons, A. (2014). Which behavioral and psychological symptoms of dementia are the most problematic? Variability by prevalence, intensity, distress ratings, and associations with caregiver depressive symptoms. *International Journal of Geriatric Psychiatry, 29*(3), 263–271.

Fisher, J. E., Drossel, C., Yury, C., & Cherup, S. (2007). A contextual model of restraint–free care for persons with dementia. In P. Sturmey (Ed.), *Functional analysis in clinical treatment* (pp. 211–238). San Diego, CA: Elsevier.

Fleming, R., Goodenough, B., Low, L. F., Chenoweth, L., & Brodaty, H. (2016). The relationship between the quality of the built environment and the quality of life of people with dementia in residential care. *Dementia, 15*(4), 663–680.

Gallagher-Thompson, D., Tzuang, Y. M., Au, A., Brodaty, H., Charlesworth, G., Gupta, R., … Shyu, Y. I. (2012). International perspectives on nonpharmacological best practices for dementia family caregivers: A review. *Clinical Gerontologist, 35*(4), 316–355.

Galvin, J. E., & Sadowsky, C. H. (2012). Practical guidelines for the recognition and diagnosis of dementia. *The Journal of the American Board of Family Medicine, 25*(3), 367–382.

Garrison-Diehn, C., Rummel, C., & Fisher, J. E. (2013). A contextual approach to dementia Care in Alzheimer's disease. In *Case studies in clinical psychological science: Bridging the gap from science to practice* (p. 279). Oxford, NY: Oxford University Press.

Geldmacher, D. S. (2003). Alzheimer's disease: Current pharmacotherapy in the context of patient and family needs. *Journal of the American Geriatrics Society, 51*(5s2), S289–S295.

Gitlin, L. N., Kales, H. C., & Lyketsos, C. G. (2012). Nonpharmacologic management of behavioral symptoms in dementia. *JAMA, 308*(19), 2020–2029.

Gitlin, L. N., Winter, L., Dennis, M. P., Hodgson, N., & Hauck, W. W. (2010). A biobehavioral home-based intervention and the Well-being of patients with dementia and their caregivers: The COPE randomized trial. *JAMA, 304*(9), 983–991.

Gnjidic, D., Hilmer, S. N., Blyth, F. M., Naganathan, V., Waite, L., Seibel, M. J., … Le Couteur, D. G. (2012). Polypharmacy cutoff and outcomes: Five or more medicines were used to identify community-dwelling older men at risk of different adverse outcomes. *Journal of Clinical Epidemiology, 65*(9), 989–995.

Goodarzi, Z. S., Mele, B. S., Roberts, D. J., & Holroyd-Leduc, J. (2017). Depression case finding in individuals with dementia: A systematic review and meta-analysis. *Journal of the American Geriatrics Society., 65*(5), 937.

Gu, J., Strauss, C., Bond, R., & Cavanagh, K. (2015). How do mindfulness-based cognitive therapy and mindfulness-based stress reduction improve mental health and wellbeing? A systematic review and meta-analysis of mediation studies. *Clinical Psychology Review, 37*, 1–12.

Hebert, L. E., Weuve, J., Scherr, P. A., & Evans, D. A. (2013). Alzheimer disease in the United States (2010–2050) estimated using the 2010 census. *Neurology, 80*(19), 1778–1783.

Hilton, L., Hempel, S., Ewing, B. A., Apaydin, E., Xenakis, L., Newberry, S., … Maglione, M. A. (2017). Mindfulness meditation for chronic pain: Systematic review and meta-analysis. *Annals of Behavioral Medicine, 51*(2), 199–213.

Holland, J. M., Currier, J. M., & Gallagher-Thompson, D. (2009). Outcomes from the resources for enhancing Alzheimer's caregiver health (REACH) program for bereaved caregivers. *Psychology and Aging, 24*(1), 190.

Hovstadius, B., & Petersson, G. (2012). Factors leading to excessive polypharmacy. *Clinics in Geriatric Medicine, 29*(2), 159–172.

Husebo, B. S., Strand, L. I., Moe-Nilssen, R., BorgeHusebo, S., Aarsland, D., & Ljunggren, A. E. (2008). Who suffers most? Dementia and pain in nursing home patients: A cross-sectional study. *Journal of the American Medical Directors Association, 9*(6), 427–433.

Jellinger, K. A., & Attems, J. (2011). Prevalence and pathology of dementia with Lewy bodies in the oldest old: A comparison with other dementing disorders. *Dementia and Geriatric Cognitive Disorders, 31*(4), 309–316.

Judge, K. S., Yarry, S. J., Looman, W. J., & Bass, D. M. (2013). Improved strain and psychosocial outcomes for caregivers of individuals with dementia: Findings from project ANSWERS. *The Gerontologist, 53*(2), 280–292.

Kales, H. C., Gitlin, L. N., & Lyketsos, C. G. (2015). State of the art review: Assessment and management of behavioral and psychological symptoms of dementia. *The BMJ, 350*, h369.

Kim, D. H., Brown, R. T., Ding, E. L., Kiel, D. P., & Berry, S. D. (2011). Dementia medications and risk of falls, syncope, and related adverse events: Meta-analysis of randomized controlled trials. *Journal of the American Geriatrics Society, 59*(6), 1019–1031.

Knapskog, A. B., Barca, M. L., & Engedal, K. (2014). Prevalence of depression among memory clinic patients as measured by the Cornell scale of depression in dementia. *Aging & Mental Health, 18*(5), 579–587.

Lambert, M. A., Bickel, H., Prince, M., Fratiglioni, L., Von Strauss, E., Frydecka, D., … Reynish, E. L. (2014). Estimating the burden of early onset dementia; systematic review of disease prevalence. *European Journal of Neurology, 21*(4), 563–569.

Lauche, R., Cramer, H., Dobos, G., Langhorst, J., & Schmidt, S. (2013). A systematic review and meta-analysis of mindfulness-based stress reduction for the fibromyalgia syndrome. *Journal of Psychosomatic Research, 75*(6), 500–510.

LoGiudice, D., & Watson, R. (2014). Dementia in older people: An update. *Internal Medicine Journal, 44*(11), 1066–1073.

Looman, W. M., Huijsman, R., Bouwmans-Frijters, C. A., Stolk, E. A., & Fabbricotti, I. N. (2016). Cost-effectiveness of the 'Walcheren integrated care Model'intervention for community-dwelling frail elderly. *Family Practice, 33*(2), 154–160.

Lopez, O. L., Becker, J. T., Wahed, A. S., Saxton, J., Sweet, R. A., Wolk, D. A., … Dekosky, S. T. (2009). Long-term effects of the concomitant use of memantine with cholinesterase inhibition in Alzheimer disease. *Journal of Neurology, Neurosurgery & Psychiatry, 80*(6), 600–607.

Lwi, S. J., Ford, B. Q., Casey, J. J., Miller, B. L., & Levenson, R. W. (2017). Poor caregiver mental health predicts mortalilty of patients with neurodegenerative disease. *Proceedings of the National Academy of Science, 201701597*. https://doi.org/10.1073/pnas.1701597114

Marcum, Z. A., Driessen, J., Thorpe, C. T., Gellad, W. F., & Donohue, J. M. (2014). Effect of multiple pharmacy use on medication adherence and drug–drug interactions in older adults with Medicare part D. *Journal of the American Geriatrics Society, 62*(2), 244–252.

Maust, D. T., Kim, H. M., Seyfried, L. S., Chiang, C., Kavanagh, J., Schneider, L. S., & Kales, H. C. (2015). Antipsychotics, other psychotropics, and the risk of death in patients with dementia: Number needed to harm. *JAMA Psychiatry, 72*(5), 438–445.

McKhann, G. M., Albert, M. S., & Sperling, R. A. (2012). Changing diagnostic concepts of Alzheimer's disease. *In Alzheimer's Disease-Modernizing Concept, Biological Diagnosis and Therapy, 28*, 115–121 Karger Publishers.

McKhann, G. M., Knopman, D. S., Chertkow, H., Hyman, B. T., Jack, C. R., Kawas, C. H., … Mohs, R. C. (2011). The diagnosis of dementia due to Alzheimer's disease: Recommendations from the National Institute on Aging-Alzheimer's association workgroups on diagnostic guidelines for Alzheimer's disease. *Alzheimer's & Dementia, 7*(3), 263–269.

Molinari, V., Chiriboga, D., Branch, L. G., Cho, S., Turner, K., Guo, J., & Hyer, K. (2010). Provision of psychopharmacological services in nursing homes. *The Journals of Gerontology Series B: Psychological Sciences and Social Sciences, 65*(1), 57–60.

Molinari, V. A. (2006). Caregiver burden. In S. M. Lobo Prabhu, V. A. Molinari, & J. W. Lomax (Eds.), *Supporting the caregiver in dementia: A guide for health care professionals* (pp. 64–81). Baltimore, MD: The Johns Hopkins University Press.

Moss, K., Scogin, F., Di Napoli, E., & Presnell, A. (2012). A self-help behavioral activation treatment for geriatric depressive symptoms. *Aging & Mental Health, 16*(5), 625–635.

Neufeld, R. R., Libow, L. S., Foley, W. J., Dunbar, J. M., Cohen, C., & Breuer, B. (1999). Restraint reduction reduces serious injuries among nursing home residents. *Journal of the American Geriatrics Society, 47*(10), 1202–1207.

Norgaard, A., Jensen-Dahm, C., Gasse, C., Hansen, E. S., & Waldemar, G. (2017). Psychotropic polypharmacy in patients with dementia: Prevalence and predictors. *Journal of Alzheimer's Disease, 56*(2), 707–716.

Odenheimer, G., Borson, S., Sanders, A. E., Swain-Eng, R. J., Kyomen, H. H., Tierney, S., … Johnson, J. (2013). Quality improvement in neurology dementia management quality measures. *Neurology, 81*(17), 1545–1549.

Paller, K. A., Creery, J. D., Florczak, S. M., Weintraub, S., Mesulam, M. M., Reber, P. J., ... O'Hara, M. (2015). Benefits of mindfulness training for patients with progressive cognitive decline and their caregivers. *American Journal of Alzheimer's Disease & Other Dementias®, 30*(3), 257–267.

Paterson, R. W., Takada, L. T., & Geschwind, M. D. (2012). Diagnosis and treatment of rapidly progressive dementias. *Neurology: Clinical Practice, 2*(3), 187–200.

Prince, M., Bryce, R., Albanese, E., Wimo, A., Ribeiro, W., & Ferri, C. P. (2013). The global prevalence of dementia: A systematic review and metaanalysis. *Alzheimer's & Dementia, 9*(1), 63–75.

Prince, M., Comas-Herrera, A., Knapp, M., Guerchet, M., & Karagiannidou, M. (2016). *World Alzheimer report 2016: Improving healthcare for people living with dementia: Coverage, quality and costs now and in the future*. London, UK: Alzheimer's Disease International (ADI).

Rahman, S. (2017). *Enhancing health and wellbeing in dementia: A person-centered integrated care approach*. London, UK: Jessica Kingsley Publishers.

Riley, K. E., & Kalichman, S. (2015). Mindfulness-based stress reduction for people living with HIV/AIDS: Preliminary review of intervention trial methodologies and findings. *Health Psychology Review, 9*(2), 224–243.

Rizzi, L., Rosset, I., & Roriz-Cruz, M. (2014). Global epidemiology of dementia: Alzheimer's and vascular types. *BioMed Research International, 2014*, 8.

Rolland, Y., Pillard, F., Klapouszczak, A., Reynish, E., Thomas, D., Andrieu, S., … Vellas, B. (2007). Exercise program for nursing home residents with Alzheimer's disease: A 1-year randomized, controlled trial. *Journal of the American Geriatrics Society, 55*(2), 158–165.

Rush, S. E., & Sharma, M. (2016). Mindfulness-based stress reduction as a stress management intervention for cancer care: A systematic review. *Journal of Evidence-Based Complementary & Alternative Medicine.*, 2156587216661467, *22*(2), 348–360.

Schneider, L. S., Dagerman, K. S., & Insel, P. (2005). Risk of death with atypical antipsychotic drug treatment for dementia: Meta-analysis of randomized placebo-controlled trials. *JAMA, 294*(15), 1934–1943.

Schultz, R., Belle, S. H., Czaja, S. J., Gitlin, L. N., Wisniewski, S. R., & Ory, M. G. (2003). Introduction to the special section on resources for enhancing Alzheimer's caregiver health (REACH). *Psychology and Aging, 18*(3), 357.

Snarski, M., Scogin, F., DiNapoli, E., Presnell, A., McAlpine, J., & Marcinak, J. (2011). The effects of behavioral activation therapy with inpatient geriatric psychiatry patients. *Behavior Therapy, 42*(1), 100–108.

Snowden, M. B., Atkins, D. C., Steinman, L. E., Bell, J. F., Bryant, L. L., Copeland, C., & Fitzpatrick, A. L. (2015). Longitudinal association of dementia and depression. *The American Journal of Geriatric Psychiatry, 23*(9), 897–905.

Tampi, R. R., Tampi, D. J., Balachandran, S., & Srinivasan, S. (2016). Antipsychotic use in dementia: A systematic review of benefits and risks from meta-analyses. *Therapeutic Advances in Chronic Disease, 7*(5), 229–245.

Tan, C. C., Yu, J. T., Wang, H. F., Tan, M. S., Meng, X. F., Wang, C., … Tan, L. (2014). Efficacy and safety of donepezil, galantamine, rivastigmine, and memantine for the treatment of Alzheimer's disease: A systematic review and meta-analysis. *Journal of Alzheimer's Disease, 41*(2), 615–631.

Teri, L., Gibbons, L. E., McCurry, S. M., Logsdon, R. G., Buchner, D. M., Barlow, W. E., … Larson, E. B. (2003). Exercise plus behavioral management in patients with Alzheimer disease: A randomized controlled trial. *JAMA, 290*(15), 2015–2022.

Thomas, P., Lalloué, F., Preux, P. M., Hazif-Thomas, C., Pariel, S., Inscale, R., … Clément, J. P. (2006). Dementia patients caregivers quality of life: The PIXEL study. *International Journal of Geriatric Psychiatry, 21*(1), 50–56.

United States Department of Health and Human Services. (2005). *Glossary: Definition of restraints*. Retrieved from http://www.medicare.gov/Glossary/ShownTerm.asp?Languge=English&term=restraints

U.S. Food and Drug Administration. (2008). *Information for Health Care Professionals: Conventional Antipsychotics*. Retrieved from https://wayback.archiveit.org/7993/20170722190727/. https://www.fda.gov/Drugs/DrugSafety/PostmarketDrugSafetyInformationforPatientsandProviders/ucm124830.htm

van der Spek, K., Gerritsen, D. L., Smalbrugge, M., Nelissen-Vrancken, M. H., Wetzels, R. B., Smeets, C. H., … Koopmans, R. T. (2016). Only 10% of the psychotropic drug use for neuropsychiatric symptoms in patients with dementia is fully appropriate. The PROPER I-study. *International Psychogeriatrics, 28*(10), 1589–1595.

Van Duijn, C. M., Clayton, D. G., Chandra, V., Fratiglioni, L., Graves, A. B., Heyman, A., … Rocca, W. A. (1994). Interaction between genetic and environmental risk factors for Alzheimer's disease: A reanalysis of case-control studies. *Genetic Epidemiology, 11*(6), 539–551.

van Hout, H. P., Vernooij-Dassen, M. J., & Stalman, W. A. (2007). Diagnosing dementia with confidence by GPs. *Family Practice, 24*(6), 616–621.

Vance, D. E., & Struzick, T. C. (2007). Addressing risk factors of cognitive impairment in adults aging with HIV: A social work model. *Journal of Gerontological Social Work, 49*(4), 51–77.

Vasudev, A., Shariff, S. Z., Liu, K., Burhan, A. M., Herrmann, N., Leonard, S., & Mamdani, M. (2015). Trends in psychotropic dispensing among older adults with dementia living in long-term care facilities: 2004–2013. *The American Journal of Geriatric Psychiatry, 23*(12), 1259–1269.

Villars, H., Oustric, S., Andrieu, S., Baeyens, J. P., Bernabei, R., Brodaty, H., … Frisoni, G. (2010). The primary care physician and Alzheimer's disease: An international position paper. *The Journal of Nutrition, Health & Aging, 14*(2), 110–120.

Wang, J., Yu, J. T., Wang, H. F., Meng, X. F., Wang, C., Tan, C. C., & Tan, L. (2014). Pharmacological treatment of neuropsychiatric symptoms in Alzheimer's disease: A systematic review and meta-analysis. *Journal of Neurology, Neurosurgery & Psychiatry, 86*(1), 101–109 jnnp-2014.

Wetzels, R. B., Zuidema, S. U., De Jonghe, J. F. M., Verhey, F. R. J., & Koopmans, R. T. C. M. (2010). Determinants of quality of life in nursing home residents with dementia. *Dementia and Geriatric Cognitive Disorders, 29*(3), 189–197.

World Health Organization. (1997). Measuring quality of life. In *Division of mental health and prevention of substance abuse*. Geneva, Switzerland: World Health Organization.

Yon, A., & Scogin, F. (2008). Behavioral activation as a treatment for geriatric depression. *Clinical Gerontologist, 32*(1), 91–103.

Yury, C. A., & Fisher, J. E. (2007). Meta-analysis of the effectiveness of atypical antipsychotics for the treatment of behavioural problems in persons with dementia. *Psychotherapy and Psychosomatics, 76*(4), 213–218.

Chapter 17
Behavioral Health and Diabetes

Rebekah J. Walker, Joni S. Williams, and Leonard E. Egede

Burden of Disease

Diabetes is a chronic disease causing tremendous burden on people worldwide. It is characterized by high levels of blood glucose due to poor or no insulin production, insulin resistance or improper use of insulin, or a combination of both (Centers for Disease Control and Prevention (CDC), 2014). In the United States, approximately 29.1 million people (9.3% of the population) have diabetes (CDC, 2014). Of those who have diabetes, over 8 million (27.8%) remain undiagnosed (CDC, 2014). In US adults 20 years of age and older, nearly 30 million have diabetes, affecting 14% of men and 11% of women (CDC, 2014). Of this same group, approximately 1.7 million new cases are diagnosed annually, and an estimated 86 million have prediabetes (CDC, 2014). Racial and ethnic minority groups in the United States including American Indians/Alaska Natives (15.9%), non-Hispanic Blacks (13.2%), Hispanics (12.8%), and Asian Americans (9.0%) have a higher disease burden of diabetes compared to non-Hispanic Whites (7.6%) (CDC, 2014).

Type 1 and type 2 diabetes are the most common forms, with type 2 diabetes accounting for 90–95% of all cases in adults (CDC, 2014). While type 1 diabetes typically has an earlier onset (mid-teens) and occurs as a result of an immune-mediated destruction of beta cells within the pancreas, type 2 diabetes occurs later in life and, often times, is preventable by eating healthy, being physically active, monitoring blood sugar levels, taking medications, reducing risks, problem solving, and coping (American Academy of Diabetes Educators (AADE), 2017; CDC, 2014). For those at risk of developing type 2 diabetes, factors such as older age,

R. J. Walker · J. S. Williams · L. E. Egede (✉)
Department of Medicine, Division of General Internal Medicine, Medical College of Wisconsin, Milwaukee, WI, USA

Center for Advancing Population Science (CAPS), Medical College of Wisconsin, Milwaukee, WI, USA
e-mail: legede@mcw.edu

M. P. Duckworth, W. T. O'Donohue (eds.), *Behavioral Medicine and Integrated Care*,
https://doi.org/10.1007/978-3-319-93003-9_17

family history, obesity, physical inactivity, race/ethnicity, and a prior diagnosis of gestational diabetes are associated with increased likelihood of developing diabetes (CDC, 2014).

Diabetes affects many organ systems within the body, accounting for significant morbidity and mortality. It is associated with heart disease and stroke, kidney disease and failure, blindness, and lower-limp amputations (CDC, 2014). Uncontrolled diabetes results in notable microvascular complications such as retinopathy, nephropathy, and neuropathy (CDC, 2014). It is the seventh leading cause of death, resulting in death rates 1.5 times higher for adults with diabetes compared to adults without diabetes (CDC, 2014). Finally, total direct and indirect costs associated with diabetes are $245 billion, where approximately $70 is due to disability, losses from work, and premature death (CDC, 2014). Average medical expenditures for people with diabetes more than double those without diabetes (CDC, 2014).

Behavioral Aspects of Diabetes

In the *2017 Standards of Medical Care for Diabetes*, the American Diabetes Association (ADA) recommends the assessment and integration of psychosocial factors such as depression and diabetes distress into initial and routine patient care to improve outcomes and overall quality of life for patients with diabetes (American Diabetes Association (ADA), 2017). The American Academy of Diabetes Educators recommends coping as one of the essential self-care behaviors needed to manage the daily challenges of diabetes. Diabetes can affect people both mentally and physically, impacting their behaviors and adherence to recommended treatment plans. Psychological conditions such as depression, distress and stress, serious psychological distress, fatalism, self-efficacy, and social support can all impact diabetes and must be considered as a part of routine care for adults with diabetes (ADA, 2017; Young-Hyman et al., 2016).

Depression

Like diabetes, depression is a major global health concern. The term "depression" can encompass an array of conditions including major or clinical depression, depressive symptoms, or depressive disorders (Egede, Grubaugh, & Ellis, 2010). Depression, or major depression, is a clinical condition characterized by the presence of a depressed mood and anhedonia within the same 2-week period and the presence of any five of the following symptoms: (1) significant unintentional weight loss or weight gain, (2) insomnia or hypersomnia, (3) psychomotor agitation or retardation, (4) poor concentration, (5) fatigue or loss of energy, (6) feelings of worthlessness or excessive guilt, and (7) suicidal ideation (Egede & Ellis, 2010b). Depressive disorders include major depression, minor depression, and dysthymia

(Egede et al., 2010), and depressive symptoms encompass a variety of signs such as mood and cognition changes, anxiety levels, sleep and eating patterns, weight changes, and energy levels (Rush et al., 1986). A history of depression, a previous or current diagnosis of depression, and the use of antidepressants are all risk factors for the development of type 2 diabetes, a risk that is compounded when other risks (i.e., positive family history, obesity, etc.) are present (ADA, 2017).

Previous evidence suggests there is a relationship between diabetes and depression, estimating that 25% of people diagnosed with diabetes also have depressive symptomatology (Fisher et al., 2012). Having a diagnosis of diabetes increases the likelihood of receiving a diagnosis of depression (Egede et al., 2016). Recent data estimates 11% of individuals with diabetes also have comorbid major depression, and 45% of adults with diabetes have undiagnosed depression (Egede et al., 2016). Similarly, more than 30% of adults with diabetes have a depressive disorder or depressive symptomatology (Egede et al., 2016). It is noteworthy to mention that the ADA now lists depression as a comorbid condition for diabetes (ADA, 2017).

Diabetes Distress and Stress

Diabetes distress results when significant and negative psychological reactions occur, specific to the burden of managing and living with diabetes, for instance, concerns about disease management, support, emotional burden, and access to care (ADA, 2017). It presents as concealed feelings and emotions that result secondary to stressing and worrying about the complexities of diabetes management (Fisher et al., 2013; Gonzalez, Fisher, & Polonsky, 2011). Often neglected by providers, since it differs from traditional psychological disorders such as clinical depression and dysthymia, diabetes distress has been linked to poor self-efficacy and self-management (Fisher et al., 2013). Evidence suggests diabetes distress significantly impacts clinical outcomes such as glycemic control and behaviors such as medication, diet, and exercise adherence, resulting in poorer glycemic control (ADA, 2017; Egede & Dismuke, 2012; Fisher et al., 2010; Fisher et al., 2010; 2013).

The prevalence of diabetes distress is estimated to be 18–45% with an incidence of 38–48% over an 18-month period (ADA, 2017). In individuals with type 2 diabetes alone, the prevalence is believed to be as high as 45% (Fisher, Hessler, Polonsky, & Mullan, 2012). Because of its distinction and association with poorer outcomes, the management of diabetes distress warrants evaluation and treatment by a mental health provider or behavioral health specialist (ADA, 2017; Fisher et al., 2013). The ADA recommends patients be informed about diabetes distress upon diagnosis, and educated about the possible impact it may have on self-management and overall health (ADA, 2017). Counseling should be provided to help distinguish it from traditional psychological conditions, and concerns associated with self-management that are responsible for higher levels of diabetes distress should be identified and addressed accordingly (ADA, 2017).

There is a widespread and common belief that stress negatively and adversely impacts health. This belief is supported by evidence suggesting stress as a barrier to effective diabetes self-management, resulting in poor outcomes (Hilliard et al., 2016; Surwit, Schneider, & Feinglos, 1992). Stress has been shown to have an environmental, psychological, and biological role in disease development and adverse outcomes (Kelly & Ismail, 2015).

Serious Psychological Distress

Serious psychological distress (SPD) is a general measure of psychological distress found to have a strong, negative association with health (Egede & Dismuke, 2012). Specifically, SPD involves severe distress and is often used as a screening mechanism for serious mental illness, such as major depression that lasts a minimum of 12 months (Winchester, Williams, Wolfman, & Egede, 2016). People with diabetes are often diagnosed with comorbid conditions such as depression and anxiety causing SPD to occur (Shin, Chiu, Choi, Cho, & Bang, 2012). Given the associated mental health problems, SPD often causes significant impairments in social, occupational, and school functioning and requires treatment (Weissman, Pratt, Miller, & Parker, 2015). SPD was associated with significantly higher health expenditures and higher utilization in US adults (Dismuke & Egede, 2011). In addition, even after controlling for depression, SPD significantly diminished quality of life in individuals with diabetes (Dismuke, Hernandez-Tejada, & Egede, 2014).

According to the data from the National Health Interview Survey between 2009 and 2013, women are more likely than men to have SPD, and middle-aged adults (45–64 years) are more likely to have SPD compared to younger (18–44 years) and older (≥65 years) adults, who have the lowest prevalence of occurrence (Weissman et al., 2015). The percentage of non-Hispanic White adults with SPD is lower than the percentage of non-Hispanic Blacks and Hispanic adults with SPD, after adjusting for age (Weissman et al., 2015). Approximately 8.7% of adults with incomes below the federal poverty level have SPD (compared to 1.2% with incomes at or above the 400% poverty level), while adults with SPD are more likely to be uninsured compared to those without SPD (Weissman et al., 2015). In addition, adults with SPD are approximately two times more likely to have diabetes and cardiovascular disease compared to adults without SPD (Shin et al., 2012; Weissman et al., 2015).

Diabetes Fatalism

Diabetes fatalism is a newer construct, conceptualized in recent years from the construct of fatalism, or the principle that events are fixed in advance, rendering human beings powerless to change them (Egede & Bonadonna, 2003; Egede & Ellis, 2010a). Diabetes fatalism is defined as "a complex psychological cycle characterized by perceptions of despair (emotional distress), hopelessness (poor coping), and powerlessness (poor self-efficacy) (Egede & Ellis, 2010a, 2010b). Similar to depression and diabetes distress, diabetes fatalism has been shown to influence diabetes outcomes, resulting in inadequate self-care, poor glycemic control, and decreased quality of life (Egede & Bonadonna, 2003; Egede & Ellis, 2010a, 2010b; Osborn, Bains, & Egede, 2010; Walker et al., 2012). A series of studies have found that accounting for depression and social support removes the significant association between diabetes fatalism and outcomes, suggesting these are important factors when considering how to decrease fatalistic attitudes in patients with diabetes (Asuzu, Walker, Williams, & Egede, 2017; Egede & Osborn, 2010; Osborn et al., 2010).

Self-Efficacy

Self-efficacy is defined as an individual's confidence in his or her abilities to perform specific behaviors needed to achieve a specified goal (Al-Khawaldeh, Al-Hassan, & Froelicher, 2012; Gao et al., 2013; Sousa, Zauszniewski, Musil, Lea, & Davis, 2005). Evidence suggests self-efficacy has an independent relationship with glycemic control (Walker, Gebregziabher, Martin-Harris, & Egede, 2014) and can be influenced by multiple psychosocial factors including depression and diabetes distress (Devarajooh & Chinna, 2017). Self-efficacy is considered a critical component for adequate self-management in diabetes care (Al-Khawaldeh et al., 2012; Gao et al., 2013) such that as self-efficacy increases, self-management improves, resulting in better glycemic control (Sousa et al., 2005). To achieve successful self-management, self-efficacy is needed to maintain healthy behaviors, improve decision-making, and promote positive well-being (Sousa et al., 2005). Previous research by Sousa et al. suggests that women, shorter disease duration, older age, non-Hispanic Black race, and a diagnosis of type 1 diabetes are associated with better self-efficacy, therefore, better diabetes-related outcomes (Sousa et al., 2005).

Social Support

Social support is a perception of acceptance, provision, and assistance from formal and informal relationships with others (Strom & Egede, 2012). It is also the realization that support is actually received from another individual (Strom & Egede, 2012). Social support can present in various ways including emotional, tangible, and informational and through companionship (Strom & Egede, 2012; van Dam et al., 2004). Emotional support occurs when feelings of validation and worth are expressed (Strom & Egede, 2012; van Dam et al., 2004). Tangible support rallies around the concept of provision such as assistance with finances, goods, and services (Strom & Egede, 2012; van Dam et al., 2004). The distribution of information, advice, and guidance to assist with problem solving, goal setting, and decision-making are perceived as informational support (Strom & Egede, 2012; van Dam et al., 2004). The sense of belonging and the presence of companions for engaging in activities describe companionship (Strom & Egede, 2012; van Dam et al., 2004). These perceptions of support can be perceived as positive (beneficial) or negative (harmful) and can be received from different sources including family members, friends and peers, providers, and organizations (Stopford, Winkley, & Ismail, 2013; Strom & Egede, 2012). Higher levels of social support are often associated with better glycemic control and outcomes, whereas lower levels of support are associated with increased mortality and adverse complications (Strom & Egede, 2012). Given the complex nature of diabetes management, evidence suggests social support serves as a facilitator for improved self-management and health outcomes in chronic diseases such as diabetes (Stopford et al., 2013; Strom & Egede, 2012) through either a buffering or direct effect (Cohen & Wills, 1985; Thoits, 1985); however, the evidence has been inconclusive.

Impact of Behavioral Aspects of Diabetes on Processes and Outcomes

Impact on Self-Care

Eating healthy, monitoring blood glucose levels, being physically active, and taking medications as prescribed are all important and necessary processes in self-care. Behavioral aspects of diabetes contribute to self-care and management, such that higher levels of depression, diabetes distress, and perceived stress, for example, typically lead to poorer self-care, while higher levels of social support and self-efficacy are often associated with better self-care (Asuzu et al., 2017; Fisher et al., 2013; Walker et al., 2012, 2014). In the *Standards of Medical Care in Diabetes*, the ADA reports that higher levels of diabetes distress significantly impact self-care behaviors such as medical adherence and are associated with poorer nutritional intake and physical activity (ADA, 2017). In a study by Fisher et al., reductions in diabetes distress resulted in significant improvements in self-care behaviors such as eating healthy, being physically active, and adhering to prescribed medication regimens (Fisher et al., 2013). Furthermore, poor medication adherence and self-care, independent of depression, have been facilitated by fatalism (Walker et al., 2012). Finally, evidence suggests patients with comorbid diabetes and SPD have higher odds of 14 or more days of limited physical activity compared to those with diabetes only (McKnight-Eily et al., 2009).

Impact on Process and Quality of Care

Quality of care is important in disease management, especially so for a chronic disease such as diabetes where patient and provider factors contribute to the complex process of management. A1c testing, cholesterol testing, annual foot examinations, and preventive services such as influenza and pneumonia vaccinations, diabetes treatment, and diabetes education classes are a few examples of processes of care that contribute to the quality of care in diabetes management (Egede et al., 2010; Walker et al., 2014). Evidence suggests that processes of care are often mediated by behavioral aspects of diabetes and have an impact on outcomes. For example, social support has been found to have a significant and indirect relationship on glycemic control, a relationship mediated by processes of care (Walker et al., 2014). In addition, adults with diabetes and depression were less likely to receive preventive care, such as mammograms, and were less likely to perceive their health as good or report being satisfied with life (Egede et al., 2010). In general, patient satisfaction has been shown to improve medication adherence, patient-provider communication, and overall health outcomes (Schoenfelder, 2012). In adults with diabetes, satisfaction has been associated with glycemic control, treatment plan management, and treatment evaluations (Williams, Pollack, & Dibonaventura, 2011).

Impact on Clinical Outcomes

Clinical outcomes such as glycosylated hemoglobin A1c (A1c), blood pressure (BP), and low-density lipoprotein cholesterol (LDL-C) are important to consider when assessing the relationship between behavioral aspects and diabetes. Measuring the A1c is particularly important in diabetes management as it offers information about glucose control over the prior 3 months of testing (ADA, 2017). Behavioral aspects of diabetes have been shown to have an impact on clinical outcomes, particularly the A1c, when assessing glycemic control in persons with diabetes. Depression has been associated with poor glycemic control in patients with both type 1 and type 2 diabetes (Egede et al., 2010). Walker et al. (2014) report that higher fatalism, higher diabetes distress, and lower self-efficacy are directly associated with lower HbA1c (Walker et al., 2014). Hilliard et al. suggest that stress is strongly associated with A1c, especially in minorities and youth, two vulnerable populations with a disproportionate stress burden (Hilliard et al., 2016).

Impact on Cost and Utilization

A comorbid diagnosis of diabetes and a psychological condition such as depression is associated with increased morbidity and mortality (Egede et al., 2016). In a study to access the association between comorbid depression and healthcare utilization and expenditures, Egede et al. report increased healthcare use and expenditures for individuals diagnosed with both depression and diabetes (Egede, Zheng, & Simpson, 2002). Simon et al. suggest that depression is associated with a 50–75% increase in healthcare expenditures for people with diabetes (Simon et al., 2005). Medical conditions including hypertension and coronary heart disease and psychological and behavioral conditions such as depression are predicted to be stronger contributors to future healthcare expenditures for adults with diabetes (Gilmer et al., 2005). Recent estimates suggest expenditures are approximately $5000 higher for symptomatic depression in adults with diabetes (Egede et al., 2016). SPD has also been associated with higher healthcare expenditures and utilization in adults with diabetes (Egede & Dismuke, 2012). Finally, individuals diagnosed with both medical and psychological conditions simultaneously often have higher utilization of services (Egede et al., 2002; Puyat, Kazanjian, Wong, & Goldner, 2017).

Pathways Linking Behavioral Health with Diabetes Outcomes

In an effort to better understand how to design care to address behavioral health of individuals with diabetes, significant work has been conducted to understand the mechanisms and pathways linking behavioral health with diabetes outcomes. These pathways include both biological and behavioral influences and link a number of psychosocial factors to diabetes self-management, glycemic control, and overall quality of life for people with diabetes.

Depression

Diabetes and depression co-occur twice as frequently as chance would predict and lead to significantly increased costs, without major improvements in outcomes (Egede, 2005; Egede et al., 2016; Holt et al., 2014a, 2014b). As such, substantial work has been done to understand the relationship both in terms of pathways linking the two diseases and the direction of causation. Epidemiologic studies show the association is bi-directional, though depression as a risk factor for diabetes is the stronger relationship (Andreoulakis, Hyphantis, Kandylis, & Iacovides, 2012; Carnethon, Kinder, Fair, Stafford, & Fortmann, 2003; Holt et al. 2014a, 2014b). Particularly in older adults, individuals who reported higher depressive symptoms or persistently high symptoms were more likely to develop diabetes, even after controlling for other risk factors (Carnethon et al., 2007). Shared biological and behavioral pathways that predispose individuals for both diabetes and depression have shifted current recommendations from focusing on the direction of association to focusing on the mechanisms common to both (Holt et al. 2014a, 2014b). Four common interrelated biological pathways have been identified, including epigenetic changes, hypothalamic-pituitary-adrenal axis dysfunction, inflammation, and sleep/circadian rhythm disruption (Holt et al., 2014b). Both the external environment, in the form of neighborhoods in which individuals live, and adversity experienced in childhood, as well as the intrauterine environment in which an individual developed, can influence the health behaviors that in turn impact these biological pathways (Holt et al., 2014b). In addition, ongoing research is focused on trying to understand how environmental factors interact with biological pathways resulting in individual vulnerability and resilience (Holt et al., 2014b).

When specifically considering patients with diabetes, independent factors associated with major depressive disorder included demographic variables such as younger age, female sex, lower income, and at least a high school education, as well as behavioral factors such as smoking and perceptions about the influence of diabetes on their health (Egede & Zheng, 2003). There are three major pathways through which comorbid depression is understood to influence diabetes outcomes (Egede, 2005; Piette, Richardson, & Valenstein, 2004). The first pathway is through directly impacting an individual's quality of life by multiplying the impact of both diseases on physical, social, and role functions (Piette et al., 2004). Diabetes is a psychologically demanding disease, requiring regular problem solving, regime maintenance, and awareness of debilitating complications associated with the disease (Piette et al., 2004). Comorbid depression may exacerbate this mental burden (Holt et al., 2014a; Egede & Zheng, 2003). For example, one study found that individuals with treated type 2 diabetes were at increased risk of developing depressive symptoms over 3 years, while those with untreated diabetes were not (Golden et al., 2008). Psychological stress associated with diabetes management, therefore, is an important factor to consider in addition to depressive symptoms, in the additive impact on outcomes (Golden et al., 2008). The presence of medical comorbidities has also been noted as a factor contributing to comorbid depression in individuals with diabetes, highlighting the psychological impact further complications may have on individuals with diabetes (Andreoulakis et al., 2012).

A second pathway through which depression impacts diabetes outcomes is through decreasing motivation to complete self-management behavior, most particularly through decreasing physical activity (Egede, 2005; Piette et al., 2004). Interventions that promote physical activity have been shown to improve both depressive- and diabetes-related symptoms, suggesting an important focus for patients with comorbid diabetes and depression (Boule, Haddad, Kenny, Wells, & Sigal, 2001). Additional self-care behaviors may also be influenced through a lack of energy, negative thought patterns, and passive coping strategies (Piette et al., 2004). Self-efficacy has been shown to significantly influence completion of self-care behaviors (Walker, Gebregziabher, Martin-Harris, & Egede, 2015). As such, treatment for depression through cognitive behavioral therapy may improve outcomes by addressing dysfunctional beliefs serving as obstacles to better self-care and improved functioning (Piette et al., 2004). Additionally, poor adherence to self-care may be a mutually reinforcing phenomenon, with poor adherence contributing to more depressive symptoms and depressive symptoms then contributing to decreased adherence (Holt et al., 2014a). In a study of individuals with diabetes followed over a 5-year period, self-care behaviors explained a significant amount of the relationship between depressive symptoms at baseline and glycemic control 5 years later (Chiu, Wray, Beverly, & Dominic, 2010). As a result, even low depressive symptoms may have long-term impacts in patients with diabetes (Chiu et al., 2010).

A third pathway involves the impact of depression on the relationship with health-care providers (Piette et al., 2004). Less satisfactory interactions with providers, including poor communication and unmet expectations, can result in less motivation to engage with the healthcare system (Piette et al., 2004). Simultaneously, providers are more likely to consider patients with depression "difficult" or "less able to cope," which can influence communication and management (Piette et al., 2004).

Diabetes Distress and Stress

Diabetes distress is common in individuals with diabetes and is both conceptually and practically distinct from depression (Fisher et al., 2010; Young-Hyman et al., 2016). The relationship between distress and the burden of diabetes is independently associated with outcomes, and, often once included in models, removes the independent relationship between depression and glycemic control (Fisher et al., 2010; Gonzalez, Shreck, Psaros, & Safren, 2015; Walker et al., 2014). In fact, in a structured equation model investigating the relationship between diabetes distress, depression, fatalism, and glycemic control, it was diabetes distress, and not depression, that served as the main pathway influencing diabetes outcomes (Asuzu et al., 2017). Distress has been found to have a direct relationship with diabetes self-care and has both a direct and indirect influence on glycemic control (Walker et al., 2014, 2015). The indirect influence has been attributed to adherence to self-care behaviors, through decreased access to patient-centered care and through decreased perceived control over diabetes (Gonzalez et al., 2015; Walker et al., 2014). Additionally, diabetes distress has an equally strong and separate relationship with self-care and glycemic control, highlighting the importance of taking both psychological and behavioral factors into account for comprehensive diabetes care (Asuzu et al., 2017). Investigation of a 12-month intervention aimed at decreasing diabetes distress found that reduction in distress was a significant pathway associated with improved self-management, including physical activity and medication adherence, as well as improved glycemic control (Hessler et al., 2014).

More general perceived stress has also been associated with adherence to self-care, and processes specific to diabetes care, such as diabetes education, but did not show a direct relationship to glycemic control (Walker et al., 2014). In addition, perceived stress may help explain the relationship between environmental factors and diabetes outcomes. For instance, higher levels of stress have been associated with socioeconomic disadvantage (Baum, Garofalo, & Yali, 1999). When investigating patients with type 1 diabetes, it was found that high diabetes-related stress linked socioeconomic disadvantage to a flatter cortisol slope, and these flatter slopes were associated with worse glycemic control (Zilioli, Ellis, Carré, & Slatcher, 2017). In addition, an investigation of pathways between discrimination and quality of life in patients with type 2 diabetes found that perceived stress served as a direct pathway with the mental component of quality of life (Achuko, Walker, Campbell, Dawson, & Egede, 2016). The impact of general stress on health was shown to occupy a central role in the way patients viewed diabetes, whereas healthcare providers and diabetes educators focused on the importance of lifestyle changes and saw stress as a regime management issue (Schoenberg, Drew, Stoller, & Kart, 2005). This difference in how patients and providers view the impact of stress on their outcomes may undermine the patient-provider relationship and limit the ability of the healthcare system to help patients adequately address psychosocial factors impacting their health (Schoenberg et al., 2005).

Mediators and Moderators of the Impact on Diabetes Outcomes

Given the influence of stress and distress on diabetes outcomes, it is not surprising that coping style is considered a possible mediator of behavioral health in individuals with diabetes. Since coping is derived from appraisal of stressors, both general and diabetes-specific stressors may influence diabetes outcomes. Using the Ways of Coping Checklist, one study showed that active coping, avoidance coping, and minimizing the situation all played a role in mediating the relationship between depressive symptoms and health-related quality of life (Huang et al., 2016). Active coping and minimizing the situation had strong negative associations with depressive symptoms; thus, patients may reduce the impact of depression on health-related quality of life through the use of these coping styles (Huang et al., 2016). In patients with type 1 diabetes followed over 1 year, avoidant coping style was shown to lead to diabetes-related distress at a later time, rather than the opposite order (Iturralde, Weissberg-Benchell, & Hood, 2017). Avoidant coping led to worse diabetes outcomes in the future, with blood glucose monitoring and glycemic control fully mediated by distress, and self-reported adherence partially mediated by distress (Iturralde et al., 2017). In a separate analysis, followed over 4 years, active coping predicted better glycemic control, which in turn predicted continued active coping (Luyckx, Seiffge-Krenke, & Hampson, 2010). Alternatively, worse glycemic control predicted avoidant coping later in time (Luyckx et al., 2010). These results suggest that coping skills are an important factor to address for long-term diabetes care.

Social support is an additional factor shown to influence psychological drivers of diabetes outcomes. Theoretical mechanisms for social support's influence on health include suppression of negative affect, improved immune system functioning, and promoting healthy lifestyle behaviors (Cohen, 1988). Social support has been found to serve as a mediator in the pathway between depression and self-care behaviors, supporting the idea of its impact on negative affect (Egede & Osborn, 2010). In an investigation of the impact of discrimination in patients with diabetes, social support had a direct and indirect effect on the mental component of quality of life (Achuko et al., 2016). The indirect effect of social support was mediated through perceived stress, suggesting social support has an influence on both perceived stress and the mental component of quality of life (Achuko et al., 2016). Social support also showed an indirect association to glycemic control in patients with diabetes, mediated through access to patient-centered care (Walker et al., 2014). And in a study of

Chinese adults with type 2 diabetes, patient-provider communication was correlated with social support, suggesting physicians may be an important aspect of support for individuals with diabetes (Gao et al., 2013). Social support's association with glycemic control has also been shown to be mediated by self-care, supporting the third theoretical mechanism hypothesized by Cohen (Gao et al., 2013). The frequency of using social support resources, both from family and friends, as well as from neighborhoods and communities, was a significant mediator of an intervention designed to increase social support on physical activity, fat consumption, and glycemic control (Barrera Jr, Toobert, Angell, Glasgow, & Mackinnon, 2006). Changes in the extensiveness of social networks also mediated the intervention's impact on physical activity (Barrera Jr et al., 2006). Interestingly the individuals' perceived availability of social support was not a mediator of this intervention (Barrera Jr et al., 2006). Contrary to Barrera's findings, a mediation analysis of the impact of a peer support intervention did not find social support to significantly mediate improvements in glycemic control (Piette, Resnicow, Choi, & Heisler, 2013). However, when investigating moderators, the intervention did have a significant impact in patients with lower social support at baseline, whereas it did not on patients with higher social support levels (Piette et al., 2013). Based on these results, while social support does not appear to have a direct influence on glycemic control, it impacts diabetes outcomes through a variety of pathways, including support received from family, friends, physicians, and communities, and may be an effective tool for improving diabetes care, particularly in those with low levels of support currently.

Models of Care to Address Behavioral Health and Diabetes Outcomes

Fragmented Care in the Context of Diabetes and Behavioral Health

One of the greatest concerns facing the increasingly complex healthcare system is fragmentation of care and lack of continuity (Egede, 2006; Frandsen, Joynt, Rebitzer, & Jha, 2015; Holt et al., 2014a; Hussey et al., 2014). Care often involves multiple providers with no central provider or organization effectively coordinating care (Egede, 2006; Frandsen et al., 2015). Lack of coordination across providers often results in poor outcomes, missed opportunities, and increased costs (Egede, 2006; Frandsen et al., 2015). In individuals with chronic disease, care fragmentation was associated with both higher costs and lower quality of care (Egede, 2006; Frandsen et al., 2015). Lack of continuity has also been associated with higher rates of hospital and emergency department (ED) use, higher rates of complications, and higher cost (Hussey et al., 2014). Even appropriate referrals to sub-specialties for patients with diabetes led to increased fragmentation and higher ED use, suggesting attention to risks and effectiveness of multiple providers is needed when designing systems of care (Liu, Einstadter, & Cebul, 2010). Without adequate coordination and integration across systems, care guidelines requiring referral to additional providers may increase patient risk and cause unnecessary confusion for patients (Liu et al., 2010).

The need for mental health treatment in the context of primary care has led to a call for integrated care systems. Despite efforts to increase integration, recognition and treatment for depression in primary care are insufficient (de Groot, Golden, & Wagner, 2016; Egede, 2006, 2007). In addition, recognition of depression does not always change treatment plans, patients often do not receive sufficient doses or duration of antidepressant medication to achieve remission, and lack of regular monitoring results in discontinuation of medication without provider knowledge or continuation of medications that are not effective (Egede, 2006, 2007; Gilbody, Sheldon, & House, 2008; Unutzer & Ratzliff, 2015).

Incorporating Psychosocial Health into Standards of Care

Healthcare professionals have an important role to play in integrating behavioral health into the care of patients with diabetes. A call for more systematic screening, with defined care pathways for patients that screen positive, has been made for years with limited uptake (de Groot et al., 2016; Egede, 2007; Holt et al., 2014a, 2014b; Piette et al., 2004). Often, screening efforts are opportunistic, rather than systematic, limiting implementation of treatment (de Groot et al., 2016). More recently, a call has been made to assess symptoms of psychosocial factors beyond depression (Young-Hyman et al., 2016). The American Diabetes Association (ADA) published a position statement on psychosocial care for people with diabetes, with a series of recommendations for incorporating psychosocial care into standard of care (Young-Hyman et al., 2016). This includes consideration of psychosocial factors across the life span, assessment of a number of psychosocial factors, and addressing psychosocial problems upon identification (Young-Hyman et al., 2016). Assessment of psychosocial factors may provide a better understanding of reasons for suboptimal glycemic control, rather than assumption. And it is based on nonadherence to self-care behaviors (Young-Hyman et al., 2016). Normalizing the idea that periodic lapses in self-management occur may help patients report problems and discuss diabetes-related and generalized psychological distress at diagnosis and when treatment changes may help ensure patients feel providers understand their lived experience (Young-Hyman et al., 2016). Increasing the recognition that mental and physical health interact and how treatment strategies need to change when dual conditions are present is important for effective care (Piette et al., 2004). Finally, providing care through a multidisciplinary team will help identify high-risk patients and deliver evidence-based therapy (Holt et al., 2014b).

Evidence-Based Integrated Care Approaches

Collaborative care, stepped care, and patient-centered medical homes (PCMH) are all evidence-based systematic efforts to improve coordination of care and satisfaction with care (Unutzer & Ratzliff, 2015). Though related, each has specific principles that define care systems.

Collaborative care has five core principles including patient-centered care incorporating shared care plans, evidence-based care based on credible research, measurement-based treatment to target requiring routine measurements of clinical outcomes and personal goals, population-based care due to each care team sharing a defined group of patients, and accountable care focused on quality care and outcomes (Unutzer & Ratzliff, 2015). Collaborative care teams include interdisciplinary cooperation and include at minimum an actively engaged patient, a primary care provider, a care manager, and a mental health professional (Petrak, Baumeister, Skinner, Brow, & Holt, 2015; Unutzer & Ratzliff, 2015). Psychiatric consults can provide a range of interaction including informal consultations, systematic case reviews, and face-to-face consultations (Unutzer & Ratzliff, 2015). Routine monitoring of outcomes and proactive follow-up with patients are overseen by a care manager, who assists in decision-making support both for the patient and providers (Petrak et al., 2015). A number of collaborative care interventions have been tested in the United States, showing increased satisfaction with care and greater improvements in depressive symptoms up to 1 year posttreatment (Katon et al., 2004; Petrak et al., 2015).

One specific clinical approach for collaborative care is stepped care, which is based on a rationale that treatment is started at low intensity and increased based on systematic reassessment (Katon et al., 2004; Stoop, Nefs, Pommer, Pop, & Pouwer, 2015; Unutzer & Ratzliff, 2015). Stepped care incorporates patient preference and different types and intensities of treatment (Katon et al., 2004). Interventions are provided sequentially based on algorithms and treatment plans with specified cutoffs for transitions to the next step (Petrak et al., 2015). For example, in treatment of comorbid depression with diabetes, if suicidal tendencies do not exist, mild depression treatment can be provided in primary care by informing patients of the link between diabetes and depression, identifying targets for intervention (such as thoughts, activity levels, social interactions, or self-care adherence), and provision of self-help materials (Petrak et al., 2015). If improvement does not occur within 2–4 weeks, treatment should be escalated to psychological or pharmacological treatment (Petrak et al., 2015). It is important to consider whether patients have a history of recurrent depression, as treatment may need to be escalated faster, or offered in combination, such as a combined pharmacological and pharmacotherapy treatment (Petrak et al., 2015). Again, response after 2–4 weeks should be monitored and escalated if improvement is not seen, highlighting the importance of having a behavioral health specialist on the multidisciplinary team to provide insight and treatment options (Petrak et al., 2015).

Patient-centered medical homes (PCMH) is a model of enhanced primary care to address fragmented care and competing interests within the healthcare system (Jortberg, Miller, Gabbay, Sparling, & Dickinson, 2012). PCMH is based on the chronic care model and focuses on patient-centered care, self-management support, patient empowerment, and team-based care (Bojadzievski & Gabbay, 2011). In the context of patients with diabetes, integration of behavioral health is necessary to address high-risk individuals and provide a way to simultaneously address mental and physical health (Jortberg et al., 2012). Similar to collaborative care, PCMH often uses a care manager to coordinate treatment regimens and assist in self-management support (Jortberg et al., 2012). By training care managers in behavioral health, they have the capacity to expand the reach of physicians and address the psychosocial aspects of diabetes care (Jortberg et al., 2012). This can be done through proactive outreach to provide follow-up, support, and scheduled appointments with providers when escalation of treatment is needed (Jortberg et al., 2012).

Training for care managers, integral in both collaborative care and PCMH models, may take multiple approaches. An implementation project to expand collaborative care initiatives found that while the intervention care manager was a diabetes nurse trained in depression care, healthcare sites implementing the program used primary care nurses, mental health professionals cross-trained in diabetes treatment guidelines, or two professionals coordinating care where one was trained to treat diabetes and the other trained to treat depression (Coleman et al., 2017). In the implementation of a collaborative care program at a safety net primary care clinic, with no additional funding for the program, it was found that investment of time and staff was required to reorganize care in order to provide a team-based approach (Chwastiak et al., 2017). A medical assistant provided support for care management by completing outreach phone calls and managing data, which allowed nurses to focus on higher-level tasks required by the patients (Chwastiak et al., 2017). Care managers then provided structured health assessments, education, brief evidence-based behavioral interventions, and conducted weekly systematic caseload reviews (Chwastiak et al., 2017). Use of a stepped care approach allowed patients with mild symptoms to be managed by the nurse case managers, while more serious disorders were primarily handled by the integrated mental health team in primary care (Chwastiak et al., 2017).

Recommendations for Integrated Care

Below are a series of recommendations for effective integrated care. The most evidence has been collected on providing care for patients with diabetes and comorbid depression, and as such, many recommendations are adapted from recommendations for integrated depression care.

First, integrated care should include (1) screening, (2) treatment, and (3) monitoring for relapse and involve a multidisciplinary team with the individual with diabetes at the center of the care process. Use of only one or two of these activities will not result in an efficient and sustainable system of care to meet the complex physical and psychosocial needs of patients with diabetes. Consistent implementation of screening is needed using standardized/validated tools, with systems in place to confirm and offer treatment based on screening results (Egede, 2007; Holt et al., 2014b; Young-Hyman et al., 2016). For example, depression can be screened for by asking if there have been changes in mood, such as little interest or pleasure in doing things or feeling down, depressed, or hopeless, during the past 2 weeks or between visits (Petrak et al., 2015; Young-Hyman et al., 2016). Stress and diabetes distress can be initially screened by asking if the patient feels overwhelmed or stressed by life or diabetes management (Young-Hyman et al., 2016). Positive responses would then be followed by standardized and validated measures, for example, use of the PHQ-9 for affirmative depression responses, use of the Diabetes Distress Scale for distress, discussion of treatment options, and referral to a behavioral health provider for assessment as needed (Petrak et al., 2015, Young-Hyman et al., 2016). Positive screening should be followed with a clear treatment pathway, and treatments should include a stepped approach where more intensive management can be offered when required (Holt et al., 2014a, b; Petrak et al., 2015). Ideally, behavioral/mental health providers should be embedded in primary care and diabetes care settings to increase care coordination; however, primary care providers can also identify behavioral/mental health providers that are knowledgeable about the psychosocial aspects of diabetes to use for referrals (Young-Hyman et al., 2016). In addition, if appropriate, identifying a support person to include in care decisions may help identify, prevent, and resolve psychosocial problems (Young-Hyman et al., 2016). Incorporating a nurse case manager in care is recommended for treatment of comorbid depression but may also assist in addressing other psychosocial concerns, such as identifying community resources and providing stress management techniques (Holt et al., 2014a; Young-Hyman et al., 2016). Finally, monitoring after treatment to prevent relapse and provide ongoing support is an important aspect of integrated care. In a study of a culturally tailored collaborative care program, relapse prevention strategies, including symptom monitoring, behavioral activation, and problem-solving plans, were credited with the sustained impact over time (Ell et al., 2011). In a study of stepped care approach, the majority of patients experienced recurrent symptoms in the monitoring phase that may have been missed without continued follow-up (Stoop et al., 2015).

Second, a number of psychosocial concerns should be included in screening, treatment, and ongoing monitoring as part of routine diabetes management, including diabetes distress, social support, and self-efficacy. Through efforts to incorporate clear guidelines on how to address these factors, healthcare professionals can better moderate the psychological burden of diabetes through psychosocial support. Based on the evidence, multiple causative pathways likely operate within the context of behavioral health and diabetes outcomes, with personal behavioral or coping styles moderating the impact on disease management and health outcomes over time (Hessler et al., 2014). Recognition of different psychosocial factors, such as perceived stress, self-efficacy, or social support resources, may help providers better understand the patient's social circumstances and their decisions to adhere or not adhere to recommendations (Schoenberg et al., 2005; Young-Hyman et al., 2016). In addition, screening for both depression and diabetes distress will help address concerns of the potential overlap between diabetes-related symptoms and depression symptoms and ensure appropriate care is planned based on results (Petrak et al., 2015). Linking treatment to community resources may also help in increasing provision of social support and addressing concerns beyond the healthcare system (Holt et al., 2014b). This more comprehensive view of the patient will then assist in better matching care recommendations to the context of the patient's life, increasing provision of truly patient-centered care.

Third, a combination of pharmacological and psychotherapy treatment approaches is recommended for effective care (Katon et al., 2004; Petrak et al., 2015). Patients may prefer either medications or psychotherapy and may accept one service, while refusing the other (Piette et al., 2004). The most effective treatment for depression and diabetes control has been seen in a combination of psychotherapeutic intervention and self-management training (Andreoulakis et al., 2012; de Groot et al., 2016; Holt et al., 2014a). Common psychological interventions include cognitive behavioral therapy (CBT), problem solving, interpersonal therapy, motivational interviewing, and counseling (de Groot et al., 2016). Cognitive behavioral treatments are particularly promising as a psychotherapy to address both behavioral health and diabetes-specific behavioral needs, as they target perceptions and behaviors likely to improve both diabetes self-care and psychological factors (Piette et al., 2004). Patients with diabetes who are struggling to maintain adequate glycemic control may be assisted through a program teaching different coping styles to help reduce depressive symptoms and address negative thought patterns that limit their ability to complete self-care behaviors (Huang et al., 2016; Piette et al., 2004). Avoidance processes inherent in avoidant coping styles are a central target in acceptance and commitment therapy (ACT) and therefore may be ideal to use with patients exhibiting avoidant coping styles (Iturralde et al., 2017). Mindfulness-based cognitive therapy has been shown to be effective in addressing anxiety and could be targeted to address diabetes-specific anxieties such as fear of complications and hypoglycemia (de Groot et al., 2016). Physical activity should also be promoted as it is an important component of effective diabetes management and has been shown to improve depressive symptoms (Holt et al., 2014b; Piette et al., 2004). Contextual factors, including cultural differences, should be taken into account given reporting of depression may vary across racial/ethnic groups, and experiences, such as discrimination, may decrease reporting of symptoms and adherence to treatment (de Groot et al., 2016; Holt et al., 2014b).

Fourth, success should be measured by a combination of physical, behavioral, and psychological outcomes (Petrak et al., 2015). Similar to research showing focus only on physical aspects of diabetes does not result in optimal outcomes, and a focus only on improvements in mental health will not likely result in optimal care (Holt et al., 2014a; Katon et al., 2004). Including monitoring of psychosocial factors and self-care behaviors will also provide a more comprehensive understanding of patient factors and inform care plans (Holt et al., 2014b; Young-Hyman et al., 2016). Stepped approaches can facilitate initial target outcomes, such as depressive symptoms or tobacco use, and followed by subsequent goals focusing on health-related quality of life, psychosocial functioning, or coping in a way that is economically sustainable (Holt et al., 2014b; Petrak et al., 2015). In addition, simultaneous consideration of cognitive factors, diabetes management, and glycemic control can improve understanding of the psychosocial needs of patients facing the demands of diabetes to ensure long-term success (Gonzalez et al., 2015; Petrak et al., 2015). Monitoring the results of treatment is necessary to ensure remission of psychological symptoms and guide stepped care approaches (Petrak et al., 2015).

Finally, new approaches that leverage the use of technology to increase reach and improve care should be investigated and implemented in clinical settings. The use of clinical information systems to offer reminders to providers and the use of mobile phone applications to offer reminders to patients can both be used to increase awareness of evidence-based guidelines (Egede, 2007). Telephone care is an effective strategy for helping patients manage both depression and diabetes and can be used for education, behavioral monitoring, and evaluation of changes (Egede, Williams, Voronca, Gebregziabher, & Lynch, 2017; Piette et al., 2004). Extending the reach of collaborative care through telemedicine, patient registries, and mHealth technologies may provide a way to address both prevention and treatment at a population level (Holt et al., 2014b; Petrak et al., 2015).

Conclusions

Psychological conditions influence diabetes-related self-management and outcomes and should be incorporated into clinical care practices, addressed in research interventions, and considered in policy implementations. These factors are important to consider as they can significantly impact glycemic control and other outcomes in adults with diabetes. Integrating behavioral and physical care for patients with diabetes will take a coordinated effort, focused on systematic screening, clear treatment pathways, and ongoing monitoring. However, efforts to integrate care have promise to better address the healthcare goals of providing patient-centered care, decreasing both morbidity and cost, and increasing satisfaction with care.

References

Achuko, O., Walker, R. J., Campbell, J. A., Dawson, A. Z., & Egede, L. E. (2016). Pathways between discrimination and quality of life in patients with type 2 diabetes. *Diabetes Technology & Therapeutics, 18*(3), 1–8.

Al-Khawaldeh, O. A., Al-Hassan, M. A., & Froelicher, E. S. (2012). Self-efficacy, self-management, and glycemic control in adults with type 2 diabetes mellitus. *Journal of Diabetes and Its Complications, 26*, 10–16.

American Academy of Diabetes Educators. (2017). AADE7 self-care behaviors. Accessible at: https://www.diabeteseducator.org/patient-resources/aade7-self-care-behaviors. Accessed 28 Apr 2017.

American Diabetes Association. (2017). Lifestyle management. Sec. 4. In standards of medical care in diabetes, 2017. *Diabetes Care, 40*(Suppl. 1), S33–S43.
Andreoulakis, E., Hyphantis, T., Kandylis, D., & Iacovides, A. (2012, July). Depression in diabetes mellitus: a comprehensive review. *Hippokratia, 16*(3), 205–214.
Asuzu, C. C., Walker, R. J., Williams, J. S., & Egede, L. E. (2017, January). Pathways for the relationship between diabetes distress, depression, fatalism and glycemic control in adults with type 2 diabetes. *Journal of Diabetes and its Complications, 31*(1), 169–174.
Barrera, M., Jr., Toobert, D. J., Angell, K. L., Glasgow, R. E., & Mackinnon, D. P. (2006, May). Social support and social-ecological resources as mediators of lifestyle intervention effects for type 2 diabetes. *Journal of Health Psychology, 11*(3), 483–495.
Baum, A., Garofalo, J. P., & Yali, A. N. N. (1999). Socioeconomic status and chronic stress: does stress account for SES effects on health? *Annals of the New York Academy of Sciences, 896*, 131–144.
Bojadzievski, T., & Gabbay, R. A. (2011). Patient-centered medical home and diabetes. *Diabetes Care, 34*(4), 1047–1053.
Boule, N. G., Haddad, E., Kenny, G. P., Wells, G. A., & Sigal, R. J. (2001). Effects of exercise on glycemic control and body mass in type 2 diabetes mellitus: a meta-analysis of controlled clinical trials. *Journal of the American Medical Association, 286*(10), 18–1227.
Carnethon, M. R., Biggs, M. L., Barzilay, J. I., Smith, N. L., Vaccarino, V., Bertoni, A. G., et al. (2007, April 23). Longitudinal association between depressive symptoms and incident type 2 diabetes mellitus in older adults: the cardiovascular health study. *Archives of Internal Medicine, 167*(8), 802–807.
Carnethon, M. R., Kinder, L. S., Fair, J. M., Stafford, R. S., & Fortmann, S. P. (2003, September). Symptoms of depression as a risk factor for incident diabetes: findings from the National Health and Nutrition Examination Epidemiologic Follow-up study, 1971–1992. *American Journal of Epidemiology, 158*(5), 416–423.
Centers for Disease Control and Prevention. (2014). *National diabetes statistics report: Estimates of diabetes and its burden in the United States, 2014*. Atlanta, GA: U.S. Department of Health and Human Services.
Chiu, C. J., Wray, L. A., Beverly, E. A., & Dominic, O. G. (2010, January). The role of health behaviors in mediating the relationship between depressive symptoms and glycemic control in type 2 diabetes: a structural equation modeling approach. *Social Psychiatry and Psychiatric Epidemiology, 45*(1), 67–76.
Chwastiak, L. A., Jackson, S. L., Russo, J., DeKeyser, P., Keifer, M., Belyeu, B., et al. (2017). A collaborative care team to integrate behavioral health care and treatment of poorly-controlled type 2 diabetes in an urban safety net primary care clinic. *General Hospital Psychiatry, 44*, 10–15.
Cohen, S. (1988). Psychosocial models of the role of social support in the etiology of physical disease. *Health Psychology, 7*, 269–297.
Cohen, S., & Wills, T. A. (1985). Stress, social support, and the buffering hypothesis. *Psychological Bulletin, 98*, 310–357.
Coleman, K. J., Magnan, S., Neely, C., Solberg, L., Beck, A., Trevis, J., Heim C, et al. (2017). The COMPASS initiative: description of a nationwide collaborative approach to the care of patients with depression and/or cardiovascular disease. *General Hospital Psychiatry, 44*, 69–76.
de Groot, M., Golden, S. H., & Wagner, J. (2016, October). Psychological conditions in adults with diabetes. *The American Psychologist, 71*(7), 552–562.
Devarajooh, C., & Chinna, K. (2017). Depression, distress and self-efficacy: the impact on diabetes self-care practices. *PLoS One, 12*(3), e0175096.
Dismuke, C. E., & Egede, L. E. (2011). Association of serious psychological distress with health services expenditures and utilization in a national sample of US adults. *General Hospital Psychiatry, 33*(4), 311–317.
Dismuke, C. E., Hernandez-Tejada, M. A., & Egede, L. E. (2014). Relationship of serious psychological distress to quality of life in adults with diabetes. *International Journal of Psychiatry in Medicine, 48*(2), 135–146.

Egede, L. E. (2005). Effect of depression on self-management behaviors and health outcomes in adults with type 2 diabetes. *Current Diabetes Reviews, 1*(3), 235–243.
Egede, L. E. (2006). Disease-focused or integrated treatment: diabetes and depression. *The Medical Clinics of North America, 90*(4), 627–646.
Egede, L. E. (2007). Failure to recognize depression in primary care: issues and challenges. *Journal of General Internal Medicine, 22*, 701–703.
Egede, L. E., Bishu, K. G., Walker, R. J., & Dismuke, C. E. (2016, May). Impact of diagnosed depression on healthcare costs in adults with and without diabetes: United States, 2004–2011. *Journal of Affective Disorders, 195*, 119–126.
Egede, L. E., & Bonadonna, R. (2003). Diabetes self-management in African Americans: An exploration of the role of fatalism. *The Diabetes Educator, 29*(1), 105–115.
Egede, L. E., & Dismuke, C. E. (2012). Serious psychological distress and diabetes: a review of the literature. *Current Psychiatry Reports, 14*, 15–22.
Egede, L. E., & Ellis, C. (2010a). Development and psychometric properties of the 12-item Diabetes Fatalism Scale. *Journal of General Internal Medicine, 25*, 61–66.
Egede, L. E., & Ellis, C. (2010b). Diabetes and depression: global perspectives. *Diabetes Research and Clinical Practice, 87*, 302–312.
Egede, L. E., Grubaugh, A. L., & Ellis, C. (2010). The effect of major depression on preventive care and quality of life among adults with diabetes. *General Hospital Psychiatry, 32*(6), 563–569.
Egede, L. E., & Osborn, C. Y. (2010, March–April). Role of motivation in the relationship between depression, self-care, and glycemic control in adults with type 2 diabetes. *The Diabetes Educator, 36*(2), 276–283.
Egede, L. E., Walker, R. J., Bishu, K., & Dismuke, C. E. (2016). Trends in costs of depression in adults with diabetes in the United States: Medical Expenditure Panel Survey, 2004–2011. *Journal of General Internal Medicine, 31*(6), 615–622.
Egede, L. E., Williams, J. S., Voronca, D. C., Gebregziabher, M., & Lynch, C. P. (2017, March). Telephone-delivered behavioral skills intervention for African American adults with type 2 diabetes: a randomized controlled trial. *Journal of General Internal Medicine, 23*. Epub ahead of print.
Egede, L. E., & Zheng, D. (2003). Independent factors associated with major depressive disorder in a national sample of individuals with diabetes. *Diabetes Care, 26*(1), 104–111.
Egede, L. E., Zheng, D., & Simpson, K. (2002). Comorbid depression is associated with increased health care use and expenditures in individuals with diabetes. *Diabetes Care, 25*, 464–470.
Ell, K., Katon, W., Xie, B., Lee, P., Kapetanovic, S., Guterman, J., & Chou, C. (2011). One-year postcollaborative depression care trial outcomes among predominantly Hispanic diabetes safety net patients. *General Hospital Psychiatry, 33*, 436–442.
Fisher, E. B., Chan, J. C., Nan, H., Sartorius, N., & Oldenburg, B. (2012). Co-occurrence of diabetes and depression: conceptual considerations for an emerging global health challenge. *Journal of Affective Disorders, 142*(Suppl), S56–S66.
Fisher, L., Glasgow, R. E., & Strycker, L. A. (2010). The relationship between diabetes distress and clinical depression with glycemic control among patients with type 2 diabetes. *Diabetes Care, 33*, 1034–1036.
Fisher, L., Hessler, D., Glasgow, R. E., Arean, P. A., Masharani, U., Naranjo, D., et al. (2013). REDEEM: a pragmatic trial to reduce diabetes distress. *Diabetes Care, 36*, 2551–2558.
Fisher, L., Hessler, D. M., Polonsky, W. H., & Mullan, J. T. (2012). When is diabetes distress clinically meaningful? Establishing cut points for the Diabetes Distress Scale. *Diabetes Care, 35*, 259–264.
Fisher, L., Mullan, J. T., Arean, P., Glasgow, R. E., Hessler, D., & Masharani, U. (2010). Diabetes distress but not clinical depression or depressive symptoms is associated with glycemic control in both cross-sectional and longitudinal analyses. *Diabetes Care, 33*, 23–28.
Frandsen, B. R., Joynt, K. E., Rebitzer, J. B., & Jha, A. K. (2015). Care fragmentation, quality and costs among chronically ill patients. *The American Journal of Managed Care, 21*(5), 355–362.

Gao, J., Wang, J., Zheng, P., Haardofer, R., Kegler, C., Zhu, Y., et al. (2013). Effects of self-care, self-efficacy, social support on glycemic control in adults with type 2 diabetes. *BMC Family Practice, 14*, 66.

Gilbody, S., Sheldon, T., & House, A. (2008). Screening and case-finding instruments for depression: a meta-analysis. *CMAJ, 178*, 997–1003.

Gilmer, T. P., O'Connor, P. J., Rush, W. A., Crain, A. L., Whitebird, R. R., Hanson, A. M., et al. (2005). Predictors of heath care costs in adults with diabetes. *Diabetes Care, 28*(1), 59–64.

Golden, S. H., Lazo, M., Carnethon, M., Bertoni, A. G., Schreiner, P. J., Diez Roux, A. V., ... Lyketsos, C. (2008, June 18). Examining a bidirectional association between depressive symptoms and diabetes. *Journal of the American Medical Association, 299*(23), 2751–2759.

Gonzalez, J. S., Fisher, L., & Polonsky, W. H. (2011). Depression in diabetes: have we been missing something important? *Diabetes Care, 34*, 236–239.

Gonzalez, J. S., Shreck, E., Psaros, C., & Safren, S. A. (2015, May). Distress and type 2 diabetes-treatment adherence: A mediating role for perceived control. *Health Psychology, 34*(5), 505–513.

Hessler, D., Fisher, L., Glasgow, R. E., Strycker, L. A., Dickinson, L. M., Arean, P. A., & Masharani, U. (2014). Reductions in regimen distress are associated with improved management and glycemic control over time. *Diabetes Care, 37*(3), 617–624.

Hilliard, M. E., Yi-Frazier, J. P., Hessler, D., Butler, A. M., Anderson, B. J., & Jaser, S. (2016). Stress and A1c among people with diabetes across the lifespan. *Current Diabetes Reports, 16*(8), 67.

Holt, R. I., de Groot, M., & Golden, S. H. (2014a, June). Diabetes and depression. *Current Diabetes Reports, 14*(6), 491.

Holt, R. I., de Groot, M., Lucki, I., Hunter, C. M., Sartorius, N., & Golden, S. H. (2014b, August). NIDDK international conference report on diabetes and depression: current understanding and future directions. *Diabetes Care, 37*(8), 2067–2077.

Huang, C. Y., Lai, H. L., Lu, Y. C., Chen, W. K., Chi, S. C., Lu, C. Y., & Chen, C. I. (2016, January). Risk Factors and Coping Style Affect Health Outcomes in Adults With Type 2 Diabetes. *Biological Research for Nursing, 18*(1), 82–89.

Hussey, P. S., Schneider, E. C., Rudin, R. S., Fox, S., Lai, J., & Pollack, C. E. (2014). Continuity and the costs of care for chronic disease. *JAMA Internal Medicine, 174*(5), 742–748.

Iturralde, E., Weissberg-Benchell, J., & Hood, K. K. (2017, March). Avoidant coping and diabetes-related distress: Pathways to adolescents' Type 1 diabetes outcomes. *Health Psychology, 36*(3), 236–244.

Jortberg, B. T., Miller, B. F., Gabbay, R. A., Sparling, K., & Dickinson, W. P. (2012). Patient-centered medical home: how it affects psychosocial outcomes for diabetes. *Current Diabetes Reports, 12*, 721–728.

Katon, W. J., Von Korff, M., Lin, E. H. B., Simon, G., Ludman, E., Russo, J., et al. (2004). The Pathways Study: a randomized trial of collaborative care in patients with diabetes and depression. *Archives of General Psychiatry, 61*, 1042–1049.

Kelly, S. J., & Ismail, M. (2015). Stress and type 2 diabetes: a review of how stress contributes to the development of type 2 diabetes. *Annual Review of Public Health, 36*, 441–462.

Liu, C. W., Einstadter, D., & Cebul, R. D. (2010). Care fragmentation and emergency department use among complex patients with diabetes. *American Journal of Managed Care, 16*(6), 413–420.

Luyckx, K., Seiffge-Krenke, I., & Hampson, S. E. (2010, July). Glycemic control, coping, and internalizing and externalizing symptoms in adolescents with type 1 diabetes: a cross-lagged longitudinal approach. *Diabetes Care, 33*(7), 1424–1429.

McKnight-Eily, L. R., Elam-Evans, L. D., Strine, T. W., Matthew, M. Z., Perry, G. S., Presley-Cantrell, L., et al. (2009). Activity limitation, chronic disease, and comorbid serious psychological distress in U.S. adults – BRFSS 2007. *International Journal of Public Health, 54*, S111–S119.

Osborn, C. Y., Bains, S. S., & Egede, L. E. (2010, November). Health literacy, diabetes self-care, and glycemic control in adults with type 2 diabetes. *Diabetes Technology & Therapeutics, 12*(11), 913–919.

Petrak, F., Baumeister, H., Skinner, T. C., Brow, A., & Holt, R. I. (2015). Depression and diabetes: treatment and health-care delivery. *The Lancet Diabetes and Endocrinology, 3*, 472–485.

Piette, J. D., Resnicow, K., Choi, H., & Heisler, M. (2013). A diabetes peer support intervention that improved glycemic control: mediators and moderators of intervention effectiveness. *Chronic Illness, 9*(4), 258–267.

Piette, J. D., Richardson, C., & Valenstein, M. (2004, February). Addressing the needs of patients with multiple chronic illnesses: the case of diabetes and depression. *The American Journal of Managed Care, 10*(2 Pt 2), 152–162.

Puyat, J. H., Kazanjian, A., Wong, H., & Goldner, E. (2017). Comorbid chronic general health conditions and depression care: a population-based analysis. *Psychiatric Services*. Epub ahead of print.

Rush, A. J., Giles, D. E., Schlesser, M. A., Fulton, C. L., Weissenburger, J., & Burns, C. (1986). The inventory for depressive symptomatology (IDS): preliminary findings. *Psychiatry Research, 18*(1), 65–87.

Schoenberg, N. E., Drew, E. M., Stoller, E. P., & Kart, C. S. (2005). Situating stress: lessons from lay discourses on diabetes. *Medical Anthropology Quarterly, 19*(2), 171–193.

Schoenfelder, T. (2012). Patient satisfaction: a valid indicator for the quality of primary care. *Primary Health Care, 2*, 4.

Shin, J. K., Chiu, Y. L., Choi, S., Cho, S., & Bang, H. (2012). Serious psychological distress, health risk behaviors, and diabetes care among adults with type 2 diabetes: the California Health Interview Survey 2007. *Diabetes Research and Clinical Practice, 95*(3), 406–414.

Simon, G. E., Katon, W. J., Ludman, E., VonKorff, M., Ciechanowski, P., & Young, B. A. (2005). Diabetes complications and depression as predictors of health service costs. *General Hospital Psychiatry, 27*(5), 344–351.

Sousa, V. D., Zauszniewski, J. A., Musil, C. M., Lea, P. J. P., & Davis, S. A. (2005). Relationships among self-care agency, self-efficacy, self-care, and glycemic control. *Research and Theory for Nursing Practice, 19*(3), 217–230.

Stoop, C. H., Nefs, G., Pommer, A. M., Pop, V. J. M., & Pouwer, F. (2015). Effectiveness of a stepped care intervention for anxiety and depression in people with diabetes, asthma, or COPD in primary care: a randomized controlled trial. *Journal of Affective Disorders, 184*, 269–276.

Stopford, R., Winkley, K., & Ismail, K. (2013). Social support and glycemic control in type 2 diabetes: a systematic review of observational studies. *Patient Education and Counseling, 93*, 549–558.

Strom, J. L., & Egede, L. E. (2012). The impact of social support on outcomes in adult patients with type 2 diabetes: a systematic review. *Current Diabetes Reports, 12*, 769–781.

Surwit, R. S., Schneider, M. S., & Feinglos, M. N. (1992). Stress and diabetes mellitus. *Diabetes Care, 15*(10), 141–1422.

Thoits, P. A. (1985). Social support and psychological well-being: theoretical possibilities. In I. G. Sarason & B. R. Sarason (Eds.), *Social support: Theory, research, and application* (pp. 52–72). Mass: Kluwer/Hingram.

Unutzer, J., & Ratzliff, A. H. (2015). Evidence base and core principles. In L. E. Raney (Ed.), *Integrated care: Working at the interface of primary care and behavioral health*. Arlington, VA: American Psychiatric Association.

van Dam, H. A., van der Horst, F. G., Knoops, L., Ryckman, R. M., Crebolder, H. F. J. M., & van den Borne, B. H. W. (2004). Social support in diabetes: a systematic review of controlled intervention studies. *Patient Education and Counseling, 59*, 1–12.

Walker, R. J., Gebregziabher, M., Martin-Harris, B., & Egede, L. E. (2014). Relationship between social determinants of health and processes and outcomes in adults with type 2 diabetes: validation of a conceptual model. *BMC Endocrine Disorders, 14*, 82.

Walker, R. J., Gebregziabher, M., Martin-Harris, B., & Egede, L. E. (2015). Quantifying direct effects of social determinants of health on glycemic control in adults with type 2 diabetes. *Diabetes Technology & Therapeutics, 17*(2), 80–87.

Walker, R. J., Smalls, B. L., Hernandez-Tejada, M. A., Campbell, J. A., Davis, K., & Egede, L. E. (2012). Effect of diabetes fatalism on medication adherence and self-care behaviors in adults with diabetes. *General Hospital Psychiatry, 34*(6), 598–603.

Weissman, J. F., Pratt, L. A., Miller, E. A., & Parker, J. D. (2015). Serious psychological distress among adults: United States, 2009–2013. *NCHS Data Brief, 203*, 1–8.

Williams, S. A., Pollack, M. F., & Dibonaventura, M. (2011). Effects of hypoglycemia on health-related quality of life, treatment satisfaction and healthcare resource utilization in patients with type 2 diabetes mellitus. *Diabetes Research and Clinical Practice, 91*(3), 363–370.

Winchester, R. J., Williams, J. S., Wolfman, T. E., & Egede, L. E. (2016). Depressive symptoms, serious psychological distress, diabetes distress and cardiovascular risk factor control in patients with type 2 diabetes. *Journal of Diabetes and its Complications, 30*, 312–317.

Young-Hyman, D., de Groot, M., Hill-Briggs, F., Gonzalez, J. S., Hood, K., & Peyrot, M. (2016, December). Psychosocial care for people with diabetes: A position statement of the American Diabetes Association. *Diabetes Care, 39*(12), 2126–2140.

Zilioli, S., Ellis, D. A., Carré, J. M., & Slatcher, R. B. (2017, April). Biopsychosocial pathways linking subjective socioeconomic disadvantage to glycemic control in youths with type I diabetes. *Psychoneuroendocrinology, 78*, 222–228.

Index

M. P. Duckworth, W. T. O'Donohue (eds.), *Behavioral Medicine and Integrated Care*,
https://doi.org/10.1007/978-3-319-93003-9

D

E

The manufacturer's authorised representative in the EU is Springer Nature Customer Service Centre GmbH, Europaplatz 3, 69115 Heidelberg, Germany. If you have any concerns regarding our products, please contact ProductSafety@springernature.com

Printed and bound by CPI Group (UK) Ltd, Croydon, CR0 4YY
25/09/2026
02222853-0009